# Integrating Technology in Positive Psychology Practice

Daniela Villani
*Università Cattolica del Sacro Cuore, Italy*

Pietro Cipresso
*Università Cattolica del Sacro Cuore, Italy & I.R.C.C.S. Istituto Auxologico Italiano, Italy*

Andrea Gaggioli
*Università Cattolica del Sacro Cuore, Italy & I.R.C.C.S. Istituto Auxologico Italiano, Italy*

Giuseppe Riva
*Università Cattolica del Sacro Cuore, Italy & I.R.C.C.S. Istituto Auxologico Italiano, Italy*

A volume in the Advances in Psychology, Mental Health, and Behavioral Studies (APMHBS) Book Series

Information Science REFERENCE
An Imprint of IGI Global

Published in the United States of America by
Information Science Reference (an imprint of IGI Global)
701 E. Chocolate Avenue
Hershey PA, USA 17033
Tel: 717-533-8845
Fax: 717-533-8661
E-mail: cust@igi-global.com
Web site: http://www.igi-global.com



Library of Congress Cataloging-in-Publication Data

Names: Villani, Daniela, 1978- editor.
Title: Integrating technology in positive psychology practice / Daniela Villani, Pietro Cipresso, Andrea Gaggioli, and Giuseppe Riva, editors.
Description: Hershey, PA : Information Science Reference, [2016] | Includes bibliographical references and index.
Identifiers: LCCN 2015050763| ISBN 9781466699861 (hardcover) | ISBN 9781466699878 (ebook)
Subjects: LCSH: Mental health promotion. | Positive psychology. | Information technology--Health aspects. | Information technology--Psychological aspects.
Classification: LCC RA790.53 .I57 2016 | DDC 616.8900285--dc23 LC record available at http://lccn.loc.gov/2015050763

This book is published in the IGI Global book series Advances in Psychology, Mental Health, and Behavioral Studies (APMHBS) (ISSN: pending; eISSN: pending)

British Cataloguing in Publication Data
A Cataloguing in Publication record for this book is available from the British Library.

All work contributed to this book is new, previously-unpublished material. The views expressed in this book are those of the authors, but not necessarily of the publisher.

For electronic access to this publication, please contact: eresources@igi-global.com.

# Advances in Psychology, Mental Health, and Behavioral Studies (APMHBS) Book Series

Bryan Christiansen
*PryMarke, LLC, USA*

ISSN: pending
EISSN: pending

Mission

The complexity of the human mind has puzzled researchers and physicians for centuries. While widely studied, the brain still remains largely misunderstood.

The **Advances in Psychology, Mental Health, and Behavioral Studies (APMHBS)** book series presents comprehensive research publications focusing on topics relating to the human psyche, cognition, psychiatric care, mental and developmental disorders, as well as human behavior and interaction. Featuring diverse and innovative research, publications within APMHBS are ideally designed for use by mental health professionals, academicians, researchers, and upper-level students.

Coverage

- Substance Abuse
- Anxiety
- Socialization
- Emotional Health
- Mental Health & Disorders
- Cognition
- Neurological Disorders
- Addiction
- Counseling & Therapy
- Treatment & Care

IGI Global is currently accepting manuscripts for publication within this series. To submit a proposal for a volume in this series, please contact our Acquisition Editors at Acquisitions@igi-global.com or visit: http://www.igi-global.com/publish/.

## Titles in this Series

*For a list of additional titles in this series, please visit: www.igi-global.com*

*Global Perspectives on Youth Gang Behavior, Violence, and Weapons Use*
Simon Harding (Middlesex University, UK) and Marek Palasinski (Liverpool John Moores University, UK)
Information Science Reference • copyright 2016 • 425pp • H/C (ISBN: 9781466699380) • US $185.00 (our price)

*Exploring the Collective Unconscious in the Age of Digital Media*
Stephen Brock Schafer (Digipen Institute of Technology, USA)
Information Science Reference • copyright 2016 • 316pp • H/C (ISBN: 9781466698918) • US $175.00 (our price)

*Psychosocial Studies of the Individual's Changing Perspectives in Alzheimer's Disease*
Cordula Dick-Muehlke (University of California, Irvine, USA) Ruobing Li (University of California, Irvine, USA) and Myron Orleans (California State University, Fullerton, USA)
Medical Information Science Reference • copyright 2015 • 434pp • H/C (ISBN: 9781466684782) • US $225.00 (our price)

*Psychological and Social Implications Surrounding Internet and Gaming Addiction*
Jonathan Bishop (Centre for Research into Online Communities and E-Learning Systems, Swansea, UK)
Information Science Reference • copyright 2015 • 335pp • H/C (ISBN: 9781466685956) • US $195.00 (our price)

*Handbook of Research on Innovations in the Diagnosis and Treatment of Dementia*
Panagiotis D. Bamidis (Aristotle University of Thessaloniki, Greece) Ioannis Tarnanas (Aristotle University of Thessaloniki, Greece) Leontios Hadjileontiadis (Aristotle University of Thessaloniki, Greece) and Magda Tsolaki (Aristotle University of Thessaloniki, Greece)
Medical Information Science Reference • copyright 2015 • 511pp • H/C (ISBN: 9781466682344) • US $245.00 (our price)

*Exploring Implicit Cognition Learning, Memory, and Social Cognitive Processes*
Zheng Jin (Zhengzhou Normal University, China & University of California, Davis, USA)
Information Science Reference • copyright 2015 • 371pp • H/C (ISBN: 9781466665996) • US $195.00 (our price)

IGI GLOBAL
DISSEMINATOR OF KNOWLEDGE
www.igi-global.com

701 E. Chocolate Ave., Hershey, PA 17033
Order online at www.igi-global.com or call 717-533-8845 x100
To place a standing order for titles released in this series, contact: cust@igi-global.com
Mon-Fri 8:00 am - 5:00 pm (est) or fax 24 hours a day 717-533-8661

# Table of Contents

# Detailed Table of Contents

a prompt response. 2) An intervention generator (IG) generates a draft response for the moderator to use, for example a positive psychology intervention. These two can help in the management of a discussion forum, supporting positive behaviours, not just dealing in situations of distress. 3) A component for synchronous support through an augmented chat system.



It is well known that physical exercise has a significant beneficial effect on mental and physical health, and elderly fitness programs are a good and widely accepted approach to prevent frailty. In this chapter, we examine what elderly people actually want and need when it comes to technologies designed to support and encourage their physical fitness. We present the ELF@Home project as a case study, and report design insights and other results from user involvement in the project. User involvement is a key component of the approach and uses methods such as interviews, focus group meetings, early component and prototype tests with users, as well as inputs from medical experts. ELF@Home is a clear example of a "Positive Technology" approach. The project proposes the adoption of new technology in everyday life from the perspective of positive psychology, approaching this aim by designing devices and systems that are actually usable and desirable in supporting extended healthy living for this target population.



This chapter focuses on how to develop tools for positive technology and more specifically, mobile e-mental health systems using a virtual stress counselor. The main objective is to develop a framework for mobile e-mental health systems reviewing existing e-mental health apps and discussing necessary system requirements. The chapter states that current e-mental health apps do not offer any facilities to promote social interaction between the counselor and the user. The proposed framework requires personalized interactions between a virtual counselor and a student. It provides personalized feedback to reduce stress level and enhances personal stress management strategies. This requires integration of technologies for facial expression detection, speech and emotion recognition as well as other psycho-physiological feedback. A prototype system for e-mental health has been developed and the components of the system architecture have been widely discussed including the need for a coping processor. Finally, conclusions are drawn regarding the tools for positive technology.

### Section 3
### Positive Interventions: Health Care



Pregnancy is a very special time in a woman's life, a time of important and complex step that can lead to the fall the previous personal balances and looking for new. This phase potentially critical, is often accompanied by anxiety, negative emotions, worries and stress about themselves, the couple's life, the baby. Among the many interventions available for the welfare of pregnant women, new technologies are playing an increasingly important role, thanks to its spread, the lower costs and its peculiar characteristics (interactivity, sociality, customizability, ubiquity, multimediality, velocity, etc). Smartphones and tablets in particular are proving excellent tools to accompany women on this journey toward a healthy motherhood.



The progressive growth of the ageing population represents opportunities as well as challenges. Consistently, the identification of effective cognitive empowerment programs in elderly population is now a worldwide health policy priority, specially for their preventive effect. In this chapter, within the paradigm of Positive Technology, the main focus will be on the use advanced technologies as effective tools for a new class of applications aimed at improving the traditional cognitive empowerment in elderly. Specifically, the attention will be devoted on how advanced technologies may be used to support elderly in reaching engaging and self-actualizing experiences. On the basis of the most recent evidence in literature, it will be discussed the possible advantages in using such advanced technologies for improving well-being in frail elderly: coupled with an increase in cognitive skills acquisition, the advantages may range increased self-efficacy and decreased subjective weakness, with a consequent improvement in both physical and cognitive performance.



With older adults living longer than ever before, more in this age demographic are seeking ways to stay engaged, happy, and healthy in the final decades of life following retirement. In this chapter, we discuss the many ways in which older adults can benefit from learning new technologies, including enjoying more functional independence, social connection, and cognitive engagement. We also discuss the barriers that prevent older adults from learning new technologies, including physical ailment and disability, skepticism over the benefits, and stereotype threat. Finally, we introduce the concept of Langerian mindfulness and how learning to be mindful as opposed to mindless can help older adults over these barriers.

## Section 4
## Positive Interventions: Games for Well-Being

# Foreword

Integrating Technology in Positive Psychology Practice opens new avenues using technology to enhance the quality of personal experiences, to increase well-being, empowerment and connectedness on the level of individuals, as well as organizations and society.

The editors of this volume have challenged their contributing authors to think beyond traditional positive psychology. They show how emerging technologies can be of added value to design interventions that engage, empower and that foster social interactions to change the capabilities of individuals and organizations to play an active role in the management of health and well-being.

The novelty of the volume's advocated approach is twofold, the use of emerging technologies to mediate personal experiences and the interdisciplinary based approach of positive psychology. Rather than considering technology as a medium or tool to exchange information and to interact in a user friendly and low-cost setting, the editors show how emerging technologies can enhance personal experiences in three ways, namely by structuring, providing a goal-oriented feedback system to focus on participation in the experience, by augmenting to achieve multimodal, interactive experiences and by replacing, using virtual realities to simulate physical presence in a synthetic world. It is at that edge, that sets this volume apart from the traditional view on technology used in positive psychology research and practice.

The technology perspective, expressed in the many chapters, reveals an interdisciplinary research and education area for positive technology that is innovative, dynamic, well thought out and at the same time critical, transcending the traditional use of technology as helpful to merely improve the accessibility, affordability and efficiency of healthcare services within the institutional contexts of care, cure and prevention. Technology has the capacity to create virtual persuasive environments that provide simultaneously multimodal cues and psycho-physiological feedback for personal change by strengthening emotional, social and physical presence. Besides technology can be used to collect and analyze data by self-tracking behaviors, emotions, thoughts presenting a quantified holistic self-concept that will shed new lights on how technology integrates in our lives, health and well-being, and how people engage each other and their environments using unobtrusive and pervasive technologies. The editors have strived to present emerging technologies not just as new devices to support health and well-being but as movements towards a new framework for positive technology and to contribute to the ongoing scientific debate on the active role of people in constructing a participatory healthy society.

The volume presents a cohesive understanding of how technology integrates in positive psychology by dividing the book into five interrelated sections. They introduce the three pillars of positive technology, empowerment, engagement and change, and how design can influence users' psychological well-being (section 1,2). The theoretical concepts that underpin the three pillars are applied in the design of positive interventions in different fields; healthcare, games for well-being and virtual realities for cognition and stress (section3-5). This organization of the volume facilitates readers to internalize novel concepts on positive technology and to understand how these concepts can be implemented in education, research and practice. The attempts to develop and unfold the ideas on how to integrate positive technology in practice run as a transversal through the volume taking readers by the hand on a journey to participate in thoughts and debate on positive technology.

The editors and contributing authors have drawn on their knowledge, experiences in research and teaching on the intersection between psychology, human interaction and machine cognition, neuroscience and emerging technologies. This has resulted in a volume that is of great value to students, healthcare workers, researchers with an interest in engineering, psychology and healthcare.

*Lisette van Gemert-Pijnen*
*University Of Twente, The Netherlands*
*November, 2015*

# Preface

Information and communication technologies have become a pervasive presence in our lives, yet its potential for improving people's wellbeing is not fully understood. Most psychological research on the impact of computers and the Internet has focused on the negative side of technology – i.e. how the use (abuse) of interactive systems, videogames can negatively affect mental health and behaviour. On the other hand, less attention has been devoted to understand how emerging technologies can promote optimal functioning at individual, group and community levels. The main motivation of this book is to explore this question, by examining what roles technology can play in the development of psychological interventions aimed at helping people to thrive.

The interest towards the scientific study of well-being has a long history, dating back to the humanistic psychology with the important concept of fully-functioning person and self-actualization proposed, respectively, by Carl Rogers (Rogers, 1961) and Abraham Maslow (Maslow, 1954). Since that moment, the past half century has seen the study of the psychological aspects of what makes life worth living recede to the background, whereas studies on disorder and damage have taken center stage. The recognition of this imbalance and a desire to address the full spectrum of human experience has led to the the birth and development of Positive Psychology (Seligman & Csikszentmihalyi, 2000), a multifaced research area interested in investigating "what makes life worth living" (Peterson & Seligman, 2004). The scientific study of optimal human functioning is pursued at three different levels of analysis: subjective, individual and social. The subjective level focuses on positive subjective states such as happiness, well-being, satisfaction with life, love, hope and optimism, as well as on the conditions under which these positive experiences occur. The individual level is concerned with the identification and cultivation of positive individual traits and engagement in absorbing activities (i.e., flow). The last level - societal - focuses on creating and maintaining meaningful positive relationships and positive institutions. The societal level is also concerned with fostering those civic virtues that are capable of promoting better citizenship, by increasing responsibility, altruism, tolerance of diversity, equality, opportunity, civility, reciprocity and moderation.

Martin Seligman, one of the pioneers of Positive Psychology, introduced the "Authentic Happiness" theory, which identifies three key components of optimal functioning (Seligman, 2002):

1. **The Pleasant Life:** Achieved through the presence of pleasure and promoted by activities that increase positive emotions;
2. **The Engaged Life:** Achieved through engagement in empowering activities and utilization of own strengths and virtues;
3. **The Meaningful Life:** Achieved by identifying and connecting with something larger than oneself.

The pleasant life is based on a hedonic definition of well-being, which is rooted in Epicurean equation of happiness with pleasure, comfort and enjoyment. Kahneman and colleagues (Kahneman et al., 1999) defined hedonic psychology, one of the two fundamental approaches of Positive Psychology (Ryan & Deci, 2001), as the study of *"what makes experiences and life pleasant and unpleasant"*. So defined, the hedonic approach poses for itself an ambitious target of research and intervention by maximizing human happiness. Although there are many ways to evaluate the pleasure continuum in human life, most study has used assessment of subjective well-being (SWB) (Diener & Lucas, 1999), that consists of three components: life satisfaction, the presence of positive mood, and the absence of negative mood. The salience of positive emotions in increasing well-being is addressed by the "broaden-and-build model" of positive emotions (Fredrickson, 2001; 2004). According to Fredrickson, first of all positive emotions provide the organism with undefined action tendencies that may lead to adaptive behavior. Secondly, positive emotions could reduce or mitigate the impact of stressful negative emotions and, finally, positive emotions have fundamental long-term effects by broadening the thought–action repertoire and by building future physical, psychological, and social resources.

The engaged life is a eudaimonic definition of well-being, that is rooted in Aristotle' ethical doctrine and its advocacy to fully realize our true nature (one's daemon), through the exercise of personal virtues in pursuit of a common good (Ryff & Singer, 2008). According to eudaimonic view, well-being consists of more than the merely satisfaction of pleasure because it involves instead the actualization of human potential (Ryan & Deci, 2001). Ryff & Keyes (1995) have introduced the concept of psychological well-being (PWB) that consists of six aspects of human experience: autonomy, personal growth, self-acceptance, life purpose, mastery, and positive relatedness. Self-determination theory (Deci & Ryan, 2000; Ryan, Huta & Deci, 2008) is an interesting perspective that has embraced the concept of self-realization as a central aspect of well-being specifying what it means to actualize the self and how that can be accomplished. Within the eudaimonic approach, Peterson and Seligman (2004) identified six universal virtues (wisdom, courage, humanity, justice, temperance, and transcendence) that are favoured by character strengths representing the psychological components of them.

The last level – the meaningful life - integrates individual well-being to social well-being by serving a purpose larger than oneself to promote connectedness between individuals, groups, and communities (Keys & Haidt, 2003). In this framework, Ryff and Singer have embraced introduced the concept of interpersonal flourishing, which could be defined as the development of positive relations with other people as a key dimension of well-being (2000).

However, more recently Seligman realized these three components were not exhaustive elements of happiness. In particular, he acknowledged three main limitations of the Authentic Happiness theory: first, it did not take into consideration the role of other key variables, such as success and the sense of control. Furthermore, according to Seligman, the term happiness itself was misleading, because it posits a superficial identification with "feeling in a good mood", while neglecting the dimensions of engagement and meaning. A further weakness was that happiness was mainly operationalized as life satisfaction and measured subjectively by self-report thus overlooking the assessment of the other two components – engagement and meaning (Seligman, 2011). To overcome the limitations of Authentic Happiness theory, in 2011 Seligman introduced the PERMA model (Seligman, 2011), an acronym for the five pillars of well-being: Positive emotions, Engagement, Relationships, Meaning, and Accomplishment. Of these components, three were inherited from the former Authentic Happiness model. The additional ones – relationships and accomplishment – refer, respectively, to the role played by significant others in helping us to face the challenges in life, and to the motivation to achieve, to have mastery, and competence.

Positive Psychology proposes a novel approach to study human behavior, which encompasses all traditional areas of psychological investigation by proposing a transversal approach to psychology, with applications in a number domains, including work, development, education, clinical, health and community (Delle Fave, Massimini, & Bassi, 2011). However, in their recent review of positive psychology McNulty and Fincham indicate the need to think beyond positive psychology (McNulty & Fincham, 2012) and an interesting suggestion comes from the shift of the focus to personal experience (Riva, 2012): how it is possible to manipulate the quality of personal experience with the goal of increasing wellness, and generating strengths and resilience in individuals, organizations and society?

To answer to this broaden question, the first step is recognize the impact of technology-mediated experiences delivered through smarthphones, tablets and other personal wearable devices. On one side, in fact, ICTs are becoming more and more popular in daily life because they are user-friendly and low-cost. On the other side, the technological sophistication has allowed the development of increasingly advanced devices.

According to Riva et al., (2012), emerging technologies could be used to manipulate personal experience in three separate, but related ways:

- *By structuring it* using a goal, rules, and a feedback system to provide individuals with a sense of purpose focusing his/her attention and orienting his/her participation in the experience;
- *By augmenting it* to achieve multimodal, mixed and interactive experiences;
- *By replacing it* with a synthetic one using VR system to simulate physical presence in a synthetic world that reacts to the action of the individual as if he/she was really there.

In order to manipulate and enhance the features of our personal experience, Positive Psychology appears to be a promising framework to develop ICT that foster positive emotions, promote engagement in empowering activities and support connectedness between individuals, groups, and communities.

## ORGANIZATION OF THE BOOK

The starting point of the book is the assumption that there is an emerging convergence of technologies, that are always more used to support our daily activities, and the search for wellbeing that is a transversal goal of the psychological discipline.

Following this perspective, the book is divided in five sections:

**Section 1:** Empowerment, Engagement, and Change: The Three Pillars of Positive Technology.
**Section 2:** Design Positive Systems.
**Section 3:** Positive Interventions: Health Care.
**Section 4:** Positive Interventions: Games for Well-being.
**Section 5:** Positive Interventions: Cognition and Stress.

*Section 1 - Empowerment, Engagement and Change: the three pillars of Positive Technology* – includes three chapters that focus on the theorethical foundations of the Positive Technology approach. In Chapter 1, Riva and colleagues describe "Positive Technology" as the approach to using of technology for improving the quality of our personal experience. On the one side, the authors suggest that our cognitive system is naturally shaped to identify and counter the experiential conflicts that are usually the main motives for change. Optimal experiences, also defined as "flow experiences", instead allow the individual to consider long-term personal goals differently and start to experiment with changing them. In other words optimal experiences, when meaningful for the individual, widen the array of thoughts and actions, facilitating generativity and behavioral flexibility. On the other side, authors explain how is possible to use technology to manipulate the quality of experience, with the goal of increasing wellness, and generating strengths and resilience in individuals, organizations and society.

Banos and colleagues in Chapter 2 focus on the connection between positive psychological interventions (PPIs) and the digital world. This chapter presents an updated review of the relationship between these two fields (PPIs and technologies), and discusses relevant considerations that should be taken into account when technologies are used to deliver PPIs, as well as the elements that can moderate their effectiveness. The final aim of the chapter is to provide readers with basic tools to make critical judgments about PPIs delivered via a technological format.

In Chapter 3, Barello and colleagues move on describing the participatory health revolution stating that consumers' health behaviors are increasingly influenced by people's desire to play an active role in promoting a positive life functioning and technologies are addressing this emerging need. This chapter describes the results of a software-assisted quali-quantitative study aimed at exploring the scientific debate about technological interventions for wellbeing in the era of participatory health. Based on the study's results, technologies for wellbeing in the participatory health era may be clustered depending on the "context of delivery," on their degree of personalization," and on their inner "conceptualization of positive interventions". A consumer health perspective may be a compass to orient the planning and delivery of technological solutions aimed to sustain positive psychological interventions by effectively engaging people in health and wellbeing management, keeping in mind a dynamic vision of a participatory health construction.

*Section 2 - Design Positive Systems* – moves the attention to the other side of the coin, that refers to the importance of taking a critical design approach and exploring how design may have an impact on the users psychological wellbeing.

In Chapter 4, Calvo and colleagues start from the idea that technology based mental health interventions can be particularly effective for young people. Amongst these, online support groups are becoming increasingly popular. This model of mental health service provision includes moderators who read posts, recognise those that need attention and provide support via online responses. However, as these groups become more popular they risk becoming more difficult to manage due to the sheer volume of posts. This challenge can be addressed through computational linguistics techniques. This chapter reports on work with a mental health organisation on three components to help scale up the number of people they can support. The design aims to go beyond helping end-users and explores how design can support the wellbeing of the moderators themselves.

In Chapter 5, Waterworth and colleagues examine what elderly people actually want and need when it comes to technologies designed to support and encourage their physical fitness. Starting from the premise that physical exercise has a significant beneficial effect on mental and physical health, and elderly fitness programs are a good and widely accepted approach to prevent frailty, authors present the ELF@ Home project as a case study, and report design insights and other results from user involvement in the project. The project proposes the adoption of new technology in everyday life from the perspective of positive psychology, approaching this aim by designing devices and systems that are actually usable and desirable in supporting extended healthy living for this target population.

In Chapter 6, Kavlaki and colleagues focus on how to develop tools for positive technology and more specifically, mobile e-mental health systems using a virtual stress counselor. The main objective is to develop a framework for mobile e-mental health systems reviewing existing e-mental health apps and discussing necessary system requirements. Current e-mental health apps do not offer any facilities to promote social interaction between the counselor and the user. The proposed framework requires personalized interactions between a virtual counselor and a student through feedback aimed to reduce stress level and enhance personal stress management strategies. This requires integration of technologies for facial expression detection, speech and emotion recognition as well as other psycho-physiological feedback. The chapter aims to describe a prototype system for e-mental health and to discuss the components of the system architecture.

*Sections 3, 4, and 5* are dedicated to describe *Positive Interventions* in three different fields, respectively *Health Care, Games for Well-Being, and Cognition and Stress.*

Concerning *Health Care,* Carissoli and colleagues present an emerging model of pregnancy care. In Chapter 7 authors investigate how it is possible to enhance women's well-being during pregnancy by taking into consideration the three levels of well-being identified by positive psychology and how actual mothers-to-be use new technologies to meet several needs. Furthermore, authors describe their Italian mobile app "BenEssere Mamma" aimed to support mothers' well-being during pregnancy.

In Chapter 8 Serino addresses the worldwide health policy priority of identification of effective cognitive empowerment programs in elderly population. Specifically she focuses on the use advanced technologies as effective tools for a new class of applications aimed at improving the traditional cognitive empowerment in elderly. The attention is devoted on how advanced technologies may be used to support elderly in reaching engaging and self-actualizing experiences. On the basis of the most recent evidence in literature, the possible advantages in using such advanced technologies for improving well-being in frail elderly are discussed.

In Chapter 9 Bercovitz and Pagnini still focus on elderly population and discuss the many ways in which older adults can benefit from learning new technologies, including enjoying more functional independence, social connection, and cognitive engagement. Authors recognize the existence of barriers that prevent older adults from learning new technologies, including physical ailment and disability, skepticism over the benefits, and stereotype threat. To help older adults in overcoming these barriers they introduce the concept of Langerian mindfulness and the importance of how learning to be mindful as opposed to mindless.

Within the *Section 4 – Positive Interventions: Games for Well-Being*, Chapter 10 introduced Serious Games (SGs) as new opportunities for human training and empowerment, imparting knowledge or skills in an engaging and motivating way to a new generation of learners. Further, they can be used to improve the quality of both individual and collective experience. In particular, SGs can nurture positive emotions promote engagement, as well as enhance social integration and connectedness. Argenton and colleagues present an in-depth analysis of each of these aspects, with the support of concrete examples and case-analysis and a game design practice.

In Chapter 11, Tichon and Tornqvist discusses a range of positive psychological effects associated with playing two genres of popular off-the-shelf video games as opposed to video games that have been constructed to specifically target education or teach health-related lessons. The positive psychological outcomes of play are especially investigated in the areas of resilience, competency, and autonomy. These outcomes have potential application across a number of areas of education and preventative health.

The interest in videogames is the object of Chapter 12, where Triberti discusses on complex emotions generated by videogames. On the one hand, video gamers may feel frustration and anger due to the difficulty of the gameplay. On the other hand, they may experience sadness, anxiety and fear due to the immersion into emotionally rich narratives. Yet, video gamers seem to appreciate gaming technologies generating negative emotions, and the research on media frequently highlights a counterintuitive positive relationship between negative affect and enjoinment/well-being outcomes. Starting from these premises, the present chapter aims to review the negative emotions typical of video games, in order to understand in what ways they can concur in generating an overall positive experience. Then, the chapter discusses implications for research on video games as positive technologies, namely technologies able to promote well-being in their users.

In Chapter 13, Diaz-Orueta provides an overview of the state-of-the-art serious games currently available as psychological interventions across popular delivery formats (virtual reality environments, online and PC videogames) and discusses their potential to complement traditional psychological interventions and improve psychological wellbeing for people of all ages.

Finally in *Section 5 - Positive Interventions: Cognition and Stress*, in Chapter 14, Villani and colleagues describe how Positive Technology can help people cope with stress in several contexts. On the one hand, thanks to the combination of traditional assessment measures of stress and the analysis of physiological correlates of this experience, it is possible to overcome limitations related to self-reported data and move towards self-tracking. On the other hand, the emerging convergence of technology and health care is offering new methods and tools not only to assess but also to cope with stress. In this view, there is growing empirical support for the use of several technologies for stress management protocols. This chapter focuses on the hedonic and eudaimonic experiences supported by technologies in terms of inducing positive affective states and supporting personal growth by teaching strategies to reduce stress and enhance well-being.

Chapter 15 explores how immersion in virtual reality (VR) evokes emotional states similar to those of the real world, and how deliberate immersion in high-stress situations can help teach individuals affective strategies to remain in control of their emotions. Affective Control Theory (ACT) proposes that affective strategies that typically strengthen and support performance are skills integral to stress management. Thus, Tichon and Mavin describe how VR experiences allow individuals the opportunity to practice coping with their emotional states while immersed in difficult scenarios.

One important task of Positive Psychology is to develop effective interventions to increase and sustain processes of mental health, subjective and psychological well-being, functional groups and flourishing institutions.

This book is not exhaustive, meaning it does not address every positive topics of inquiry, but it attempts to take a first step in what we hope will be an ongoing rigorous and dynamic multidisciplinary journey towards the integration of technologies in positive psychology practice.

*Daniela Villani*
*Università Cattolica del Sacro Cuore, Italy*

*Pietro Cipresso*
*Università Cattolica del Sacro Cuore, Italy & I.R.C.C.S. Istituto Auxologico Italiano, Italy*

*Andrea Gaggioli*
*Università Cattolica del Sacro Cuore, Italy & I.R.C.C.S. Istituto Auxologico Italiano, Italy*

*Giuseppe Riva*
*Università Cattolica del Sacro Cuore, Italy & I.R.C.C.S. Istituto Auxologico Italiano, Italy*

## REFERENCES

Deci, E., & Ryan, R. (2000). The What and Why of Goal Pursuits: Human Needs and the Self- Determination of Behavior. *Psychological Inquiry: An International Journal for the Advancement of Psychological Theory*, *11*, 227–268.

Delle Fave, A., Massimini, F., & Bassi, M. (2011). Hedonism and Eudaimonism in Positive Psychology. In A. Delle Fave (Ed.), *Psychological Selection and Optimal Experience Across Cultures* (Vol. 2, pp. 3–18). New York: Springer.

Diener, E., & Lucas, R. E. (1999). Personality and subjective well-being. In D. Kahneman, E. Diener, & N. Schwarz (Eds.), *Well-Being: The Foundations of Hedonic Psychology* (pp. 213–229). Russell Sage Foundation.

Fredrickson, B. L. (2001). The role of positive emotions in positive psychology: The broaden-and-build theory of positive emotions. *The American Psychologist*, *56*, 218–226.

Fredrickson, B. L. (2004). The Broaden-and-Build Theory of Positive Emotions. *Philosophical Transactions of the Royal Society of London. Series B, Biological Sciences*, *359*, 1367–1377.

Kahneman, D., Diener, E., & Schwarz, N. (1999). *Well-being: the foundations of hedonic psychology*. New York: Russell Sage Foundation.

Keyes, C. L. M., & Haidt, J. (2003). *Flourishing: Positive Psychology and the Life Well-Lived*. Washington, DC: American Psychological Association.

Maslow, A. H. (1954). *Motivation and personality*. New York: Harper.

McNulty, J. K., & Fincham, F. D. (2012). Beyond Positive Psychology? Toward a contextual view of psychological processes and well-being. *The American Psychologist*, *67*(2), 101–110.

Peterson, C., & Seligman, M. E. P. (2004). *Character strengths and virtues: A handbook and classification*. Washington, DC: American Psychological Association.

Riva, G. (2012). Personal experience in positive psychology may offer a new focus for a growing discipline. *The American Psychologist*, *67*(7), 574–575.

Riva, G., Banos, R. M., Botella, C., Wiederhold, B. K., & Gaggioli, A. (2012). Positive technology: Using interactive technologies to promote positive functioning. *Cyberpsychology, Behavior, and Social Networking*, *15*, 69–77.

Rogers, C. (1961). *On becoming a person: A therapist's view of psychotherapy*. London: Constable.

Ryan, R., & Deci, E. (2001). On Happiness and Human Potentials: A Review of Research on Hedonic and Eudaimonic Well-Being. *Annual Review of Psychology*, *52*, 141–166.

Ryan, R. M., Huta, V., & Deci, E. (2008). Living well: A self-determination theory perspective on eudaimonia. *Journal of Happiness Studies*, *9*, 139–170.

Ryff, C. D., & Keyes, C. L. (1995). The structure of psychological well-being revisited. *Journal of Personality and Social Psychology*, *69*, 719–727.

Ryff, C. D., & Singer, B. (2000). Interpersonal flourishing: A positive health agenda for the new millennium. *Personality and Social Psychology Review*, *4*, 30–44.

Ryff, C. D., & Singer, B. (2008). Know thyself and become what you are: A eudaimonic approach to psychological well-being. *Journal of Happiness Studies*, *9*, 13–39.

Seligman, M. E. P. (2002). *Authentic happiness: using the new positive psychology to realize your potential for lasting fulfillment*. New York: Free Press.

Seligman, M. E. P. (2011). *Flourish: a visionary new understanding of happiness and well-being*. New York: Free Press.

Seligman, M. E. P., & Csikszentmihalyi, M. (2000). Positive psychology. An introduction. *The American Psychologist*, *55*(1), 5–14.

# Section 1

# Empowerment, Engagement, and Change:

## The Three Pillars of Positive Technology

# Chapter 1
# Positive Technology:
## The Use of Technology for Improving and Sustaining Personal Change

**Giuseppe Riva**
*Università Cattolica del Sacro Cuore, Italy & I.R.C.C.S. Istituto Auxologico Italiano, Italy*

**Pietro Cipresso**
*Università Cattolica del Sacro Cuore, Italy & I.R.C.C.S. Istituto Auxologico Italiano, Italy*

**Daniela Villani**
*Università Cattolica del Sacro Cuore, Italy*

**Andrea Gaggioli**
*Università Cattolica del Sacro Cuore, Italy & I.R.C.C.S. Istituto Auxologico Italiano, Italy*

## ABSTRACT

*This chapter describes and discusses the "Positive Technology" approach: the scientific and applied approach for the use of technology in improving the quality of our personal experience through its structuring, augmentation and/or replacement - as a way for improving and sustaining personal change. On one side, we suggest that our cognitive system is naturally shaped to identify and counter the experiential conflicts that are usually the main motives for change. Optimal experiences, also defined as "flow experiences", instead allow the individual to consider long-term personal goals differently and start to experiment with changing them. In other words optimal experiences, when meaningful for the individual, widen the array of thoughts and actions, facilitating generativity and behavioral flexibility. On the other side we claim that it is possible to use technology to manipulate the quality of experience, with the goal of increasing wellness, and generating strengths and resilience in individuals, organizations and society.*

## INTRODUCTION

Emerging technologies – the Internet, mobile devices, virtual reality, etc. – have greatly improved our lives (Castelnuovo, Gaggioli, Mantovani, & Riva, 2003; Preziosa, Grassi, Gaggioli, & Riva, 2009; Riva & Mantovani, 2012a). However, integration of technology in every sphere of our life is also changing us. But how is it changing us and why?

Cyberpsychology is a recent branch of psychology that is trying to answer these questions. Cyberpsychology originated in human sciences, and is driven by the quest to help humans deal with their digital environments. The object of study in cyberpsychology, as it is for much Human-Computer Interaction research, is the change introduced by the technology and not the technology itself. In particular, it aims

DOI: 10.4018/978-1-4666-9986-1.ch001

at the understanding, forecasting and activation of the different processes of change related to the use of new technologies.

But, how do we lastingly change our lives for the better? This chapter presents a possible answer to this question by focusing on the concept of personal change. As underlined by recent research in psychology and neuroscience, personal change is a complex process depending on the person, the issues, and the situation. However, by merging the ideas of two influential transdiagnostic models of change - the Perceptual Control Theory and the TransTheoretical Model of Behavior Change - it is possible to describe a process of personal change that moves from an expressed desire for change to a recovery from inevitable relapses. Even if these characteristics of personal change are now shared by many of the leading approaches to psychotherapy, many of us experience psychological change without the help of any form of treatment. But how does this happen and why?

In this chapter we suggest that our cognitive system is naturally shaped to identify and counter the experiential conflicts that are usually the main motives for change. This is achieved through a specific cognitive process – presence - whose goal is the control of the activity of the individual: I am present in a real or virtual space if I manage to put my intentions into action (enacting them). Specifically presence *provides the self with a feedback about the status of its activity*: the self perceives the variations in the feeling of presence (*breakdowns* and *optimal experience*) and tunes its activity accordingly. The role of breakdowns in personal change is clear: to push individuals towards it. By perceiving a conflict (awareness) between different goals the subject is pushed to resolve the conflict between them.

Optimal experiences, also defined as "flow experiences", instead allow the individual to consider long-term personal goals differently and start to experiment with changing them. In other words optimal experiences, when meaningful for the individual, widen the array of thoughts and actions, facilitating generativity and behavioral flexibility. Within this view, we defined *transformation of flow* as a person's ability to draw upon an optimal experience and use it to marshal new and unexpected psychological resources and sources of involvement.

In this chapter we will focus on the possible role of technology in this process. Specifically, we will introduce and describe the "Positive Technology" approach - the scientific and applied approach to the use of technology for improving the quality of our personal experience through its structuring, augmentation and/or replacement - as a way of framing a suitable object of study in the field of personal change (Graffigna, Barello, Wiederhold, Bosio, & Riva, 2013; Riva, 2012c; Riva, Banos, Botella, Wiederhold, & Gaggioli, 2012; Wiederhold & Riva, 2012). Specifically, we suggest that it is possible to use technology to influence three specific features of our experience - affective quality, engagement/actualization and connectedness - that promote optimal experiences inducing adaptive behaviors and personal change (Graffigna, Barello, & Riva, 2013a, 2013c). In this framework, positive technologies are classified according to their effects on a specific feature of personal experience. Moreover, for each level we have identified critical variables that can be manipulated to guide the design and development of positive technologies.

## UNDERSTANDING PERSONAL CHANGE

How do we lastingly change our lives for the better? There is not an easy answer to this question. As noted by Higginson and Mansell (2008): "The mechanism of psychological change is not fully understood. This is clear in research demonstrating the efficacy of different therapeutic approaches and the significant rates of natural recovery." (p. 326).

On one side it is well known that different therapies can all facilitate psychological change (Stiles, Barkham, Mellor-Clark, & Connell, 2008; Stiles, Barkham, Twigg, Mellor-Clark, & Cooper, 2006). On the other side, it is also true that some people experience psychological change without the help of any form of treatment (Higginson & Mansell, 2008).

However, due to the advances in psychology and neuroscience we now have a better view of personal change that is not limited to a specific viewpoint. In particular, the emergence of integrative and transdiagnostic accounts suggests that change is contextual, depending on the person, the issues, and the situation (Kottler, 2014). Moreover, personal change is a process, happening in discontinuous and nonlinear ways, following life transitions and traumatic events (Hayes, Laurenceau, Feldman, Strauss, & Cardaciotto, 2007).

## The Models of Change

Between the transdiagnostic models of change, one of the most influential is the TransTheoretical Model of Behavior Change - TTC (Prochaska & DiClemente, 1982, 1983; Prochaska, DiClemente, & Norcross, 1992). In this model change implies phenomena occurring over time. However, this aspect is largely ignored by many theories of change. To overcome this issue, TTC describes personal change as a progression through a series of five stages: precontemplation, contemplation, determination, action, and maintenance (see Table 1 for a detailed description of these stages). These stages represent a temporal dimension that allows both the individuals and the persons supporting them to understand when particular shifts in attitudes, intentions, and behaviors occur.

Another influential transdiagnostic model of change is the Perceptual Control Theory – PCT (Higginson, Mansell, & Wood, 2011; Vancouver & Putka, 2000). According to PCT at the core of human

*Table 1. The TransTheoretical Model of behavior change*

| | Definition | Subjective Experience |
|---|---|---|
| Precontemplation | The stage at which there is no intention to change behavior in the foreseeable future. | "I do not have a problem": the individual is not ready to change his/her behavior |
| Contemplation | The stage at which there is the recognition of the problem but it is still missing the commitment to take action. | "I know I have a problem and need to change. I will do something about it, one day": The individual is considering change, but he/she is not yet committed to it |
| Determination | The stage at which there is the decision to do something. | "Yes I have a problem and I need to do something to change - now": This stage opens for a limited time-period. If the individual moves into action, the process continues. If not, they lapse back into contemplation. |
| Action | The stage at which individuals modify their behavior, experiences, or environment in order to overcome their problems | "I am doing something to change my behavior now": This stage involves the most overt behavioral changes and requires considerable commitment of time and energy |
| Maintenance | The stage in which individuals work to prevent relapse and consolidate the gains attained during action. | "I do not stop my work to prevent myself from losing the obtained gains": This stage requires more and more practice to transform the new behaviors into habits. |

Adapted from Prochaska & DiClemente, 1982, 1983; Prochaska, DiClemente, & Norcross, 1992.

nature is the process of control (Higginson et al., 2011): "life is a constant process of comparing how things are with how we want things to be and if they do not match doing something to get closer to how we want things to be." (p. 250).

In this view control is a process of reducing the distance between what we want and what we are (*error*). Interestingly, the source of errors is both *within* and *between* individuals (Gianakis & Carey, 2011; Higginson et al., 2011). Specifically, PCT suggests that a possible source of error is internal: the coherence between goals and subgoals of the individual (*conflict*).

To eliminate a conflict, the individual must direct his or her awareness to the experience that is creating the conflict. Then, a reorganization is required: a trial and error process which modifies the characteristics or the conflicting goals (Higginson & Mansell, 2008). A summary of the key concepts expressed by PCT is reported in Table 2.

As noted by Kottler (2014), by merging these theories we can describe a process of change that basically follows this sequence (pp. 19-20):

1. There is an expressed desire for change that is triggered by a crisis, trauma, or developmental transition;
2. A level of pain and discomfort is reached that can't any longer be ignored or denied;
3. There is an awareness or insight that something different must be done;
4. There is a gradual process of applying what was realized or learned into constructive action;
5. There is recovery from inevitable relapses.

Within this process a critical milestone is the passage between stage 2 and 3. In general it occurs through an intense focus on the particular instance or experience creating the conflict (Wolfe, 2002). By exploring this experience as thoroughly as possible, the individual can relive all of the significant elements associated with it (i.e., conceptual, emotional, motivational, and behavioral) and make them available for reorganization.

Within this general model, different psychotherapies suggested specific approaches for exploring and modifying the conflicting experience: we can find the insight-based approach of psychoanalysis, the schema-reorganization goals of cognitive therapy, the functional analysis of behavioral activation, the interpersonal relationship focus of interpersonal therapy, and the enhancement of experience awareness in experiential therapies.

*Table 2. The Perceptual Control Theory*

| | Definition |
|---|---|
| Control | Keeping a variable within fixed limits despite outside disturbances. |
| Error | The difference between what we want and what we are currently experiencing. |
| Goals | What we want. Goals are set inside the individuals and are organized in a range of subgoals. |
| Conflict | The experience of incompatible subgoals for the individual's immediate experience. |
| Reorganization | A trial-and-error learning process that alters the way that we perceive our environment and set our goals until we manage to achieve them in the long term. |
| Awareness | The ability to perceive, or to be conscious of personal goals. For reorganization to be effective in the long term, awareness must be directed and sustained at personal higher level goals. |

Adapted from Higginson, Mansell, & Wood, 2011; Vancouver & Putka, 2000.

What are the differences between them? According to Safran and Greenberg (1991) behind the specific therapeutic approach there are two different models of change: bottom-up and top-down. Bottom-up processing begins with a specific emotional experience and leads eventually to change at the behavioral and conceptual level; top-down change usually involves exploring and challenging tacit rules and beliefs that guide the processing of emotional experience and behavioral planning.

These two models of change are focused on two different cognitive systems, one for information transmission and one for conscious experience, both of which may process sensory input (Brewin, 1989; Kahneman, 2002). Stanovich and West (2000) noted that in the last forty years, different authors from different disciplines suggested a two-process theory of reasoning. Even if the details and specific features of these theories do not always match perfectly, nevertheless they share the following properties:

- Intuitive operations are faster, automatic, effortless, associative, and difficult to control or modify.
- Rational operations, instead, are slower, serial, effortful, and consciously controlled.

The differences between the two systems are described in Table 3.

In sum we can identify some important properties of personal change:

- The focus of personal change is reducing the distance between goals and reality;
- This reduction is achieved through:
    - An intense focus on the particular experience creating the conflict;
    - A reorganization of this experience.
- The focus and reorganization of the experience may happen both at the intuitive and at the rational level;
- This reduction requires a complex process based on different stages.

*Table 3. Differences between the rational and the intuitive systems*

| | Rational System | Experiential/Intuitive System |
|---|---|---|
| Main Features | • **Rational:** Conscious, deliberative and affect-free<br>• **Abstract:** Encodes reality in symbols, words, and numbers<br>• **Analytic:** Connections by cause-and-effect relations<br>• **Slower Processing:** Capable of long delayed action<br>• **Less Resistant to Change:** Can change with speed of thought<br>• **More Highly Differentiated:** nuanced thinking<br>• **More Highly Integrated:** Organized in part by cross-situational principles<br>• **Experienced Actively and Consciously:** We believe we are in control of our thoughts<br>• **Not Self-Evident:** Requires justification via logic and evidence | • **Intuitive:** Preconscious, automatic, and intimately associated with affect<br>• **Concrete:** Encodes reality in images, metaphors, and narratives<br>• **Associative:** Connections by similarity and contiguity<br>• **Rapid Processing:** Oriented toward immediate action<br>• **Resistant to Change:** Changes with repetitive or intense experience<br>• **Differentiated:** Broad generalization gradient; categorical thinking<br>• **Integrated:** Situationally specific; organized in part by cognitive-affective modules<br>• **Experienced Passively and Preconsciously:** We are seized by our emotions<br>• **Self-Evidently Valid:** "Experiencing is believing" |
| How it works | • Operates by reality principle (what is logical and supported by evidence)<br>• Acquires its beliefs by conscious learning and logical inference<br>• More process oriented<br>• Behavior mediated by conscious appraisal of events | • Operates by hedonic principle (what feels good)<br>• Acquires its schemas by learning from experience<br>• Outcome oriented<br>• Behavior mediated by "vibes" from past experience |

As noted by different authors, these characteristics of personal change are now shared by many of the leading approaches to psychotherapy, including psychodynamic and cognitive behavioral therapy (Higginson et al., 2011; Kottler, 2014).

However, many people experience psychological change without the help of any form of treatment. How does this happen and why?

To answer these questions, our main tenets are:

- *Our cognitive system is naturally shaped to identify and counter experiential conflicts*;
- *This is achieved through a specific cognitive process – presence - whose goal is the control of the activity of the individual.* I am present in a real or virtual space if I manage to put my intentions into action (enacting them);
- *There is a link between presence and the effectiveness of an action.* The greater level of presence a subject experiences in an activity, the greater the individual's involvement in the activity will be, and this increases the probability of the activity ending well (the transformation of the intention into action);
- *There are "optimal experiences" in which both the individual experiences the maximum feeling of presence, and he/she is able to change/produce creative work more easily.*

In the following paragraphs we will endeavor to justify these claims. In order to do so, we will begin with the analysis of the transformations which are characterizing cognitive sciences.

## PERSONAL CHANGE: THE VISION OF COGNITIVE SCIENCES

Different recent discoveries from cognitive sciences are suggesting that human cognition - rather than being centralized, abstract, and sharply distinct from peripheral input and output modules - has instead deep roots in sensorimotor processing.

An example of this trend is the recent discovery of neuronal resonance processes activated by the simple observation of actions. Rizzolatti and colleagues found that a functional cluster of premotor neurons (F5c-PF) contains two groups of "bimodal" neurons in which sensory and motor faculties are linked (Gallese, Fadiga, Fogassi, & Rizzolatti, 1996; Rizzolatti, Fadiga, Gallese, & Fogassi, 1996).

- **The First Group of Neurons (F5ab-AIP):** Known as "canonical" neurons, are activated when the individual sees an object with which he/she can potentially interact;
- **The Second Group of Neurons (F5c-PF):** Known as "mirror" neurons, are activated when the individual sees another subject performing the same action.

The existence of bimodal neurons suggests that action and perception are more closely linked than has traditionally been assumed. Specifically, for the *Common Coding Theory* (Hommel, Müsseler, Aschersleben, & Prinz, 2001), the cognitive representations for perceived events (perception) and intended or to-be generated events (action) are formed by a common representational domain: actions are coded in terms of the perceivable effects they should generate. For example, "canonical" neurons permit an immediate and intuitive (pre-reflexive) understanding of opportunities for interaction which various objects may offer (in the case of the handle of a coffee cup, the possibility of being taken hold of if the subject wants to drink).

For this reason, when an effect is intended, the movement that produces this effect as perceptual input is automatically activated, because actions and their effects are stored in a common representational domain: the sight of a red apple is believed to activate a simulation of the motor functions necessary to pick it up.

In simpler words, the brain has its own virtual reality system that is used in both action planning and action understanding. But how can the subject know whether his or her intention has really been transformed into an effective action? We shall try to answer this question in the following paragraph by introducing the concept of presence.

## Presence: An Introduction

The concept of "presence" originated from and was diffused by a technological scientific community at the same time as the introduction of a unique piece of communication technology, teleoperators: robots controlled from a distance by a human operator (Heeter, 1992). In this case the term telepresence refers to the human operator's sensation of being present in the remote location in which the teleoperator is situated (Held & Durlach, 1992). But am I present only when I'm experiencing a telepresence system or a virtual reality environment?

Obviously the answer is no. This is why recent neuropsychological studies suggest that presence has a key role in our cognitive processes: it can be described as the outcome of an intuitive metacognitive process that allows us to control our actions through the comparison between intentions and perceptions (Riva & Mantovani, 2012d).

According to Gamberini, Spagnolli and Mantovani, the sense of presence is linked to a subject's capacity for action and his ability to position himself within his physical and social space (Spagnolli & Gamberini, 2005). More precisely, for Spagnolli and Gamberini (2005): "Presence is the feature of the agent which is manifested through the creation of a space during action" (p. 8).

A similar, but broader view, was recently outlined by Riva and Waterworth (Riva, Waterworth, Waterworth, & Mantovani, 2011; Waterworth, Waterworth, Mantovani, & Riva, 2010). The idea proposed by the two authors is the following: presence can be described as a selective and adaptive mechanism which allows the Self to define the boundaries of action by means of the distinction between "internal" and "external" within the sensory flow (Riva & Mantovani, 2012a, 2012d). In other words, the subject is "present" in a space if he/she can act in it. Moreover, the subject is "present" in the space – real or virtual – where he/she can act in (Waterworth et al., 2010). Interestingly, what we need for presence are both the affordance for action (the possibility of acting) and its enaction (the ability of successfully acting).

To sum up, we can define presence as the pre-reflexive sensation of "being" in an environment, real or virtual, which results from the capacity to carry out intuitively one's intentions within that environment.

## Presence and Intentions

An important consequence of this framework is the need to understand more what "acting successfully" means. We can start from the definition of "Agency": "the power to alter at will one's perceptual inputs" (Russell, 1996). But how can we define our will? A simple answer to this question is: through intentions.

Following this line of reasoning, presence can be defined as "the non-mediated (prereflexive) perception of using the body to successfully transform intentions into actions (enaction)" (Riva, 2008).

A possible criticism to this definition is the following (Riva, 2009a): "I may be asked to repair a computer, and I may be unable to fix it. This does not mean that I am not present in the environment (real or virtual) where the computer and I are."

This objection makes sense if we use the folk psychology definition of intention: the intention of an agent performing an action is his/her specific purpose in doing so. However, the latest cognitive studies clearly show that, as also suggested by the Perceptual Control Theory discussed in the introduction, any behavior is the result of a complex intentional chain that cannot be analyzed at a single level (Pacherie, 2006; Searle, 1983).

According to the *Activity Theory* introduced by Leontjev and disseminated by Kaptelinin, & Nardi (Kaptelinin & Nardi, 2006; Leontjev, 1978), and to the *Dynamic Theory of Intentions* presented by Pacherie (Pacherie, 2006, 2008; Pacherie & Haggard, 2010) repairing a computer is driven by an above objective (e.g., obtaining the money for paying a new car) and is the result of lower-level operations (e.g., removing the hard disk or the CPU, cleaning them, etc.) each driven by specific purposes.

So, for an intention that failed (repairing the computer) many others were successful (removing the hard disk, cleaning it, etc.) inducing Presence (Riva, 2009a, 2010).

Specifically, the *Dynamic Theory of Intentions* identifies three different "levels" or "forms" of intentions (Figure 1), characterized by different roles and contents: distal intentions (D-intentions), proximal intentions (P-intentions) and motor intentions (M-intentions):

- **D-Intentions (Future-Directed Intentions):** These high-level intentions act both as intra- and interpersonal coordinators, and as prompters of practical reasoning about means and plans: in the activity "obtaining a Ph.D. in psychology" described in Figure 1, "helping others to solve problems" is a D-intention, the object that drives the activity of the subject.
- **P-Intentions (Present-Directed Intentions):** These intentions are responsible for high-level (conscious) forms of guidance and monitoring. They have to ensure that the imagined actions

*Figure 1. The intentional chain*
*From Riva and Mantovani, 2012.*

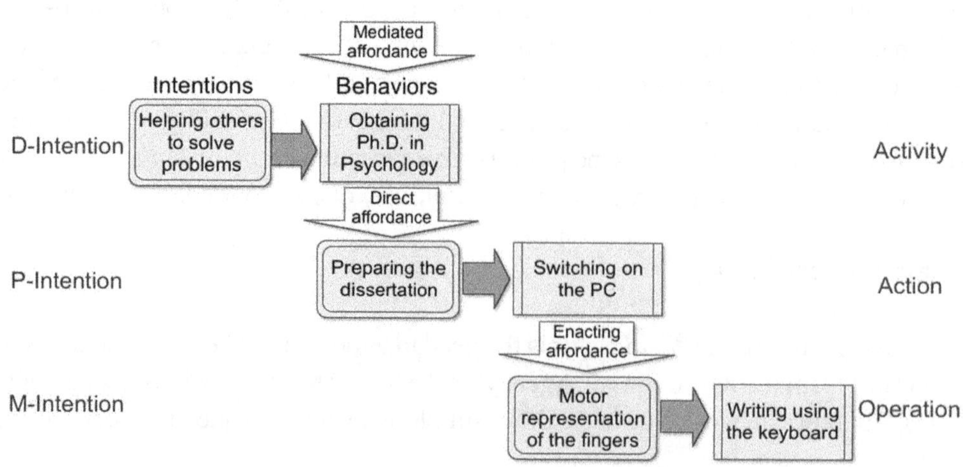

become current through situational control of their unfolding: in the activity described in Figure 1, "preparing the dissertation" is a P-intention.

- **M-Intentions (Motor Intentions):** These intentions are responsible for low-level (unconscious) forms of guidance and monitoring: we may not be aware of them and have only partial access to their content. Further, their contents are not propositional: in the activity described in Figure 1, the motor representations required to write using the keyboard are M-intentions.

Any intentional level has its own role: the rational (D-intentions), situational (P-Intention) and motor (M-Intention) guidance and control of action. They form an intentional cascade (Pacherie, 2006, 2008) in which higher intentions generate lower intentions.

Even if presence is a unitary feeling, the hypothesis formulated by Riva and Waterworth (Riva & Waterworth, 2003; Riva, Waterworth, & Waterworth, 2004) suggests that, on the process side, it can be divided into three phylogenetically different layers/subprocesses, that correspond reasonably well to the three levels of intentions identified by Pacherie (Figure 2 and Table 4):

1. **Proto Presence:** Motor Intentions (Self vs. non Self);
2. **Core Presence:** Proximal Intentions, directed towards the Present (Self vs. actual external world);
3. **Extended Presence:** Distal Intentions, directed towards the Future (Self vs. possible/future external world).

In practice, the Self evolves by extending the boundaries of its actions through the acquisition higher levels of intentional ability.

*Figure 2. Presence in the intentional chain*
*Adapted from Riva and Mantovani, 2012.*

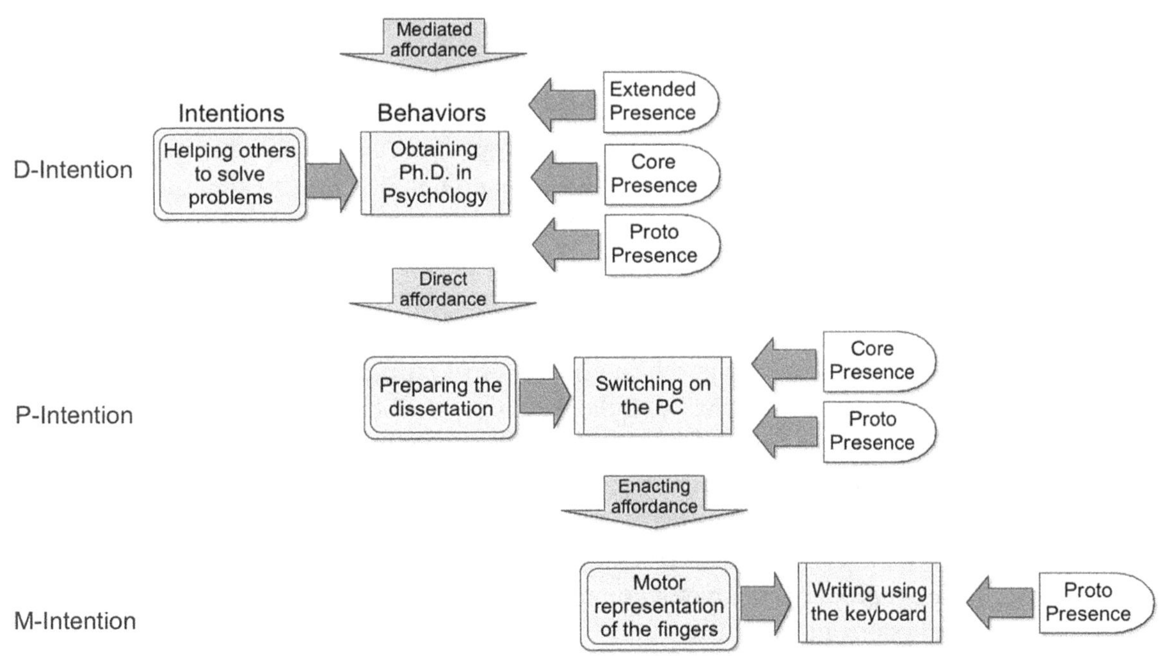

*Table 4. The layers of presence*

| Concept | Definition |
|---|---|
| Presence | A selective and adaptive mechanism which allows the Self to define the boundaries of action by means of the distinction between "internal" and "external" within the sensory flow. The feeling of presence is the outcome an intuitive metacognitive process that allows us to control our actions through the comparison between intentions and perceptions. Although presence is a unitary feeling, on the process side it can be divided into three different layers/subprocesses, phylogenetically different, and strictly related to the evolution of self. |
| Proto Presence | The first subprocess of Presence is related to the emergence of proto-self: the intuitive perception of successfully differentiating the self from the external world through action. It depends on the level of perception-action coupling (Self vs. non Self). |
| Core Presence | The second subprocess of Presence is related to the emergence of core-self: the intuitive perception of successfully acting in the external world towards a present Object. It depends on the level of vividness (Self vs. Present External World). |
| Extended Presence | The third subprocess of Presence is related to the emergence of extended-self: the intuitive perception of successfully acting in the external world towards a possible Object. It depends on the level of relevance (Self vs. Possible External World). |

In fact, the three levels of intention are differentiated by the limits to the actions which the subject is able to perform. The boundaries of the actions resulting from motor intentions are defined by the relationship between body and mind: I can only move my body. The boundaries of the actions resulting from proximal intentions depend upon the relationship between the mind and the physical world: I can only interact with the objects which are present around me. The boundaries of the actions resulting from distal intentions are given by the relationship between the mind and the possible world: I can try to do everything that I can imagine doing.

This view suggests that when the subject is present during agency – he/she is able to successfully enact his/her intentions – he/she locates him/herself in the physical and cultural space in which the action occurs.

Moreover, it also suggests that the feeling of presence will be different according to the ability of the subject to enact his/her intentions within an external environment. For instance, in the movie "Pretty Woman" Julia Robert is in a restaurant for a formal dinner with Richard Gere, but she doesn't know how to use the snail tongs and the snail forks she has nearby her dish. In this situation Julia is physically there, but the lack of knowledge puts her outside, at least partially, from the social and cultural space of the "formal dinner". The result is reduced presence and a limitation in her agency: she is not able to enact her intention (opening an escargot) using the snail forks, and this puts her in an embarrassing situation (she launches the escargot across the restaurant).

In conclusion, from an evolutionary point of view, presence has three functions:

- To permit the subject to position himself in a space – real, virtual or social – through the distinction between "internal" and "external" and the definition of a boundary;
- To check the efficacy of the subject's actions through the comparison of intention and the result of the action. From a computational viewpoint, the experience of presence is achieved through a forward-inverse model (Figure 3) that is similar to the negative feedback loop described by Perceptual Control Theory to reduce errors:
    - First, the agent produces the motor command for achieving a desired state given the current state of the system and the current state of the environment;

   - Second, an efference copy of the motor command is fed to a forward dynamic model that generates a prediction of the consequences of performing this motor command;
   - Third, the predicted state is compared with the actual sensory feedback. Errors derived from the difference between the desired state and the actual state can be used to update the model and improve performance.
- To allow its own evolution through the identification of "optimal experiences" (Flow) and the incorporation of the artifacts – physical and social – linked to it.

## Understanding Intentions using Social Presence

The concept of presence concerns the subject and the ability to act his or her intentions in the world: I am present in a real or virtual space if I am able to put my intentions into action. But how does one connect to others? How do others become present for the subject?

To answer this question we will analyze the implications of the "mirror" neurons discover (Riva & Waterworth, 2014; Riva, Waterworth, & Murray, 2014). These neurons, discovered in the ventral pre-motor cortex of apes (area F5), have, amongst other qualities, that of activating not only when the animal performs a given action, but also when the animal sees another animal – man or ape – performing the same action (Rizzolatti et al., 1996; Rizzolatti & Sinigaglia, 2006). Therefore, the individual who observes is able to put himself in the shoes of the actor: I am able to understand what another is doing because when I watch him I experience, completely intuitively, the same neuron activity as when *I* perform that action.

*Figure 3. The experience of presence*
*Adapted from Riva, 2009.*

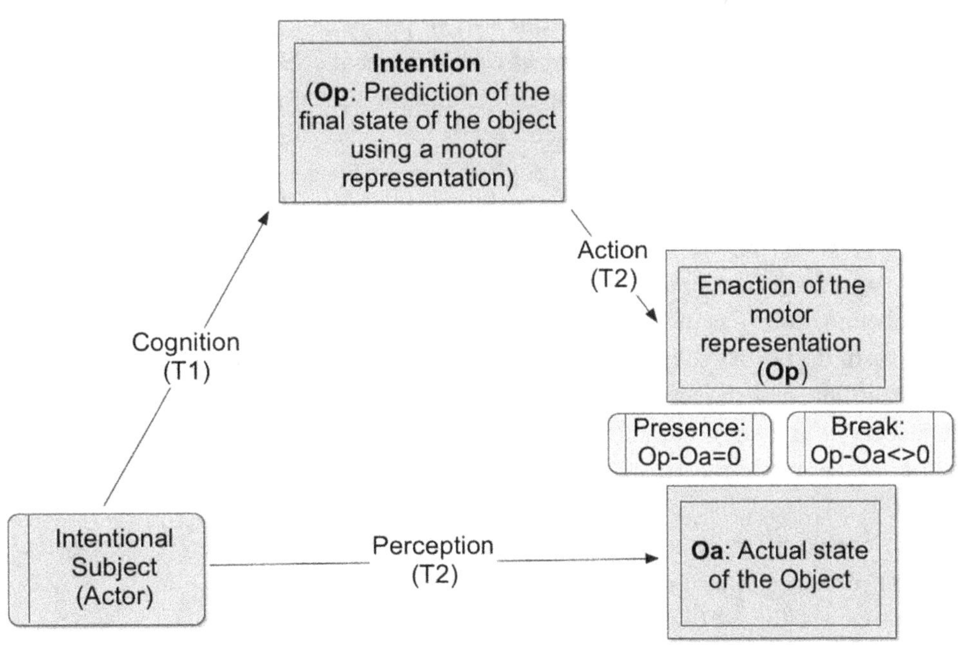

The result is the creation of neural representations which are shared on two levels (Gallagher & Jeannerod, 2002):

- On the one hand, execution and observation share the same neural substratum in one individual subject;
- On the other, when a subject observes another subject's action, the same representations are simultaneously active in the brains of both subjects.

This means that at neural level, the action performed and the action observed are codified in a multi-subjective format, which does not recognize actor or observer. This process is, however, effective if the subject is capable of distinguishing between an action performed and an action perceived. At the moment in which the subject is able, through presence, to distinguish between him or herself and another, "an I and an Other are created". The "Other similar to the Self" thus becomes, together with the Self, one of the two relevant elements which the organism is able to identify within its perceptive flow.

This suggests the existence of a second selective and adaptive mechanism, social presence, which enables the Self to identify and interact with the Other by understanding his intentions. In other words, from an evolutionary point of view, social presence has three functions:

- To enable the subject to identify the Other and to attribute to him an ontological status – "the Other similar to the Self" – different from the other objects perceived,
- To allow interaction and communication through the understanding of the Other's intentions; From the computational viewpoint, it happens using the same approach used by Presence:
    - First, the agent recognizes a motor intention, and identify the actor as another intentional self (Other);
    - Second, an efference copy of the motor command is fed to a forward dynamic model that generates a prediction of the consequences of performing this motor command (goal);
    - Third, the predicted state is compared with the actual sensory feedback. Errors derived from the difference between the predicted state and the actual state (break) can be used to update the model and improve performance.
- To permit the evolution of the Self through the identification of "optimal shared experiences" (Networked Flow) and the incorporation of artifacts – physical and social – linked to them.

In summary, we can define social presence (Biocca, Harms, & Burgoon, 2003; Riva, 2008; Riva, Davide, & IJsselsteijn, 2003) as the sensation of "being with other selves" in a real or virtual environment, resulting from the ability to intuitively recognize Others' intentions in our surroundings.

The study of infants and the analysis of their ability of understanding and interacting with people (Meltzoff & Decety, 2003) suggest that also Social Presence, on the process side, includes three different layers/subprocesses phylogenetically different, but mutually inclusive (Riva, 2008) (see Table 5):

- Other's Presence (Other vs the Self - M-Intentions);
- Interactive Presence (Other toward the Self – P-Intentions);
- Shared Presence (Other is like the Self - D-Intentions).

*Table 5. The layers of social presence*

| Concept | Definition |
|---|---|
| Social Presence | A selective and adaptive mechanism which allows the Self to identify and interact with Others by understanding their intentions. The feeling of social presence is the the outcome of an intuitive metacognitive process that allows us to understand the actions of an enacting Other through the comparison between his/her expected intentions and perceptions. Although social presence is a unitary feeling, on the process side it can be divided into three different layers/subprocesses, phylogenetically different, and strictly related to the evolution of self. |
| Other's Presence | The first subprocess of Social Presence is related to the ability of recognizing motor intentions in other individuals. This capacity allows the Self to recognize an intentional Other (the Other in opposition to the Self). |
| Interactive Presence | The second subprocess of Social Presence is related to the ability of recognizing motor and proximal intentions in other individuals. This capacity allows the Self to identify the Other whose intention is directed towards him (the Other towards the Self). |
| Shared Presence | The third subprocess of Social Presence is related to the ability of recognizing motor, proximal and distal intentions in other individuals. This capacity allows the Self to identify Another whose intentions correspond to his/her own. (the Other like the Self). |

The first level of imitative skills – the ability to imitate a human being – corresponds to "Other's Presence", the ability to recognize motor intentions, which allows the Self to recognize an intentional Other: the better the subject is able to *recognize within the sensorial flow the stimuli which relate to "another similar to the self"*, the better he/she is able to carry out an intention, and thus increases his/her chances of survival (the Other in opposition to the Self).

The second level of imitative skills – the ability to identify a human being who is imitating me – corresponds to "Interactive Presence", the ability to recognize motor and proximal intentions which allows the Self to identify the Other whose intention is directed towards him/her: the better the subject is able to *recognize within the sensorial flow the intention direct towards hi/her by "an Other similar to the self"*, the greater the chances of successfully carrying out an action, and therefore the greater the chances of survival (the Other towards the Self).

The third level of imitative skills – the ability to recognize the intentions and emotions of a human being – corresponds to "Shared Presence", the ability to recognize motor, proximal and distal intentions, which enables the Self to identify Another whose intentions correspond to his/her own: the better the subject is able to *recognize within the sensorial flow an "Other similar to the self" with intentions the same as his/her own,* the better he/she will be able to successfully initiate collaborative interaction or communication, increasing his chances of survival (the Other like the Self).

Shared presence permits the subject to feel empathy, *the capacity to see oneself in another person, to get inside another's thoughts and state of mind.* During the experience of empathy, the subject separates himself from his own intentional and emotional state, and identifies with that of another person (the Other merges with the Self).

What is the link between the three levels of social presence? As with presence, the three levels are evolutionarily organized: from the lowest to the highest. However, unlike presence, the levels of social presence are not functionally separate but mutually inclusive. This leads to two consequences. The superior levels also include the inferior levels: if the subject is able to understand distal intentions (shared presence), he is also capable of understanding motor intentions (other's presence). At the same time, it is impossible to activate the higher levels of social presence if the lower levels are not activated first: if

I am unable to understand a subject's proximal intentions (interactive presence) then I will not be able to understand his distal intentions (shared presence).

The three levels of social presence are linked by *simultaneous influences on the subject's capacity for social interaction:* the way in which the interaction is experienced changes depending on the level of social presence experienced by the subject. It is important to note that, as with presence, the subject is unaware of the role of social presence in determining the characteristics of his actions. He/she is, however, evolutionarily programmed to perceive the shift from one level of social presence to another in social interactions. Furthermore, if this shift offers a valuable opportunity, the subject can act to increase his level of social presence. If a girl starts staring at me at a party, I immediately become aware of the shift from other's presence (the girl is at the same party as me) to interactive presence (the girl is looking at me). If the girl is interesting, I can approach her and talk to her in order to understand her intentions: is she looking at me because she likes me or because I have a stain on my jacket?

## Presence and Optimal Experiences

At this point, a possible question from the readers of the chapter is this one: interesting stuff, but how can it help me in sustaining personal change?

An important consequence of the considerations made in the preceding paragraphs, is the existence of certain "optimal experiences", *in which the individual experiences the maximum feeling of presence and/or social presence at each of the three levels* (Waterworth & Riva, 2014; Waterworth & Waterworth, 2012, 2014).

The highest level of presence, when associated with a positive emotional state (it is also possible to experience the maximum feeling of presence in emotionally negative situations, such as during an escape), is defined as "flow experience" (Csikszentmihalyi, 1990, 1994). This state is characterized by a high level of concentration and participation in the activity, by the balance of the perception of the difficulties of the situation and the *challenge*, and personal *skills,* by the distortion of the sense of time (the internal clock slows down, whilst the external one speeds up), and by a natural interest in the process which produces a sense of pleasure and satisfaction. More, flow has been associated to creativity and emotional wellbeing (Csikszentmihalyi, 1997) (see Table 6).

*Table 6. Optimal experiences*

| Concept | Definition |
|---|---|
| Optimal Experiences | Specific individual (Flow) and social (Networked Flow) situations in which the individual experiences *the maximum feeling of presence.* |
| Flow | There are exceptional situations – e.g., a tennis player who goes to the right (proto presence) before the ball bounces on the court to swing a winning forehand ground stroke (core presence) on a second set-point at the Wimbledon final (extended presence) - in which the activity of the subject is characterized by a high level of presence in all the three different subprocesses (Maximal Presence). When this experience is associated with a positive emotional state, it constitutes a flow state. |
| Networked Flow | There are exceptional social situations in which a group of subjects in a liminality phase (a state of transition, in which the earlier *positive* condition is no longer present, and the future *positive* condition has not yet come into) experiences the maximum level of social presence (the feeling of sharing objectives and emotions with others) and the feeling of being able through the their collective action of exiting from liminality (maximum level of presence). |

Similar considerations can also be made concerning the concept of social presence. There is a specific optimal experience for social presence – *"networked flow"* – the result of the association between (Gaggioli, Mazzoni, Milani, & Riva, 2015; Gaggioli, Milani, Mazzoni, & Riva, 2011, 2013; Gaggioli & Riva, 2014):

- **The Maximum Level of Social Presence:** The feeling of sharing objectives and emotions with others;
- **The Group Members' Perception of Being in a Phase of Liminality:** A state of transition, of being "about to…", in which the earlier *positive* condition is no longer present, and the future *positive* condition has not yet come into being.
- **The Shared Recognition of a Possible Common Strategy for Exiting from Liminality:** Everybody working towards a shared objective, which the group can change.
- **The Maximum Level of Presence:** The feeling of being able, through the personal involvement in the group, of successfully transforming intentions – both individual and collective - in actions.

In this case, the maximum level of presence and social presence permits the subject to increase their self-efficacy and to find the motivation for change within the shared group activity (Gaggioli et al., 2015).

This concept shares a number of similarities with the concept of the "nascent state" proposed by Alberoni. Subjects who go through this have a strange experience which causes them to develop an alternative interpretation of existence (Alberoni, 1977). *Nascent state is an exploration of the boundaries of the possible, given a certain type of social system, with the goal of maximizing what is realizable within that experience and solidarity for oneself and others in that moment in time. The group of men amongst whom a nascent state is created will always attempt to construct a way of living which is completely different from the everyday institutional norm (p. 31).* Alberoni's ideas highlight how the simultaneous union between high levels of presence and social presence make *networked flow* a *state of transition* which constitutes the specific conditions for social transformation. It is at this moment that the subjective intention becomes collective (we-intention).

Another important consequence of this model is that we can develop technologies – "Positive Technologies" - that are able to improve the quality of our personal experience by enhancing the level of presence and social presence experienced interacting with them (Graffigna, Barello, et al., 2013c; Graffigna, Barello, Wiederhold, et al., 2013; Riva, 2012c). In the next paragraph we will explore and discuss this claim.

## POSITIVE TECHNOLOGIES: POSITIVE PSYCHOLOGY IN PRACTICE

The recent discoveries of cognitive sciences suggest the possibility of a new paradigm -*Positive Technology* (Riva, 2012c; Riva et al., 2012) – whose main objective is to use technology to manipulate and enhance the features of our personal experience, by manipulating presence and social presence, for increasing wellness, and generating strength and resilience in individuals, organizations and society (Wiederhold & Riva, 2012).

This concept has many similarities with the concept of *Positive Computing* (Calvo & Peters, 2012, 2014): "The research and development of technology to support wellbeing and human potential" (p. 2). In particular Positive Technology shares with it the methodological approach to the technology design for wellbeing (Calvo & Peters, 2014): the identification of key factors from existing theories of wellbeing and their use for prevent detriments of wellbeing (prevention), actively integrated promotional design (action) and the development of technologies aimed specifically at promoting well-being (creation).

The main difference, however, is in the focus: Calvo and Peters focus their analysis on the concept of wellbeing, while Positive Technology focuses its analysis on the concept of personal experience.

What is behind this difference? Wellbeing is a subjective experiene, and for this reason cannot be defined in a unique way, with the risk of being too vague to be useful within a scientific research program: What is wellbeing for me and you?

In their book the two authors are aware of this problem and present and discuss three different definitions of wellbeing (Calvo & Peters, 2014):

- **Medical:** The absence of illnesses;
- **Hedonic:** An aggregate of pleasurable experiences;
- **Eudaimonic:** Finding meaning in life and fulfilling one's greatest potential.

This choice is clearly explained in the text: "For designers of technology, the underlying philosophical standpoint is perhaps less important than the strategies arising from these theories that have been proven to improve wellbeing in practice" (p. 14). And, as reported in Table 7, they focused their efforts in the identification of the possible factors involved in wellbeing and in the strategies to strengthen them.

To address this issue we will define Positive Technology starting from the concept of experience (Riva, 2012a). According to the Merriam Webster Dictionary, it is possible to define experience both as "a) the fact or state of having been affected by or gained knowledge through direct observation or participation" (personal experience), and "b) direct observation of or participation in events as a basis of knowledge" (subjective experience)

These definitions underline the two connected faces of our experience: on one side, we can intentionally control the contents of our experience (subjective experience); on the other side, its contents define our future emotions and intentions (personal experience). In other words, we both shape and are shaped by it.

However, there is a critical difference between subjective experience and personal experience. If subjective experience is the experience of being a subject (experience as subject,, the "I" described by William James), personal experience is the experience affecting a particular subject (experience as object, the "Me" described by William James).

This simple shift suggests that, independently from the subjectivity of any individual, it is possible to alter the features of our experience from outside. In other words, personal experience becomes the dependent variable that may be manipulated and studied by external researchers. In particular cognitive and positive psychology identified three determinants of personal experience: emotional quality, engagement/actualization and connectedness (Inghilleri, Riva, & Riva, 2015).

In the proposed framework (see Figures 4 and 5), positive technologies are classified according to their effects on the above features of personal experience (Botella et al., 2012):

- **Hedonic (Emotional Quality):** Technologies used to induce positive and pleasant experiences.
- **Eudaimonic (Engagement/Actualization):** Technologies used to support individuals in reaching engaging and self-actualizing experiences.
- **Social/Interpersonal (Connectedness):** Technologies used to support and improve social integration and/or connectedness between individuals, groups, and organizations.

See also Table 8 for a list of the key factors influencing the three variables determining personal experience.

*Table 7. Well being factors for positive computing*

| | Wellbeing Factor | Literature and Theory | Strategies | Methods and Measures |
|---|---|---|---|---|
| Self (Intrapersonal) | Positive Emotions | • Hedonic Psychology (Kahneman); • Subjective Wellbeing (Deiner); • Building & Broadening Effect (Fredrickson). | Savouring; Positive ruminating; Reframing Compassion & meditation. | PANAS scales; General wellbeing measures such as SWB, SWLS and QoL scales. |
| | Motivation & Engagement | • Self-determination Theory (Ryan & Deci); • Flow Theory (Csikszentmihalyi). | Intrinsic and extrinsic rewards. | The Motivation and Engagement Scale; Self-Regulation Questionnaires. |
| | Self-Awareness | • Cognitive Behavioral Therapy (Aaron Beck); • Emotional Intelligence (Mayer & Salovey). | Life summary; Online CBT study; Technology Mediated Reflection. | Emotional Intelligence measures (e.g. MSCEIT); Wellbeing measures such as Life Satisfaction. |
| | Mindfulness | • Mindfulness based Stress Reduction (Kabat Zinn); • Mindfulness based Cognitive Therapy (Segal, Williams & Teasdale). | Mindfulness meditation; MBSR strategies; MBCT strategies. | MAAS; Freiburg Mindfulness Inventory. |
| | Resilience | • Psychology of resilience (Seligman, Keyes); • Building & Broadening Effect (Fredrickson). | Positive psychology interventions; SuperBetter. | Resilience Scale. |
| Social (Interpersonal) | Gratitude | Psychology of Gratitude (Emmons & McCullough). | Gratitude visit; Gratitude journal. | Gratitude Questionnaire. |
| | Empathy | • Emotional Intelligence (Salovey & Mayer; Goleman); • Affective and Cognitive empathy (Gerdes et al; Singer); • Compassion Focused Therapy (Paul Gilbert). | Role playing; Perspective taking; Emotion recognition training. | EQ; Interpersonal Reactivity Index; Children's Empathic Attitudes Questionnaire. |
| | Compassion | Compassion Focused Therapy (Paul Gilbert). | Compassion; Meditation. | Self-compassion Scale; Prosocial Orientation Scale; Hostile Attribution Bias Questionnaire. |
| | Altruism | Empathy Altruism (Bateson). | Prosocial games; Role playing helping behavior. | |

Adapted from Calvo and Peters, 2014.

*Figure 4. Positive technology levels*
*Adapted from Riva et al. 2012.*

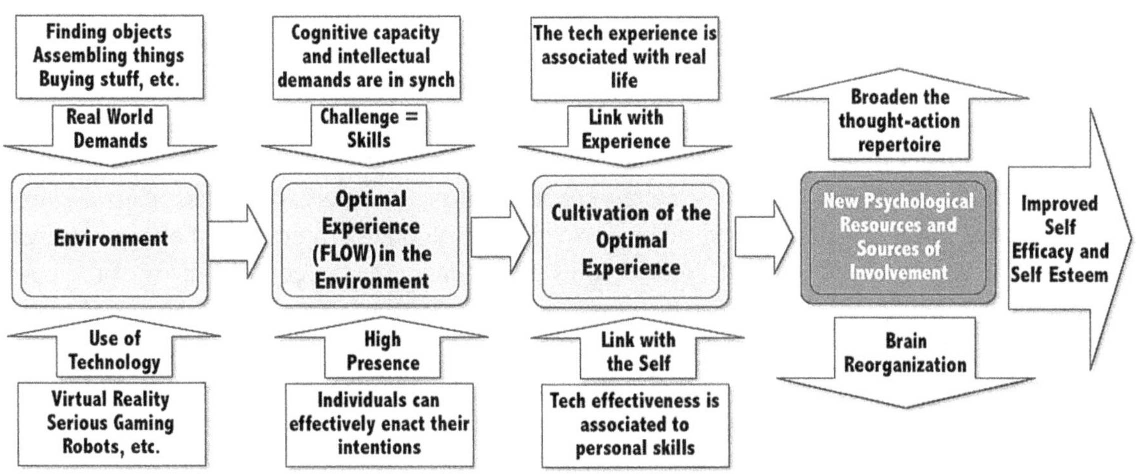

*Figure 5. Transformation of flow*

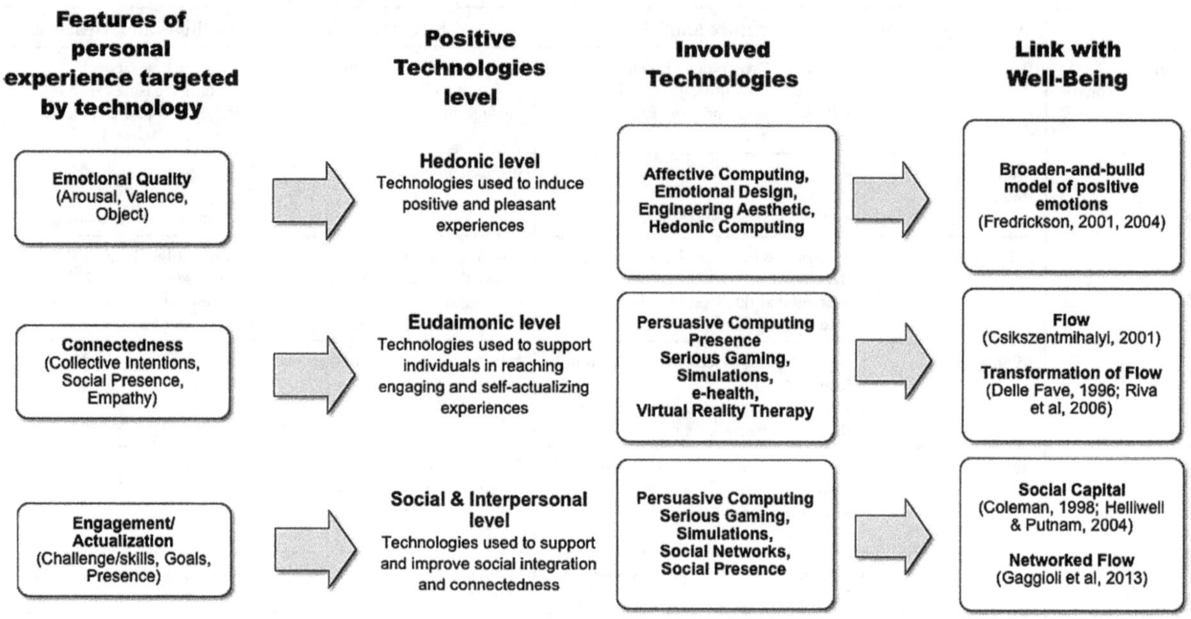


## Hedonic Technologies: Using Technology to Foster Positive Emotional States

The first dimension of Positive Technology concerns how to use technology to foster positive emotional states. According to the model of emotions developed by James Russell (2003) it is possible to modify the affective quality of an experience through the manipulation of "core affect", a neurophysiological category corresponding to the combination of valence and arousal levels that endow the subjects with a kind of "core knowledge" about the emotional features of their experience.

The "core affect" can be experienced as freefloating (mood) or attributed to some cause (and thereby begins an emotional episode). In this view, an emotional response is the attribution of a change in the core affect given to a specific object (affective quality). Simply put, a positive emotion is achieved by increasing the valence (positive) and arousal (high) of core affect (affect regulation) and by attributing this change to the contents of the proposed experience (object).

Key arguments for the usefulness of positive emotions in increasing well-being have been recently provided by Fredrickson (Fredrickson, 2001, 2004) in what she called the "broaden-and-build model" of positive emotions. According to Fredrickson, positive emotions provide the organism with nonspecific action tendencies that can lead to adaptive behavior (Fredrickson, 2001). For example, in children joy is associated with the urge to play, whereas interest sparks the urge to explore; in adults, positive emotions make them more likely to interact with others, provide help to others in need, and engage in creative challenges. The second proposition of Fredrickson's model concerns the consequences of the positive emotions: by broadening an individual's awareness and thought–action repertoire, they build upon the resultant learning to create future physical, psychological and social resources (Fredrickson, 2004).

In literature it is possible to find many different approaches to hedonic technologies. For example, Riva and colleagues (2007) investigated how the content of interactive media, in particular virtual reality (VR), can be manipulated to induce specific emotional responses, including positive moods. The results

*Table 8. Personal experience factors for positive technology*

| Determinants of Personal Experience | Key Factors | Literature and Theory | Strategies (Augmentation, Structuration and Replacement) | Methods and Measures |
|---|---|---|---|---|
| Emotional Quality (Hedonic Level) | Positive Emotions | • Building & Broadening Effect (Fredrickson);<br>• Writing Therapy (Pennebaker)<br>• Hedonic Psychology (Kahneman); | Writing Therapy; Exposure Therapy and Relaxation; Savouring; Positive ruminating; Reframing Compassion & meditation. | PANAS scales; General measures such as STAI, BDS, SWLS and QoL scales. |
| | Mindfulness | • Mindfulness based Stress Reduction (Kabat Zinn); | Mindfulness meditation; MBSR strategies; MBCT strategies. | MAAS; Freiburg Mindfulness Inventory. |
| | Resilience | • Psychology of resilience (Seligman, Keyes);<br>• Building & Broadening Effect (Fredrickson). | Positive psychology interventions; SuperBetter. | Resilience Scale. |
| Engagement & Actualization (Eudaimonic Level) | Engagement & Presence | • Flow Theory (Csikszentmihalyi).<br>• Presence (Riva & Waterworth)<br>• Patient Engagement (Graffigna, Barello & Riva) | Challenge and Skills; Intrinsic and extrinsic rewards; | Flow Scales; Experiential Sampling Method |
| | Self-Efficacy & Motivation | • Self-Efficacy (Bandura)<br>• Transtheoretical Model of change (Prochaska & DiClemente)<br>• Self-determination Theory (Ryan & Deci); | Life summary; Online CBT study; Technology Mediated Reflection. | General Self-Efficacy Scale; Transtheoretical Model Questionnaire. |
| Connectedness (Social/ Interpersonal level) | Networked Flow | • Networked Flow (Gaggioli & Riva)<br>• Psychological Selection (Delle Fave, Inghilleri, Massimini) | Presence and Social Presence Transformation of Flow | Social Network Analysis |
| | Gratitude | Psychology of Gratitude (Emmons & McCullough). | Gratitude visit; Gratitude journal. | Gratitude Questionnaire. |
| | Empathy | • Emotional Intelligence (Salovey & Mayer; Goleman);<br>• Affective and Cognitive empathy (Gerdes et al; Singer);<br>• Compassion Focused Therapy (Paul Gilbert). | Role playing; Perspective taking; Emotion recognition training. | EQ; InterpersonalReactivity Index; Children's Empathic Attitudes Questionnaire. |
| | Altruism | Empathy Altruism (Bateson). | Prosocial games; Role playing helping behavior. | Self-compassion Scale; Prosocial Orientation Scale; Hostile Attribution Bias Questionnaire. |

suggested the efficacy of VR as an affective medium: the interaction with “anxious” and “relaxing” virtual environments produced anxiety and relaxation.

In a subsequent study, Villani and colleagues (Villani, Lucchetta, Preziosa, & Riva, 2009; Villani, Riva, & Riva, 2007) compared the efficacy of structured experiences provided through different technologies (video, audio and VR) for inducing relaxing states. The results of this experiment showed a significant reduction in anxiety and a significant improvement in positive emotional states, measured through self-report questionnaires and physiological parameters, but no difference among the media conditions. However, findings highlighted a significant correlation between changes in emotional states and factors related to the sense of presence felt by participants during media exposure.

Different studies have also shown that a possible path for improving positive emotions is the use of meditation, in particular mindfulness (Epel, Daubenmier, Moskowitz, Folkman, & Blackburn, 2009; Pagnini, Di Credico, et al., 2014; Pagnini, Phillips, & Langer, 2014). Mindfulness is a psychological mindset that is focused on being aware of novelty in personal experience and perceiving differences in contexts and events, disrupting stress pathways and possibly having direct beneficial effects on physiological arousal systems (Phillips & Pagnini, 2014).

Epel and colleagues, in their review of the effects of mindfulness, suggested that meditative practices improve the endocrine balance toward positive arousal (high DHEA, lower cortisol) and decrease oxidative stress, slowing the rate of cellular aging (Epel et al., 2009). They concluded: "Thus, meditation practices may promote mitotic cell longevity both through decreasing stress hormones and oxidative stress and increasing hormones that may protect the telomere" (p. 49).

In this process, the role of technology is quite simple, i.e., to facilitate meditation. Our team developed different immersive (computer-based) and non-immersive (smarphone and tablet-based) experiences to improve meditation abilities in untrained individuals (Carissoli, Villani, & Riva, 2015; Grassi, Gaggioli, & Riva, 2011; Manzoni et al., 2006; Manzoni et al., 2009; Preziosa et al., 2009; Simona Raspelli et al., 2011). The feeling of presence and the immersive visual cue provided by virtual reality (VR) are known to facilitate relaxation, reduce stress, and improve positive emotional states (Serino et al., 2014; Villani, Lucchetta, Preziosa, & Riva, 2006; Villani, Preziosa, Riva, & Riva, 2006; Villani et al., 2007).

For example, in the "Green Valley" experience, different narratives were presented together with a very relaxing virtual environment showing a mountain landscape around a calm lake. After being immersed in the Green Valley, participants were asked to walk around the lake, to observe nature, and, after few minutes, to virtually sit on a comfortable deck chair and relax (Manzoni et al., 2006; Manzoni et al., 2009; Riva, Manzoni, Villani, Gaggioli, & Molinari, 2008).

When aimed at relaxation, VR lends itself to be associated with biofeedback training (Cipresso et al., 2012; Riva, 2009e). Biofeedback is a coaching and training technique that helps people learn how to change their physiological response patterns in order to improve their mental and emotional functioning (Repetto et al., 2009). The person is connected to psychophysiological biosensors and uses the information provided as feedback to increase awareness or consciousness of the changes in the functioning of the body/mind (Riva, Algeri, et al., 2010).

## Eudaimonic Technologies: Using Technology to Promote Engagement and Self-Empowerment

The second level of Positive Technology is strictly related to the eudaimonic concept of well-being, and consists of investigating how technologies can be used to support individuals in reaching engaging and self-actualizing experiences.

The theory of flow, developed by Positive Psychology pioneer Mihaly Csikszentmihalyi (1990), provides a useful framework for addressing this challenge. Flow or optimal experience is a positive and complex state of consciousness that is present when individuals act with total involvement. The basic feature of this experience is the perceived balance between high environmental opportunities for action (challenges) and adequate personal resources in facing them (skills). Additional characteristics are deep concentration, clear rules in and unambiguous feedback from the task at hand, loss of self-consciousness, control of one's actions and environment, positive affect and intrinsic motivation.

The theory of flow has been extensively used to study user experience with information and communication technologies. Ghani (Ghani & Deshpande, 1994) identified three factors that influence the occurrence of flow in human-computer interaction: perceived control, fitness of task (i.e., the difference between challenges and skills), and cognitive spontaneity ("playfulness"). According to Ghani's model, the experience of flow can produce positive cognitive effects in users, such as an augmented focus on the process, increased creativity, and enhanced learning.

Among the different types of interactive technologies investigated so far by flow researchers, immersive systems such as VR are considered the most capable of supporting the emergence of this experience (Gaggioli, Bassi, & Delle Fave, 2003; Riva, Castelnuovo, & Mantovani, 2006; Riva, Raspelli, et al., 2010). Research conducted thus far highlights some key characteristics of this technology as a source of flow: (a) opportunities for action (goals and rules) – due to its flexibility, VR provides designers with the possibility of creating a wide range of increasingly challenging situations and tasks, (b) feedback – VR systems can offer multimodal feedback to individuals' actions and behavior (Gaggioli, 2004; Gaggioli et al., 2003). Some researchers have drawn parallels between the experience of flow in VR and the sense of presence, defined as the subjective perception of "being there" in a virtual environment (Heeter, 2003; Riva, 2009c; Riva et al., 2004; Riva et al., 2011; Zahoric & Jenison, 1998). From the phenomenological viewpoint, both experiences have been described as absorbing states, characterized by a merging of action and awareness, loss of self-consciousness, a feeling of being transported into another reality, and an altered perception of time (J.A. Waterworth et al., 2010). Further, both presence and optimal experience are associated with high involvement, focused attention and high concentration on the ongoing activity (Marsh, 2003). In particular, Riva and Waterworth (Riva et al., 2011; J.A. Waterworth et al., 2010) have argued that there is a correspondence between "maximal" presence and optimal experience. Drawing on Damasio's (1999) three-fold model of self (proto-self, core-self, and extended self), these authors have suggested that "optimal presence" arises when the three components of the self are combined with an abnormally tight focus on the same content, so that intentions and action are directed exclusively towards the current external situation.

Starting from these theoretical premises, Riva and colleagues (Riva, 2009e; Riva et al., 2006; Riva & Gaggioli, 2009) suggested the possibility of using VR for a new type of applications in positive mental health for the ageing based on a strategy defined as "transformation of flow." This strategy is based on a person's ability to draw upon an optimal experience induced by technology and use it to promote new and unexpected psychological resources and sources of involvement.

The proposed approach consists of the following activities (Figure 5). First, using positive technologies to offer an enriched environment that contains *functional*, real-world demands (e.g., finding objects, assembling things, and buying stuff); second, using the technology to provide tasks (challenges) that are to matched to the cognitive capacity of the individual (skills) and to enhance the level of Presence (the feeling of being "inside" the technological experience (Riva & Mantovani, 2012a, 2012d)) to induce an optimal experience; third, allowing cultivation by linking this optimal experience to the actual experience and skills of the subject (Riva & Gaggioli, 2009). The expected effect is a functional reorganization of the brain produced by the broadening of the thought-action repertoire associated with improved self-esteem and self-efficacy.

The first proposed claim, i.e., the possibility of using positive technologies for creating enriched environments offering real world demands, is demonstrated by the Virtual Multiple Errand Test (V-MET) (Pedroli et al., 2013; S. Raspelli et al., 2012). The V-MET is a VR version of the Multiple Errands Test (Fortin, Godbout, & Braun, 2003), which is usually performed at a real shopping mall or in a hospital environment and involves the completion of various tasks with rules that must be followed within a specified time frame. The VR version enables the active exploration of a virtual supermarket in which individuals are requested to select and buy various products presented on shelves. Correlations between

Virtual Multiple Errands Test variables (e.g., errors and execution time) and some traditional executive functions measures provide preliminary support for the ecological and construct validity of the VMET. In addition, the performances obtained with the Virtual Multiple Errands Test provided the ability to distinguish between clinical and healthy populations and between two age-related control groups (Pedroli et al., 2013; S. Raspelli et al., 2012).

The second proposed claim – the possibility of using positive technologies for fostering optimal experiences in the elderly – was demonstrated by the "V-STORE Project" (Castelnuovo, Lo Priore, Liccione, & Cioffi, 2003; Lo Priore, Castelnuovo, & Liccione, 2003). The researchers investigated the quality of experience and the feeling of Presence in a group of 10 patients with frontal lobe syndrome involved in VR-based cognitive rehabilitation (Castelnuovo, Lo Priore, et al., 2003). They used the ITC-Sense of Presence Inventory Test (Lessiter, Freeman, Keogh, & Davidoff, 2001) to evaluate the feeling of Presence induced by the VR sessions. The findings highlighted the association of VR sessions with both positive affect and a high level of Presence.

The third claim – the use of transformation of flow for producing some form of functional reorganization in the elderly who are able to improve their cognitive abilities – received preliminary support by the work of Optale and his team (Optale et al., 2001; Optale et al., 2010). These authors investigated the experience of elderly individuals with memory deficits engaged in a six-month, virtual-reality, rehabilitative experience, including auditory stimulation and path-finding. The study also included a control group that had equivalent, face-to-face training sessions using music therapy. Only the VR group showed significant improvements in the memory tests, especially in long-term recall with an effect size of 0.7 and in several other aspects of cognition. Thus, the results that were showed that this approach was able to improve memory function (Optale et al., 2001; Optale et al., 2010).

## Social Technologies: Using Technology to Promote Social Integration and Connectedness

The final level of Positive Technology - the social and interpersonal one - is concerned with the use of technologies to support and improve the connectedness between individuals, groups, and organizations. However, an open challenge is to understand how to use technology to create a mutual sense of awareness, which is essential to the feeling that other participants are there, and to create a strong sense of community at a distance. Short et al., (1976) define 'social presence' as the "degree of salience of the other person in a mediated communication and the consequent salience of their interpersonal interactions" (p. 65). Conventional computer-mediated communicative tools, such as email or text-based chat, are regarded as having lower social presence and social context cues when compared to face-to-face communication. However, different authors have suggested that it is possible to manipulate the technological experience to enhance social presence and thereby improve different mediated activities (Park, 2010) such as online learning (Joyce, 2009), e-commerce (Swamynathan, Wilson, Boe, Almeroth, & Zhao, 2008) and health care (Boulos & Wheeler, 2007).

Riva and colleagues (2010) recently suggested that a subject is present within a virtual group if he is able to put his own intentions (presence) into practice and to understand the intentions of the other group members (social presence). This implies that to sustain social optimal experiences (networked flow), the technology has to provide the virtual group with the possibility of expressing itself and of understanding what each individual member is doing (Riva, 2004). More, Gaggioli and colleagues (Gaggioli et al., 2011) argued that optimal group state is achieved when the team develops a "we-intention", in which the actions of the individuals and of the collective are merged, and the group acts as an autonomous, self-organizing entity.

An interesting example of this approach is the use of technologies to improve inter-generational reminiscence (Gaggioli et al., 2014). Inter-generational reminiscence offers the potential for reducing existing barriers between generations by transmitting the heritage of folk traditions and by triggering the interest of younger people concerning their roots (Webster & McCall, 1999). To facilitate this process Gaggioli and colleagues used an interesting approach: a) the elderly narrated their life experiences they liked most or that they found more meaningful to share with their young audience; b) during storytelling, children were encouraged to express their interest towards specific aspects of the reminiscence and ask questions; c) the older adults were asked to collect material (photographs, letters, newspaper articles, etc.) that could help them document the aspects of their memories selected by the young audience; d) to allow further discussion and sharing, older and younger participants reported the content of the most interesting reminiscences in a website, by integrating texts with multimedia objects. Different examples of collected reminiscences are available on the project's website Nostalgia Bits (http://nobits.it/).

Analyses of pre- and post-intervention measures showed that even three two-hour sessions of group reminiscence activities had a positive impact on elderly psychosocial wellbeing: they reported significantly over values of loneliness and an increase in perceived Quality of life. Further, results indicated that following their participation in the program the children's attitude towards the elderly positively changed in a positive way (Gaggioli et al., 2014).

In a different study, Auburn University's Harrison School of Pharmacy created a Facebook page – Countryside Diabetes (http://goo.gl/ZPqsSE) - to provide ongoing education and support for elderly people affected by diabetes. As reported by the authors, membership and participation to Facebook page continue to grow among the senior population (Lee & Whitley, 2014).

Following this vision Morris (2005) has recently described how social-networking and pervasive computing technologies can be effectively used to help reduce feelings of social isolation and depression in elderly individuals. In their approach, sensor data measuring phone calls and visits are used to derive public displays of social interactions with relatives and friends, which they introduced into selected elders' homes. These ambient displays, which reflect data on remote and face-to-face interaction gathered by wireless sensor networks, are intended to raise awareness of social connectedness as a dynamic and controllable aspect of well-being. According to findings, this strategy was effective in reducing the feeling of social isolation of elderly users.

Key arguments for the usefulness of connectedness in increasing well-being have been presented by Ryff and Singer (2000). The authors argued that interpersonal flourishing (the development of positive relations with other people) is a key dimension of well-being, which is stable across different cultures and time. Furthermore, in a recent paper, Mauri and colleagues (2011) used a variety of physiological data - skin conductance, blood volume pulse, electroencephalogram, electromyography, respiratory activity, and pupil dilation – to evaluate the affective experience evoked by the use of Facebook. The biological signals revealed that Facebook use can evoke a psychophysiological state characterized by high positive valence and high arousal (Core Flow State). These findings support the hypothesis that the successful spread of social networks might be associated with a specific positive affective state experienced by users when they use their account.

Finally, the concept of "social capital" underlines the value of social relationships for the society as a whole: relations among persons facilitate activity and promote well-being (Coleman, 1988; Helliwell & Putnam, 2004). Despite the fact that creating and maintaining social relationships is considered a major indicator of well-being and a protective factor for health (House, Landis, & Umberson, 1988), Western society is characterized by increasing levels of loneliness and lack of social integration. The need of social integration is higher in specific social groups, such as adolescents, disabled, and elderly people. As a consequence, healthcare policies have become increasingly interested in supporting mental health and rehabilitation programs aimed at overcoming social isolation. Information and communication technologies can play a key role in improving these programs.

## CONCLUSION: POSITIVE TECHNOLOGY FOR PERSONAL CHANGE

How do we lastingly change our lives for the better? What is the role played by technology in this process? The chapter presented a possible answer to this question by focusing on the concepts of personal change and Positive Technology.

As underlined by recent research in psychology and neuroscience, personal change is a complex process depending on the person, the issues, and the situation. However, by merging the ideas of two influential transdiagnostic models of change - the Perceptual Control Theory (Higginson et al., 2011; Vancouver & Putka, 2000) and the TransTheoretical Model of Behavior Change (Prochaska & DiClemente, 1982, 1983; Prochaska et al., 1992) - it is possible to describe a process of personal change (Kottler, 2014) following this sequence (pp. 19-20):

1. There is an expressed desire for change that is triggered by a crisis, trauma, or developmental transition;
2. A level of pain and discomfort is reached that can't any longer be ignored or denied;
3. There is an awareness or insight that something different must be done;
4. There is a gradual process of applying what was realized or learned into constructive action; and there is recovery from inevitable relapses.

Even if these characteristics of personal change are now shared by many of the leading approaches to psychotherapy, many of us experience psychological change without the help of any form of treatment. How and why?

In the chapter we suggested that our cognitive system is naturally shaped to identify and counter the experiential conflicts that are described in the points 1 and 2 of the above list.

This is achieved through a specific cognitive process – presence – the goal of which is to control the activity of the individual: I am present in a real or virtual space if I manage to put my intentions into action (enacting them).

On one side, there is a link between presence and the effectiveness of an action: the greater level of presence a subject experiences in an activity, the greater the individual's involvement in the activity will be, and this increases the probability of the activity ending well (the transformation of the intention into action). On the other side, presence provides the self with a feedback about the status of its activity. Specifically, the self perceives the variations in the feeling of presence (breakdowns and optimal experience) and tunes its activity accordingly.

The role of breakdowns in personal change is clear: to push individuals towards it. By perceiving a conflict (awareness) between different goals the subject is pushed to resolve the conflict between them.

Optimal experiences, also defined as "flow experiences", instead allow the individual to consider their long-term personal goals differently and start to experiment with changing them. In other words optimal experiences, when meaningful for the individual, widen the array of thoughts and actions, facilitating generativity and behavioral flexibility. Within this view, we defined *transformation of flow* a person's ability to draw upon an optimal experience and use it to marshal new and unexpected psychological resources and sources of involvement.

An important consequence of this model is that we can develop technologies that are able to improve the quality of our personal experience by enhancing the level of presence and social presence experienced interacting with them (Graffigna, Barello, et al., 2013c; Graffigna, Barello, Wiederhold, et al., 2013; Riva, 2012c).

Following this claim we introduced and described the "Positive Technology" approach: the scientific and applied approach to the use of technology for improving the quality of our personal experience as a way of framing a suitable object of study in the field of personal change (Graffigna, Barello, Wiederhold, et al., 2013; Riva, 2012c; Riva et al., 2012; Wiederhold & Riva, 2012).

Firstly, we have classified positive technologies according to their effects on these three features of personal experience (Figure 2):

- **Hedonic:** Technologies used to induce positive and pleasant experiences.
- **Eudaimonic:** Technologies used to support individuals in reaching engaging and self-actualizing experiences.
- **Social/Interpersonal:** Technologies used to support and improve the connectedness between individuals, groups, and organizations.

Additionally, for each level we have identified critical variables – affect regulation for the Hedonic, flow and presence for the Eudaimonic; social presence, collective intentions and networked flow for the Social/Interpersonal – that can be manipulated and controlled (Table 7) to guide the design and development of positive technologies.

Finally, the different examples show that technology can be used to manipulate the features of an experience in three separate but related ways (Figure 6):

- *By structuring it* using a goal, rules and a feedback system (McGonigal, 2011): The goal provides subjects with a sense of purpose focusing attention and orienting his/her participation in the experience. The rules, by removing or limiting the obvious ways of getting to the goal, push subjects to see the experience in a different way. The feedback system tells players how close they are to achieving the goal and provides motivation to keep trying.
- *By augmenting it* to achieve multimodal and mixed experiences. Technology allows multisensory experiences in which content and its interaction is offered through more than one of the senses. It is even possible to use technology to overlay virtual objects onto real scenes (Rosenblum, 2000).
- *By replacing it* with a synthetic one. Using VR it is possible to simulate physical presence in a synthetic world that reacts to the action of the subject as if he/she was really there. Moreover, the replacement possibilities offered by technology even extend to the induction of an illusion of ownership over a virtual arm or a virtual body (Slater, Spanlang, Sanchez-Vives, & Blanke, 2010).

*Figure 6. Positive technology tools*
*Adapted from Botella et al., 2012.*

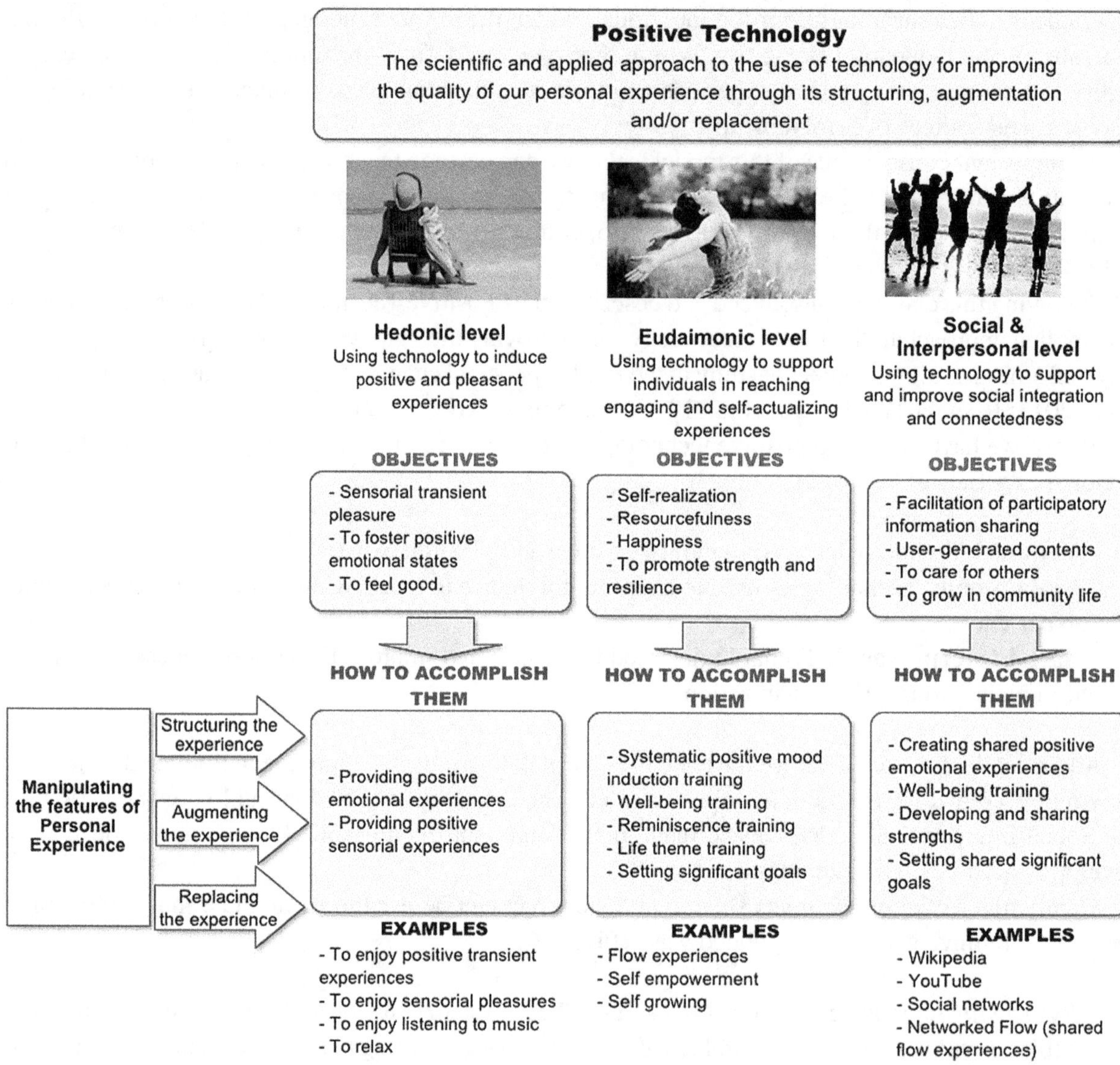


Even if Positive Technology tools can be used for clinical change, too, there is a relevant difference: to be effective, they have to adapt to the specific stage of the change process that the patient is in. More, Positive Technologies are successful for clinical change only if they are able to sustain the patient engagement within the provided experience. Recently, Graffigna and colleagues (Graffigna, 2009; Graffigna, Barello, et al., 2013a; Graffigna, Barello, Wiederhold, et al., 2013) defined "patient engagement" as the experience resulting from the conjoint conative (act), cognitive (think) and emotional (feel) enactment of individuals in their *care & cure* management.

These different experiential dimensions play different (but complementary) driving roles, as key factors for promoting patients' advancement in this sense-making process. The unachieved synergy among the different subjective dimensions inhibits patients from engaging in their *care and cure* management, limiting their potential for obtaining the greatest benefit from the offered Positive Technologies.

## REFERENCES

Biocca, F., Harms, C., & Burgoon, J. K. (2003). Toward a more robust theory and measure of social presence: Review and suggested criteria. *Presence (Cambridge, Mass.)*, *12*(5), 456–480.

Botella, C., Riva, G., Gaggioli, A., Wiederhold, B. K., Alcaniz, M., & Banos, R. M. (2012). The present and future of positive technologies. *Cyberpsychology, Behavior, and Social Networking*, *15*(2), 78–84. doi:10.1089/cyber.2011.0140 PMID:22149078

Boulos, M. N. K., & Wheeler, S. (2007). The emerging Web 2.0 social software: An enabling suite of sociable technologies in health and health care education. *Health Information and Libraries Journal*, *24*(1), 2–23. doi:10.1111/j.1471-1842.2007.00701.x PMID:17331140

Brewin, C. R. (1989). Cognitive Change Processes in Psychotherapy. *Psychological Review*, *96*(3), 379–394. doi:10.1037/0033-295X.96.3.379 PMID:2667012

Calvo, R. A., & Peters, D. (2012). Positive computing: Technology for a wiser world. *Interactions (New York, N.Y.)*, *19*(4), 28–31. doi:10.1145/2212877.2212886

Calvo, R. A., & Peters, D. (2014). *Positive Computing: Technology for Wellbeing and Human Potential.* Cambridge, MA: MIT Press.

Carissoli, C., Villani, D., & Riva, G. (2015). Does a meditation protocol supported by a mobile application help people reduce stress? Suggestions from a controlled pragmatic trial. *Cyberpsychology, Behavior, and Social Networking*, *18*(1), 46–53. doi:10.1089/cyber.2014.0062 PMID:25584730

Castelnuovo, G., Gaggioli, A., Mantovani, F., & Riva, G. (2003). New and old tools in psychotherapy: The use of technology for the integration of traditional clinical treatments. *Psychotherapy (Chicago, Ill.)*, *40*(1-2), 33–44. doi:10.1037/0033-3204.40.1-2.33

Castelnuovo, G., Lo Priore, C., Liccione, D., & Cioffi, G. (2003). Virtual Reality based tools for the rehabilitation of cognitive and executive functions: The V-STORE. *PsychNology Journal*, *1*(3), 311–326. Retrieved from http://www.psychnology.org/pnj311(313)_castelnuovo_lopriore_liccione_cioffi_abstract.htm

Cipresso, P., Gaggioli, A., Serino, S., Raspelli, S., Vigna, C., & Pallavicini, F. et al.. (2012). Inter-Reality in the Evaluation and Treatment of Psychological Stress Disorders: The INTERSTRESS Project. *Studies in Health Technology and Informatics*, *181*, 8–11. PMID:22954818

Coleman, J. S. (1988). Social Capital in the creation of human capital. *American Journal of Sociology*, *94*, S95–S120. doi:10.1086/228943

Csikszentmihalyi, M. (1990). *Flow: The psychology of optimal experience.* New York: HarperCollins.

Csikszentmihalyi, M. (1994). *The evolving self.* New York: Harper Perennial.

Csikszentmihalyi, M. (1997). *Creativity: Flow and the Psychology of Discovery and Invention*. New York: Harper Perennial.

Damasio, A. (1999). *The Feeling of What Happens: Body, Emotion and the Making of Consciousness*. San Diego, CA: Harcourt Brace and Co, Inc.

Epel, E., Daubenmier, J., Moskowitz, J. T., Folkman, S., & Blackburn, E. (2009). Can meditation slow rate of cellular aging? Cognitive stress, mindfulness, and telomeres. *Annals of the New York Academy of Sciences*, *1172*(1), 34–53. doi:10.1111/j.1749-6632.2009.04414.x PMID:19735238

Fortin, S., Godbout, L., & Braun, C. M. J. (2003). Cognitive structure of executive deficits in frontally lesioned head trauma patients performing activities of daily living. *Cortex*, *39*(2), 273–291. doi:10.1016/S0010-9452(08)70109-6 PMID:12784889

Fredrickson, B. L. (2001). The role of positive emotions in positive psychology. The broaden-and-build theory of positive emotions. *The American Psychologist*, *56*(3), 218–226. doi:10.1037/0003-066X.56.3.218 PMID:11315248

Fredrickson, B. L. (2004). The broaden-and-build theory of positive emotions. *Philosophical Transactions of the Royal Society of London. Series B, Biological Sciences*, *359*(1449), 1367–1378. doi:10.1098/rstb.2004.1512 PMID:15347528

Gaggioli, A. (2004). Optimal Experience in Ambient Intelligence. In G. Riva, F. Vatalaro, F. Davide, & M. Alcañiz (Eds.), Ambient Intelligence: The evolution of technology, communication and cognition towards the future of human-computer interaction (pp. 35–43). Amsterdam: IOS Press. Retrieved from http://www.emergingcommunication.com/volume6.html

Gaggioli, A., Bassi, M., & Delle Fave, A. (2003). Quality of Experience in Virtual Environments. In G. Riva, W. A. IJsselsteijn, & F. Davide (Eds.), Being There: Concepts, effects and measurement of user presence in synthetic environment (pp. 121–135). Amsterdam: Ios Press. Retrieved from http://www.emergingcommunication.com/volume5.html

Gaggioli, A., Mazzoni, E., Milani, L., & Riva, G. (2015). The creative link: Investigating the relationship between social network indices, creative performance and flow in blended teams. *Computers in Human Behavior*, *42*, 157–166. doi:10.1016/j.chb.2013.12.003

Gaggioli, A., Milani, L., Mazzoni, E., & Riva, G. (2011). Networked Flow: A Framework for Understanding the Dynamics of Creative Collaboration in Educational and Training Settings. *The Open Education Journal, 4*(Suppl 2:M2), 107-115.

Gaggioli, A., Milani, L., Mazzoni, E., & Riva, G. (2013). *Networked Flow: Towards an Understanding of Creative Networks*. Dordrecht: Springer. doi:10.1007/978-94-007-5552-9

Gaggioli, A., Morganti, L., Bonfiglio, S., Scaratti, C., Cipresso, P., Serino, S., & Riva, G. (2014). Intergenerational Group Reminiscence: A Potentially Effective Intervention to Enhance Elderly Psychosocial Wellbeing and to Improve Children's Perception of Aging. *Educational Gerontology*, *40*(7), 486–498. doi:10.1080/03601277.2013.844042

Gaggioli, A., & Riva, G. (2014). Psychological treatments: Smart tools boost mental-health care. *Nature, 512*(7512), 28. doi:10.1038/512028b PMID:25100471

Gallagher, R., & Jeannerod, M. (2002). From action to interaction. *Journal of Consciousness Studies, 9*, 3–26.

Gallese, V., Fadiga, L., Fogassi, L., & Rizzolatti, G. (1996). Action recognition in the premotor cortex. *Brain, 119*(2), 593–609. doi:10.1093/brain/119.2.593 PMID:8800951

Ghani, J. A., & Deshpande, S. P. (1994). Task characteristics and the experience of optimal flow in Human-Computer Interaction. *The Journal of Psychology, 128*(4), 381–391. doi:10.1080/00223980.1994.9712742

Gianakis, M., & Carey, T. A. (2011). An interview study investigating experiences of psychological change without psychotherapy. *Psychology and Psychotherapy: Theory, Research and Practice, 84*(4), 442–457. doi:10.1111/j.2044-8341.2010.02002.x PMID:22903885

Gorini, A., Capideville, C. S., De Leo, G., Mantovani, F., & Riva, G. (2010). The Role of Immersion and Narrative in Mediated Presence: The Virtual Hospital Experience. *Cyberpsychology, Behavior, and Social Networking*. doi:10.1089/cyber.2010.0100 PMID:20649451

Graffigna, G. (2009). *Interpersonal exchanges about HIV-Aids through different media: A cross-cultural comparison*. Saarbrücken: VDM Verlag.

Graffigna, G., Barello, S., & Riva, G. (2013a). How to make health information technology effective: The challenge of patient engagement. *Archives of Physical Medicine and Rehabilitation, 94*(10), 2034–2035. doi:10.1016/j.apmr.2013.04.024 PMID:24075414

Graffigna, G., Barello, S., & Riva, G. (2013c). Technologies for patient engagement. *Health Affairs (Project Hope), 32*(6), 1172. doi:10.1377/hlthaff.2013.0279 PMID:23733998

Graffigna, G., Barello, S., Wiederhold, B. K., Bosio, A. C., & Riva, G. (2013). Positive technology as a driver for health engagement. *Studies in Health Technology and Informatics, 191*, 9–17. PMID:23792833

Grassi, A., Gaggioli, A., & Riva, G. (2011). New technologies to manage exam anxiety. [Randomized Controlled Trial]. *Studies in Health Technology and Informatics, 167*, 57–62. PMID:21685642

Hayes, A. M., Laurenceau, J. P., Feldman, G., Strauss, J. L., & Cardaciotto, L. (2007). Change is not always linear: The study of nonlinear and discontinuous patterns of change in psychotherapy. *Clinical Psychology Review, 27*(6), 715–723. doi:10.1016/j.cpr.2007.01.008 PMID:17316941

Heeter, C. (1992). Being There: The subjective experience of presence. *Presence (Cambridge, Mass.), 1*(2), 262–271. doi:10.1162/pres.1992.1.2.262

Heeter, C. (2003). Reflections on real presence by a virtual person. *Presence (Cambridge, Mass.), 12*(4), 335–345. doi:10.1162/105474603322391587

Held, R. M., & Durlach, N. I. (1992). Telepresence. *Presence (Cambridge, Mass.), 1*(1), 109–112. doi:10.1162/pres.1992.1.1.109

Helliwell, J. F., & Putnam, R. D. (2004). The social context of well-being. *Philosophical Transactions of the Royal Society of London. Series B, Biological Sciences*, *359*(1449), 1435–1446. doi:10.1098/rstb.2004.1522 PMID:15347534

Higginson, S., & Mansell, W. (2008). What is the mechanism of psychological change? A qualitative analysis of six individuals who experienced personal change and recovery. *Psychology and Psychotherapy: Theory, Research and Practice*, *81*(3), 309–328. doi:10.1348/147608308X320125 PMID:18588749

Higginson, S., Mansell, W., & Wood, A. M. (2011). An integrative mechanistic account of psychological distress, therapeutic change and recovery: The Perceptual Control Theory approach. *Clinical Psychology Review*, *31*(2), 249–259. doi:10.1016/j.cpr.2010.01.005 PMID:20171771

Hommel, B., Müsseler, J., Aschersleben, G., & Prinz, W. (2001). The Theory of Event Coding (TEC): A framework for perception and action planning. *Behavioral and Brain Sciences*, *24*(5), 849–937. doi:10.1017/S0140525X01000103 PMID:12239891

House, J. S., Landis, K. R., & Umberson, D. (1988). Social relationships and health. *Science*, *241*(4865), 540–545. doi:10.1126/science.3399889 PMID:3399889

Inghilleri, P., Riva, G., & Riva, E. (Eds.). (2015). Enabling Positive Change. Flow and Complexity in Daily Experience. Berlin: De Gruyter Open. Retrieved from http://www.degruyter.com/view/product/449663 doi:10.2478/9783110410242

Joyce, K. M. (2009). Enhancing Social Presence in Online Learning: Mediation Strategies Applied to Social Networking Tools. *Online Journal of Distance Learning Administration*, *12*(4). Retrieved from http://www.westga.edu/~distance/ojdla/winter124/joyce124.html

Kahneman, D. (2002). Maps of Bounded Rationality: A Perspective on Intuitive Judgment and Choice. In T. Frängsmyr (Ed.), *The Nobel Prizes 2002* (pp. 449–489). Stockholm: Nobel Foundation.

Kaptelinin, V., & Nardi, B. (2006). *Acting with Technology: Activity Theory and Interaction Design*. Cambridge, MA: MIT Press.

Kottler, J. A. (2014). *Change: What really leads to lasting personal transformation*. New York, NY: Oxford University Press.

Lee, R., & Whitley, H. P. (2014). Use of Social Media to Support Patients with Diabetes Mellitus. *The Consultant Pharmacist*, *29*(1), 53–57. doi:10.4140/TCP.n.2014.53 PMID:24413015

Leontjev, A. N. (1978). Activity, consciousness, and personality. Englewood, NJ: Prentice-Hall; Retrieved from http://marxists.org/archive/leontev/works/1978/ch3.htm

Lessiter, J., Freeman, J., Keogh, E., & Davidoff, J. (2001). A Cross-Media Presence Questionnaire: The ITC-Sense of Presence Inventory. *Presence (Cambridge, Mass.)*, *10*(3), 282–297. doi:10.1162/105474601300343612

Lo Priore, C., Castelnuovo, G., Liccione, D., & Liccione, D. (2003). Experience with V-STORE: Considerations on presence in virtual environments for effective neuropsychological rehabilitation of executive functions. *Cyberpsychology & Behavior*, *6*(3), 281–287. doi:10.1089/109493103322011579 PMID:12855084

Manzoni, G. M., Cesa, G. L., Villani, D., Castelnuovo, G., Molinari, E., & Riva, G. (2006). VR-enhanced treatment of anxiety in obese subjects: A follow-up study on trait-anxiety, psychological symptornatology, and generalized self-efficacy. *Cyberpsychology & Behavior*, *9*(6), 699–700.

Manzoni, G. M., Pagnini, F., Gorini, A., Preziosa, A., Castelnuovo, G., Molinari, E., & Riva, G. (2009). Can relaxation training reduce emotional eating in women with obesity? An exploratory study with 3 months of follow-up. *Journal of the American Dietetic Association*, *109*(8), 1427–1432. doi:10.1016/j.jada.2009.05.004 PMID:19631051

Marsh, T. (2003). Staying there: an activity-based approach to narrative design and evaluation as an antidote to virtual corpsing. In G. Riva, F. Davide, & W. A. IJsselsteijn (Eds.), *Being There: Concepts, effects and measurements of user presence in synthetic environments* (pp. 85–96). Amsterdam: IOS Press.

Mauri, M., Villamira, M., Cipresso, P., Balgera, A., & Riva, G. (2011). Why Is Facebook So Successful? Psychophysiological Measures Describe a Core Flow State While Using Facebook. *Cyberpsychology, Behavior, and Social Networking*, *14*(12), 723–731. doi:10.1089/cyber.2010.0377 PMID:21879884

McGonigal, J. (2011). *Reality Is Broken. Why games make us better and how they can change the world.* New York: The Penguin Press.

Meltzoff, A. N., & Decety, J. (2003). What imitation tells us about social cognition: A rapprochement between developmental psychology and cognitive neuroscience. *Philosophical Transactions of the Royal Society*, *358*(1431), 491–500. doi:10.1098/rstb.2002.1261 PMID:12689375

Morris, M. E. (2005). Social networks as health feedback displays. *IEEE Internet Computing*, *9*(5), 29–37. doi:10.1109/MIC.2005.109

Optale, G., Capodieci, S., Pinelli, P., Zara, D., Gamberini, L., & Riva, G. (2001). Music-enhanced immersive virtual reality in the rehabilitation of memory-related cognitive processes and functional abilities: A case report. *Presence (Cambridge, Mass.)*, *10*(4), 450–462. doi:10.1162/1054746011470217

Optale, G., Urgesi, C., Busato, V., Marin, S., Piron, L., Priftis, K., & Bordin, A. et al. (2010). Controlling Memory Impairment in Elderly Adults Using Virtual Reality Memory Training: A Randomized Controlled Pilot Study. *Neurorehabilitation and Neural Repair*, *24*(4), 348–357. doi:10.1177/1545968309353328 PMID:19934445

Pacherie, E. (2006). Toward a dynamic theory of intentions. In S. Pockett, W. P. Banks, & S. Gallagher (Eds.), *Does consciousness cause behavior?* (pp. 145–167). Cambridge, MA: MIT Press. doi:10.7551/mitpress/9780262162371.003.0009

Pacherie, E. (2008). The phenomenology of action: A conceptual framework. *Cognition*, *107*(1), 179–217. doi:10.1016/j.cognition.2007.09.003 PMID:17950720

Pacherie, E., & Haggard, P. (2010). What are intentions? In L. Nadel & W. Sinnott-Armstrong (Eds.), *Conscious Will and Responsibility. A tribute to Benjamin Libet* (pp. 70–84). Oxford: Oxford University Press. doi:10.1093/acprof:oso/9780195381641.003.0008

Pagnini, F., Di Credico, C., Gatto, R., Fabiani, V., Rossi, G., Lunetta, C., & Amadei, G. et al. (2014). Meditation training for people with amyotrophic lateral sclerosis and their caregivers. *Journal of Alternative and Complementary Medicine (New York, N.Y.)*, *20*(4), 272–275. doi:10.1089/acm.2013.0268 PMID:24328393

Pagnini, F., Phillips, D., & Langer, E. (2014). A mindful approach with end-of-life thoughts. *Frontiers in Psychology*, *5*, 138. doi:10.3389/fpsyg.2014.00138 PMID:24600429

Park, H. (2010). The Effect Of Activities In Virtual Worlds As A Communication Environment To Understand Each Other. *Journal of Cyber Therapy and Rehabilitation*, *3*(1), 71–82.

Pedroli, E., Cipresso, P., Serino, S., Pallavicini, F., Albani, G., & Riva, G. (2013). Virtual multiple errands test: Reliability, usability and possible applications. *Studies in Health Technology and Informatics*, *191*, 38–42. PMID:23792839

Phillips, A., & Pagnini, F. (2014). A mindful approach to chronic illness. In A. Le, C. T. Nguoumen, & E. Langer (Eds.), *The Wiley-Blackwell Handbook of Mindfulness* (pp. 852–863). London: Wiley-Blackwell. doi:10.1002/9781118294895.ch43

Preziosa, A., Grassi, A., Gaggioli, A., & Riva, G. (2009). Therapeutic applications of the mobile phone. *British Journal of Guidance & Counselling*, *37*(3), 313–325. doi:10.1080/03069880902957031

Prochaska, J. O., & DiClemente, C. C. (1982). Transtheoretical therapy: Toward a more integrative model of change. *Psychotherapy (Chicago, Ill.)*, *19*(3), 212–216.

Prochaska, J. O., & DiClemente, C. C. (1983). Stages and processes of self-change in smoking toward an integrative model of change. *Journal of Consulting and Clinical Psychology*, *5*(3), 390–395. doi:10.1037/0022-006X.51.3.390 PMID:6863699

Prochaska, J. O., DiClemente, C. C., & Norcross, J. C. (1992). In search of how people change. *The American Psychologist*, *47*(9), 1102–1114. doi:10.1037/0003-066X.47.9.1102 PMID:1329589

Raspelli, S., Pallavicini, F., Carelli, L., Morganti, F., Pedroli, E., Cipresso, P., & Riva, G. et al. (2012). Validating the Neuro VR-based virtual version of the Multiple Errands Test: Preliminary results. *Presence (Cambridge, Mass.)*, *21*(1), 31–42. doi:10.1162/PRES_a_00077

Raspelli, S., Pallavicini, F., Grassi, A., Cipresso, P., Balgera, A., & Meazzi, D. et al.. (2011). Validation of a narrative as an emotional-induction technique through different non-invasive psychophysiological monitoring devices: Preliminary results. *Journal of Cybertherapy and Rehabiliation*, *4*(2), 261.

Repetto, C., Gorini, A., Vigna, C., Algeri, D., Pallavicini, F., & Riva, G. (2009). The use of biofeedback in clinical virtual reality: The INTREPID project. *Journal of Visualized Experiments*, November, 33. PMID:19915521

Riva, G. (2004). The psychology of Ambient Intelligence: Activity, situation and presence. In G. Riva, F. Davide, F. Vatalaro, & M. Alcañiz (Eds.), Ambient Intelligence: The evolution of technology, communication and cognition towards the future of the human-computer interaction (pp. 19–34). Amsterdam: IOS Press. Retrieved from http://www.emergingcommunication.com/volume6.html

Riva, G. (2008). Enacting Interactivity: The Role of Presence. In F. Morganti, A. Carassa, & G. Riva (Eds.), Enacting Intersubjectivity: A cognitive and social perspective on the study of interactions (pp. 97–114). Amsterdam: IOS Press. Retrieved from http://www.emergingcommunication.com/volume10.html

Riva, G. (2009a). Is presence a technology issue? Some insights from cognitive sciences. *Virtual Reality (Waltham Cross), 13*(3), 59–69. doi:10.1007/s10055-009-0121-6

Riva, G. (2009c). Presence as Cognitive Process. In D. Benyon, M. Smyth, & I. Helgason (Eds.), *Presence for everyone: A short guide to presence research* (pp. 29–31). Edinburgh, UK: Napier University.

Riva, G. (2009e). Virtual reality: An experiential tool for clinical psychology. *British Journal of Guidance & Counselling, 37*(3), 337–345. doi:10.1080/03069880902957056

Riva, G. (2010). Dall'intenzione, all'azione, all'interazione: il ruolo di "presenza" e "presenza sociale". In F. Morganti, A. Carassa, & G. Riva (Eds.), *Intersoggettività e Interazione: Un dialogo fra scienze cognitive, scienze sociali e neuroscienze* (pp. 136–177). Torino: Bollati Boringhieri.

Riva, G. (2012a). Personal experience in positive psychology may offer a new focus for a growing discipline. *The American Psychologist, 67*(7), 574–575. doi:10.1037/a0029955 PMID:23046310

Riva, G. (2012c). What is Positive Technology and its impact on CyberPsychology. *Studies in Health Technology and Informatics, 181*, 37–41. PMID:22954824

Riva, G., Algeri, D., Pallavicini, F., Repetto, C., Gorini, A., & Gaggioli, A. (2010). The use of advanced technologies in the treatment of psychological stress. *Journal of Cyber Therapy and Rehabilitation, 2*(2), 169–171.

Riva, G., Banos, R. M., Botella, C., Wiederhold, B. K., & Gaggioli, A. (2012). Positive technology: Using interactive technologies to promote positive functioning. *Cyberpsychology, Behavior, and Social Networking, 15*(2), 69–77. doi:10.1089/cyber.2011.0139 PMID:22149077

Riva, G., Castelnuovo, G., & Mantovani, F. (2006). Transformation of flow in rehabilitation: The role of advanced communication technologies. *Behavior Research Methods, 38*(2), 237–244. doi:10.3758/BF03192775 PMID:16956100

Riva, G., Davide, F., & IJsselsteijn, W. A. (Eds.). (2003). Being There: Concepts, effects and measurements of user presence in synthetic environments. Amsterdam: Ios Press. Retrieved from http://www.emergingcommunication.com/volume5.html

Riva, G., & Gaggioli, A. (2009). Rehabilitation as Empowerment: The Role of Advanced Technologies. *Studies in Health Technology and Informatics, 145*, 3–22. PMID:19592783

Riva, G., & Mantovani, F. (2012a). Being There: Understanding the Feeling of Presence in a Synthetic Environment and its Potential for Clinical Change. In C. Eichenberg (Ed.), Virtual Reality in Psychological, Medical and Pedagogical Applications (pp. 3–34). New York: InTech. Retrieved from http://www.intechopen.com/books/virtual-reality-in-psychological-medical-and-pedagogical-applications/being-there-understanding-the-feeling-of-presence-in-a-synthetic-environment-and-its-potential-for-c doi:10.5772/46411

Riva, G., & Mantovani, F. (2012d). From the body to the tools and back: A general framework for presence in mediated interactions. *Interacting with Computers*, *24*(4), 203–210. doi:10.1016/j.intcom.2012.04.007

Riva, G., Mantovani, F., Capideville, C. S., Preziosa, A., Morganti, F., Villani, D., & Alcañiz, M. et al. (2007). Affective interactions using virtual reality: The link between presence and emotions. *Cyberpsychology & Behavior*, *10*(1), 45–56. doi:10.1089/cpb.2006.9993 PMID:17305448

Riva, G., Manzoni, M., Villani, D., Gaggioli, A., & Molinari, E. (2008). Why you really eat? Virtual reality in the treatment of obese emotional eaters. *Studies in Health Technology and Informatics*, *132*, 417–419. PMID:18391333

Riva, G., Raspelli, S., Algeri, D., Pallavicini, F., Gorini, A., Wiederhold, B. K., & Gaggioli, A. (2010). Interreality in practice: Bridging virtual and real worlds in the treatment of posttraumatic stress disorders. *Cyberpsychology, Behavior, and Social Networking*, *13*(1), 55–65. doi:10.1089/cyber.2009.0320 PMID:20528294

Riva, G., & Waterworth, J. A. (2003). Presence and the Self: A cognitive neuroscience approach. *Presence-Connect, 3*(1). Retrieved from http://presence.cs.ucl.ac.uk/presenceconnect/articles/Apr2003/jwworthApr72003114532/jwworthApr72003114532.html

Riva, G., & Waterworth, J. A. (2014). Being present in a virtual world. In M. Grimshaw (Ed.), *The Oxford Handbook of Virtuality* (pp. 205–221). New York: Oxford University Press.

Riva, G., Waterworth, J. A., & Murray, D. (Eds.). (2014). Interacting with Presence: HCI and the sense of presence in computer-mediated environments. Berlin: De Gruyter Open. Retrieved from http://www.presence-research.com doi:10.2478/9783110409697

Riva, G., Waterworth, J. A., & Waterworth, E. L. (2004). The Layers of Presence: A bio-cultural approach to understanding presence in natural and mediated environments. *Cyberpsychology & Behavior*, *7*(4), 405–419. doi:10.1089/cpb.2004.7.402 PMID:15331027

Riva, G., Waterworth, J. A., Waterworth, E. L., & Mantovani, F. (2011). From Intention to Action: The role of Presence. *New Ideas in Psychology*, *29*(1), 24–37. doi:10.1016/j.newideapsych.2009.11.002

Rizzolatti, G., Fadiga, L., Gallese, V., & Fogassi, L. (1996). Premotor cortex and the recognition of motor actions. *Brain Research. Cognitive Brain Research*, *3*(2), 131–141. doi:10.1016/0926-6410(95)00038-0 PMID:8713554

Rizzolatti, G., & Sinigaglia, C. (2006). *So quel che fai. Il cervello che agisce e i neuroni specchio*. Milano: Raffaello Cortina.

Rosenblum, L. (2000). Virtual and Augmented Reality 2020. *IEEE Computer Graphics and Applications*, *20*(1), 38–39. doi:10.1109/38.814551

Russell, J. A. (1996). *Agency: Its role in mental development*. Hove: Erlbaum.

Russell, J. A. (2003). Core Affect and the psychological construction of Emotion. *Psychological Review*, *110*(1), 145–172. doi:10.1037/0033-295X.110.1.145 PMID:12529060

Ryff, C. D., & Singer, B. (2000). Interpersonal flourishing: A positive health agenda for the new millennium. *Personality and Social Psychology Review*, *4*(1), 30–44. doi:10.1207/S15327957PSPR0401_4

Safran, J. D., & Greenberg, L. S. (1991). *Emotion, psychotherapy, and change*. New York: The Guilford Press.

Searle, J. (1983). *Intentionality: An essay in the philosophy of mind*. New York: Cambridge University Press. doi:10.1017/CBO9781139173452

Serino, S., Triberti, S., Villani, D., Cipresso, P., Gaggioli, A., & Riva, G. (2014). Toward a validation of cyber-interventions for stress disorders based on stress inoculation training: A systematic review. *Virtual Reality (Waltham Cross)*, *18*(1), 73–87. doi:10.1007/s10055-013-0237-6

Short, J., Williams, E., & Christie, B. (1976). *The social psychology of telecommunications*. London: Wiley.

Slater, M., Spanlang, B., Sanchez-Vives, M. V., & Blanke, O. (2010). First person experience of body transfer in virtual reality. *PLoS ONE*, *5*(5), e10564. doi:10.1371/journal.pone.0010564 PMID:20485681

Spagnolli, A., & Gamberini, L. (2005). A Place for Presence. Understanding the Human Involvement in Mediated Interactive Environments. *PsychNology Journal*, *13*(1), 6–15. Retrieved from http://www.psychnology.org/index.php?page=abstract---volume-13---spagnolli PMID:16190023

Stanovich, K. E., & West, R. F. (2000). Individual differences in reasoning: Implications for the rationality debate? *Behavioral and Brain Sciences*, *23*(5), 645–665, discussion 665–726. doi:10.1017/S0140525X00003435 PMID:11301544

Stiles, W. B., Barkham, M., Mellor-Clark, J., & Connell, J. (2008). Effectiveness of cognitive-behavioural, person-centred, and psychodynamic therapies in UK primary-care routine practice: Replication in a larger sample. *Psychological Medicine*, *38*(5), 677–688. doi:10.1017/S0033291707001511 PMID:17825124

Stiles, W. B., Barkham, M., Twigg, E., Mellor-Clark, J., & Cooper, M. (2006). Effectiveness of cognitive-behavioural, person-centred and psychodynamic therapies as practised in UK National Health Service settings. *Psychological Medicine*, *36*(4), 555–566. doi:10.1017/S0033291706007136 PMID:16476185

Swamynathan, G., Wilson, C., Boe, B., Almeroth, K., & Zhao, B. Y. (2008). Do social networks improve e-commerce?: a study on social marketplaces. *Paper presented at the First Workshop on Online Social Networks*, New York, USA. doi:10.1145/1397735.1397737

Vancouver, J. B., & Putka, D. J. (2000). Analyzing Goal-Striving Processes and a Test of the Generalizability of Perceptual Control Theory. *Organizational Behavior and Human Decision Processes*, *82*(2), 334–362. doi:10.1006/obhd.2000.2901 PMID:10891301

Villani, D., Lucchetta, M., Preziosa, A., & Riva, G. (2006). Narrative versus environment: The role of media content in emotional induction. *Cyberpsychology & Behavior*, *9*(6), 724–725.

Villani, D., Lucchetta, M., Preziosa, A., & Riva, G. (2009). The role of affective media features on the affective response: A virtual reality study. *e-Minds. International Journal of Human-Computer Interaction*, *1*(5), 35–55.

Villani, D., Preziosa, A., Riva, F., & Riva, G. (2006). Presence enhances relaxation: A preliminary controlled study. *Cyberpsychology & Behavior*, *9*(6), 723–724.

Villani, D., Riva, F., & Riva, G. (2007). New technologies for relaxation: The role of presence. *International Journal of Stress Management*, *14*(3), 260–274. doi:10.1037/1072-5245.14.3.260

Waterworth, J. A., & Riva, G. (2014). *Feeling Present in the Physical World and in Computer-Mediated Environments*. Basingstoke, UK: Palgrave Macmillan. doi:10.1057/9781137431677

Waterworth, J. A., & Waterworth, E. L. (2012). Presence as a dimension of communication: Context of use and the person *Emerging Communication. Studies in New Technologies and Practices in Communication*, *9*, 80–95.

Waterworth, J. A., & Waterworth, E. L. (2014). Altered, expanded and distributed embodiment: the three stages of interactive presence. In G. Riva, J. A. Waterworth, & D. Murray (Eds.), Interacting with Presence: HCI and the sense of presence in computer-mediated environments (pp. 36–50). Berlin: De Gruyter Open. Retrieved from http://www.presence-research.com

Waterworth, J. A., Waterworth, E. L., Mantovani, F., & Riva, G. (2010). On Feeling (the) Present: An evolutionary account of the sense of presence in physical and electronically-mediated environments. *Journal of Consciousness Studies*, *17*(1-2), 167–178.

Webster, J. D., & McCall, M. E. (1999). Reminiscence functions across adulthood: A replication and extension. *Journal of Adult Development*, *6*(1), 73–85. doi:10.1023/A:1021628525902

Wiederhold, B. K., & Riva, G. (2012). Positive technology supports shift to preventive, integrative health. *Cyberpsychology, Behavior, and Social Networking*, *15*(2), 67–68. doi:10.1089/cyber.2011.1533 PMID:22320253

Wolfe, B. E. (2002). The Role of Lived Experience in Self- and Relational Observation: A Commentary on Horowitz (2002). *Journal of Psychotherapy Integration*, *12*(2), 147–153. doi:10.1037/1053-0479.12.2.147

Zahorik, P., & Jenison, R. L. (1998). Presence as being-in-the-world. *Presence (Cambridge, Mass.)*, *7*(1), 78–89. doi:10.1162/105474698565541

## KEY TERMS AND DEFINITIONS

**Eudaimonic Technologies:** Technologies used to support individuals in reaching engaging and self-actualizing experiences.

**Flow:** There are exceptional situations – e.g., a tennis player who goes to the right (proto presence) before the ball bounces on the court to swing a winning forehand ground stroke (core presence) on a second set-point at the Wimbledon final (extended presence) - in which the activity of the subject is characterized by a high level of presence in all the three different subprocesses (Maximal Presence). When this experience is associated with a positive emotional state, it constitutes a flow state.

**Hedonic Technologies:** Technologies used to induce positive and pleasant experiences.

**Networked Flow:** There are exceptional social situations in which a group of subjects in a liminality phase (a state of transition, in which the earlier *positive* condition is no longer present, and the future *positive* condition has not yet come into) experiences the maximum level of social presence (the feeling of sharing objectives and emotions with others) and the feeling of being able through the their collective action of exiting from liminality (maximum level of presence).

**Optimal Experiences:** Specific individual (Flow) and social (Networked Flow) situations in which the individual experiences the maximum feeling of presence.

**Patient Engagement:** The experience resulting from the conjoint conative (act), cognitive (think) and emotional (feel) enactment of individuals in their *care & cure* management.

**Positive Computing:** The research and development of technology to support wellbeing and human potential.

**Positive Technology:** The use of technology to manipulate and enhance the features of our personal experience, by manipulating presence and social presence, for increasing wellness, and generating strength and resilience in individuals, organizations and society.

**Presence:** A selective and adaptive mechanism which allows the Self to define the boundaries of action by means of the distinction between "internal" and "external" within the sensory flow.

**Social Presence:** A selective and adaptive mechanism which allows the Self to identify and interact with Others by understanding their intentions.

**Social/Interpersonal Technologies:** Technologies used to support and improve social integration and/or connectedness between individuals, groups, and organizations.

**Transformation of Flow:** The person's ability to draw upon an optimal experience induced by technology and use it to promote new and unexpected psychological resources and sources of involvement.

# Chapter 2
# Positive Psychological Interventions and Information and Communication Technologies

**Rosa M. Baños**
*University of Valencia, Valencia, Spain*

**Alba Carrillo-Vega**
*University of Valencia, Valencia, Spain*

**Ernestina Etchemendy**
*Instituto Carlos III, Valencia, Spain*

**Cristina Botella**
*University Jaume I, Spain*

## ABSTRACT

*Since the advent of Positive Psychology there has been a connection between positive psychological interventions (PPIs) and the digital world. The development of PPIs, especially those delivered online, is becoming widespread within and outside the scientific field. Therefore, there is currently a need for accurate information that provides a critical view of all the interventions currently available. This chapter presents an updated review of the relationship between these two fields (PPIs and technologies), and discusses relevant considerations that should be taken into account when technologies are used to deliver PPIs, as well as the elements that can moderate their effectiveness. The final aim of the chapter is to provide readers with basic tools to make critical judgments about PPIs delivered via a technological format.*

## INTRODUCTION

Positive Psychological Interventions (PPIs) can be defined as interventions or intentional activities designed to cultivate positive feelings, cognitions and behaviours (Sin & Lyubomirsky, 2009). Since the establishment of the basic principles and objectives of Positive Psychology, increasing and relevant knowledge, both empirical and theoretical, has been produced in this field, demonstrating the efficacy of these interventions for improving well-being and reducing clinical symptomatology (specially depressive). Some examples of this idea come from the two meta-analyses carried out by Sin and Lyubomirsky (2009) and Bolier, Haverman, Westerhof, Riper, Smit and Bohlmeijer (2013). In the latter, the authors concluded that most of the analysed PPIs had a self-applied format, sometimes with face-to-face support, but most were delivered online (Bolier et al., 2013).

DOI: 10.4018/978-1-4666-9986-1.ch002

The connection between PPIs and Information and Communication Technologies (ICTs), especially with the development of the World Wide Web (WWW), has been present since their inception. Positive Psychology emerged at the same time as the expansion of the digital era; from the beginning it has taken advantage of many of the possibilities offered by ICTs, especially the Internet. In fact, one of the first studies to assess the efficacy of different PPIs was carried out over the Internet by recruiting a sample of people who had visited the webpage https://www.authentichappiness.sas.upenn.edu/ (Seligman, Steen, Park & Peterson, 2005).

Most of PPIs are brief and simple exercises or activities that can be implemented as part of one's daily routine, and where both commitment and daily practice become essential elements of their efficacy (Sheldon & Lyubomirsky, 2006). ICTs (especially mobile devices with Internet access) are being introduced exponentially in our daily lives. They can be very useful tools for designing, introducing and managing the intervention naturally as part of a routine, taking advantage of the growing number of innovative resources they offer, which can make the intervention more attractive and flexible. Moreover, the Internet provides accessibility that allows that these interventions reach a population that otherwise would not have access to them (Andersson, 2009; Andrews, Cuijpers, Craske, McEvoy & Titov, 2010; Bolier, et al., 2014). The current technological advances not only offer a new way to provide treatment, they also open up new possibilities for assessment and intervention. For example, sensorisation systems, currently available through mobile technologies, allow to monitor an intervention, patient's parameters, and environmental indicators, with a degree of ecological validity not previously achieved in the field of Psychology (where the main sources of information were self-reports and retrospective information). There are also examples of the potential benefits of other ICTs. Virtual Reality and Augmented Reality offer high-quality simulations of environments at an increasingly affordable cost, making them powerful tools for therapeutic change. Video games are also presented as innovative learning methods aimed at improving adherence and motivational components, both important variables for increasing treatment efficiency and efficacy. It is not surprising that the potential of ICTs has promoted most developed countries to consider them as the basis for health-care solutions.

This work aims to further examine and describe the associations between PPIs and ICTs. First, the current definitions of the relationships between the two fields will be clarified, and a summary of the PPIs using ICTs for which scientific evidence exists, including several technological applications developed by our group, will be described. Then, relevant considerations to be taken into account when technologies are used to deliver PPIs, as well as the elements that can moderate their effectiveness and their relationship with technologies will be considered. Finally, information from existing scientific literature regarding who consumes technology-based PPIs will be provided.

## RELATIONSHIP BETWEEN PPIs AND ICTs: DEFINITIONS

The application of technology to the field of PPIs has led to the emergence of different terms and definitions that try to capture this interaction. The terms are summarised below:

- **Online Psychological Interventions (OPIs):** These are defined by Ritterband, Gonder-Frederock, Cox, Clifton, West and Borowitz (2003) as interventions focused on behavioural aspects designed to modify and establish certain behaviours and subsequent improvement in symptomatology.

Generally, they refer to customisable and interactive interventions that fit the individual's own pace and use the multimedia format offered by the Internet.

- **Technological Behavioural Interventions (TBIs):** Mohr, Burns, Schueller, and Klinkman (2013) proposed this term for technological apps specifically designed to intervene on behavioural, cognitive and emotional aspects, in order to improve physical and psychological health and well-being. TBIs use different devices and technological developments (for example, smartphones, computers, virtual reality, videogames, social networks) for self-assessment, monitoring, psycho-education, goal setting, skills training, and feedback among others.
- **Positive Technologies (PTs):** This term was proposed by Botella, Riva, Gaggioli, Wiederhold, Alcañiz and Baños (2012) and Riva, Baños, Botella, Wiederhold and Gaggioli (2012) to refer to the scientific and applied approach focused on the study of the use of technology to improve the quality of personal experiences. It is a perspective that seeks to promote the use of technology to foster personal growth and the development of human virtues and strengths, thus contributing to social and cultural development.

As can be seen, there are overlaps between these definitions. Some definitions are more general than others, emphasising either the intervention or the technology used. In this chapter, the focus will be on the definition of PTs proposed by Botella et al. (2012a) and Riva et al. (2012), as it is the only definition that establishes a classification of technologies based on conceptualisations of subjective, psychological and social well-being (Diener, 1984; Kahneman, Diener & Schwarz, 1999; Ryff, 1989; Keyes, 1998; Ryan, Huta & Deci, 2008). According to Botella et al. (2012a), each level of wellbeing includes different goals (hedonic level: emotion regulation; eudaimonic level: flow and presence; and social level: community aims and social connections), and different technological applications can be designed to influence each level. Examples of hedonic PTs would be those that induce a positive and enjoyable experience, such as a virtual reality environment of joy/relax induction (e.g. Alcañiz, Baños, Botella & Rey, 2003; Baños et al., 2004, 2006). Eudaimonic PTs include technologies that help people achieve experiences focused on the search for a full and meaningful life (e.g., Botella et al., 2012b, Mira et al., 2012b). Social PTs include technologies that support and enhance communication and cooperation among individuals, groups and organisations (e.g., Botella et al., 2011).

## PPIs AND ICTs

As previously mentioned, in recent years there has been a significant rise in the number of interventions aimed at increasing positive emotions, behaviours and thoughts that contribute to improved well-being and happiness. Currently, a set of PPIs has already shown efficacy in increasing well-being and reducing depressive symptoms. Despite these advances, it is still necessary to carry out further rigorous work, especially regarding the effectiveness of PPIs (Bolier et al., 2013). This section first summarises those PPIs that have received greater empirical evidence. For each type of PPI, some currently available applications will be listed as examples. Then, technological applications developed by our group, as well as other PTs with evidence-based effectiveness, will be described.

## 1. PPIs

- **Savouring:** this activity is designed to intensify and prolong pleasurable experiences (Peterson, 2006). Several studies have shown the effectiveness of savouring in increasing positive mood and happiness (Bryant, 2003). The savouring intervention can be used with a sensory experience, such as eating an ice cream or feeling the sunshine on one's face, and also with memories. The variants within this intervention can be grouped into two categories: 1) the ones that teach and promote the practice of savouring in general; and 2) the ones that teach a specific savouring skill and promote its use. The first group usually includes asking the person to stop every day for at least 2-3 minutes and direct his/her attention to the present moment, focusing on the details and trying to prolong the pleasure of the activity as much as possible. For example, in the case of drinking hot chocolate, the person might focus on the taste, texture or temperature, then on the different sensations experienced when drinking it, and then on the mixture of flavours it leaves in the mouth. This same strategy can be applied at different times or in different situations, for example, walking to work or sitting on the bus, taking the same trip one takes every day. By contrast, the second group involves more structured training, so that people remember pleasant aspects of their lives, for example, being in a specific time and scenario, remembering what the temperature was, who they were with, or why it was a good time. In this case, participants use savouring techniques anchored in positive reminiscence work in order to re-edit a past moment and re-experience an event that has already occurred or even discover new positive feelings about it. The "Live Happy" (Parks, Della Porta, Pierce, Zilca, & Lyubomirsky, 2012) application is an example of transferring several PPIs to an online format; the app includes two savouring exercises. "Remembering happy days" is focused on creating a personal photo album to remember good times, where the user must also write a short description of that special moment. Thus, the exercise uses savouring while activating past experiences and recovering the original emotions and feelings. In the other exercise, "Savouring the moment", the user must take a picture of something beautiful and meaningful and write a brief paragraph that describes the value of the image and what he/she notices when watching it.
- **Gratitude:** This is one of the most used PPIs and with more empirical evidence compared to other PPIs (Bolier et al., 2013; Parks & Biswas-Diener, 2013). It involves doing activities to cultivate gratitude, either reflexively and following structured guidelines, or by carrying out a specific activity. These interventions have proved their effectiveness in increasing well-being, positive affect and physical health, and in reducing negative symptoms. However, literature has also pointed out the need for caution when prescribing this type of intervention. For example, Seligman, Steen, Parks and Peterson (2005) showed the usefulness of gratitude activities in people suffering from mild to moderate depression. In addition, Sergeant and Mongrain (2011) examined the effects of a gratitude intervention in depressed people with different styles of functioning (e.g., people with a greater need for support from others, or people with a self-critical functioning style). They found that people with a greater need for support and stronger feelings of helplessness about their goals did not benefit from the intervention, or, in some cases, even worsened when they did the activity.

One of the strategies focusing on a "more reflective" gratitude is the "Journal of gratitude". In this case, participants are asked to record once a week, for several weeks, at least five things for which they are grateful (Emmons & McCullough, 2003; Lyubomirsky, Sheldon & Schkade, 2005). Another exercise to cultivate gratitude is the intervention designed by Seligman and his team (Seligman et al., 2005), entitled

"Three blessings". Every night, participants should think for 10 minutes and write down in a journal three events about which they feel grateful and why. This exercise is not designed to record important or unusual events, but rather to focus on those small things that are part of their daily routine and make them feel good. Unlike the "Journal of gratitude", which deals with general functioning areas such as family, friends, work, studies, etc., the "Three Blessings" exercise focuses on situations that occur throughout the day. Regarding implementing specific activities, one example is "The visit of Gratitude". In this case, the participant is asked to write a letter of appreciation to someone about some detail or event that he/she has not had a chance to thank that person for, listing the details and/or situations that reflect the feeling of gratitude. Some authors recommend delivering this letter (Seligman et al., 2005), while others say it is not necessary (Lyubomirsky, Dickerhoof, Boehm & Sheldon, 2011). Regarding online interventions using this technique, one example is "Day to Day" (https://intellicare.cbits.northwestern.edu/#apps), an intervention delivered over smartphones that includes among its activities an exercise designed to cultivate gratitude. For seven days the user receives on his/her phone a simple exercise that must be done throughout the day. In addition, short simple messages explaining the importance of this exercise are sent, and the person is encouraged to follow the received guidelines. "Day to Day" also includes other exercises to increase connectedness, the frequency of pleasant moments, flexibility of thinking and problem solving. Each exercise lasts for seven days and maintains the same structure: at the beginning of the day, the user receives the activity to be done, brief messages of explanation and reinforcement are sent, the user is asked if he/she thinks the prescribed exercise will be positive for him/her, and at the end of the seventh day, two short questionnaires assessing levels of depression and anxiety are administered.

The "Live Happy" application also includes gratitude exercises. In the "Gratitude Journal" exercise, the user records something that happened during the day and why he/she is grateful. In another version of the exercise, the person chooses somebody to whom he/she wants to express gratitude.

- **Kindness**: In any of their variants, in general all these PPIs are aimed at getting the person involved to perform acts of kindness in his/her daily activities. The intention is to produce an interaction between the feelings aroused by doing something for someone and the feeling of gratitude, thus generating a reciprocity between giving and receiving that can lead to increased levels of happiness and well-being. An example of this procedure is the one developed by Lyubomirsky, Tkach and Sheldon (2004), in which the person must commit to five daily acts of kindness for 6 weeks. Another variant of interventions to foster kindness, although based on pro-social behaviour, proposes spending money on another person (Dunn, Aknin, & Norton, 2008). Regarding the number of acts of kindness, the important thing is that the person strives to do more actions of this kind than usual during his/her daily routine. "Live Happy" also includes a diary for recording acts of kindness and nurturing kindness in daily routines through making contact with a friend, relative, etc. With this exercise, "Live Happy" seeks to improve the quality of the user's social interactions.
- **Promoting Positive Social Relationships:** This PPI includes interventions focused on increasing social contacts and the quality of the interactions. One of the PPIs designed to meet this goal is "Respond actively and constructively" (Gable, Reis, Impett & Asher, 2004), which aims to train the user to respond actively and constructively to good things that happen and/or that someone is sharing with him/her. The user is asked to try to respond with happiness and genuine interest when asking about the event or situation. The purpose of the intervention is to transform neutral (or negative) styles of social interaction into positive interactions and generate new positive social interactions. These new interactions can range from a simple greeting in the morning when

encountering someone to fostering genuine relationships with people with whom there is a deep bond of friendship. An example of PPI that includes interventions of this type is one of the exercises proposed by the "Day to Day" app, previously mentioned. In this case, for a period of one week the user receives a daily pattern of positive social interactions to perform. The app tells what, how and how many interactions should be performed every day. The exercise is designed to increase social connectivity and improve the quality of the connections by strengthening ties with close links (e.g., friends) and with people with no bonds or distant links (e.g., salesman, etc.).

- **Search for Meaning:** These interventions help a person build meaning and goals in life that contribute to happiness. An example of these interventions is the "Best Possible Self". This technique is based on the work of King (2001), who proposed the therapeutic activity of writing about future objectives in life in order to achieve greater awareness and define life goals. The exercise requires the individual to write about a future where he/she has worked hard and, as a result, achieved all of his/her objectives and developed his/her full potential. Then, the assignment is to visualise this version of the self at least three minutes a day for a week (Sheldon & Lyubomirsky, 2006).

A similar exercise for building meaning is the "Summary of Life", proposed by Seligman, Rashid and Parks (2006). In this case, the person is prompted to write one or two pages reflecting how he/she expects to live day to day, and think about whether he/she can imagine actively working to achieve the objectives described in the narrative.

As we have seen, in general PPIs that promote the construction and search for meaning have narrative content. However, a study conducted by Lyubomirsky, Sousa and Dickerhoof (2006) warns of the differences in working on positive and negative material to generate increases in emotional well-being. When working with the memory of past experiences, it is preferable to work on the negative material analytically, using questions (e.g., why, how) that will lead to its restructuring. In these cases, the construction of written or oral narratives is very useful, as they involve a systematic, step-by-step process, providing coherence and an explanation for the negative event. The positive material, however, should be worked on without this type of analysis, without trying to make sense of it through written or oral narratives. The repetitive, circular and disorganised nature of experiences that "presumably" remains when remembering the event in private would be more beneficial to increasing well-being, as it would lead to reliving, savouring and capitalising on the experience (Langston, 1994; Quoidbach, Berry, Hansenne & Mikolajczak, 2010). This type of intervention is currently spreading, and there are numerous studies that evaluate this exercise in different clinical and non-clinical populations (Lyubomirsky et al., 2011; Meevissen, Peters & Alberts, 2011; Peters, Meevissen, & Hanssen, 2013). An example of this type of intervention is "Live Happy", which includes an exercise based on the "Best Possible Self" designed to promote optimism.

- **Personal Strengths:** Although there are some variations in their applications, in general the activities associated with this PPI attempt to identify, use and develop a personal strength. From the perspective of Seligman (2002), a personal strength is a positive personality trait with the following characteristics: the feeling that it is something one owns, a sense of excitement about showing it off, a fast learning curve when practicing it for the first time, a longing to find new ways to use it, the inability to prevent its use, a more energetic feeling when using it, the creation and pursuit of personal projects that revolve around it, and a feeling of joy, excitement and even ecstasy when using it (Seligman, 2002). It is possible to identify one's personal strengths through the VIA

(Values In Action) Strengths Inventory (Peterson & Park, 2009), which evaluates 24 strengths grouped into six virtues: "wisdom and knowledge", "courage", "humanity and love" "justice", "temperance", and "transcendence". Usually interventions on personal strengths ask people to identify their 5 main strengths, and then they have to exercise one or more of them in a new way for a week, whether at work, at home or during leisure time. Several important issues should be considered in the training: to clearly define the way the located strength must be practiced, the individual must record how he/she felt before, during and after doing it. It is also important that the individual assess whether the activity was stimulating and easy, whether time passed quickly, and whether he/she planned to repeat the activity. Thus far we have described the PPIs most used and with the most empirical evidence, some of which have been adapted to be delivered through the Internet and mobile devices. Next we will focus on interventions that were initially designed to be applied through ICTs.

## 2. Positive Technologies to Deliver PPIs

Below, we present a brief description of various positive technologies developed by our team (EARTH of Well-being, Butler system, and Smiling is fun), as well as other applications with evidence-based effectiveness in improving well-being.

- **EARTH of Well-Being (Baños et al., 2014):** This is a self-applied system that includes three modules with activities for working on different aspects of positive affect and hedonic and eudaimonic well-being. A module called "Well-being Park" includes two virtual reality environments and is designed to induce two emotional states (joy and relaxation) by using widely validated emotional induction methods (Lang, Bradley, & Cuthbert, 1995; Velten, 1968). Another module, "Well-being in Nature", also includes two virtual reality environments and different PPIs activities to induce joy and relaxation (savouring, slow breathing and positive reminiscence). The third and final module, the "Book of Life", works like a personal diary and includes 16 exercises focused on the past or the future. The former are directed at recalling past experiences related to different topics (e.g., "A happy moment", "The best place", "Important people", "An achievement", "Courage", "Optimism", "Gratitude", and "Passion"), and the latter involve defining objectives and positive future goals (e.g., in relation to oneself, family, friends, work, and life in general). All exercises have the same structure: a general instruction that explains the overall objective of the exercise and a series of secondary guidelines to aid in writing the narrative. In addition, the user can add multimedia resources (videos, pictures and music) to each chapter. Some of the exercises proposed have been validated in different populations: students (Baños et al, 2014.), people with adjustment disorders (Andreu-Mateu et al., 2012), cancer patients (Baños et al., 2014), and older adults (Baños et al., 2012), among others. EARTH of Well-being was initially developed for the Mars-500 project as a self-guided system to generate positive experiences for astronauts during a simulated Mars mission (Botella, Baños, Etchemendy, García-Palacios & Alcañiz, submitted), and it was then tested with Spanish university students. Both studies showed that the system was effective in increasing positive mood and decreasing negative emotions (Farfallini, 2014).
- **BUTLER System (Botella et al., 2011):** This is a positive technology (PT) designed to influence social well-being, but it also has resources aimed at promoting hedonic and eudaimonic well-being. Butler is a social and e-health technological platform based on web technology and virtual

reality. It is aimed mainly toward older adults with no experience with ICTs and includes tools to support formal and informal caregivers, families, etc. Its main objectives are to improve users' emotional state, empower the social support network through the use of ICTs, and provide activities that help improve quality of life of the older population (Botella, et al., 2011). The system was designed based on both the Active Aging and Positive Psychology perspectives. Butler's structure includes three types of users (older adults, formal caregivers and relatives/friends of an older adult), and the structure has tools for each of these profiles. In addition, two ways of functioning have been generated (leisure and professional), but they share the same users flow (the older adults). The two types of functioning are described below:

  - **Butler-Leisure** (www.mundomayordomo.com)**:** This function offers tools for older adults and their relatives/friends, and is designed to improve the social use of the platform. Butler-Leisure is a completely open access platform that can be used from any computer with Internet access and works as any e-social network currently available on the Internet (e.g., Facebook, Twitter), where each user obtains and administers his/her own account and enjoys the system. Butler-Leisure offers an e-mailbox, videoconference, a search for friends in the Butler net, and the Book of Life (blog) where the users can write and later share their writing with friends from Butler net. There is also a digital library with multimedia elements (photos, music, videos) and easy access to the Internet with favourites links and access to two virtual environments to generate positive emotions (joy and relaxation).
  - **Butler-Clinical:** This function includes the three user profiles above mentioned (older adults, formal caregivers and family or friends), and each user profile has different tools available. Its main feature is that the caregiver is the main administrator of the e-social and e-health tools. Therefore, Butler-Clinical is not an open platform like Butler-Leisure, as a caregiver must generate access to this type of use. Regarding older adult users, the social tools are the same as in Butler-Leisure. In the case of e-health tools, Butler-Clinical adds the Therapeutic Book of Life, which applies a training program of specific positive events from the autobiographical memory, based on the Review of Life Therapy (Haight & Webster, 1995; Serrano, Latorre, Gatz, & Montañez, 2004). For formal caregivers, the main goal of Butler-Clinical is to facilitate and optimise professional work through daily mood assessment tools, as well as a database with all the user's daily emotional information. In addition, an alarm system is included to send a warning to the professional in charge when the user's score reaches a certain clinical level. The system also restricts user access to social or clinical tools when this is therapeutically recommended. Last, this option allows older adults to share their book of life with relatives and friends and contact them using the e-mail and videoconference tools.

An interdisciplinary team consisting of psychologists, engineers and programmers monitored the development of Butler. The function has been tested in different seniors' profiles in different contexts. All the studies found positive results regarding efficacy in increasing positive mood states and decreasing negative ones, and it also has shown a high degree of acceptance (satisfaction, usefulness, difficulty of use) in older adult users (Baños et al., 2012, Botella et al., 2009; Castilla et al., 2011; Etchemendy et al., 2011, Preschl et al., 2012).

- **Smiling is Fun (Mira, 2014):** This is another example of a eudaimonic technological development. It is an Internet-based, multimedia (video, image, etc.) interactive programme that allows the individual to learn and practice adaptive ways to cope with depressive symptoms and confront daily problems. *Smiling is fun* trains a range of skills based on the Positive Psychology approach and seeks to break the vicious cycle of stress, isolation, depressive or anxiety symptoms, poor coping, and poor functioning (self-efficacy). Specifically, the programme was designed to promote activity and positive emotions, enhance social support, and work on meaningful goals and values. It has several modules complemented by transversal tools that accompany the user throughout implementation. These tools provide useful feedback that is important for participants' motivation and reinforcement:

- ◦ The "Activity Report" for self-monitoring provides feedback to users, showing them that their mood is related to the activities performed, and the benefits of being active. First, users are asked about their coping ability, mood state and stress level on a scale from 0 to 10. Then, they are asked about their degree of satisfaction with each activity performed during the past 24 hours and to what extent these activities are related to their own goals and values in life. Furthermore, users are asked about the percentage of the day that they have been active or involved in their lives for the past 24 hours.
- ◦ The "Calendar" allows users to know what step they are on throughout the program, and provides information about homework and tasks already completed, reminding users about those still outstanding. Furthermore, the "Calendar" shows which days the participant has filled in the activity report.
- ◦ "How am I?" offers a set of graphs and feedback to visualise the user's progress. It shows the evolution of information about activity level, emotional distress (anxiety and sadness), positive emotionality (active, enthusiastic, energetic, etc.) and negative emotionality (angry, fearful, stressed, tense, moody, etc.). With this tool, participants can graphically see the relationship between their activity level, mood state, stress and coping ability.

The system has been tested in different studies with different sample profiles (Botella et al., 2012b; Mira, et al., 2012a; Mira 2014). Results showed that *Smiling is fun* is effective in improving clinical status and decreasing depressive symptomatology. Currently, a large-scale study designed to compare the effectiveness of *Smiling is fun* with treatment as usual is in progress. Thus far, the results obtained are promising.

- **Live Happy:** We have commented about this technological application in the previous section. It is one of the few evidence-based applications for mobile devices, and its use has been shown to improve users' happiness (Parks et al., 2012). The application was developed using the research approaches of Lyubomirsky, and it includes 8 interventions, all of which have been shown in previous studies to be effective in improving well-being and reducing depressive symptoms: 1) savouring, 2) reminiscence, 3) journal of kindness, 4) strengthening social relations, 5) evaluation and monitoring of objectives, 6) journal of gratitude, 7) expressing gratitude and 8) optimistic thinking.
- **Psyfit.nl (Bolier, et al., 2013):** A completely self-applied online intervention with no support from a therapist, developed to improve well-being and reduce depressive symptoms. The intervention was designed based on the principles of Positive Psychology, focusing on positive experiences, personal strengths and skills rather than mental health problems and deficiencies. It includes

6 modules, each with exercises and evidence-based content: setting life goals, positive emotions, positive relationships, mindfulness, optimistic thinking and mastery of life. Each module includes 4 lessons to be taught once a week, and each lesson provides some brief psycho-education and an exercise. In addition, Psyfit.nl includes self-administered questionnaires for monitoring mood, levels of happiness, and well-being, as well as videos of experts, a personal action plan, and an online community where participants can share their experiences.

- **Happiness Coach (Vansteenwegen, 2011):** Is an intervention developed following the same pattern as Psyfit.nl. In this case, the programme uses a subway ride as a metaphor for the interventions. A map emulates different subway tracks and indicates different strategies to improve happiness levels given the different objectives and progress. The programme includes information, advice and interactive exercises to generate behavioural changes.
- **Better Days (Drozd, Mork, Nielsen, Raeder, Bjokli, 2014):** Is an online intervention designed to be used through the mobile phone and aimed at improving daily lives and well-being. It consists of 13 sessions lasting 10 minutes each distributed over 4 weeks. Each session contains some initial psycho-education and an exercise. The available exercises include: gratitude, acts of kindness, optimism, coping strategies, living in the present moment, and strengths. Recently, a controlled study showed an increase in the level of happiness of its users (Drozd et al., 2014).

As described above, different PPIs have shown their effectiveness in improving well-being. In addition, due to the simplicity and ease of use of these interventions, the vast majority have been adapted to a technological format. At present, there is a broad range of applications developed and available on the network that are based on the precepts of Positive Psychology. However, not all technology-based PPIs rely on empirical evidence or have been tested to evaluate effectiveness. For this reason, it is important to mention the Beacon website (www.beacon.anu.edu.au), which offers rigorous assessment by experts and researchers, various online interventions, and apps developed for different physical and emotional disorders. For each intervention, there is a brief description, login information and a summary of the accumulated scientific evidence. Although the Positive Psychology category includes few interventions, Beacon is a good example and tool for the dissemination and use of ICT-based PPIs.

Another recent initiative worth mentioning is the *Center for behavioral intervention technologies* (Cbits; webpage http://www.cbits.northwestern.edu/), opened in 2011 and directed by David Mohr (Northwestern University Feinberg School of Medicine, Chicago). The purpose of this institute, formed by an interdisciplinary team of researchers (computer experts, psychologists, engineers, doctors, etc.), is to develop technological applications that promote behavioural changes in order to improve physical, mental and emotional health. Currently, it has technological developments for smartphones, virtual reality, websites, or phone therapy. The practical use of Cbits is a good example of evidence-based technological developments. Its applications can be downloaded from the Internet, and they also give access to scientific studies that test the effectiveness of each system developed (https://intellicare.cbits.northwestern.edu/#apps). Specifically related to PPIs, "Day to day", "Aspire" or "My mantra" are worth mentioning.

## SOME CONSIDERATIONS ON PPIs, EFFECTIVENESS, AND ICTs

As mentioned earlier, the connection between PPIs and ICTs offers a number of benefits and improvements that help to reinforce the spread of PPIs. ICTs are considered powerful resources in the field of

PPIs: the progress made in the digital era makes it possible to detect, evaluate, investigate, monitor and intervene in a way that had never been seen before in the disciplines that study human behaviour (Miller, 2012). However, PPIs also present difficulties and limitations that must be acknowledged, in order to make an effort to further improve them. Below, some of these difficulties are highlighted.

## Motivation and Commitment

Adherence is a key element in the effectiveness and efficiency of any psychological intervention. Lack of motivation, low levels of commitment and dropout rates are some of the main difficulties in any treatment. Unfortunately, online interventions are not exempt from these problems, which may even be greater in this area (Eysenbach, 2005). Studies show that dropout rates that occur with the traditional format are lower than those observed with the online format. If we also consider online interventions that are delivered outside the scientific field, which are not included in the studies, or those that are simply available on the Internet or through mobile applications, the dropout rates are even higher because there is less pressure to stay on task when there is no previous commitment (Christensen, Griffiths, & Farrer, 2009; Parks, 2014). Therefore, this problem is by no means a minor issue, thus justifying the fact that a significant part of the research efforts at the moment are directed to try to resolve it. Some of the resources being used and analysed in order to maintain the person's commitment and adherence are: message reminders, positive reinforcement sent via mobile, daily emails, gamification of the intervention process, the possibility of publishing results in social networks, and frequent feedback on progress. There is a large body of literature about the factors that promote engagement and prevent neglect. However, when it comes to technology-based interventions, it is necessary to learn how to adapt to the connection between the two fields.

According to Rogers (1983), it is important to abandon the naive idea that technological innovations that involve some degree of improvement in efficiency and will be directly adopted by users, and that they will easily obtain more positive results than previous options. Instead, Roger explains that the process of accepting the adoption of improved technology is much more complex, and he proposes five qualities that would influence the adoption rate of an innovation ("comparative advantage", "support", "observability" "complexity" and "experimentation"). Table 1 provides a brief explanation of each of the qualities and its relationship with PPIs. Taking these qualities into account when designing, analysing and selecting a PPI can contribute to solving the problem of the attrition rate, the lack of motivation, and adherence.

## Variety and Doses

The vast majority of the PPIs that have shown effectiveness generally come from studies with only one intervention (gratitude, best possible self, etc.). However, the literature suggests that when users practice PPIs outside the scientific field (that is, naturally in the real world context), they prefer to use a wide variety of activities (Parks et al., 2012). In addition to the fact that the implementation of interventions in empirical studies is often disconnected from the users' preferences in a real context, the literature has also indicated that offering variability in interventions has a positive impact on motivation and adherence and increases effectiveness (Parks et al., 2012).

Another element to consider in PPIs is the hedonic adaptation, a phenomenon inherent to almost all positive changes. Along time, an action that once produced an increase in positive emotions and happiness loses its strength until becoming ineffective (Lyubomirsky, 2011). This adaptation also occurs with

*Table 1. Qualities that influence the adoption of an innovation and their relationship with PPIs*

| Definition by Rogers (1983) | Connection with PPIs |
|---|---|
| **Comparative Advantage:** The degree to which an innovation is perceived as better than the idea it replaces. The nature of the innovation will determine the specific type of relative advantage it should have (whether social, economic, political, etc.). | Finding out the opinions of other users regarding the user experience, having a ranking based on the scores given by other users, including videos of experts and participants explaining the advantages of its use, etc. are all aspects that would facilitate this quality. |
| **Compatibility:** The degree to which an innovation is perceived as consistent with existing values, past experiences, and needs of potential users. A compatible innovation is the one that is less uncertain for the potential user. In this sense, an innovation can be compatible or incompatible with social values and beliefs, with previous ideas, with needs, and so on. | At these levels it is important to have information on user preferences and whether the intervention is suitable for them. Moreover, given the flexibility offered by current technologies, being able to customise aspects of the intervention would also contribute to this quality. |
| **Observability:** The degree to which the results of an innovation are visible to users. The results of some ideas are easily observed and reported by others, while some innovations are difficult to describe. | Giving users constant feedback about their progress, making this information visible through graphs, ratings, messages, etc. helps to make the results of the intervention visible to users. |
| **Complexity:** The degree to which an innovation is perceived as relatively difficult to understand and use. Any idea can be located on the complexity-simplicity continuum. Some innovations have a clear meaning to potential users, while others do not. Studies suggest that the complexity of an innovation is negatively related to the rate of adoption. | In this case it is important to consider what PPIs are being prescribed to what user, taking into account their age, degree of immersion in technology, etc. Some online interventions are simple, while others include many more functions. It is not advisable to give a PPI with many options to a person who is not familiar with technology or, conversely, offer something oversimplified to someone with a high technological profile. |
| **Experimentation:** Refers to the degree to which an innovation can be experienced on a limited basis. New ideas that can be tested in parts are generally accepted more quickly than innovations that are not visible. In other words, an innovation that can be experienced by prospective users is less uncertain for them and would facilitate its adoption. | Currently there is a widespread dissemination of free or very affordable apps. This aspect helps to promote experimentation. |

Rogers, 1983.

PPIs. If a person is carrying out only one activity for a long time, it will probably become saturating and boring and, therefore, disable the benefit pursued by the intervention. The literature suggests that one way to deal with hedonic adaptation, either avoiding it or delaying it, is to offer several activities and not just one (Layous & Lyubomirsky, 2012). However, this does not mean that more is always better. A recent study shows that when two, four and six interventions were compared, the combination of four interventions showed greater efficacy (Schueller & Parks, 2012).

Another curious aspect related to the intervention doses, but equally relevant, has to do with the time required by PPIs. While scientific studies point to reducing them to the shortest possible time, in the natural context, outside of empirical studies, people spend an average of 1 hour a day on activities aimed at increasing happiness (Parks et al., 2012).

In conclusion, doses and variability are major issues in the effectiveness of PPIs. These factors need to be consider when prescribing a PPI, given that all these minor changes can undermine motivation and adherence, two crucial elements for a PPI to be effective in increasing well-being. These cautions are even more relevant in the context of research, since attempts to highly standardise the procedures and to guarantee internal validity could reduce the effectiveness of a PPI by making them less attractive.

## Customising Interventions

It is important for people to perform activities that suit their preferences and profiles. For instance, the study by Schueller (2012) concludes that introverts and extroverts benefited from different interventions. For extroverts, the best results were shown by the "gratitude visit" and "savouring" exercises, while introverts benefited more from the responding actively and constructively and "strengths" interventions and the "three blessings" exercise. Another finding from the same study showed that when participants focused on the "visit of gratitude", whether in person, by mail or by telephone, extraverts benefited most from the visit in person, while this variation was not the best solution for introverts.

In a similar vein, another study also conducted previously by Schueller (2010) investigated whether preferences for some exercises were related to preferences for other exercises. The results showed three preference groups: a group that preferred savouring and responding actively and constructively, another group that favoured three blessings and summary of life, and a third group that preferred the visit of gratitude and strengths. Regarding this grouping, Schueller also found that the participants' preferences were related to a greater probability of completing both the intervention and its matching intervention.

Therefore, it is important to take into account the preferences and adjustment to the interventions. However, again it is imperative to be careful not to oversimplify the findings from the literature and conclude that just because people like to perform a prescribed procedure, the procedure would be sufficient to increase their well-being. The study by Parks et al. (2012), in which participants could choose what activity to perform, showed that the strategies they chose to increase happiness were not necessarily the most effective. For example, two of the most popular activities, "Goal evaluation and tracking" and "Savouring the moment", were not associated with increased happiness and mood. This finding highlights an important issue: individuals' opinions when choosing what is good for them may be wrong. Therefore, deciding which intervention should be prescribed based only on the participant's choice would over-simplify the decision and not lead to more effective results.

The types of mistakes people make when engaging in emotional predictions have been widely demonstrated by theorists who study "Affective Forecasting" (Wilson & Gilbert, 2003). The literature shows that people tend to make mistakes and are not necessarily accurate in predicting the intensity and duration of their emotional responses. Therefore, their decision-making about the activities they can do to increase their levels of happiness and well-being might not be related to reality, especially in people who have difficulties with emotional regulation (Halpern & Arnold, 2008).

## Identified Profiles of Consumers of ICT-Based PPIs

Currently, a PPIs without any technological elements are almost inexistent, the access to interventions is faster, free and very easy. In fact, there are numerous interventions divulgated daily through social networks as Facebook, Twitter, etc. In addition, a large number of studies are realised through calls via Internet that seek people that want to be happier. Nevertheless, there are not enough data about the profile of people who use or seek ICT-based PPIs. This means that samples and data obtained could be biased. So, to identify and analyse the different PPIs consumers' profiles and the effects of interventions is important. In our search we have found some relevant but still few studies addressing this question. Parks et al. (2012) carried out three studies focused in consumers of online interventions. The first one shows the non-homogeneity of the people who use PPIs; two clusters of people were found. The first, "non-distressed", showed lower rates of depression, adequate levels of satisfaction with life, a balance between positive and negative affect, and happiness. The second, "distressed", showed clinical depression rates, low life satisfaction, improper balance of positive-negative affect, and low levels of happiness. The second study was focused on finding out how people increased their levels of happiness and well-being naturally in everyday life, that is, outside of experimental procedures that prescribe who, what, for how long and how often to do the exercise. The results showed that, in a real context, people use between 7 and 8 activities at once, that the hedonic adaptation that is produced in any intervention does not occur until "several months" after beginning an activity, and that the most meaningful activity for them was practiced several times a week and at least one hour a day. That is, there are relevant differences between the procedures being used in the experimental field and spontaneous behaviours that people perform in their daily lives. Finally, the third study, conducted with the Live Happy application and focused on the activities undertaken to increase happiness, showed that in the real world people use, like, and obtain benefits for their mood and happiness by using the same activities that are being used in experimental studies. A variety of preferences were found, as the most preferred activity was "Goal evaluation and tracking", and the least preferred one was the "Acts of kindness journal". Finally, the people who used the application reported a greater increase in well-being.

## FUTURE RESEARCH DIRECTIONS

ICTs have much to offer, but the digital world develops and spreads at a much greater rate than the scientific field can keep up with. One of the first consequences involved, which surely cannot be avoided, is that not all the currently available exercises were developed through an evidence-based method. For this reason, it is important to improve the effectiveness of Positive Technology through evidence-based practices as randomized controlled trials in order to discern between "good" and "bad" practices. It is crucial for people (clinicians and users) to have information that allows them to discern between interventions, so they can choose critically which interventions they want to use, knowing whether they are supported by the scientific literature.

On the other hand, the ease and simplicity that characterise PPIs might suggest that any exercise can be effective in increasing these variables. However, this is far from reality. A growing body of literature shows the importance of certain variables that are critical to the effectiveness of these interventions. Some of these variables are: the characteristics of the activity, previous well-being levels, the intervention dose, users' motivation, hedonic adaptation, the match between the activity prescribed and the person, personality characteristics, and the technological user profile, among others. For this reason, the effectiveness of PPIs cannot be taken for granted. It is important to further deepen the knowledge about the profiles of people who use PPIs, their daily practices and preferences, in order to promote a rigorous dissemination of positive psychology over the Internet.

## CONCLUSION

ICTs are making it possible to redesign the forms, scope and quality of psychological interventions. They offer significant advantages without sacrificing the quality of the intervention, and they allow an accessibility to interventions that was unviable in the traditional format. At the same time, given their simplicity, PPIs are presented as very good candidates to be adapted to and delivered in digital format. This union has led to a great expansion of PPIs in digital format and to different lines of research on the effectiveness of these interventions, the promotion of rigorous and evidence-based practice, and the study of the different factors that contribute to increasing PPIs' effectiveness when delivered digitally.

As a consequence, the number of apps, webpages, or online exercises that "sell happiness" increases exponentially day by day. It should be kept in mind that most PPIs, due to their simplicity, are mainly designed to be self-administered, and ICTs offer a format and advantages that make their use in this area convenient. However, as mentioned above, the technological offer grows so quickly that makes it impossible to ensure the reliability of all its contents and to all its users, and, in fact, a number of applications and exercises currently available were not developed through rigorous studies that show their effectiveness in increasing happiness and well-being.

As stated, Positive Psychology was born during the digital revolution, thus the union between the two fields has been present since its inception. This union certainly will grow and improve in the future. The 21st century represents a new era in which PPIs and technology can interact synergistically. Future technologies allow for constant monitoring, sensing and feedback (at the pace that the user wants) and this one will help to increase the efficacy and effectiveness of PPIs. In addition, future technological strategies (such as artificial intelligence or augmented reality) will be able to provide either new enhanced experiences. These new mixed ICT tools might evolve into experts in "increasing well-being" in all its facets (hedonic, eudaimonic, and social-interpersonal). Nevertheless, given that the expansion and growth of ICT developments will be faster than the psychological scientific evidence, it is necessary to improve and disseminate PPIs with the help of ICTs. But we cannot forget that "not everything works"; "not everything works for everyone" and "not everything works with everything". This "growth with caution" is one of the most important challenges of Positive Technology based in evidence.

## REFERENCES

Alcañiz, M., Baños, R., Botella, C., & Rey, B. (2003). The EMMA project: Emotions as a determinant of presence. *Psychology Journal, 1*(2), 141–150.

Andersson, G. (2009). Using the Internet to provide cognitive behaviour therapy. *Behaviour Research and Therapy, 47*(3), 175–180. doi:10.1016/j.brat.2009.01.010 PMID:19230862

Andreu-Mateu, S., Botella, C., Quero, S., Guillén, V., & Baños, R. (2012). La utilización de la realidad virtual y estrategias de psicología positiva en el tratamiento de los trastornos adaptativos. *Behavioral Psychology/Psicología Conductual, 20*(2), 323-348.

Andrews, G., Cuijpers, P., Craske, M., McEvoy, P., & Titov, N. (2010). Computer therapy for the anxiety and depressive disorders is effective, acceptable and practical health care: A meta-analysis. *PLoS ONE, 5*(10), 131–196. doi:10.1371/journal.pone.0013196 PMID:20967242

Baños, R., Etchemendy, E., Farfallini, L., García-Palacios, A., Quero, S., & Botella, C. (2014). EARTH of Well-Being system: A pilot study of an Information and Communication Technology-based positive psychology intervention. *The Journal of Positive Psychology, 6*(9), 482–488. doi:10.1080/17439760.2014.927906

Baños, R. M., Botella, C., Alcañiz, M., Liaño, V., Guerrero, B., & Rey, B. (2004). Immersion and emotion: Their impact on the sense of presence. *Cyberpsychology & Behavior*, *7*(6), 734–741. doi:10.1089/cpb.2004.7.734 PMID:15687809

Baños, R. M., Etchemendy, E., Castilla, D., García-Palacios, A., Quero, S., & Botella, C. (2012). Positive mood induction procedures for virtual environments designed for elderly people. *Interacting with Computers*, *24*(3), 131–138. doi:10.1016/j.intcom.2012.04.002

Baños, R. M., Liaño, V., Botella, C., Alcañiz, M., Guerrero, B., & Rey, B. (2006). Changing Induced Moods via Virtual Reality. In W. Ijsselsteijn, Y. de Kort, C. Midden, B. Eggen & E. van dem Hoven (Eds.), Persuasive Technology, LNCS (Vol. 3962, pp. 7-15). Berlin/Heilderberg: Springer-Verlag.

Bolier, L., Haverman, M., Kramer, J., Westerhof, G. J., Riper, H., Walburg, J. A., & Bohlmeijer, E. et al. (2013). An Internet-based intervention to promote mental fitness for mildly depressed adults: Randomized controlled trial. *Journal of Medical Internet Research*, *15*(9), e200. doi:10.2196/jmir.2603 PMID:24041479

Bolier, L., Haverman, M., Westerhof, G. J., Riper, H., Smit, F., & Bohlmeijer, E. (2013). Positive psychology interventions: A meta-analysis of randomized controlled studies. *BMC Public Health*, *13*(1), 119. doi:10.1186/1471-2458-13-119 PMID:23390882

Bolier, L., Majo, C., Smit, F., Westerhof, G. J., Haverman, M., Walburg, J. A., & Bohlmeijer, E. et al. (2014). Cost-effectiveness of online positive psychology: Randomized controlled trial. *The Journal of Positive Psychology*, *9*(5), 460–471. doi:10.1080/17439760.2014.910829

Botella, C., Baños, R., Etchemendy, E., Castilla, D., García-Palacios, A., & Alcañiz, M. (2011). An e-health system for promoting wellbeing in elderly: The Butler System. In Å. Smedberg (Ed.), *E-Health Communities and Online Self-Help Groups: Applications and Usage* (pp. 57–71). Hershey, PA, USA: IGI Global. Doi:10.4018/978-1-60960-866-8

Botella, C., Baños, R. M., Etchemendy, E., García-Palacios, A., & Alcañiz, M. (in press). Psychological countermeasures in manned space missions: "EARTH" system for the Mars-500 project. *Computers in Human Behavior*.

Botella, C., Etchemendy, E., Castilla, D., Baños, R. M., García-Palacios, A., Quero, S., … Lozano, J. A. (2009). An e-health system for the elderly (Butler Project): a pilot study on acceptance and satisfaction. *Cyberpsychology & Behavior: the impact of the Internet, multimedia and virtual reality on behavior and society, 12*(3), 255-262.

Botella, C., Mira, A., Garcia-Palacios, A., Quero, A., Navarro, M. V., Riera López del Amo, T., & Baños, R. M. et al. (2012b). Smiling is fun: A coping with stress and emotion regulation program. Annual Review of Cybertherapy and Telemedicine 2012. Advanced Technologies in the Behavioral. *Social Neuroscience*, 2012, 123–128.

Botella, C., Riva, G., Gaggioli, A., Wiederhold, B. K., Alcaniz, M., & Baños, R. M. (2012a). The present and future of positive technologies. *Cyberpsychology, Behavior, and Social Networking*, *15*(2), 78–84. doi:10.1089/cyber.2011.0140 PMID:22149078

Bryant, F. B. (2003). Savoring beliefs inventory (SBI): A scale for measuring beliefs about savouring. *Journal of Mental Health (Abingdon, England)*, *12*(2), 175–196. doi:10.1080/0963823031000103489

Castilla, D., García-Palacios, A., Bretón-López, J., Etchemendy, E., Farfallini, L., & Botella, C. (2011). Process of design and usability evaluation of a technology web and virtual reality system for the elderly: Butler. *International Journal of Human-Computer Studies*, *71*(3), 350–362. doi:10.1016/j.ijhcs.2012.10.017

Christensen, H., Griffiths, K. M., & Farrer, L. (2009). Adherence in internet interventions for anxiety and depression. *Journal of Medical Internet Research*, *11*(2), e13. doi:10.2196/jmir.1194 PMID:19403466

Diener, E. (1984). Subjective well-being. *Psychological Bulletin*, *95*(3), 542–575. doi:10.1037/0033-2909.95.3.542 PMID:6399758

Drozd, F., Mork, L., Nielsen, B., Raeder, S., & Bjørkli, C. A. (2014). Better Days – A randomized controlled trial of an internet-based positive psychology intervention. *The Journal of Positive Psychology*, *9*(5), 377–388. doi:10.1080/17439760.2014.910822

Dunn, E. W., Aknin, L. B., & Norton, M. I. (2008). Spending money on others promotes happiness. *Science*, *319*(5870), 1687–1688. doi:10.1126/science.1150952 PMID:18356530

Emmons, R. A., & McCullough, M. E. (2003). Counting blessings versus burdens: An experimental investigation of gratitude and subjective well-being in daily life. *Journal of Personality and Social Psychology*, *84*(2), 377–389. Retrieved from http://www.ncbi.nlm.nih.gov/pubmed/12585811 doi:10.1037/0022-3514.84.2.377 PMID:12585811

Etchemendy, E., Baños, R. M., Botella, C., Castilla, D., Alcañiz, M., Rasal, P., & Farfallini, L. (2011). An e-health platform for the elderly population: The Butler system. *Computers & Education*, *56*(1), 275–279. doi:10.1016/j.compedu.2010.07.022

Eysenbach, G. (2005). The law of attrition. *Journal of Medical Internet Research*, *7*(1), e11. doi:10.2196/jmir.7.1.e11 PMID:15829473

Farfallini, L. (2014). Validación de una Intervención Positiva auto-aplicada orientada al bienestar: EARTH of Wellbeing [Doctoral thesis]. Universitat Jaume I.

Gable, S. L., Reis, H. T., Impett, E. A., & Asher, E. R. (2004). What do you do when things go right? The intrapersonal and interpersonal benefits of sharing positive events. *Journal of Personality and Social Psychology*, *87*(2), 228–245. doi:10.1037/0022-3514.87.2.228 PMID:15301629

Haight, B. K., & Webster, J. D. (1995). *The art and science of reminiscing: Theory, research method, and applications*. Washington, DC: Taylor & Francis.

Halpern, J., & Arnold, R. M. (2008). Affective forecasting: An unrecognized challenge in making serious health decisions. *Journal of General Internal Medicine*, *23*(10), 1708–1712. doi:10.1007/s11606-008-0719-5 PMID:18665428

Kahneman, D., Diener, E., & Schwarz, N. (1999). *Well-being. The foundations of hedonic psychology*. New York, NY: Russell Sage.

Keyes, C. L. M. (1998). Social Well-being. *Social Psychology Quarterly*, *61*(2), 121–140. doi:10.2307/2787065

King, L. A. (2001). The Health Benefits of Writing about Life Goals. *Personality and Social Psychology Bulletin*, *27*(7), 798–807. doi:10.1177/0146167201277003

Lang, P. J., Bradley, M. M., & Cuthbert, B. N. (1995). *International affective picture system (IAPS): Technical manual and affective ratings*. Gainesville: NIMH Center for the Study of Emotion and Attention, University of Florida.

Langston, C. A. (1994). Capitalizing on and coping with daily-life events: Expressive responses to positive events. *Journal of Personality and Social Psychology*, *67*(6), 1112–1125. doi:10.1037/0022-3514.67.6.1112

Layous, K., & Lyubomirsky, S. (2012). The how, who, what, when, and why of happiness: Mechanisms underlying the success of positive interventions. In J. Gruber & J. Moscowitz (Eds.), *The light and dark side of positive emotions* (pp. 473–495). New York, NY: Oxford University Press.

Lyubomirsky, S. (2011). Hedonic adaptation to positive and negative experiences. In S. Folkman (Ed.), *Oxford handbook of stress health and coping* (pp. 200–224). New York, NY: Oxford University Press.

Lyubomirsky, S., Dickerhoof, R., Boehm, J. K., & Sheldon, K. M. (2011). Becoming happier takes both a will and a proper way: An experimental longitudinal intervention to boost well-being. *Emotion (Washington, D.C.)*, *11*(2), 391–402. doi:10.1037/a0022575 PMID:21500907

Lyubomirsky, S., Sheldon, K. M., & Schkade, D. (2005). Pursuing happiness: The architecture of sustainable change. *Review of General Psychology*, *9*(2), 111–131. doi:10.1037/1089-2680.9.2.111

Lyubomirsky, S., Sousa, L., & Dickerhoof, R. (2006). The costs and benefits of writing, talking, and thinking about life's triumphs and defeats. *Journal of Personality and Social Psychology*, *90*(4), 692–708. doi:10.1037/0022-3514.90.4.692 PMID:16649864

Lyubomirsky, S., Tkach, C., & Sheldon, K. M. (2004). Pursuing sustained happiness through random acts of kindness and counting one's blessings: Tests of two six-week interventions [Unpublished data]. Department of Psychology, University of California, Riverside.

Meevissen, Y. M. C., Peters, M. L., & Alberts, H. J. E. M. (2011). Become more optimistic by imagining a best possible self: Effects of a two week intervention. *Journal of Behavior Therapy and Experimental Psychiatry*, *42*(3), 371–378. doi:10.1016/j.jbtep.2011.02.012 PMID:21450262

Miller, G. (2012). The Smartphone Psychology Manifesto. *Perspectives on Psychological Science*, *7*(3), 221–237. doi:10.1177/1745691612441215 PMID:26168460

Mira, A. (2014). Eficacia diferencial de un programa de intervención auto-aplicado a través de Internet para la prevención y el tratamiento de la depresión leve o moderada con apoyo y sin apoyo por parte del terapeuta. [Doctoral thesis]. Universitat Jaume I. Retrieved from http://hdl.handle.net/10803/284396

Mira, A., Botella, C., García-Palacios, A., Bretón-López, J., Moragrega, I., & Riera-López del Amo, A., ... Baños, R. M. (2012a). Coping with stress: A program for the prevention of depression. *Proceedings of the 1st Workshop on ICT applied to Mental Health* (pp. 48-52).

Mira, A., Botella, C., García-Palacios, A., Riera, A., Quero, S., Alcañiz, M., & Baños, R. (2012b). An internet-based program to cope with regulating stress and emotion: An example of positive technology. *Cybertherapy & Rehabilitation, 2*(1), 22-23.

Mohr, D. C., Burns, M. N., Schueller, S. M., Clarke, G., & Klinkman, M. (2013). Behavioral intervention technologies: Evidence review and recommendations for future research in mental health. *General Hospital Psychiatry, 35*(4), 332–338. doi:10.1016/j.genhosppsych.2013.03.008 PMID:23664503

Parks, A. C. (2014). A case for the advancement of the design and study of online positive psychological interventions. *The Journal of Positive Psychology, 9*(6), 502–508. doi:10.1080/17439760.2014.936969

Parks, A. C., & Biswas-Diener, R. (2013). Positive Interventions: Past, Present, and Future. In T. Kashdan & J. Carriochi (Eds.), *Bridging Acceptance and Commitment Therapy and Positive Psychology: A Practitioners's Guide to a Unifying Framework*. Oakland, CA: New Harbinger.

Parks, A. C., Della Porta, M. D., Pierce, R. S., Zilca, R., & Lyubomirsky, S. (2012). Pursuing happiness in everyday life: The characteristics and behaviors of online happiness seekers. *Emotion (Washington, D.C.), 12*(6), 1222–1234. doi:10.1037/a0028587 PMID:22642345

Peters, M. L., Meevissen, Y. M. C., & Hanssen, M. M. (2013). Specificity of the Best Possible Self intervention for increasing optimism: Comparison with a gratitude intervention. *Terapia Psicológica, 31*(1), 93–100. doi:10.4067/S0718-48082013000100009

Peterson, C. (2006). *A Primer in Positive Psychology*. New York, NY: Oxford University Press.

Peterson, C., & Park, N. (2009). Classifying and Measuring Strengths of Character. In C. R. Snyder & S. J. Lopez (Eds.), *Handbook of Positive Psychology*. New York, NY: Oxford University Press. doi:10.1093/oxfordhb/9780195187243.013.0004

Preschl, B., Maercker, A., Wagner, B., Forstmeier, S., Baños, R. M., Alcañiz, M., & Botella, C. et al. (2012). Life review therapy with computer supplements for depression in the elderly: A randomized controlled trial. *Aging & Mental Health, 16*(8), 964–974. doi:10.1080/13607863.2012.702726 PMID:22788983

Quoidbach, J., Berry, E. V., Hansenne, M., & Mikolajczak, M. (2010). Positive emotion regulation and well-being: Comparing the impact of eight savoring and dampening strategies. *Personality and Individual Differences, 49*(5), 368–373. doi:10.1016/j.paid.2010.03.048

Ritterband, L. M., Gonder-Frederick, L. A., Cox, D. J., Clifton, A. D., West, R. W., & Borowitz, S. M. (2003). Internet interventions: In review, in use, and into the future. *Professional Psychology, Research and Practice, 34*(5), 527–534. doi:10.1037/0735-7028.34.5.527

Riva, G., Baños, R. M., Botella, C., Wiederhold, B. K., & Gaggioli, A. (2012). Positive technology: Using interactive technologies to promote positive functioning. *Cyberpsychology, Behavior, and Social Networking, 15*(2), 69–77. doi:10.1089/cyber.2011.0139 PMID:22149077

Rogers, E. M. (1983). *Diffusion of Innovations*. New York, NY: Free Press.

Ryan, R. M., Huta, V., & Deci, E. L. (2008). Living well: A self-determination theory perspective on eudaimonia. *Journal of Happiness Studies, 9*(1), 139–170. doi:10.1007/s10902-006-9023-4

Ryff, C. D. (1989). Happiness is everything, or is it? Explorations on the meaning of psychological well-being. *Journal of Personality and Social Psychology*, *57*(6), 1069–1081. doi:10.1037/0022-3514.57.6.1069

Schueller, S. M. (2010). Preferences for positive psychology exercises. *The Journal of Positive Psychology*, *5*(3), 192–203. doi:10.1080/17439761003790948

Schueller, S. M. (2012). Personality Fit and Positive Interventions: Extraverted and Introverted Individuals Benefit from Different Happiness Increasing Strategies. *Psychology (Savannah, Ga.)*, *3*(12), 1166–1173. doi:10.4236/psych.2012.312A172

Schueller, S. M., & Parks, A. C. (2012). Disseminating self-help: Positive psychology exercises in an online trial. *Journal of Medical Internet Research*, *14*(3), e63. doi:10.2196/jmir.1850 PMID:22732765

Seligman, M. E. P. (2002). *Authentic Happiness: Using the New Positive Psychology to Realize Your Potential for Lasting Fulfillment*. New York, NY: Free Press.

Seligman, M. E. P., Rashid, T., & Parks, A. C. (2006). Positive psychotherapy. *The American Psychologist*, *61*(8), 774–788. doi:10.1037/0003-066X.61.8.774 PMID:17115810

Seligman, M. E. P., Steen, T. A., Park, N., & Peterson, C. (2005). Positive psychology progress: Empirical validation of interventions. *The American Psychologist*, *60*(5), 410–421. doi:10.1037/0003-066X.60.5.410 PMID:16045394

Sergeant, S., & Mongrain, M. (2011). Are positive psychology exercises helpful for people with depressive personality styles? *The Journal of Positive Psychology*, *6*(4), 260–272. doi:10.1080/17439760.2011.577089

Serrano, J. P., Latorre, J. M., Gatz, M., & Montanes, J. (2004). Life review therapy using autobiographical retrieval practice for older adults with depressive symptomatology. *Psychology and Aging*, *19*(2), 272–277. doi:10.1037/0882-7974.19.2.272 PMID:15222820

Sheldon, K. M., & Lyubomirsky, S. (2006). How to increase and sustain positive emotion: The effects of expressing gratitude and visualizing best possible selves. *The Journal of Positive Psychology*, *1*(2), 73–82. doi:10.1080/17439760500510676

Sin, N. L., & Lyubomirsky, S. (2009). Enhancing well-being and alleviating depressive symptoms with positive psychology interventions: A practice-friendly meta-analysis. *Journal of Clinical Psychology*, *65*(5), 467–487. doi:10.1002/jclp.20593 PMID:19301241

Vansteenwegen, D. (2011). *Onderzoeksrapport De gelukscoach - een online programma om meer uit je leven te halen en te werken aan geluk (Research report happiness coach)*. Leuven: ISW Limits.

Velten, E. Jr. (1968). A laboratory task for induction of mood states. *Behaviour Research and Therapy*, *6*(4), 473–482. doi:10.1016/0005-7967(68)90028-4 PMID:5714990

Wilson, T., & Gilbert, D. (2003). In M. Zanna (Ed.), *Affective forecasting* (pp. 345–411). Advances in experimental social psychology New York, NY: Elsevier.

## KEY TERMS AND DEFINITIONS

**Eudaimonic Positive Technologies:** Technologies that help people to achieve experiences focused on the search for a full and meaningful life.

**Hedonic Adaptation:** Along time, an action that once produced an increase in positive emotions and happiness loses its strength until becoming ineffective.

**Hedonic Positive Technologies:** Technologies that induce a positive and enjoyable experience, such as a virtual reality environments of joy or relax induction.

**Online Positive Psychological Interventions:** Customizable and interactive interventions offered by the Internet and focused on behavioural aspects, designed to improve symptomatology.

**Positive Psychology Interventions:** Interventions or intentional activities designed to cultivate positive feelings, cognitions and behaviours.

**Positive Psychology Intervention's Effectiveness Moderators:** The different variables that influence on the effectiveness of these interventions such as the characteristics of the activity, personal characteristics of the users, the intervention dose, elements that contribute to motivation, variety, etc.

**Positive Technologies:** Technologies designed to improve the quality of personal experiences, foster personal growth and develop human virtues and strengths.

**Social Positive Technologies:** Technologies that support and enhance communication and cooperation among individuals, groups and organizations.

**Technological Behavioural Interventions:** Technological apps specifically designed to intervene on behavioural, cognitive and emotional aspects, in order to improve physical and psychological health and well-being.

# Chapter 3
# Technologies for Participatory Wellbeing: A Consumer Health Analysis of the Ongoing Scientific Debate

**Serena Barello**
*Università Cattolica del Sacro Cuore, Italy*

**Julia Menichetti**
*Università Cattolica del Sacro Cuore, Italy*

**Guendalina Graffigna**
*Università Cattolica del Sacro Cuore, Italy*

## ABSTRACT

*The participatory health revolution is shaping consumers' health behaviors that are increasingly influence by people's desire to play an active role in promoting a positive life functioning. Technologies are addressing the emerging needs of the participatory health, as they favor a proactive users' attitude. This chapter describes the results of a software-assisted quali-quantitative study aimed at exploring the scientific debate about technological interventions for wellbeing in the era of participatory health. Based on the study's results, technologies for wellbeing in the participatory health era may be clustered depending on the "context of delivery," on their degree of personalization," and on their inner "conceptualization of positive interventions". According to a consumer health engagement perspective, those technologies are not mutually exclusive but can coexist based on the specific wellness needs and health engagement expectations of their users.*

## INTRODUCTION

We are assisting to a radical shift in the health conceptualization, more linked to a positive approach to wellness and life that is strongly influencing people's expectations of health and care services. Indeed, a new set of values is framing healthcare services and their demand. New values are changing the criteria for assessing services received, affecting clients' decision-making and satisfaction post fruition. These values are determined by the people's desire to take an active role in building the best health and well-

DOI: 10.4018/978-1-4666-9986-1.ch003

ness benefits experiences and promoting a positive life and health functioning (Riva et al., 2012). This phenomenon, known as "participatory health," constitutes an actual revolution in shaping consumers' health behaviours (Graffigna, Barello, & Triberti, 2015; Phillips et al., 2014). This shift has followed the trends of increasing consumerism (Greener, 2012), significant technological breakthroughs in health and care (Street, Gold, & Manning, 2013), and revolutionary transformation in information gathering using the Internet (Cline & Haynes, 2001). New and different contexts and targets are shaping the use and design of technologies, and new and varied consumers' needs and expectations for participation are modeling them. Consequently, in this introductory section, we briefly provide an outlook of the ways in which new positive technological solutions are boosting and supporting a new demand for participatory wellbeing. Indeed, as presented in the following sections, we are moving towards a changing healthcare landscape, where health is increasingly assuming a new and wider conceptualization and value, and consumers are increasingly asking for a more active participation in health and care choices. In this sense, we conclude the introduction by introducing a consumer health engagement perspective as roadmap to properly analyse the societal movements towards the use of technologies to meet the needs of consumers' participation in health and wellbeing experiences.

Moving from these premises discussed in the following paragraphs, and by considering a consumer health perspective of analysis, this chapter tries to systematize the scientific and applicative debate about the delivery of technologies for wellbeing in the era of participatory health. The aim is to provide an integrated overview of the features of various technologies aimed at achieving wellbeing/wellness and to offer a critical overview of the ways in which the active role of individuals in these interventions is depicted.

## BACKGROUND

### New Positive Technological Solutions: A Booster for a Participatory Wellbeing

Technologies are optimally accompanying and addressing the emerging needs of the participatory health due to their innate potential to favour a proactive attitude in their users (Kvedar, Coye, & Everett, 2014). Let us think about the effect of ICT on information seeking, social exchanges, and contents sharing. In recent years, a user-centered philosophy – where users are actively involved from the design to the technologies' delivery (Gulliksen et al., 2003) - has been gaining increasing attention in order to co-create highly personalized wellness experiences able to generate a nourishing mutual relationship between the user and the technological tool, and consequently between the user and the wellbeing goal. Particularly, it is well known that the use of new technologies has extraordinary potentialities in engaging individuals and patients. Indeed, technology modifies our experience of everyday tasks and activities, allows us to perform actions that would not be available based on our biological resources only, and gives us sensations and emotions beyond our natural perception. In general, it is possible to say that technologies improve the quality of our experience. However, the effect of new media and new technologies on our wellbeing is still a controversial topic. Moreover, the application of new technologies to complex fields, such as the patients' experience, is still inconsistent and maybe confounding. In the healthcare context, new technologies are currently used both in "micro" and "macro" applications.

"Micro" refers to the implementation of technologies to support single patients in fostering the quality of their experience and in improving their wellbeing. Indeed, some technological applications in healthcare do not focused on the mere disease treatment. On the contrary, their objective is to help patients manage the personal and emotional discomfort associated with the illness experience. For example, virtual reality and videogames are currently used for rehabilitation purposes. Currently, virtual rehabilitation has been adopted for the treatment of several types of disabilities, comprising the ones caused by stroke (Laver, George, Thomas, Deutsch, & Crotty, 2011; Saposnik & Levin, 2011; Subramanian et al., 2007), musculo-skeletal and orthopedic disabilities (Burdea, Popescu, Hentz, & Colbert, 2000; Girone, Burdea, Bouzit, Popescu, & Deutsch, 2000) and cognitive or psychological impairments (Riva, Mantovani, & Gaggioli, 2004). In this context, the patient is provided with a virtual simulation that motivates him/her to test and improve the residual (or even currently lacking) abilities in a secure environment monitored by the professionals. In this way, a technological resource is designed to allow patients to regain the highest possible level of autonomy and quality of life.

Diversely, "macro" refers to the use of new technologies at an organizational level. Indeed, health organizations can use internet-related technologies to not only improve the administration of care plans, but also consider patients' personal needs and issues. For example, EHR (Electronic Health Records), which has been designed to include information about patients' values, health goals, and action plans, proved to be particularly efficient in reporting positive behavioural changes in the patients (Chunchu, Mauksch, Charles, Ross, & Pauwels, 2012). Similar technological solutions offer the potential to share medical information with the patients, thereby promoting mindful self-care planning in them (Grant et al., 2006).

In this sense, the Positive Technology paradigm constitutes a scientific and applied approach to the use of new technologies to structure, augment, or replace personal experience. Indeed, using new technologies allows people to (1) generate/promote positive emotions (Hedonic Technologies); (2) achieve positive and self-actualizing experiences (Eudaimonic Technologies); and (3) promote connectedness and social integration, as a dynamic and controllable aspect of well-being (Social/Interpersonal Technologies).

## The Evolving Values of Health: From Disease Resolution to Active Wellness

The continuous development of technological and bio-medical solutions is not only increasing the life expectancy, but also augmenting people's expectation for a higher quality of life in all its stages – from childhood to the old age (Diener, Shu, Lucas, & Smith, 1999). Similarly, new models in the health and care settings are shaping the ways in which health, wellness, and wellbeing are lived and conceptualized. Generally, people expect to be active for a longer time of their lives (Walker, 2002). They want to be healthy and they evaluate the degree of their quality of life not only in terms of the absence of disease and symptoms, but also in terms of positive functioning and ability to enact a productive role in the community to which they belong. Moreover, they desire to be active constructors of their own life trajectories by building unique wellbeing experiences (Miller & Iris, 2002). In other words, "health" is linked more to a complex and articulated representation that goes beyond the mere request of "the absence of disease a condition." Individuals are representationally reconfiguring health as wellness, namely the positive balance of physical, mental, and social wellbeing (Edelman, Mandle, & Kudzma, 2013). This conceptualization goes beyond the traditional definition of health, embracing choices and activities aimed at achieving good or satisfactory condition of existence characterized by the presence of positive emotions and moods, physical vitality, mental alacrity a sense of accomplishment, satisfaction with life, fulfillment and positive functioning (Andrews & Withey, 2012; Diener, 2000; Diener, Suh, & Oishi, 1997; Veenhoven, 2008; Naci & Ioannidis, 2015). Health and disease are mutually exclusive, but disease is can be compatible with wellness. For instance, a patient suffering from cancer with a poor prognosis evidently lacks a good health status but he may still find new ways of enjoying life and experiencing wellness.

The expectation is to receive services that not only treat the disease in its acute manifestation, but also improve the quality of life and the possibility of keeping some satisfactory private or community activities, even in the presence of a chronic condition (Haber, 2013). Thus, people are interested predominantly in health and wellness and expect to play a key role in shaping the health and wellness offer of services according to their expectations and needs. However, most health studies and services still focus on disease rather than health. The discrepancy is evident if we think at the various research advancements in defining disease causes, and, on the other hand, at the lack of information about what affects wellness.

New collaboration models between all key healthcare players are essential to address these paradigmatic changes and to fill these gaps. To improve health, researchers, industry, policy makers and regulators increasingly understand the need to involve patients and citizens in managing their diseases to enhance the effectiveness of research and healthcare provisioning. It is time to find ways to engage people in deciding how to manage and improve their own wellness as well as in determining how this can be studied.

## The Challenges and Opportunities of Consumers' Participation in Health and Care

After the mid-1970s, specific government policies aimed at increasing professional accountability and promoting the vision of patients as active consumers of healthcare able to adjudicate and evaluate its content, features, and quality encouraged the shift away from the disease-centred vision of health to negotiated pathways of care (Herrick, 2005; Moran 1999; Wilcox, 2015). However, more fundamentally, this shift occurred because of a move towards an increasing trend of enrolling the patient in health pathways in ways that reduced the growing strain on the epistemological authority of medical knowledge (Lupton, 1994).

In this context, the shift in terminology, such as "patient trust" and "patient satisfaction" as proxies for quality of care in medicine (and also to different ways of conceptualizing, assessing and quantitatively measuring these), can be seen not simply as a technical move towards improving the quality of care, but also as an ideological move that set out the frame in which negotiation between clinician and patient in the consultation can be understood. Consumerism also contributed to modification of the patient's role in the treatment process (Robinson et al., 2005). The role of the patient is starting to shift from being a minimally informed advice recipient to an active participant, instigating collaborator, information sharer, peer leader and self-tracker engaged in participative medicine. This reflects a transition that is underway from paternalistic health care to partnership models where patients are considered as consumers of healthcare services (Herrick, 2005).

According to this new role, individuals are becoming increasingly engaged in self-management of conditions, symptoms, genomics and blood biomarkers, behaviours and personal environmental factors. Like any consumer, the patient may demand quality services. By continuously evaluating the service and sometimes have complaints about it, the patient-consumer can improve the health care system.

These changes are at the basis of a further shift in the care framework, along with the patient now being considered a critical consumer of healthcare services. This supports the need for a client-centred or consumer-directed model of care aimed at grasping the complex system of exchanges that occur between the patient ("the demand") and the healthcare system ("the supply") (Graffigna, Barello, Riva, & Bosio, 2014; Hardyman, Daunt, & Kitchener, 2014). Skyrocketing health care costs and quality deficits can only be addressed through a broad approach of quality-based benefit design. Consumer-directed health plans that are built around better consumer information tools hold the promise of making consumers the protagonists of their care and are thus at the centre of this model of care (Buntin et al., 2006). Comparative and interactive consumer information tools, coupled with provider performance transparency and payment reform, are crucial for advancing accountability, and they support consumers in getting the right care at the right time (Hardyman, Daunt, & Kitchener, 2014).

According to this paradigmatic change, individuals have shifted from being considered passive recipients of healthcare interventions to autonomous, active, or collaborative consumers able to construct various pathways to personal wellbeing.

The idea of a participatory process of health and care underlines a strong democratization of the exchange between physician and patient as well as between demand and supply of health services. From this prospective, the different actors are considered bearer of their subjectivities and their different skills in order to promote virtuous forms of dialogue and improve the use of health services and structures. The existing literature has adopted several conceptualizations to define the active role of patients in the health and care process - such as patient "activation", "involvement", "participation", and the concept of "engagement" (often used as synonymous in the scientific debate). These terms focus on different levels of the exchange between the demand and supply of healthcare services, and they show a new important role of the patient in defining healthcare services that would optimally promote health trajectories (Menichetti, Libreri, Lozza & Graffigna, 2014; Murray, Charles, & Gafni, 2006; Thompson, 2007). The basic shared idea is that an active and engaged individual is able to become not only an aware consumer of the traditional form of health services, but also a good promoter of best practices of health promotion in his/her social context (for example, by sharing care practices in online forums and communities, by advocating for patients' right at the institutional level or becoming founding member of patient's associations…) and an innovator able to personalize his/her own healthcare paths.

Therefore, a consumer health-engagement perspective seems to fit the technology-driven demand of citizens for wellbeing promotion and for high participation level in the health care.

Considering this framework, a better understanding of how technologies can foster the participatory attitude of individuals when achieving positive life experiences might guide the development and delivery of technologies for wellbeing.

## METHODS

In line with the study's aims, we performed a software-based narrative literature review of scientific papers on technologies for wellbeing/wellness published from 2000 to 2015 within the framework of participatory health. Article retrieval was conducted using the following search strategy launched in SCOPUS on 20th May 2015: "technolog*" AND ("well*being" OR "wellness") AND ("involvement" OR "engagement" OR "participation" OR "activation"). We chose to search for terms related to the active role of individuals in health management based on the most frequently used terms within the current literature (Menichetti et al., 2014; Barello et al., 2014). We chose to exclude in the search strategy terms strictly anchored to the situation of patient's disease management and those that do not consider a wider and democratized context of exchange between provider and client that constitutes the participatory health culture (i.e., "self-management", "adherence", "compliance", "shared decision-making"). The search was limited to the titles/abstracts/keywords and to the English-written literature because of the interest in mapping the international debate on the theme. The search was limited to the last 15 years, as the theme of interest is quite recent. After the initial screening of the retrieved sources (N=183), we carried out a lexical analysis of the whole corpus of titles and abstracts considered eligible according to their relevance to the study's aims (N=118) using the software T-LAB (version 7.1). We chose to focus on titles and abstracts because they should reflect the articles' contents. The T-LAB software is a mixed-method tool that allows performing a set of linguistic and statistical analysis on a collection of texts (Lancia, 2004; 2012). During the importation stage, the software automatically divides the corpus of texts into elementary contexts units (ECUs) that are used for subsequent analysis. ECUs are portions of text, delimited by punctuation, that correspond to one or more statements.

Specifically, a thematic analysis of elementary contexts (TAEC) was performed to obtain a representation of the corpus content through few significant thematic clusters (Gambetti & Quigley, 2012). The clusters obtained are represented by a unique set of elementary contexts – sentences and paragraphs – characterized by the same patterns and significances. In this way, clusters are depicted by lemmas and variables are distinctive of the elementary contexts. For this study, we categorized each abstract by years of publication coded categorically as follows: 2000-2005; 2006-2010; and 2011-2015. Thereafter, elementary contexts of each cluster were used to extract the articles contained in each cluster. These were qualitatively analysed to identify specific features and contents of the emerging clusters. Finally, the spatial dimension where clusters were set up were used to identify clusters, allowing us to qualitatively interpret relationships among clusters. To strengthen the methodological validity of this analysis, two independent investigators (SB; JM) conducted the data analysis and the qualitative interpretation of the T-Lab outputs.

## TECHNOLOGIES FOR PARTICIPATORY WELLBEING: EXPLAINING THE FACTORIAL PLAN ILLUSTRATING THE LITERATURE DEBATE

Looking at the factorial plan where clusters are projected, we could identify three main factors (see Figure 1). The first factor (32.0% of inertia explained), labelled "context of delivery," opposes technologies used in the "daily environment" versus those delivered in the "healthcare organization". It is illustrated on the horizontal axis, showing a substantial polarization between the first and fourth clusters on one side and the second and third clusters on the other side. The first two clusters (1 and 4) focus more on health technologies delivered in the organizational context of the healthcare (hospital or HCS); on the other hand, clusters 2 and 3 are geared more towards the technological delivery within the daily life environment (community or home).

The second factor (41.5% of inertia explained), named "degree of technology personalization", opposes 'fixed technologies" versus "client-driven technologies" (Figure 1). It is represented on the vertical axis and particularly polarizes clusters 1 and 2 and clusters 3 and 4. In other words, there is a substantial polarization between technological solutions designed and delivered through a top-down approach where few degrees of personalization are allowed and technologies the configuration of which is guided by the users' unique needs and contingencies. Fixed solutions mainly collapse in the field to enable technologies the main aim of which is to repair or compensate damaged/limited functions (such as in the case of mental or physical disabilities) and/or reduce social inequalities (such as in the case of marginalized

*Figure 1. The three-axes explanatory plan of clusters*

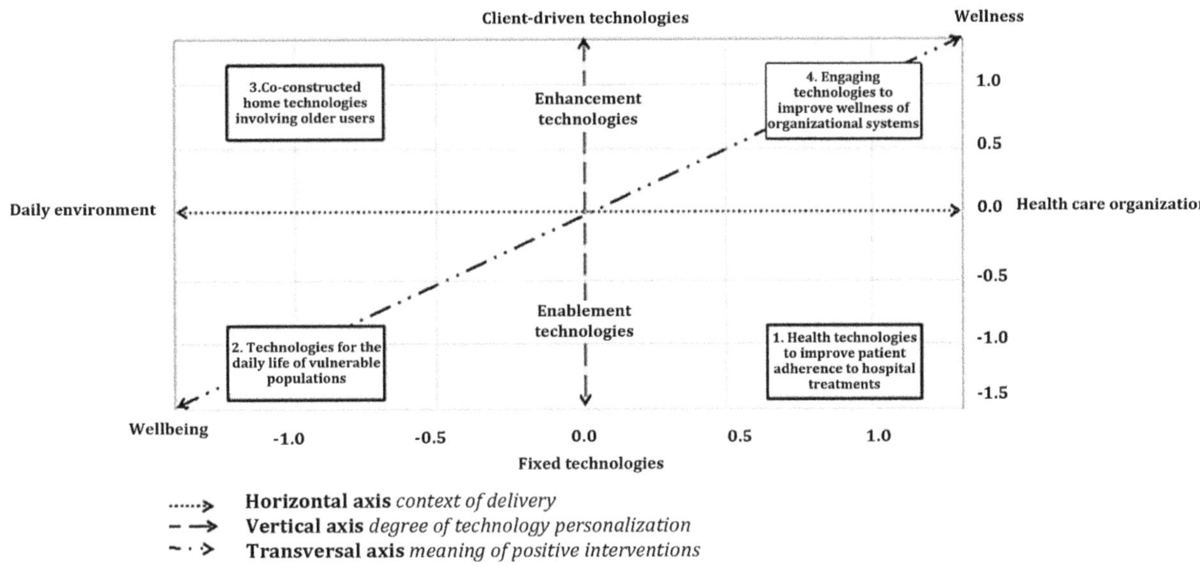


or stigmatized populations). In this case, the approach used to develop technologies and interventions implied an a priori diagnosis of the users' needs and problems and a top-down prefiguration of the best technological solution to address them.

On the other hand, client-driven solutions refer mainly to the field of enhancement technologies aimed at improving and empowering users' skills and resources to foster positive life experiences and reduce health risks. According to this vision of the technologies' goal, such solutions imply a high involvement of users in shaping their features and in configuring them based on the users' specificities and requirements. In this sense, those kinds of solutions are driven and co-constructed with the individuals who use them.

According to this framework, as represented by the third axis (26.5% of inertia explained) labelled "meaning of positive interventions" in Figure 1, technologies are related to different conceptualizations of positive life experiences depending on their contexts and aims of delivery. This axis opposes clusters 1 and 2 and clusters 3 and 4, according to their implicit vision of positive interventions ("wellness" versus "wellbeing"). Interventions featuring technologies in the healthcare contexts are more closed to a vision of wellness promotion where the main concern of interventions is to empower individuals and potentiate their existing inner resources. This vision is strictly connected to a medical conceptualization of health where the aim is to prevent health risks and reduce possible disease relapses to prolong life. Interventions featuring technologies in the daily environment are aimed at supporting individual's wellbeing by managing people vulnerabilities and strengthening their quality of life despite those vulnerabilities.

## CLUSTERING TECHNOLOGIES FOR WELLBEING IN THE PARTICIPATORY ERA: INSIGHT FROM THE LITERATURE DEBATE

Thematic Analysis of Elementary Context (TAEC) of the text corpus identified four thematic clusters (total ECUs= 769) explaining, respectively, 24.45%, 24.32%, 28.48%, and 22.76% of the total inertia.

*Table 1. Weights and lemmas included in each thematic cluster*

| | Clusters | | | |
|---|---|---|---|---|
| | Cluster 1 | Cluster 2 | Cluster 3 | Cluster 4 |
| Weights (%) | 188 (24.45%) | 187 (24.32%) | 219 (28.48%) | 175 (22.76%) |
| Lemmas (Chi-squared value)* | • Patient (159.5)<br>• Treatment (73.9)<br>• Intervention (64.7)<br>• Care (46.6)<br>• Cancer (42.7)<br>• Group (41.0)<br>• Foot (40.6)<br>• Trial (40.3)<br>• Ankle (31.3)<br>• Practice (26.9)<br>• Individual (25.4)<br>• PHS (25.3)<br>• Psychosocial (24.9)<br>• University (22.5)<br>• Control (19.7)<br>• Work (19.6)<br>• Patient-centred (18.7)<br>• Family (17.8)<br>• Healthy (17.4) | • Dementia (102.7)<br>• People (76.5)<br>• Person (48.2)<br>• Wellbeing (46.7)<br>• Social (41.2)<br>• Disability (40.5)<br>• Participation (39.3)<br>• Connection (37.2)<br>• Interaction (36.4)<br>• House (33.4)<br>• Assistive (33.2)<br>• Nature (29.5)<br>• Environment (26.3)<br>• Carer (26.3)<br>• Collective (26.2)<br>• Innovation (25.9)<br>• Development (23.6)<br>• Sustainability (22.7) | • Older (211.8)<br>• User (106.8)<br>• Adult (94.2)<br>• Game (54.5)<br>• Smart (40.9)<br>• Learning (40.3)<br>• Education (36.0)<br>• Sensor (26.4)<br>• Divide (25.2)<br>• TV (25.2)<br>• Elderly (24.7)<br>• Age (24.4)<br>• Digital (23.1)<br>• Inclusion (20.9) | • Health (118.6)<br>• Wellness (102.7)<br>• Program (53.5)<br>• Plan (51.1)<br>• Employee (49.4)<br>• Risk (45.9)<br>• Incentive (44.5)<br>• Promotion (32.9)<br>• Survey (28.8)<br>• Google (26.8)<br>• Health-related (25.7)<br>• E-mail (24.4)<br>• Medicine (24.4)<br>• Platform (22.9)<br>• Enrolees (21.9)<br>• CDHP (21.9)<br>• Personalize (21.7)<br>• Management (21.1)<br>• Company (20.4) |

* Chi-squared test results from the intersections of the contingency table "words × clusters" that derives from the thematic analysis of elementary contexts.

The clusters were labelled according to the typical vocabulary (i.e., lemmas) of the Elementary Contexts (see Table 1), and were categorized considering:

1. The target population involved in the intervention;
2. The context where the technologies were employed;
3. The technology type;
4. The role of individuals in the technology's development and/or use.

Clusters' features are summarized in Table 2. In Figure 2, a graphic representation of the clusters resulting from the thematic analysis is provided. In the following paragraphs, we provide an in-depth description of each cluster.

**Cluster N° 1:** "Health technologies to improve patient adherence to hospital treatments".

This cluster – comprising the literature published between 2005 and 2010 - denotes the application of technology in hospital-based care practices for disease-management (cancer, ankle, foot). The main context in which technologies are delivered is the healthcare organization or public health services (PHS), and the privileged targets for technologies are the patients and persons in their lives (e.g., professionals, families). Health technologies are used to deliver treatment interventions or trials to patients (individual or group) manage their disease and improve the quality of care by adopting standardized methods to control procedures and minimize errors. The word patient-centred indicates, with its focus on individual needs, the framework of reference of this cluster and the renewed attention in healthcare to the patient's

*Table 2. Clusters' features basing on qualitative analysis of the included abstract*

| Features | Cluster N | | | |
|---|---|---|---|---|
| | Cluster 1 | Cluster 2 | Cluster 3 | Cluster 4 |
| Main target | Patient | People | User | Consumer |
| Context of application | Healthcare organization | Daily environment | Daily environment | Health system |
| Technology type | • Telemedicine<br>• EHR<br>• Internet | • Assistive<br>• Smart home | • Gaming<br>• Virtual reality<br>• ICT<br>• Mobile<br>• Smart home<br>• Smart textile | • Mobile<br>• PHR<br>• Online<br>• Web<br>• Social media |
| Individuals' role | Adherent | Participant | Actively involved | Fully engaged |

*Figure 2. Clusters' representation as resulting from thematic analysis*

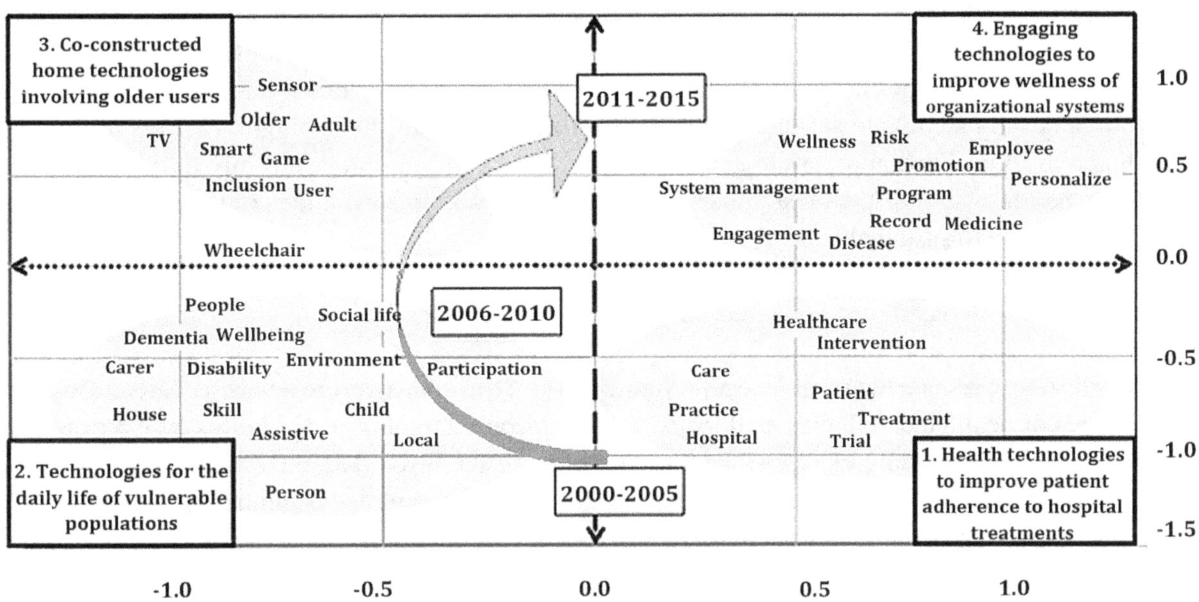


voice and to the psychosocial aspects of dealing with physical health problems. Calls for patient-centred care have often led to technological changes, such as electronic health records and advanced access scheduling, which are likely to strengthen the patient-clinician relationship and thus foster better health outcomes,. These practices are necessary to move medical care into the 21st century. Considering the Elementary Context and articles featuring this cluster, examples of such technological innovations include telemedicine, which influences the organization of doctor-patient communication (Miller, 2003); electronic health records, which provide quantified information regarding patients' condition (Dimaras et al., 2012); or internet-based technologies that support the needs- or skills-based treatments of patients and their caregivers (Hu et al., 2014; Page et al., 2005; Wakefield et al., 2015). Contributions in this area describe the users of technologies as passive recipients. Consequently, the target is expected to effectively adhere to the technological interventions without considering its preferences and expectations.

**Cluster N° 2:** "Technologies for the daily life of vulnerable populations".

The second cluster's literature pertained to the period between 2005 and 2010. Words expressing vulnerable or minority populations - such as people with dementia, disabled, or children – describe this cluster, which incorporates the technologies used to enable and assist those persons in their daily environment. Thus, the main context of technological delivery is the daily social life outside the healthcare organization (house, social environment, local), and the main target are people or persons who need assistance with accomplishing tasks due to their chronic condition (e.g., dementia, disability, obesity) or status of a vulnerable or marginalized population (e.g., children, women, students). According to this goal, technologies are mostly assistive. Examples are potential intelligent power wheelchair for navigation assistance (Dahlia Kairy et al., 2014), computer-based assistive technologies for children with disabilities to access various activities (Chantry & Dunford, 2010), and videoconferencing to connect remote communities and individuals to mental health services (Gibson, et al., 2011). Through enabling people to perform various tasks, minority populations are also motivated to improve their connection and interaction with the social environment, promoting wellbeing of these individuals. Therefore, a collective culture is sustained, where boundaries determined by health inequalities are overstepped and targets of such technologies are expected to participate in their use and delivery. Particularly terms like innovation, development, and sustainability characterize this cluster, indicating the efforts to promote overall access to new and appropriate technologies with an aim to improve steadily living conditions, which can be lifesaving for the most vulnerable populations, and to ensure the commitment of technological innovation to sustainable development.

**Cluster N° 3:** "Co-constructed home technologies: Involving older users".

This cluster represents the most recent literature (2011-2015) considering a new recently introduced role of users of health technologies, and focusing on a specific target of users, in this case represented by older people (older, adult, elderly). The presence of a cluster devoted to older users indicates its relevance in the health technologies' discourse and probably reflects a global health scenario governed by the need to find effective and sustainable solutions to manage increasingly aging population (Menichetti, Cipresso, Bussolin, & Graffigna, 2015). In the same way, it suggests the importance of personalizing, such a health technological strategies, for specific segments of population. The lemmas "education", "divide", and "learning" express the specific need to train this type of users in the use of technologies, which would allow them to participate in an increasingly technology-based society. Such solutions aim to help older people live independently by creating sustainable conditions for self-determined lifestyles and performing tasks that are difficult to accomplish. As shown by the frequencies of the words "game" and "smart", gaming and smart home/textile solutions are preferred solutions to accomplish the mentioned goals. Their examples include improvements in the visualization system of smart home data that is subsequently integrated into a wellness framework (Le, Reeder, Yoo, Aziz, Thompson, & Demiris, 2015), the design of flexibility sensors to promote independence and wellbeing of older users (Wu, Xue, & Hu, 2014), or tests/designs of games to increase the physical exercise of older citizens (Leinonen et al., 2012; Miller et al., 2014; Proffitt & Lange, 2013). Thus, the preferred context of the use of technologies in this cluster is the user's home, which becomes a place where technologies could be embedded to overcome age-related barriers and foster inclusion of older citizens in social life.

Finally, analysing the Elementary Contexts and articles within this cluster, three main type of articles emerge: articles explaining the process of working with older people to develop technological solutions (Proffitt & Lange, 2013; Leinonen et al., 2012), articles testing the acceptability or effectiveness of detected solutions (Le Thai et al., 2015; Ballesteros et al., 2014; Grindrod et al., 2014), and theoretical articles underlying psychological frameworks for such technological solutions (Argenton et al., 2014; Hill et al., 2015; Riva et al., 2014). Those topics reflect a two-ways process of matching the demands of needy and not technologically literate targets, which is a fundamental process of involving older persons both in technology design and in the goals of the solutions. In this sense, older users are expected to be involved in the health solution's use and development to increase "the importance and personal relevance of a system to the user" (Barki & Hartwick, 1989, p. 53) and consequently improve acceptance, usability, and health outcomes.

**Cluster N° 4:** "Engaging technologies to improve wellness of organizational systems".

This cluster, discussed mainly within the current scientific literature (2011-2015), is represented by words expressing the technologies' potential to engage the different actors of the healthcare system in promoting and managing their own health and wellness. The technologies' main goal is to enhance the employees and consumers' ability to manage wellness and prevent health-related risk. In this cluster, professionals and patients (defined respectively as employees and consumers) play an active role in a wider system (and not merely as individuals), and they are both considered potential targets of positive health programs. This reflects a new managerial approach to healthcare, the sustainability of which depends strictly on the wellness of the whole system. This features highly personalized technologies sponsored particularly by public health policies, which are aimed at sustaining long-term wellness plans able to improve the quality of life of health companies and of the actors who are engaged with them. Typical technologies characterizing this cluster are social media, personalized health record (PHR), and mobile tools. Technological tools in this area aim to support workplace wellness or personalized medicine plans by preventing disease and improving the individual's health status. The Elementary Context and articles within this cluster include mobile and social media platforms to enhance health and wellness management (Mitra & Padman, 2014); new personal health record to predict risk factors, enable preventative responses, and personalize a participatory medicine for maintain wellness and limit disease (Happonen et al., 2009; Mora, 2012; Yoediono & Snyderman, 2008); and social media- or interactive web-based wellness programs to empower employees to proactively assess health risks and promote wellness in workplace (Goetzel et al., 2008; 2013; Loeppke et al., 2013; Mattila et al., 2013). In this sense, the users of technologies are here expected to fully engage in the entire delivery process (from the design to the use) to sustain long-term health outcomes.

## DISCUSSION

In this chapter, we tried to answer the question "How technologies for wellbeing can address the requirements of a participatory health era." Many healthcare professionals, managers, and policy makers are today struggling with this question to develop positive psychology interventions able to address the individuals' increasing demands of health and wellness experiences. Based on the results of our analysis, it is possible to highlight that

1. Patient identity has different implicit conceptualizations, and thus its role in the technological process varies, and
2. Such conceptualizations are linked to a specific temporal development.

The four main clusters detected in the contemporary landscape of technologies for wellbeing, indeed, unveil different conceptualizations of the individuals' role in the technological and healthcare process. Specifically, the clusters move from a passive conception of the users of technologies (i.e., the first and second clusters: "technology for patient adherence", "technologies for the daily life of vulnerable populations") to a culture where users, on the one hand, actively engage, drive, and shape the technologies' delivery and use (i.e., the third clusters "Co-constructed home technologies: involving older users"), and, on the other hand, benefit from the enriching possibilities of engagement and wellness offered by technologies (i.e. the fourth cluster "engaging technologies to improve wellness of organizational systems"). These clusters are also related to different ways of conceptualizing the active role of health consumer. From our perspective, the conception of an individual engaged with technology in his/her care and wellness overarches other conceptualizations, such as patient adherence, patient involvement, and patient participation, as well as goes beyond the traditional conception of "patient" and "doctor" by considering them equal partners in the health and care delivery. Adherence refers specifically to the effective application of technological interventions for health management by each individual. This construct moves from a hierarchical vision of the healthcare relationship, where the healthcare provider (i.e., the expert) prescribes to individuals (i.e., the lay actor) the rules to manage his/her health condition better. This concept does not fully acknowledge the theme of healthcare process negotiation. "Adherence" implies an evaluation of the health providers against a patient more or less good, more or less able to respond adequately to the expert's requirements (Vlasnik, Aliotta, & DeLor, 2005). The concepts of "involvement" and "participation" in this case refer to a more active vision of persons and users. In detail, "participation" is used to denote the inclusion of vulnerable populations in programs/ interventions aimed at repairing a diagnosed lack of mental and/or physical functioning; whereas "involvement" implies a direct inclusion of users both in the development and in the usage of technological solutions for improving the quality of life and wellbeing in the daily environment. Finally, the concept of "engagement" is related to a broader and systemic exchange between demand and supply of health services, where wellness achieved by using technological programs strictly depends on the active inclusion of consumers in long-term health plans.

Furthermore, when observing the temporal trends featuring the contributions analyzed in this work from a consumer health perspective, it is possible to note that we are progressively moving from passive users of technologies to active users who become increasingly involved in innovation, or as labelled by the more recent literature innosumer (Peine, 2014). Indeed, literature has shown that participatory culture is a new trend that is offering a renewed perspective on the individuals' roles in societies, from being merely recipients of services to individuals who inter-act with the supply of such services and who contribute to it (prosumers) (Toffler, 1980). Looking at the technological field, let us think at recent advances in technologies, which have enabled individuals to develop media, such as personal computers and Internet. This new culture has been described as Web 2.0, and it has supported the paradigmatic participatory shift away from producer hegemony to audiences or consumers (Miller, 2011). Thus, since producers are individuals who create contents and objects, and consumers are the audiences or purchasers of those objects, "prosumers" are those who use technological tools and, at the same time, have an active role in shaping their design and delivery (Miller, 2011). This "allows for more consumer influence over the production of goods" (Miller, 2011, p.87). The recently introduced term of innosumer in the field of gerotechnology highlights an emerging type of consumer who not merely completes designs tasks already foreseen by producers of technology (Humphreys & Grayson, 2008), but actively engages in configuring modifiable technological tools by adding a great and creative technological change (Peine, 2014). This captures a more fundamental shift in the distribution of tasks between users and producers, creating technology-literate, intelligent informed and learning consumers who become innovators capable of configuring the technological environments they deem desirable.

Following these suggestions, technologies for positive life experiences are increasingly evolving from a Web 1.0 culture with an unidirectional movement between technological deliverers and users, where subjects are patients or persons expected to adhere to and participate in the technological interventions through a Web 2.0 culture with a bidirectional movement between producers and consumers of technologies, to a Web 3.0 culture where users actively engage, drive, and shape the technologies' delivery and use (see Figure 3).

## FUTURE RESEARCH DIRECTIONS

In light of the discussion presented in this chapter, we discovered that the consumer health perspective may provide a compass to read the complexity of the use and delivery of technologies for participatory wellbeing, thus allowing new technological solutions to appropriately meet the consumers' needs, expectations, and characteristics. Further studies are needed to better define and analyse the complex bidirectional relationship between technologies and different participatory needs in the health and care

*Figure 3. The temporal and conceptual evolution of the patients' role in the technological innovation for participatory wellbeing*

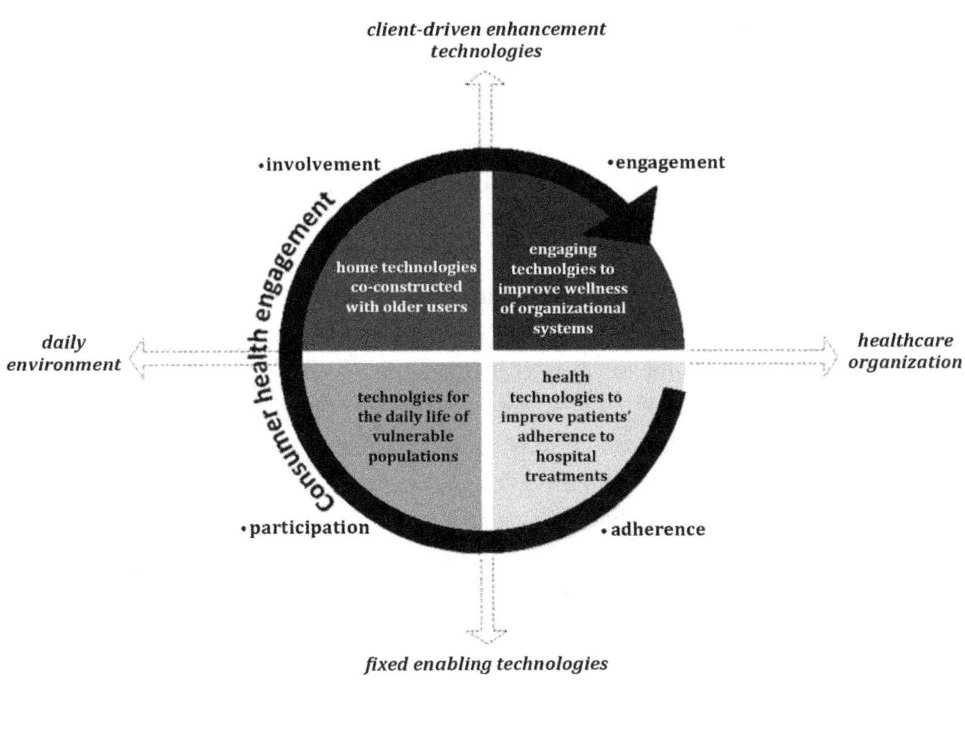

contexts. In particular, further studies are required to help technologies developers understand the participatory requirements of consumers and to check whether technologies are properly responding to those needs. Finally, since consumers have an increasing need to take an active role in constructing their own wellbeing trajectories, we found lack of technological interventions that would address the participatory needs of consumers. It is necessary to develop technological solutions that would be directly grounded in people's expectation of participation in health and care contexts to effectively engage people in the management of their own wellness, which could potentially improve the health in our societies.

## CONCLUSION: A CONSUMER HEALTH FRAMEWORK OF TECHNOLOGIES FOR PARTICIPATORY WELLBEING

Various conceptualizations of new technological solutions to sustain and foster participatory wellbeing described in the literature require a conceptual perspective that would be able to embrace a similar complexity. This is further complicated by the multitude of wellness experiences and health trajectories that individuals encompass during their life. In our opinion, a consumer health framework may fit those requirements, functioning as theoretical compass to orient the planning and delivery of health and wellness actions aimed at sustaining consumer health engagement while at the same time facilitating the assessment of the level of engagement of a target population to personalize those solutions. As an umbrella framework and dynamic compass, the consumer health perspective may help moving into the changing and multifaceted offer of technological solutions for wellbeing, identifying positive psychology interventions able to make consumers active carriers of innovation by fully engaging them in positive life trajectories (Graffigna et al., 2014; Graffigna, Barello, & Triberti, 2015).

Consumer health psychology is a well-established discipline that seeks to unveil the basic subjective processes that rule individuals' decision-making and choice behaviours in different domains of daily life. Consumer health psychology's theoretical frameworks have shown their effectiveness not only in diagnosing consumers' healthcare behaviours, but also in orienting managerial practices aimed to improve exchanges between "demand" and "offers" for healthcare services (Graffigna, Barello, Bonanomi, & Lozza, 2015). Consumer health psychology, applied to healthcare research and health technologies development, may offer important clues to unveil the roots of individual's care and cure preferences (Barello et al., 2015), the way in which they make decisions among wellness options (Barello & Graffigna, 2015), and the reasons why they act or do not act concerning specific ways of health management. In other words, consumer health psychology may help understand the "whys" behind individuals' ways of reasoning, behaving, and feeling in relation to their health and wellbeing paths.

In this light, a consumer health perspective may cast light on the subjective complexity of the health experience and offer concrete insight to support technological solutions aimed at fostering participatory wellbeing. Health engagement, indeed, cannot be simply conceived as an "on-off" status. Health engagement is a process-like experience that may (or may not) evolve; it has a processual and dynamic nature that depends on the unique needs that feature each phase of its development (Graffigna, Barello, Libreri, & Bosio, 2014). To achieve this goal, grounding health and care delivery into the ecological understanding of individuals' experiences, preferences, and needs may be the only concrete answer to innovate health services in the direction of a sensitive consumer engagement approach. Health management behaviours enacted by individuals are only the outcomes of a complex intertwining of cognitive and emotional elaboration processes.

In this sense, enabling technologies - aimed mainly at promoting individuals' adherence to and constant participation in top-down interventions in order to guarantee their effectiveness - are mostly preferable when target populations need a strong guide to manage their problems (such as disabilities or illness conditions) and recover a positive functioning. On the contrary, enhancement technologies –aimed mainly at fostering individuals' strengths and empowering them in building their own wellness - are mostly preferable when users have developed an increased awareness of their wellness needs and want a motivator to easily put in practice their own desires. These kinds of technologies obviously require a more active user involvement and a high engagement in healthcare to meet individuals' expectations.

On these basis, a consumer health perspective may be a compass to orient the planning and delivery of technological solutions aimed to sustain positive psychological interventions by effectively engaging people in health and wellbeing management, keeping in mind a dynamic vision of a participatory health construction (Graffigna, Barello, Bonanomi, & Lozza, 2015).

## REFERENCES


Andrews, F. M., & Withey, S. B. (2012). *Social indicators of well-being: Americans' perceptions of life quality*. New York, NY: Springer Science & Business Media.

Argenton, L., Triberti, S., Serino, S., Muzio, M., & Riva, G. (2014). Serious games as positive technologies for individual and group flourishing. In A. L. Brooks et al. (Eds.), *Technologies of Inclusive Well-Being* (pp. 221–244). Berlin, Heidelberg: Springer. doi:10.1007/978-3-642-45432-5_11

Barello, S., & Graffigna, G. (2015). Engaging patients to recover life projectuality: An Italian cross-disease framework. *Quality of Life Research: An International Journal of Quality of Life Aspects of Treatment, Care and Rehabilitation*, *24*(5), 1087–1096. doi:10.1007/s11136-014-0846-x PMID:25373927

Barello, S., & Graffigna, G. (2015). Patient engagement in healthcare: Pathways for effective medical decision-making. *Neuropsychogical Trends*, *17*, 53–65. doi:10.7358/neur-2015-017-bare

Barello, S., Graffigna, G., & Vegni, E. (2012). Patient engagement as an emerging challenge for healthcare services: Mapping the literature. *Nursing Research and Practice*, *2012*, 905-934. doi:10.1155/2012/905934 PMID:23213497

Barello, S., Graffigna, G., Vegni, E., Savarese, M., Lombardi, F., & Bosio, A. C. (2015). 'Engage me in taking care of my heart': A grounded theory study on patient–cardiologist relationship in the hospital management of heart failure. *BMJ Open*, *5*(3), e005582. doi:10.1136/bmjopen-2014-005582 PMID:25776041

Barki, H., & Hartwick, J. (1989). Rethinking the concept of user involvement. *Management Information Systems Quarterly*, *13*(1), 53–63. doi:10.2307/248700

Bosio, C. A., & Graffigna, G. (2014). People Health Engagement: Fra mainstream e nuovo paradigma. *Psicologia della Salute*, *11*(3), 5–10. doi:10.3280/PDS2014-003001

Breslow, L. (1972). A quantitative approach to the World Health Organization definition of health: Physical, mental and social well-being. *International Journal of Epidemiology*, *1*(4), 347–355. doi:10.1093/ije/1.4.347 PMID:4669083

Buntin, M. B., Damberg, C., Haviland, A., Kapur, K., Lurie, N., McDevitt, R., & Marquis, M. S. (2006). Consumer-directed health care: Early evidence about effects on cost and quality. *Health Affairs*, *25*(6), 516–530. doi:10.1377/hlthaff.25.w516 PMID:17062591

Burdea, G., Popescu, V., Hentz, V., & Colbert, K. (2000). Virtual reality-based orthopedic telerehabilitation. *IEEE Transactions on* Rehabilitation Engineering, *8*(3), 430–432.

Chantry, J., & Dunford, C. (2010). How do computer assistive technologies enhance participation in childhood occupations for children with multiple and complex disabilities? A review of the current literature. *British Journal of Occupational Therapy*, *73*(8), 351–365. doi:10.4276/030802210X12813483277107

Chunchu, K., Mauksch, L., Charles, C., Ross, V., & Pauwels, J. (2012). A patient centered care plan in the EHR: Improving collaboration and engagement. *Families, Systems & Health*, *30*(3), 199–209. doi:10.1037/a0029100 PMID:22866953

Cline, R. J., & Haynes, K. M. (2001). Consumer health information seeking on the Internet: The state of the art. *Health Education Research*, *16*(6), 671–692. doi:10.1093/her/16.6.671 PMID:11780707

Diener, E. (2000). Subjective well-being: The science of happiness and a proposal for a national index. *The American Psychologist*, *55*(1), 34–43. doi:10.1037/0003-066X.55.1.34 PMID:11392863

Diener, E., Suh, E., & Oishi, S. (1997). Recent findings on subjective well-being. *Indian Journal of Clinical Psychology*, *24*(1), 25–41.

Diener, E., Suh, E. M., Lucas, R. E., & Smith, H. L. (1999). Subjective well-being: Three decades of progress. *Psychological Bulletin*, *125*(2), 276–302. doi:10.1037/0033-2909.125.2.276

Dimaras, H., Kimani, K., Dimba, E. A., Gronsdahl, P., White, A., Chan, H. S., & Gallie, B. L. (2012). Retinoblastoma. *Lancet*, *379*(9824), 1436–1446. doi:10.1016/S0140-6736(11)61137-9 PMID:22414599

Edelman, C. L., Mandle, C. L., & Kudzma, E. C. (2013). *Health Promotion Throughout the Life Span*. Elsevier Health Sciences.

Finfgeld-Connett, D. (2014). Use of content analysis to conduct knowledge-building and theory-generating qualitative systematic reviews. *Qualitative Research*, *14*(3), 341–352. doi:10.1177/1468794113481790

Gambetti, R., & Quigley, S. (Eds.). (2012). *Managing Corporate Communication: A Cross-cultural Approach. Palgrave*. Macmillan.

Garside, R. (2013). Systematic review and synthesis of qualitative research. In Ziebland S., Coulter A., Calabrese J.D., & Lokock L. (Ed.), Understanding and using health experiences: Improving Patient Care (104-135). USA: Oxford Scholarship Online. doi:10.1093/acprof:oso/9780199665372.003.0011

Gibson, K. L., Coulson, H., Miles, R., Kakekakekung, C., Daniels, E., & O'donnell, S. (2011). Conversations on telemental health: Listening to remote and rural First Nations communities. *Rural and Remote Health*, *11*(2), 1656–1674. PMID:21553998

Girone, M., Burdea, G., Bouzit, M., Popescu, V., & Deutsch, J. E. (2000). Orthopedic rehabilitation using the" Rutgers ankle" interface. *Studies in Health Technology and Informatics*, 2000, 89–95. PMID:10977590

Goetzel, R. Z., & Ozminkowski, R. J. (2008). The health and cost benefits of work site health-promotion programs. *Annual Review of Public Health*, *29*(1), 303–323. doi:10.1146/annurev.publhealth.29.020907.090930 PMID:18173386

Goodman, C. A., Jimison, H. B., & Pavel, M. (2002). Participatory design for home care technology. *Proceedings of the Second Joint* (Vol. 3, pp. 1873-1874). Houston, USA: IEEE.

Graffigna, G., Barello, S., Bonanomi, A., & Lozza, E. (2015). Measuring patient engagement: Development and psychometric properties of the Patient Health Engagement (PHE) scale. *Frontiers in Psychology*, March, 6. PMID:25870566

Graffigna, G., Barello, S., Libreri, C., & Bosio, C. A. (2014). How to engage type-2 diabetic patients in their own health management: Implications for clinical practice. *BMC Public Health*, *14*(1), 648. doi:10.1186/1471-2458-14-648 PMID:24966036

Graffigna, G., Barello, S., & Riva, G. (2013). How to make health information technology effective: The challenge of patient engagement. *Archives of Physical Medicine and Rehabilitation*, *94*(10), 2034–2035. doi:10.1016/j.apmr.2013.04.024 PMID:24075414

Graffigna, G., Barello, S., & Riva, G. (2013). Technologies for patient engagement. *Health Affairs*, *32*(6), 1172–1172. doi:10.1377/hlthaff.2013.0279 PMID:23733998

Graffigna, G., Barello, S., Riva, G., & Bosio, A. C. (2014). Patient Engagement: The Key to Redesign the Exchange Between the Demand and Supply for Healthcare in the Era of Active Ageing. *Studies in Health Technology and Informatics*, *203*, 85–95. PMID:26630515

Graffigna, G., Barello, S., & Triberti, S. (2015). *Patient Engagement: A consumer-centered model to innovate healthcare*. Warsaw, Poland: De Gruyter Open. doi:10.1515/9783110452440

Graffigna, G., Barello, S., Triberti, S., Wiederhold, B. K., Bosio, A. C., & Riva, G. (2014). Enabling eHealth as a pathway for patient engagement: A toolkit for medical practice. *Studies in Health Technology and Informatics*, *199*, 13–21. PMID:24875682

Graffigna, G., Barello, S., Wiederhold, B. K., Bosio, A. C., & Riva, G. (2013). Positive technology as a driver for health engagement. *Studies in Health Technology and Informatics*, *191*, 9–17. PMID:23792833

Greener, I. (2012). Consumerism in Health Policy: Where Did it comes from and how can it work. In A. Hann (Ed.), *Health Policy and Politics* (pp. 57–81). Aschgate, UK: Ashgate.

Gulliksen, J., Göransson, B., Boivie, I., Blomkvist, S., Persson, J., & Cajander, Å. (2003). Key principles for user-centred systems design. *Behaviour & Information Technology*, *22*(6), 397–409. doi:10.1080/01449290310001624329

Haber, D. (2013). *Health promotion and aging: Practical applications for health professionals*. New York, NY: Springer Publishing Company Heesen.

Happonen, A. P., Mattila, E., Kinnunen, M. L., Ikonen, V., Myllymäki, T., Kaipainen, K., & Korhonen, I. (2009, April). P4Well concept to empower self-management of psychophysiological wellbeing and load recovery. *Paper presented at the 3rd International Conference on Pervasive Computing Technologies for Healthcare*, London, UK. doi:10.4108/ICST.PERVASIVEHEALTH2009.6037

Hardyman, W., Daunt, K. L., & Kitchener, M. (2014). (in press). Value Co-Creation through Patient Engagement in Health Care: A micro-level approach and research agenda. *Public Management Review*.

Herrick, D. M. (2005). *Consumer driven health care: the changing role of the patient*. Retrieved from http://www.ncpa.org/pub/st276/

Hu, C., Kung, S., Rummans, T. A., Clark, M. M., & Lapid, M. I. (2015). Reducing caregiver stress with internet-based interventions: A systematic review of open-label and randomized controlled trials. *Journal of the American Medical Informatics Association*, *22*(e1), e194–e209. PMID:25125686

Humphreys, A., & Grayson, K. (2008). The Intersecting Roles of Consumer and Producer: A Critical Perspective on Co-production, Co-creation and Prosumption. *Social Compass*, *2*(3), 963–980. doi:10.1111/j.1751-9020.2008.00112.x

Humphreys, A., & Grayson, K. (2008). The intersecting roles of consumer and producer: A critical perspective on co-production, co-creation and presumption. *Social Compass*, *2*(3), 963–980. doi:10.1111/j.1751-9020.2008.00112.x

Insel, P. A., Amara, S. G., & Blaschke, T. F. (2015). Introduction to the Theme "Precision Medicine and Prediction in Pharmacology". *Annual Review of Pharmacology and Toxicology*, *55*(1), 11–14. doi:10.1146/annurev-pharmtox-101714-123102 PMID:25562643

Kairy, D., Rushton, P. W., Archambault, P., Pituch, E., Torkia, C., El Fathi, A., & Gourdeau, R. (2014). Exploring powered wheelchair users and their caregivers' perspectives on potential intelligent power wheelchair use: A qualitative study. *International Journal of Environmental Research and Public Health*, *11*(2), 2244–2261. doi:10.3390/ijerph110202244 PMID:24566051

Kvedar, J., Coye, M. J., & Everett, W. (2014). Connected health: A review of technologies and strategies to improve patient care with telemedicine and telehealth. *Health Affairs*, *33*(2), 194–199. doi:10.1377/hlthaff.2013.0992 PMID:24493760

Lancia, F. (2004). *Strumenti per l'Analisi di Testi. Introduzione all'Uso di T-LAB* [Tools for Text Analysis. An Introduction to the Use of T-LAB]. Milano, Italy: Angeli.

Lancia, F. (2012a). *T-LAB 8.0 – User's Manual*. Retrieved from http://www.tlab.it/en/download.php

Lancia, F. (2012b). *T-LAB pathways to thematic analysis*. Retrieved from http://www.tlab.it/en/tpatways.php

Laver, K., George, S., Thomas, S., Deutsch, J. E., & Crotty, M. (2011). Virtual reality for stroke rehabilitation. *Stroke*, *43*(2), e20–e21. doi:10.1161/STROKEAHA.111.642439

Le, T., Reeder, B., Yoo, D., Aziz, R., Thompson, H. J., & Demiris, G. (2015). An Evaluation of Wellness Assessment Visualizations for Older Adults. *Telemedicine Journal and e-Health*, *21*(1), 9–15. doi:10.1089/tmj.2014.0012 PMID:25401414

Leinonen, M., Koivisto, A., Sirkka, A., & Kiili, K. (2012, October). Designing games for well-being; Exergames for elderly people. *Paper presented at the 6th European Conference on Games Based Learning*, Cork, Ireland.

Loeppke, R. R., Schill, A. L., Chosewood, L. C., Grosch, J. W., Allweiss, P., Burton, W. N., & Larson, P. W. et al. (2013). Advancing workplace health protection and promotion for an aging workforce. *Journal of Occupational and Environmental Medicine*, *55*(5), 500–506. doi:10.1097/JOM.0b013e31829613a4 PMID:23657074

Lupton, D. (1997). Consumerism, reflexivity and the medical encounter. *Social Science & Medicine*, *45*(3), 373–381. doi:10.1016/S0277-9536(96)00353-X PMID:9232732

Mattila, E., Orsama, A. L., Ahtinen, A., Hopsu, L., Leino, T., & Korhonen, I. (2013). Personal health technologies in employee health promotion: Usage activity, usefulness, and health-related outcomes in a 1-year randomized controlled trial. *Journal of Medical Internet Research*, *1*(2), e16. PMID:25098385

Menichetti, J., Cipresso, P., Bussolin, D., & Graffigna, G. (2015). Engaging older people in healthy and active lifestyles: A systematic review. *Ageing and Society*, *1*, 1–25. doi:10.1017/S0144686X15000781

Menichetti, J., Libreri, C., Lozza, E., & Graffigna, G. (2014). Giving patients a starring role in their own care: A bibliometric analysis of the on-going literature debate. *Health Expectations*, *4*(11), 1369–7625. PMID:25369557

Miller, A. M., & Iris, M. (2002). Health promotion attitudes and strategies in older adults. *Health Education & Behavior*, *29*(2), 249–267. doi:10.1177/1090198102029002009 PMID:11942718

Miller, E. A. (2003). The technical and interpersonal aspects of telemedicine: Effects on doctor–patient communication. *Journal of Telemedicine and Telecare*, *9*(1), 1–7. doi:10.1258/135763303321159611 PMID:12641885

Miller, K. J., Adair, B. S., Pearce, A. J., Said, C. M., Ozanne, E., & Morris, M. M. (2014). Effectiveness and feasibility of virtual reality and gaming system use at home by older adults for enabling physical activity to improve health-related domains: A systematic review. *Age and Ageing*, *43*(2), 188–195. doi:10.1093/ageing/aft194 PMID:24351549

Miller, V. (2011). Convergence and the Contemporary Media Experience. In D. M. Berry (Ed.), *ED.) Understanding Digital Culture* (pp. 72–94). London, UK: Sage.

Mitra, S., & Padman, R. (2012). Exploring social media for health and wellness: A health plan case study. *Journal of Cases on Information Technology*, *14*(2), 42–64. doi:10.4018/jcit.2012040104

Mora, F. (2012). The demise of Google Health and the future of personal health records. *International Journal of Healthcare Technology and Management*, *13*(5/6), 363–377. doi:10.1504/IJHTM.2012.052563

Murray, E., Charles, C., & Gafni, A. (2006). Shared decision-making in primary care: Tailoring the model to fit the context of general practice. *Patient Education and Counseling*, *62*(2), 205–211. doi:10.1016/j.pec.2005.07.003 PMID:16139467

Page, R. C., Martin, J. A., & Loeb, C. F. (2005). The Oral Health Information Suite (OHIS): Its use in the management of periodontal disease. *Journal of Dental Education*, *69*(5), 509–520. PMID:15897333

Peine, A., Faulkner, A., Jæger, B., & Moors, E. (2014). Science, technology and the "grand challenge" of ageing – Understanding the socio-material constitution of later life. *Technological Forecasting and Social Change*, *93*, 1–9. doi:10.1016/j.techfore.2014.11.010

Peine, A., Rollwagen, I., & Neven, L. (2014). The rise of the "innosumer" - Rethinking older technology users. *Technological Forecasting and Social Change*, *82*, 199–214. doi:10.1016/j.techfore.2013.06.013

Phillips, N. M., Street, M., & Haesler, E. (2014). Measuring patient participation in health care: A comprehensive systematic review protocol. *The JBI Database of Systematic Reviews and Implementation Reports*, *12*(3), 68–88. doi:10.11124/jbisrir-2014-1380

Proffitt, R., & Lange, B. (2015). Considerations in the efficacy and effectiveness of virtual reality interventions for stroke rehabilitation: Moving the field forward. *Physical Therapy*, *95*(3), 441–448. doi:10.2522/ptj.20130571 PMID:25343960

Riva, G., Banos, R. M., Botella, C., Wiederhold, B. K., & Gaggioli, A. (2012). Positive technology: Using interactive technologies to promote positive functioning. *Cyberpsychology, Behavior, and Social Networking*, *15*(2), 69–77. doi:10.1089/cyber.2011.0139 PMID:22149077

Riva, G., Castelnuovo, G., & Mantovani, F. (2006). Transformation of flow in rehabilitation: The role of advanced communication technologies. *Behavior Research Methods*, *38*(2), 237–244. doi:10.3758/BF03192775 PMID:16956100

Riva, G., & Gaggioli, A. (2009). Rehabilitation as empowerment: The role of advanced technologies. *Studies in Health Technology and Informatics*, *145*, 3–22. PMID:19592783

Riva, G., Mantovani, F., & Gaggioli, A. (2004). Presence and rehabilitation: Toward second-generation virtual reality applications in neuropsychology. *Journal of Neuroengineering and Rehabilitation*, *1*(1), 9. doi:10.1186/1743-0003-1-9 PMID:15679950

Riva, G., Marsan, P. A., & Grassi, C. (2014). *Active Ageing and Healthy Living: A Human Centered Approach in Research and Innovation as Source of Quality of Life*. Amsterdam, The Netherlands: IOS Press.

Robinson, J. C. (2005). Managed consumerism in health care. *Health Affairs*, *24*(6), 1478–1489. doi:10.1377/hlthaff.24.6.1478 PMID:16284020

Salzer, M. S. (1997). Consumer empowerment in mental health organizations: Concept, benefits, and impediments. *Administration and Policy in Mental Health and Mental Health Services Research*, *24*(5), 425–434. doi:10.1007/BF02042724 PMID:9239946

Saposnik, G., & Levin, M. (2011). Virtual reality in stroke rehabilitation a meta-analysis and implications for clinicians. *Stroke*, *42*(5), 1380–1386. doi:10.1161/STROKEAHA.110.605451 PMID:21474804

Seligman, M. E. P. (2002). Positive psychology, positive prevention, and positive therapy. In *Handbook of positive psychology* (pp. 3–9). USA: Oxford University Press.

Seligman, M. E. P. (2002). *Authentic Happiness*. New York, USA: Atria Books.

Seligman, M. E. P., & Csikszentmihalyi, M. (2000). Positive psychology: An introduction. *The American Psychologist*, *55*(1), 5–14. doi:10.1037/0003-066X.55.1.5 PMID:11392865

Serino, S., Cipresso, P., Gaggioli, A., & Riva, G. (2013). The potential of pervasive sensors and computing for positive technology: the interreality paradigm. In S. Mukhopadhyay & O. Postolache (Eds.), *Pervasive and Mobile Sensing and Computing for Healthcare* (pp. 207–232). New York, USA: Springer.

Serino, S., Triberti, S., Villani, D., Cipresso, P., Gaggioli, A., & Riva, G. (2013). Toward a validation of cyber-interventions for stress disorders based on stress inoculation training: A systematic review. *Virtual Reality (Waltham Cross)*, 2013, 237–236.

Stephens-Reicher, J., Metcalf, A., Blanchard, M., Mangan, C., & Burns, J. (2011). Reaching the hard-to-reach: How information communication technologies can reach young people at greater risk of mental health difficulties. *Australasian Psychiatry*, *19*(1), S58–S61. doi:10.3109/10398562.2011.583077 PMID:21878021

Street, R. L., Gold, W. R., & Manning, T. R. (2013). *Health promotion and interactive technology: Theoretical applications and future directions*. London, UK: Routledge.

Subramanian, S., Knaut, L. A., Beaudoin, C., McFadyen, B. J., Feldman, A. G., & Levin, M. F. (2007). Virtual reality environments for post-stroke arm rehabilitation. *Journal of Neuroengineering and Rehabilitation*, *4*(1), 20. doi:10.1186/1743-0003-4-20 PMID:17587441

Tariman, J. D., Berry, D. L., Cochrane, B., Doorenbos, A., & Schepp, K. (2010). Preferred and actual participation roles during health care decision making in persons with cancer: A systematic review. *Annals of Oncology*, *21*(6), 1145–1151. doi:10.1093/annonc/mdp534 PMID:19940010

Thompson, G. (2007). The meaning of patient involvement and participation in health care consul-tations: A taxonomy. *Social Science & Medicine*, *64*(6), 1297–1310. doi:10.1016/j.socscimed.2006.11.002 PMID:17174016

Toffler, A. (1980). *The Third Wave*. London, UK: Pan Books.

Veenhoven, R. (2008). Sociological theories of subjective well-being. In M. Eid & R. J. Larsen (Eds.), *The science of subjective well-being* (pp. 44–61). New York: Guilford Press.

Vlasnik, J. J., Aliotta, S. L., & DeLor, B. (2005). Medication adherence: Factors influencing compliance with prescribed medication plans. *The Case Manager*, *16*(2), 47–51. doi:10.1016/j.casemgr.2005.01.009 PMID:15818344

Wakefield, C. E., Sansom-Daly, U. M., McGill, B. C., McCarthy, M., Girgis, A., Grootenhuis, M., & Cohn, R. J. (2015). Online parent-targeted cognitive-behavioural therapy intervention to improve quality of life in families of young cancer survivors: Study protocol for a randomized controlled trial. *Trials*, *16*(1), 153. doi:10.1186/s13063-015-0681-6 PMID:25872773

Walker, A. (2002). A strategy for active ageing. *International Social Security Review*, *55*(1), 121–139. doi:10.1111/1468-246X.00118

Wiederhold, B. K., Riva, G., & Graffigna, G. (2013). Ensuring the best care for our increasing aging population: Health engagement and positive technology can help patients achieve a more active role in future healthcare. *Cyberpsychology, Behavior, and Social Networking*, *16*(6), 411–412. doi:10.1089/cyber.2013.1520 PMID:23751102

Wilcox, A. B. (2015). Patient Engagement and Consumerism. In P. R. O. Payne & P. J. Embi (Eds.), *Translational Informatics* (pp. 153–161). London, UK: Springer.

Wu, Y. C., Xue, Y., & Hu, F. (2014). Embedded Smart Textile Detecting Equipment Base on Flexibility Sensors. *Applied Mechanics and Materials*, *670*, 1218–1221.

Yoediono, Z., & Snyderman, R. (2008). Proposal for a new health record to support personalized, predictive, preventative and participatory medicine. *Personalized Medicine*, *5*(1), 47–54. doi:10.2217/17410541.5.1.47

## KEY TERMS AND DEFINITIONS

**Consumer Health Psychology:** Discipline that seeks to unveil the basic subjective processes that rule individuals' decision-making and choice behaviours in different domains of daily life. Consumer health psychology's theoretical frameworks have shown their effectiveness not only in diagnosing consumers' healthcare behaviours, but also in orienting managerial practices aimed to improve exchanges between "demand" and "offers" for healthcare services.

**E-Health:** Emerging field in the intersection of medical informatics, public health and business, referring to health services and information delivered or enhanced through the Internet and related technologies. In a broader sense, the term characterizes not only a technical development, but also a state-of-mind, a way of thinking, an attitude, and a commitment for networked, global thinking, to improve health care locally, regionally, and worldwide by using information and communication technology.

**Healthy Ageing:** Process of optimizing opportunities for good health, so that older people can take an active part in society and enjoy an independent and high quality of life.

**Participatory Medicine:** A model of medical care in which networked patients shift from being mere passengers to responsible and engaged drivers of their health, and in which care providers encourage and value them as full partners in the care process.

**Patient Engagement:** Process-like and multi-dimensional experience, resulting from the conjoint cognitive (think), emotional (feel), and conative (act) enactment of individuals toward their health management. In this process, patients go through four subsequent positions (i.e., blackout, arousal, adhesion, and eudaimonic project). The unachieved synergy among the different subjective dimensions (think, feel, act) at each stage of the process may inhibit patients' ability to engage in their care.

**Positive Psychology:** Branch of psychology that uses scientific understanding and effective intervention to aid in the achievement of a satisfactory life, rather than treating mental illness. The focus of positive psychology is on personal growth rather than on pathology, as is common among other frameworks within the field of psychology.

**Wellbeing:** Condition of an individual or group, for example their social, economic, psychological, spiritual or medical state; a high level of well-being means in some sense the individual or group's experience is positive, while low well-being is associated with negative happening.

Section 2

# Design Positive Systems

# Chapter 4
# Augmenting Online Mental Health Support Services

**Rafael A. Calvo**
*The University of Sydney, Australia*

**M. Sazzad Hussain**
*The University of Sydney, Australia & Health and Biosecurity, CSIRO, Australia*

**David Milne**
*The University of Sydney, Australia*

**Kjartan Nordbo**
*The University of Sydney, Australia*

**Ian Hickie**
*The University of Sydney, Australia*

**P. Danckwerts**
*ReachOut, Australia*

## ABSTRACT

*The Internet allows mental health organisations to provide services to more people via new models of care. Amongst these, online support groups are becoming increasingly popular. This model of mental health service provision includes moderators who read posts, recognise those that need attention and provide support via online responses. However, as these groups become more popular they risk becoming more difficult to manage due to the sheer volume of posts. This challenge can be addressed through computational linguistics techniques. This chapter reports on work with a mental health organisation on three components to help scale up the number of people they can support. The design aims to go beyond helping end-users and explores how design can support the wellbeing of the moderators themselves. The design of the three components is discussed: 1) A triage component automatically detects posts that need a prompt response. 2) An intervention generator (IG) generates a draft response for the moderator to use, for example a positive psychology intervention. These two can help in the management of a discussion forum, supporting positive behaviours, not just dealing in situations of distress. 3) A component for synchronous support through an augmented chat system.*

## INTRODUCTION

Strong evidence supports the idea that technology based mental health interventions can be effective (Griffiths, Farrer, & Christensen, 2010), particularly for young people, the focus of this chapter. For example, 21% of 12–17 year-olds and 34% of 18–25 year-olds reported searching the Internet for information to help themselves, with 78% of them feeling that the internet had helped; 85% would recom-

DOI: 10.4018/978-1-4666-9986-1.ch004

mend it to a friend or family member; and 94% felt somewhat or very satisfied with the information they received (Burns et al., 2010).

The broad e-health ecosystem includes different services such as psycho-educational websites, interactive self-guided interventions, online counseling and psychotherapy, online support groups and blogs, mobile apps and new media such as virtual reality (Collin et. al. 2011). Psycho-educational interventions generally deliver generic and static information and resources on websites about mental health without any human interaction from the service provider. Self-guided interventions include web-based Cognitive Behavioral Therapy (CBT) (Van Bilsen, 2013), and positive psychology interventions (e.g. Shuller & Parks, 2012). The online counseling and psychotherapy (e.g. by clinicians) includes the use of technology to move one-to-one human support to the online world, for example, through computer mediated interactions (video conferencing, chat, email, etc.)

In this chapter we report on our development for ReachOut Australia, a mental health organization focused on young people. ReachOut offers resources on wellbeing (e.g. staying healthy, relationships, social skills) and mental health issues (e.g. addiction, bullying, grief, etc.) to 15-25 year olds. The focus of the first two components discussed later was on their discussion forums where help-seekers can meet and discuss their problems (Eysenbach, Powell, Englesakis, Rizo, & Stern, 2004; Webb et al., 2008). The development aimed to explore two problems:

1. How new technologies could be used to improve the quality of moderation in peer-support groups, and
2. How these technologies can be designed to support the moderators' wellbeing.

The first aim is driven by the recognition that the Internet has the potential to help young people with mental illness (e.g. by reducing stigma or providing access to care). It can also be used for health promotion interventions by targeting positive emotions, behaviors and cognitions as proposed by positive psychology. Amongst Internet-based interventions into peer-to-peer communities are considered amongst the most promising forms of e-health support (Eysenbach, Powell, Englesakis, Rizo, & Stern, 2004). For example, the feedback received by peer-supporters on social media can help individuals reflect on their thoughts, which offer a type of mental health intervention through the feedback loop (Grohol, Anthony, Nagel, & Goss, 2010; Hoyt & Pasupathi, 2008). However, these interventions are not without their limitations - as they are also vulnerable to the quality of the feedback being offered. In general the evaluation of the peer-support groups is challenging because they typically include other types of interventions or interaction with health professionals (Eysenbach, Powell, Englesakis, Rizo, & Stern, 2004). There are also different types of online communities: they can be unmoderated (i.e. purely peer-to-peer) or be provided with a more structured support where trained moderators intervene in the conversations. The trained moderators in these forums are responsible for identifying people at risk and responding with resources (e.g. links to mental health related information and motivation). Although the work discussed generalizes to any online moderated support group, this chapter focuses—as a case study—on ReachOut (ReachOut's forums and other online resources can be visited at www.reachout.com), (Collin et.al, 2011) an online mental health service that aims to help young people through health and wellbeing issues, from relationship problems to dealing with stress at school. Their website is focused on Australian young people, and receives about 1.5 million unique visitors every year.

The goal of a peer-support group is to foster an environment in which visitors help each other, and that supports self-efficacy and pro-social behaviors. ReachOut's forum, for example, is carefully curated by a team of paid and volunteer moderators. Distressing posts are identified and quickly responded to, and occasionally removed and addressed in private, through one-on-one conversations. This strategy is intended to ensure that ReachOut remains a positive place to be, despite the difficult content matter it frequently addresses. The efforts at ReachOut reflect the ethos that people who seek help need to be able to find those who are trained and equipped to provide it. According to Kummervold et al. (2002) this is an opinion that is held by the majority of people who use these services. Their survey of online mental health forums found that only 3% of respondents felt that professionals should be excluded from the forums; the majority (68%) felt they should instead take an active part, and the remainder felt they should passively monitor them.

Our first goal was to support the moderators' work in the forums. In particular, when online support groups require moderation they risk becoming unsustainable as their popularity increases (Liu, Calvo, Davenport, & Hickie, 2013). Moderators are required to spend significant amount of time reading posts, identifying members at risk, and communicating useful information compassionately and persuasively. Furthermore, difficulty maintaining the quality of feedback and complying with duty of care can be challenging even with small communities, but are likely to become more so as the number of users increases. One approach to managing increased traffic in peer-to-peer support groups is to recruit and train volunteers, creating a community of moderators that can help each other, but such a loop may not keep pace with user demand. Only a small proportion of help-seekers make suitable volunteer moderators because the work required is often very confronting and requires a great deal of personal resilience and commitment. This chapter describes efforts to address the likely future crisis of scale in the online peer support mental health services. To meet increased demand and retain service quality, we describe the use of a combination of automation of tasks and augmentation of the moderators' abilities.

Our second goal was to investigate how designing these systems could be informed by considering the impact on the psychological wellbeing of all its users, including moderators. In particular the chapter considers the trade-offs between using automation and augmentation in e-health systems, and how the principles of positive computing can inform their design (Calvo. & Peters, 2014). The features described are designed to support basic psychological needs studied by Self-Determination Theory (SDT), namely autonomy, competence and relatedness (Ryan & Deci 2000; Gagné, 2014). Other wellbeing design approaches for helping end-users include those described by (Botella et al., 2012; Giuseppe Riva, Banos, Botella, Wiederhold, & Gaggioli, 2012; G. Riva, Calvo, & Lisetti, 2015).

Before touching on any technical details, we first describe the basic concepts of Self-Determination Theory, then the broader challenges faced by mental health services in Australia and abroad. In the context of the ReachOut case study we describe three components designed to help moderators better serve their online community. The first two components focus on the peer-support groups: *Triage*, uses text classification techniques to identify concerning posts so that moderators can prioritize them; *Intervention Generator* (Hussain et al., 2015; Liu et al., 2013) uses natural language generation to help moderators construct appropriate, tailored responses more efficiently. Finally, *Cybermate* provides synchronous one-on-one support through an augmented chat component.

## SELF-DETERMINATION THEORY

Self-determination theory (Ryan & Deci 2000; Gagné, 2014) studies factors that hinder or support intrinsic and extrinsic motivation. In its beginning SDT focused on intrinsic motivation based in the inherent satisfaction we get from certain actions. Ryan and Deci (2000) and other researchers have provided evidence of how a person's sense of autonomy and competence support intrinsic motivation.

- **Autonomy:** Has been identified as critical to wellbeing by various wellbeing theories. It has been defined as, "a state of being independent or self-governing" (Spear & Kulbok, 2001), "a capacity for thinking and acting independently" (Littlewood, 1996), and more narrowly, in the context of SDT as "an internal perceived locus of causality" (Ryan & Deci, 2000). Within HCI, these theories have been used to describe the sense of agency required for enjoyable gameplay and the self-regulation users are seeking to enhance through the use of behavior change, healthcare and learning technologies.

Calvo, Peters, Johnson and Rogers (2014) have explored with the HCI community ways in which autonomy can be promoted in technology design. At this level, autonomy can be grouped in four spheres. In the narrowest sense, design can support a feeling of freedom and control within a software environment, for example through choice over tasks and goals. Design for autonomy in this sphere is familiar to game designers (Ford et.al, 2012) and might be related to measures of presence and intuitive controls (Ryan et.al, 2006). We often design technologies that give people greater autonomy in daily life (for example assistive technologies, life-tracking, productivity tools, etc.), removing obstacles or augmenting capabilities, allowing people to pursue self-determined goals more fluently. A third sphere of autonomy is developed through kits and frameworks that allow users to feel empowered by designing their own technologies (Rogers and Marsden, 2013). Finally, and perhaps most significantly, there is the potential to design technologies that foster autonomy as an overarching characteristic of psychological development and flourishing. In other words, how can technologies (e.g. educational, health management or behavior change tools) be designed to help users develop autonomy (and related concepts like self-efficacy, independence and self-regulation) over time as a trait, characteristic or capacity?

Ryan et al. (2006) showed how perceived autonomy in video games can lead to game enjoyment, preferences and short-term wellbeing (they did not explore the impact of game playing in the long term). Some of the instruments used to measure sense of autonomy come from the psychology literature. For example, the Index of Autonomous Functioning (Weinstein et. al., 2012) is designed to measure dispositional autonomy using three characteristics (i.e., authorship/congruence, interest-taking, and non-susceptibility to being controlled).

- **Competence:** Or the need for a challenge and sense of being the locus of causality, is the second psychological need as defined by SDT. There are certain factors that have shown to enhance the sense of competence including being optimally challenged, receiving positive feedback and opportunities for further learning. These are all factors that can be taken into account in the design of new technologies.
- **Relatedness:** Described as "Belongingness and connectedness with others; a secure relational base … relatedness is core to most, if not all, theories of wellbeing" (Reis & Gable, 2003) and more recent research has shown that the impact of positive relationships. Since relationships are mediated by technology, and digital experience is increasingly social, this is a critical area of wellbeing literature for designers.

## REACHOUT AND AUSTRALIAN YOUTH

Every year, one in five young Australians aged 16 to 24 years' experience a mental health problem with only 25% of them seeking or receiving professional help (Slade, Johnston, Oakley Browne, Andrews, & Whiteford, 2009). These statistics are common for most countries ("The World health report," 2001), therefore the global need for effectively addressing mental health problems is well established. ReachOut is an Australian non-profit organisation established in 1996 with a mission to help young people lead happier lives.

Despite high rates of mental illness in the community, mental health care has long been neglected (Burns et al., 2010; Clarke & Yarborough, 2013; Strecher, 2007). Key reasons for this neglect include, but are not limited to:

- Lack of appropriate recognition and diagnosis by health professionals,
- Inappropriate help seeking in the general population,
- Strong stigmatisation of mental illness,
- High costs,
- For some communities, multiculturalism and language barriers.

Internet based platforms like ReachOut overcome some of these traditional barriers to seeking and receiving mental health support in the community. For example, features that facilitate help seeking include the anonymous nature of interaction through the Internet, which can make help seeking process more encouraging (Ybarra & Eaton, 2005). Internet-based platforms can also be an alternative to face-to-face care, making the treatment more flexible, quicker, time saving and cost effective (Currell, Urquhart, Wainwright, & Lewis, 2000; Doherty, Coyle, & Sharry, 2012) and not limited by geophraphical constraints.

ReachOut's services include online resources on topics, such as sex and relationships, school, family, bullying and mental health. These resources describe a topic (e.g. mindfulness), how it influences wellbeing, and often describes techniques that can be used. Besides these psychoeducational resources, ReachOut also has a strong community, both online and offline. Within the ReachOut service, the online forums are a moderated digital space where 14-25 year olds can discuss their personal experiences following a few rules that aim to make it a safe and positive environment. The rules include behaviours to make the environment safer (e.g. do not disclose your real identity and do not engage in illegal activities) as well as to make the social environment more positive (e.g. respect others, give credit) and with a focus on solutions (e.g. "what can you learn from a negative situation?"). The moderators ensure that they carefully collect, read and understand the comments posted on the forum by members. Moderators stay alert for posts in the forums that might reflect certain mental health issues as well as ideas on self-help options. They respond with resources (e.g. links) from ReachOut as well as other national sources based on the issue of the post. The moderators are also encouraged to share any personal experiences related to the members concern and to maintain an ongoing dialogue with the members. The moderation task in ReachOut depends much on peer moderators who volunteer. They are aged 16 to 25 years and are recruited through ReachOut, via announcements on their website and forums. The selected peer moderators complete face-to-face training in ReachOut with the Community Managers and senior moderators (also known as the Mod Squad).

The moderation task in organizations and forums like ReachOut can be very challenging since given the limited number of volunteers only a handful of moderators can be engaged in the support process at any given time. The turnover of moderators also means that at any point in time many of them would lack experience providing feedback. Furthermore, some of the volunteers may have suffered mental health issues themselves, and while this helps them understand what the person posting is going through and connect to them, they might lack the resilience required and extra care must be taken to keep them safe.

Despite these issues there is the potential for integrating systems with the ability to detect some of the issues from the forums and provide template-based responses. The technical augmentation can help automatically in detecting people in need, and improve the quality and efficiency of providing feedback while also supporting the moderators with features that contribute to their wellbeing. It is important to note that because of the sensitive nature of the content (mental health concerns), it is our view that full automation is inappropriate. Instead augmentation is more desirable, where human moderators can administer, personalize, edit contents detected and generated by machines.

Our design supports a process with automated detection / triaging of posts followed by an augmented (i.e. scaffolded) feedback generation process. One of the design briefs was to take into account productivity and efficacy. We expect that this approach has the potential to reduce the moderators' workload and improve the quality of their feedback. Another design goal was to support the moderators' wellbeing with features and design alternatives that positively influence what Self-Determination Theory calls the satisfaction of psychological needs, particularly their sense of autonomy, competence and relatedness (Ryan and Deci, 2001). Using this and other positive psychology theories engineers can start to design applications that take into account their impact on psychological wellbeing.

## TRIAGE: IDENTIFYING AND PRIORITIZING POSTS

Managing online traffic requires that moderators spend their time wisely, identifying and responding to help-seekers expressing the most urgent need. This section introduces a system called *Triage* that was designed to facilitate the identification and prioritization of posts. As the name implies, Triage separates critical cases from other less urgent or non-urgent posts that can be adequately addressed by the wider community of peers. The Triage system monitors every new post made within ReachOut online communities. Text classification algorithms are applied to these posts to identify those containing distressing content. Those meeting criteria for distressing content are passed directly to the moderator for response.

### Gathering Training Data for Classification

The machine-learned classifiers require training data; in the current application the data are sentences manually annotated with the labels ReachOut's moderators are most concerned with. This data was collected in an annotation study of 4,583 posts from three peer-support groups: one hosted on Facebook, another on LiveJournal, and the last from ReachOut. Sentences from these posts that contained evidence for one of the labels were manually identified and labeled by psychology interns ($N$=38) into one or more of 16 mental health categories, such as depression, anxiety, self-harm, suicide, drug/alcohol use, bullying, violence, medication/treatment, psychosis, bipolar, eating disorder, personality disorder, sleep, accessing help, positive emotion, and self-care.

Initially, inter-rater agreement and definitions for the 16 mental health categories were developed by two psychologists and a psychiatrist. Psychology interns were then recruited and trained face-to-face by a psychiatrist to classify the 16 mental health categories and to complete the annotation task. The final annotation task completed by the interns involved labeling text segments (i.e. a sentence, a sentence segment or a key phrase) from the posts into one or more of the 16 categories, which would then be used to train machine leaning classifiers (discussed in the previous section).

In order to ensure consistency between interns, concordance of response was examined using a sub-sample of posts completed by interns during the face-to-face training. Any differences in the agreement were resolved through additional training and group discussion. Once agreement was established, interns were each allocated 350 posts to annotate, which were completed over a period of four weeks. The corpus annotation study provided a total of 12,640 unique sentences that were labeled into one or more of the 16 categories.

## Classifying Concerning Posts

The main technical challenge of Triage is to identify and label the concerning posts automatically. To do so it relies on a suite of rule-based and machine learned classifiers. An otherwise un-troubling post that contains one single suicidal statement is nevertheless of great concern, so the classifiers operate on one sentence at a time. Each classifier corresponds to a single label (e.g. depression, anxiety, self-harm) and makes a binary decision about whether that label is relevant or not to the given sentence. It also provides a confidence score for each judgment. These are summed to provide a confidence score for each label over the entire post. A tunable threshold makes the final decision for whether or not the label applies to the post as a whole.

There are multiple approaches to develop each binary classifier, and Triage combines these in an ensemble, where the score for a sentence is the maximum score given by any of the various classifiers. The most basic classifier simply consults lists of key terms and phrases that are known to be relevant to each label (e.g. "sad"), and scores posts when these key terms are found. The lists are maintained by the moderators, and can be updated via the triage interface. More sophisticated classifiers were developed using machine-learning algorithms, specifically Multinomial Naïve Bayes, Logistic Regression and Support Vector machines. The data used to train these algorithms is described in the next section.

## The Triage Interface

When designing Triage, it was important as part of the goal to improve quality and productivity, to minimize the effort required for moderators to engage with the system. Consequently it appears not as a stand-alone system, but as a small side-bar (visible only to moderators) in the existing ReachOut webpage (see Figure 1). Here the moderator can see a list of cases that have been identified by our algorithms as urgent (i.e. concerning). Each is tagged with one or more labels, such as *depression*, *self-harm*, *anxiety* and so on. Classifiers that identify three types of positive behaviors ('accessing help', 'positive emotions', and 'self care') have been trained but not yet integrated into the production system. These can eventually be used for supporting users through positive reinforcement.

Moderators can either view *my cases* (posts they have personally taken responsibility for) or—as is shown in the figure—those that still need to be claimed. The ordering encourages moderators to treat

*Figure 1. Viewing pending triage cases*

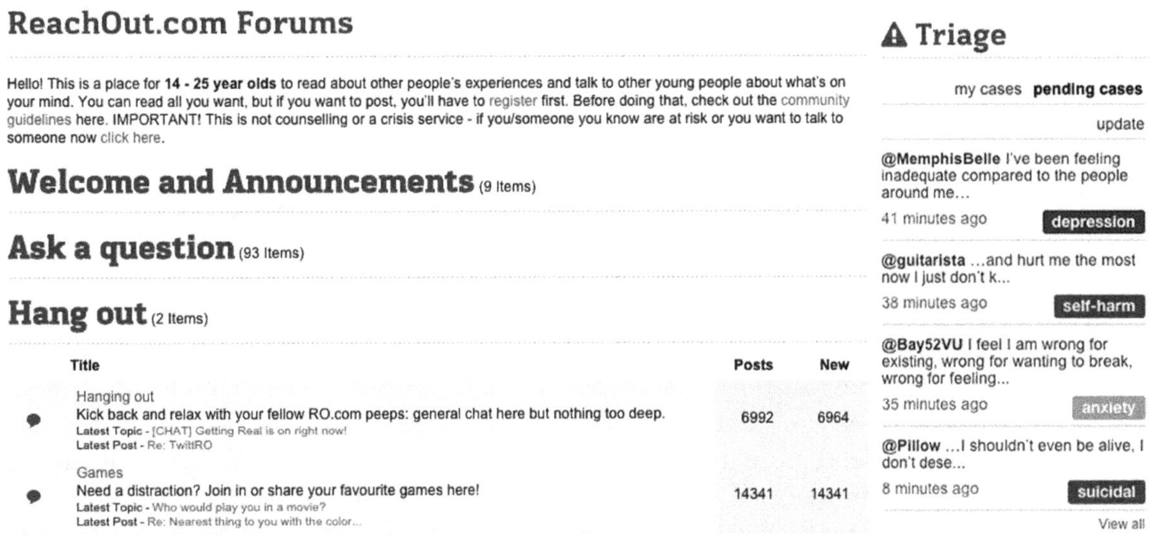


cases like a queue, and deal with the oldest items first. Any of these cases can be clicked to navigate directly to the relevant post.

As part of addressing our second goal, of considering moderators' wellbeing using SDT we first considered the different ways to manage the moderation processes and how it could impact the moderators' sense of autonomy. The allocation of cases could be done in different ways:

1. Automatically, for example assigning the same number of posts to each moderator, or to assign new posts to the last moderator to login.
2. Manually, by a manager who might assign posts based on his/her knowledge of moderators' experience on the topic of the post.
3. Manually, by allowing the moderators to themselves pick the posts they would like to respond to.

Each design imposes different requirements on moderators. We also believe that each of these designs will have a different impact on the moderators' sense of autonomy and sense of control of the situation: it is expected that the fully automated design offers the least sense of autonomy, while the self-allocated one the most. This is a consequence of design rarely studied yet we consider it important since autonomy support has been shown to have positive correlation with wellbeing and job satisfaction (Ryan and Deci, 2001).

The list of cases in Figure 1 is visible whenever the moderator browses the ReachOut forum. If they navigate down to a specific thread or post, the sidebar changes to display only details pertinent to it, as shown in Figure 2. For example, here the forum user *MemphisBelle* has shared her struggles with self-esteem, and the classifier has correctly labeled it as relating to *depression.* Moderator *Blithe* has taken ownership, and committed to seeing her through her current troubles. Blythe can respond as she normally would, and will eventually mark the case as resolved (at which point it would disappear from the case list) or as something she does not feel comfortable resolving (which would move it from *my cases* to *pending cases*, where someone else could take ownership). There is also room for moderators to chat privately about each case, to coordinate their efforts or offer encouragement and advice to each other. This we hope will have a positive impact on their sense of relatedness with others, particularly supporting a feeling of belonging to a community of moderators. Relatedness has also been linked to psychological wellbeing (Ryan and Deci, 2001).

A second way in which the interface can have an impact on moderators is their sense of competence. Algorithms, like humans, may mislabel posts. In our design the moderators have the last word and are able to overwrite any computer generated labeling. A more detailed sidebar (but similar to Figure 2) is available for every post, not just those that the algorithm identified as concerning. The moderators are free to add and remove new labels, so they are always able to correct the judgments made by the algorithms and add new cases that were missed.

These design decisions may have an impact on the mental state, and wellbeing, of the moderators. In particular, when an algorithm makes a mistake the human moderator may interpret it in different ways. Some may understand the error as a natural aspect of technology, and correct it as described above. However, others might not recognize it as a computer error and instead question their own judgment. This could have a negative impact on their sense of competence at mastering their task, an effect known to have a negative impact people's wellbeing (Ryan and Deci, 2001). Although the feedback from the moderators has not shown evidence of such impact, we are comparing different designs that can minimize its likelihood. Allowing moderators' to always have the last word is maybe the most important one.

*Figure 2. Resolving a single triage case*

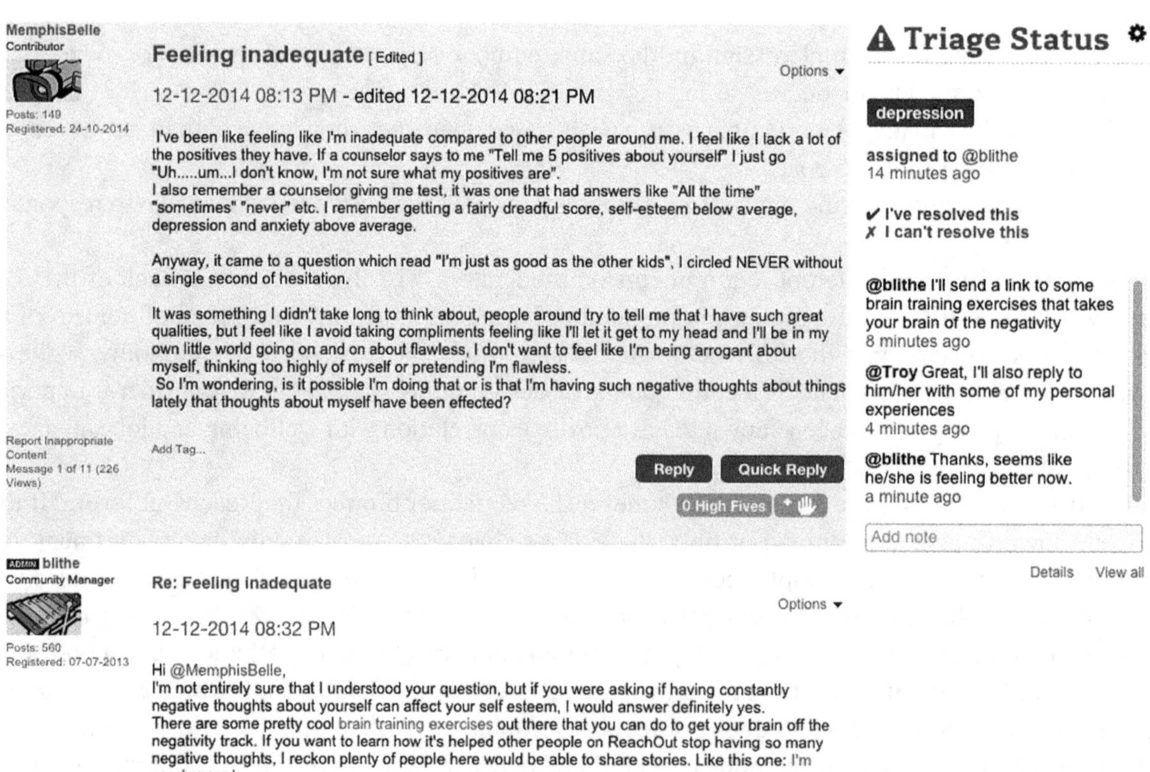

ReachOut moderators have very few opportunities to meet face to face. Most of the interactions happen online through email or in the forums they moderate. Another way in which the interface can have a positive impact on moderators' wellbeing is by helping them connect to each other, for example, to discuss a particular post. In order to support relatedness we added a feature where they can discuss a post that the triage system has identified as important. Through this feature, when a post appears moderators can discuss 'behind the scenes' what is the best way or who should respond to the post. Although this may delay responses we expect it would improve their sense of community and the quality of the feedback provided, specially from less experienced moderators.

### Future Opportunities for Text Classification

Currently, Triage's classifiers are built using *n*-gram features (a sequence of *n* words from a post). There are many opportunities to improve their performance by considering other features, such as forum structure and the past behavior of the post author, or the way the other peers respond to them. Additionally, the classifiers were training exclusively on the dataset described above. In future, we plan to use online classifiers (Bordes et.al, 2005) that continue learning from the manual corrections made by moderators as they use the system, to maintain a feedback loop that ensures it remains up-to-date.

Beyond improving the classifiers, there are also opportunities to retrain them to detect other types of content. For example, they might be retrained (via another annotation experiment) to detect forms of content describing positive behaviors and outcomes that could be showcased in a community-wide positive psychology intervention. Alternatively, the same technology might be used to weigh cases by difficulty (as opposed to urgency) and assign lower-scoring items to more junior moderators and peers. Ideally, every genuine help-seeker in a peer support forum will receive the undivided attention of someone qualified to assist them. The Triage system described above helps somewhat, by enabling moderators to spend their time with the people who need them most.

## GENERATING RESPONSES AND SUGGESTING RESOURCES

While identifying urgent posts for moderators to prioritize their responding will streamline some of the challenges of moderating peer-supported online communities, what happens when even this filtered workload of urgent cases becomes too great?

This section introduces *Intervention Generator*, a system that applies natural language generation techniques to automatically construct appropriate responses that are tailored to each individual post, thereby greatly reducing the time required for a moderator to resolve each case. Introducing such a system may appear impersonal for peer-supported formats, however it is worth considering that problems are not unique even if people are. The same advice can be given more than once, and so even the most caring moderator can become formulaic in their responses to all but the most difficult of cases. Thus, there is some room for automation, as long as its impact on users is carefully considered.

*Figure 3. Sample of automated draft interventions that the moderator could select, edit and submit*

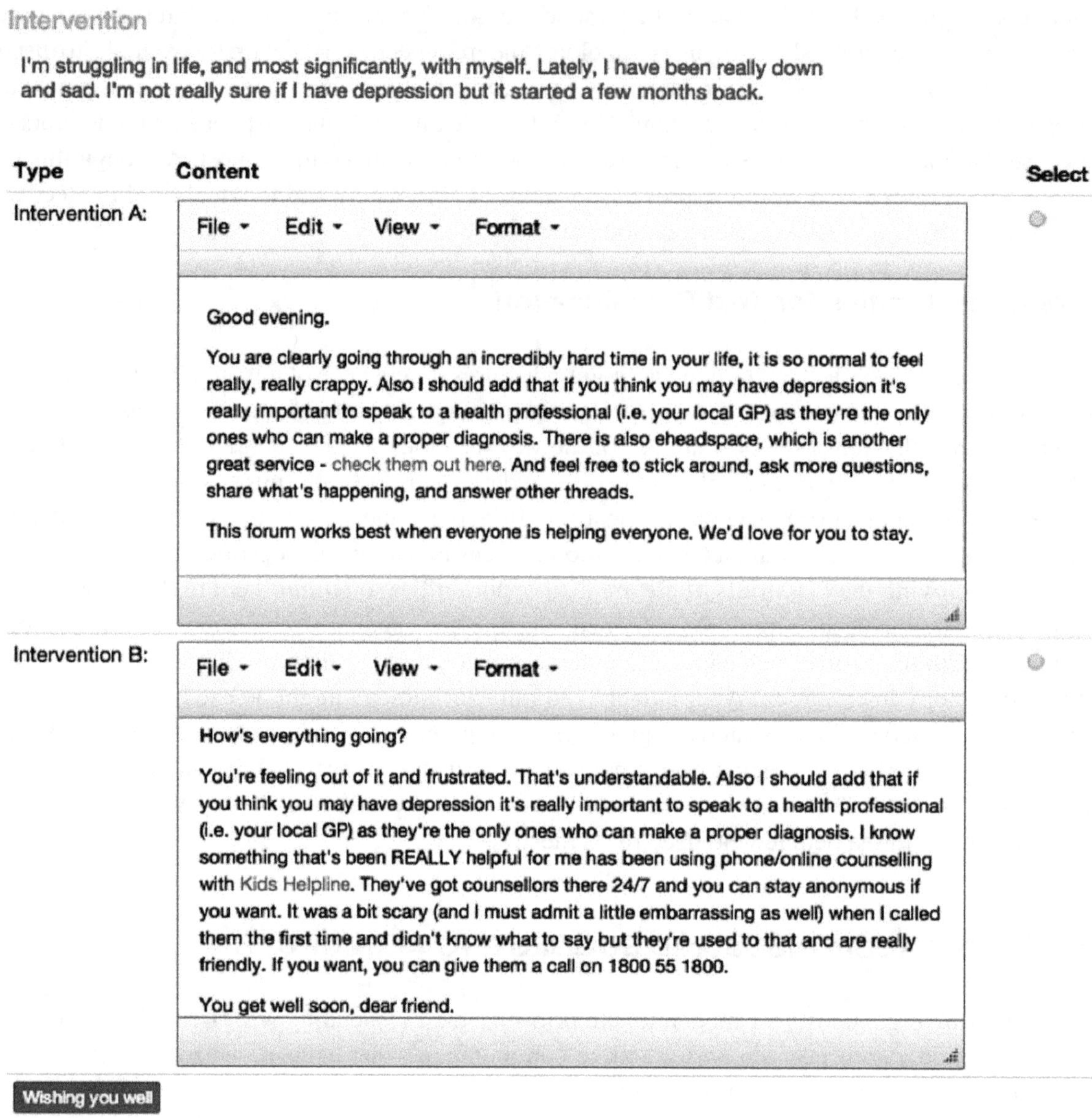


## The Intervention Generator Interface

We are considering a number of design alternatives for the interface of the intervention (response) generator. In general they provide a 2 or 3 options based in different types of interventions (e.g. cognitive behavioral, positive psychology or psychoeducation). Figure 3 shows two complete interventions from which the moderator can choose for the post at the top. Features like the "Wishing you well" (rather than the "submit") button aim to remind moderators of the purpose of their activity, and reduce the chance of them seeing it as an administrative task. In order to help maintain the sense of autonomy of the moderators, and because the natural language generation (NLG) algorithms make mistakes, all the designs we are considering allow the moderators to edit the response before it is sent to the end-user.

## The Intervention Generator Algorithm

The main technical challenge is to generate a selection of relevant responses for each post. The simplest approach would be to rely on a pre-constructed library of responses, one or more of which would be automatically selected based on keywords found within the triggering text. However, such an approach is unlikely to be received well if it becomes widely relied-upon, because it would result in the forum being flooded with very similar replies. The readers' feelings of connection and trust in the moderators—and what they have to say—is likely to be diminished. In interviews with stakeholders at ReachOut it has become clear that using canned responses is not a viable approach.

A more sophisticated approach is to use NLG techniques (Reiter, Dale, & Feng, 2000) to produce dynamic human-like, personalized sentence structures suitable for various contexts. NLG is a subfield of artificial intelligence and computational linguistics and gained diversity in the late 1990s with its adaptation in a growing number of real-word applications such as marketing and health. Despite being used to generate interventions in the physical health domain (DiMarco et al., 2007; Ehud & Reiter, 1999; Varges et al., 2012), the use of NLG for personalized interventions in the mental health is new.

In the context of mental health, high quality interventions (i.e. responses) can be generated by incorporating psychological approaches (Van Bilsen, 2013; Wiemer-Hastings, Janit, Wiemer-Hastings, Cromer, & Kinser, 2004) and strategies practiced by trained mental health moderators based on the information extracted from posts, such as the classifier predicted mental health categories and information specific to the author of the post (e.g. age, social habits).

Although a fully automated approach could be used in both Moderator Assistant and Cybermate, our conversations with stakeholders indicated that an augmentation approach, where the system helps the human accomplish their tasks rather than doing it all, would be more appropriate. The first reason is the accuracy of the system: it is not yet reliable enough so that the intervention could be sent to an end user without the moderators' intervention. Beyond human moderators add valuable life experiences that are most useful to the users'. These past experiences make the moderators' input irreplaceable. Finally, when a moderator provides feedback the benefits arguably go both ways: the user benefits from receiving help, but helping behaviors can also help build the resilience of those who provide it.

The interventions generated by the system can become draft responses aimed at providing template-based information to moderators. The contents of each response is then customized to each target user. This design approach, where moderators can overwrite the computers' writing contributes to the sense of autonomy discussed previously.

There are several architectures for NLG systems, however Reiter and Dale's (2000) has proven suitable with many applications. This architecture includes three main components connected together into a pipeline: *Document Planner*, *Microplanner*, and *Surface Realiser* with the input and output of each component represented by *Message*, *Document Plan* and *Text Specification*. Figure 4 gives the overview of the proposed NLG architecture for mental health interventions.

The first step is *Content Determination*, where the extracted mental health categories (from text-classifiers) are mapped into corresponding information to construct *Messages*. Each *Message* represents a chunk of information that is grouped together to express a specific meaning (e.g. greeting, comforting, suggestion, encouragement, etc.).

*Figure 4. Overview of NLG architecture for mental health interventions*
*Hussain et al., 2015.*

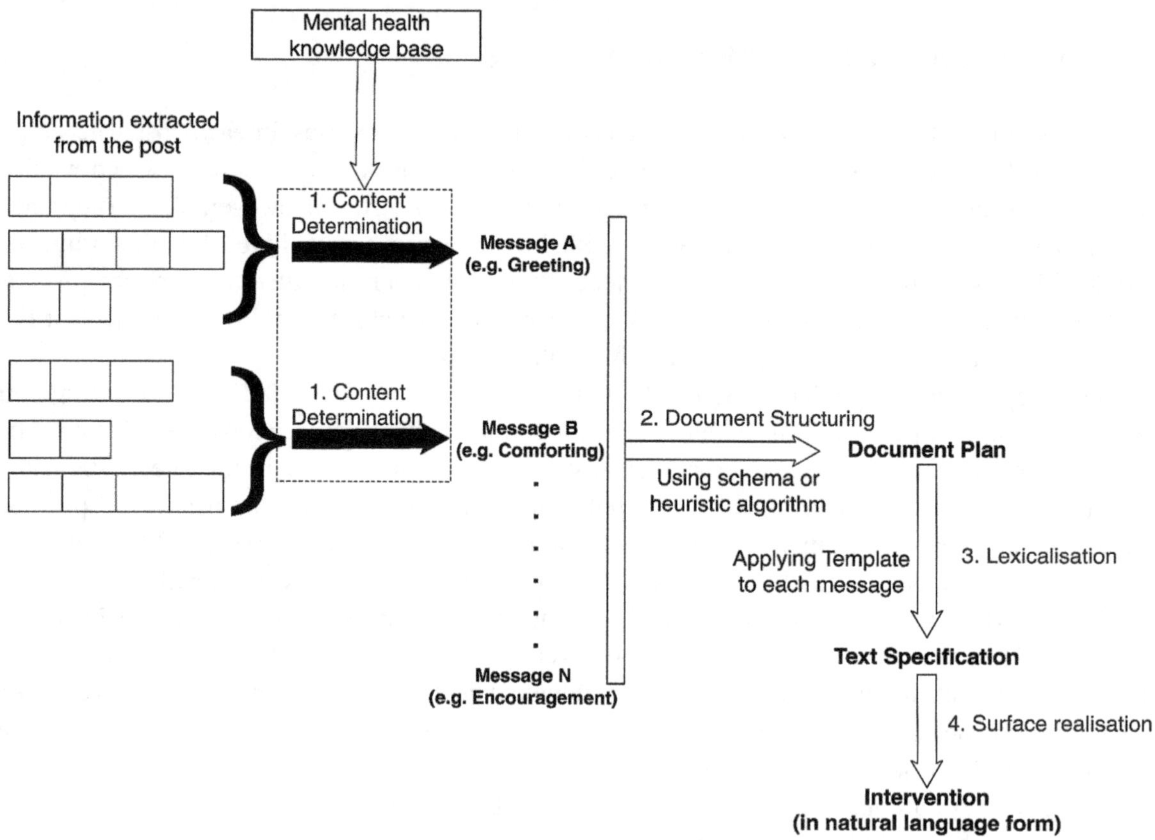


The second step is *Document Structuring*, where the *Messages* are combined using schema and heuristic algorithm to obtain a *Document Plan*. Following this the *Text Specification* is achieved by the *Lexicalization* and *Aggregation* process, which contains all the information and the sentence structure. The *Text Specification* is then passed to the *Surface Realiser*, to obtain the real text from the abstract representations. The final outcome of the process will provide the complete interventions.

Intervention templates for each of the mental health categories were collected from mental health professionals (e.g. psychologists, trained moderators) for the *Content Determination* phase. The clinical and moderator based intervention templates will provide well-formed and well-structured sentences for *Messages* in the *Content Determination* stage (Hussain et al., 2015).

## Future Opportunities for Generating Interventions

Beyond NLG, there are other techniques we can draw on to augment a moderator's ability to quickly craft appropriate responses. One is to employ a recommendation engine (Resnick and Varian, YEAR) to identify appropriate external resources for moderators to share and link to. For example, the moderator responding to *MemphisBelle* in Figure 2 might naturally provide a fact sheet about self-esteem or refer her to other, more specialized online services. At the very bottom of the figure *Blythe* has inserted a link to a brain training activity. The time and effort required to build these links could be greatly reduced by a recommendation engine that analyzes a help-seeker's language use and past behavior, and the behavior of similar users. It is likely that the triage classifiers described previously—which essentially provide a high-level diagnosis of the poster's needs—would provide valuable input to the recommender.

There is also an opportunity to apply the same text similarity measures commonly employed to combat plagiarism (Clough, 2003). In this context they could warn a moderator that the response they are currently crafting is excessively similar to previous responses, and encourage them to carefully consider what makes the current case unique. This would be most useful when tailoring the automatically generated responses like the ones shown in Figure 3, but could also be relevant when moderators construct replies from scratch; even humans can become formulaic.

Finally we are exploring how tracking the impact of the interventions, by counting the number of times people click through a link to a resource, may help moderators' understand the positive impact of their work. Understanding the positive impact of an altruistic behavior is known to support resilience and more willingness to help others (Peters and Calvo, 2014). Resilience may also help to reduce burnout and improve moderators' wellbeing.

## SUPPORTING SYNCHRONOUS ONE-ON-ONE CONVERSATIONS

The *Triage* and *Intervention Generator* systems described above both augment ReachOut's existing services. Our third system, *Cybermate*, is a chatbox where users can have conversations with trained moderators. Cybermate opens up an entirely new mode of service that is increasingly used in customer service, yet is not common for mental health support services. By allowing visitors to engage in private, one-on-one conversations with the volunteer moderators, they can receive help in a way we expect will be more engaging and effective.

Figure 5 shows a new widget that allows visitors to initiate chatting with ReachOut moderators. Here the (fictitious) visitor is taking the chat seriously, and the moderator will be able to help them by guiding them to appropriate materials. However, many other visitors might be less genuine, or might have expectations that the moderators cannot meet. While these moderators have a great deal of experience communicating with youth and detailed knowledge of the resources available, they are not psychologists; it is important for ReachOut to ensure that the peer-support is not a substitute for professional medical assistance.

Before looking for ways to automate and augmentate the work of the moderators using Cybermate, we are exploring how it could benefit end users, and support the cost-benefit analysis for the organisation. We have not yet attempted to support one-on-one chats at scale, but have instead focused on efficiently answering some key questions:

- Do ReachOut visitors want one-on-one interaction? What are they looking for when they engage? This will be useful to understand if this type of immediate help, may for example, be sought for the positive psychology type interventions available in Reachout or if these users require immediate care not offered by the organisation.
- Do ReachOut moderators want to provide it? Is it within their scope to provide it?
- How much time does this one-on-one support require? Can it scale? What can we do to make the moderator's job easier?

*Figure 5. The Cybermate chat widget*

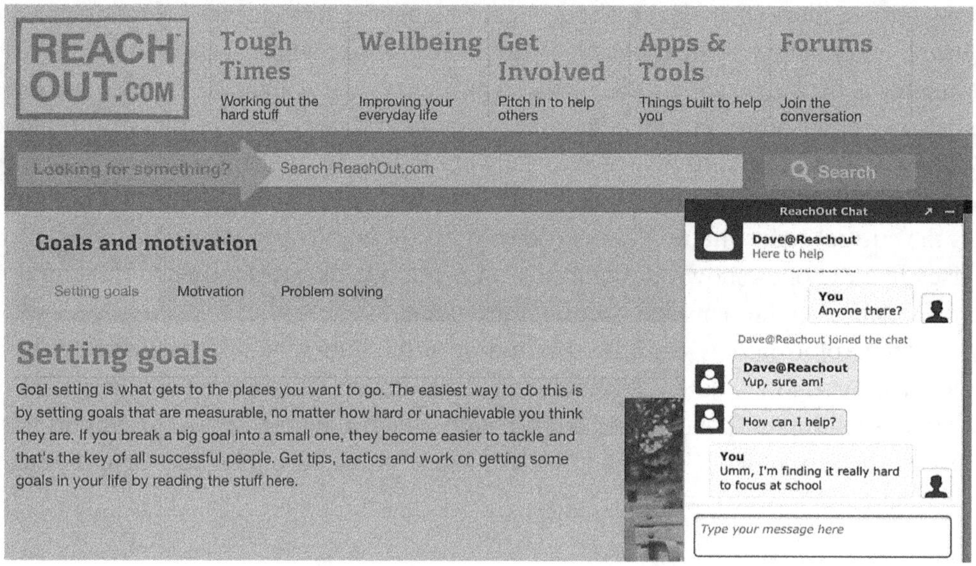


- What types of duty of care issues might come up? How will we handle an interaction with, for example, a person considering suicide?

To begin answering our questions, the chat widget has been introduced to the site provisionally during low volume periods. All activity is collected in the analytics platform presented in Figure 6. Here we have a summary of several chats, where each chat transcript is paired with feedback from both parties; the visitor and the moderator. The moderator follows a script to assess the visitor's eligibility (based on age), gain their informed consent for the data collection, and to deal with any visitors who appear to be in crisis. The decisions they make while following the script are stored, along with responses to a short survey in which the moderator assesses whether the chat was a worthwhile use of their time. Visitors who are eligible, consent to participate, and who are not in crisis are also asked to complete a short survey, which captures their feelings before and after the chat.

The collected data gives us a clear idea of how much effort is expended in the chat, and how each party feels about it. So far the resulting data is encouraging; a good proportion of visitors are genuine, and have needs that can be met by ReachOut staff. We have not yet encounteredanyone in crisis, and almost all visitors are comfortable with the collection of anonymized data for research purposes. Each chat is time-consuming, but the experiment is already collecting the data we need to support the mod-

*Figure 6. The Cybermate chat log*

| Started | Visitor | Transcript | Visitor Feedback | Moderator Feedback |
|---|---|---|---|---|
| 3 months ago | Visitor 88164291 | 47 messages in 20 minutes | started fine and left better | worthwhile |
| 4 months ago | Visitor 46399352 | 45 messages in 37 minutes | not applicable | in crisis |
| 4 months ago | Visitor 19553285 | 36 messages in 35 minutes | started anxious and left better | worthwhile |
| 4 months ago | Visitor 74813905 | 4 messages in 7 minutes | not applicable | ineligable |

erators with suggested responses. In future we hope to conduct a range of Natural Language Processing and Recommendation experiments, such as:

- Automatically diagnosing the needs and mood of the visitor,
- Recommending links to relevant resources, for the moderator to share,
- Autosuggesting messages for the moderator, based on Natural Language Generation and similar chat discussions from the past.

These opportunities for augmentation are very similar to those presented previously in the section about Moderator Assistant. In some ways, Cybermate's private chats are a more forgiving venue for augmentation than the public many-to-many conversations addressed by Triage and Intervention Generator. Here each conversation is seen by a single visitor, so there is less danger that repetition will be detected across them. However, the real-time nature of the conversations will add pressure; in our experience users become frustrated if the moderator (or algorithm) takes longer than a minute or two to reply.

## DISCUSSION

### Automation vs. Augmentation

We have mentioned the design trade-offs between an automation and augmentation focus to online moderator support software. These trade-offs are common, yet not always acknowledged in technology projects. ReachOut is not the only organisation with the challenge of providing services to more people, while maintaining the quality, and existing resource levels. One design approach is to automate as much of the process as possible, replacing unnecessary human effort with computational approaches (Davenport, 2013). For example, interactive voice response systems allow people to get support by navigating a set of menu options using their voice (e.g., over the phone) and have been used in the management and treatment of chronic disease - see Piette (2000) for a review. Mundt (1997) for example, argued that such systems should be used as a cost-efficient part of mental health services. One could foresee using this approach in mental health services that allow users to provide information and find resources without having to speak, or write to, an actual human. These approaches might have some benefits beyond the obvious cost reduction. There is evidence for example, that some people (e.g. those with social anxiety) may be more candid when interacting with a computer than with another human. Yet, some people may feel the need to reach out to others in difficult times, often when they feel lonely and vulnerable. There is the risk that an automated response system could feel unsatisfactory and dehumanising during a time when an individual may be seeking out human contact/support. Despite this risk, automation design approaches are persistently popular approach because they are cost efficient.

In many projects a more helpful organic/suitable approach is to augment human abilities. In the case study provided here, we would argue that, helping employees and volunteers in mental health services respond to more people more accurately and efficiently improves service delivery but does not compromise the quality of the peer-support model of ReachOut. Humans are better than computers at social interactions, but computers are better than humans at processing large amounts of data. For example, log files that point to the amount of times a user has accessed a service, the time and the type of language they used (something known to reflect their mood). This information can be utilized to inform peer interventions highlighting the history of an individual unknown to them, identifying people at risk and generating interventions (e.g. canned or template responses to posts/emails). Technologies can also help connect people, e.g. the service providers, in new and more efficient ways, and these connections can be used to enhance the quality of services offered.

## Principles of Positive Computing

The automation vs. augmentation trade-offs can be taken into account in the design of a system by considering how they impact different determinants of wellbeing. Positive Computing (Calvo. & Peters, 2014) provides a theoretical framework to do so. In the previous sections we discussed how different design decisions have an impact on the moderators sense of competence, autonomy and relatedness: how the classification/labeling of the texts may influence moderator's sense of competence when it is different to their own; how the discussions between moderators may affect their sense of belonging to a community; and how the assignment of tasks may affect their sense of autonomy. Our interpretations of the impact of different designs are based on research from psychology, in particular Self-Determination Theory (Ryan and Deci, 2001). It is already known that introducing new systems, or adapting existing ones, within an organization will often have an impact on the behavior and psychology (e.g. autonomy, competence, relatedness, job satisfaction, etc.) of the workforce (Calvo. & Peters, 2014; Gagné, 2003). For example, it has been reported that implementation of enterprise systems influence employee's job characteristics such as job demand, job control and job satisfaction (Bala & Venkatesh, 2013). These considerations are critical for ReachOut and similar organizations, because:

1. The helping nature of the work, where the moderators must deal with distressing content, increases the likelihood of burnout and trauma (Conrad, 2006) and
2. The risk maybe higher because moderators are often volunteers who have themselves suffered mental illness.

In this chapter we have described a first approach on how to design a tool to improve productivity and efficacy while taking into consideration these two important concerns. Regrettably we still lack definitive results about the impact the features described have had on users autonomy, competence and relatedness.

We see *Positive Computing* (Calvo. & Peters, 2014) as a way of bringing positive psychology principles to the design of all technologies. Considering these trade-offs can help engineers and designers think of new ways to go beyond supporting the recovery of end users, and also contribute to the moderators' ongoing wellbeing. In future work we plan to look for ways to support their resilience, for example by using behavioral analytics and visualizations that allow moderators to see when people read their posts and follow their advice. These and other ways to track the impact of the interventions they provide shows that their efforts are having an impact (Peters & Calvo, 2014).

A limitation to the current discussion is that we are still in the process of evaluating the impact of such design choices on factors known to affect workplace wellbeing including autonomy, competence and relatedness.

## CONCLUSION

We have described three new systems that support moderators of online peer-support groups. Although we wanted to improve efficiency and productivity it is important to take a critical design approach and explore how design may have an impact on the psychological wellbeing of *all* users, including the moderators of the forums.

We have discussed two designs approaches for mental health services: automation, where the computer is aimed at reducing the need for human effort to reduce time and cost, and augmentation, where the computer is instead aiming to enhance human abilities. These two design approaches rarely come individually, i.e. many systems would have features of both, so the distinction is for the purpose of identifying design principles only.

Furthermore, we hypothesize that each design approach (automation and augmentation) will influence the stakeholders in different ways. In one design, where automation is considered paramount, automated responses can be sent (at least technically) directly to users. As many have argued this can reduce costs and time, but it also means trusting that the algorithms interpreted correctly the need of the user and that the generated intervention is appropriate and useful. Furthermore, when this approach is taken we should ask important questions such as: how would the recipient feel when the system makes a mistake? Or should the user even be told the message was computer generated?

In augmented support, these responses can be edited, corrected and administered by human volunteers who then deliver them to individuals through social media or online forums. In this scenario, the computer aims to help the human provide a better intervention. For example, an information extraction phase can provide a way to triage people at risk of mental health issues, and highlight issues that the human moderator might have missed.

## ACKNOWLEDGMENT

Calvo is supported by an ARC Future Fellowship and Milne by an ARC Linkage Project. This project is funded by the Young and Well Cooperative Research Centre, an Australian-based international research centre that unites young people with researchers, practitioners, innovators and policy-makers from over 70 partner organisations. Together we explore the role of technology in young people's lives, and how it can be used to improve the mental health and wellbeing of young people aged 12-25. The Young and Well CRC is established under the Australian Government's Cooperative Research Centres Program.

## REFERENCES

Bala, H., & Venkatesh, V. (2013). Changes in employees' job characteristics during an enterprise system implementation: A latent growth modeling perspective. *Management Information Systems Quarterly*, *37*(4), 1113–1140.

Barak, A., & Grohol, J. M. (2011). Current and future trends in internet-supported mental health interventions. *Journal of Technology in Human Services*, *29*(3), 155–196. doi:10.1080/15228835.2011.616939

Bordes, A. et al.. (2005). Fast kernel classifiers with online and active learning. *Journal of Machine Learning Research*, *6*, 1579–1619.

Botella, C., Riva, G., Gaggioli, A., Wiederhold, B. K., Alcaniz, M., & Baños, R. M. (2012). The present and future of positive technologies. *Cyberpsychology, Behavior, and Social Networking*, *15*(2), 78–84. doi:10.1089/cyber.2011.0140 PMID:22149078

Burns, J. M., Davenport, T. A., Durkin, L. A., Luscombe, G. M., & Hickie, I. B. (2010). The internet as a setting for mental health service utilisation by young people. *The Medical Journal of Australia*, *192*(11), S22–S26. PMID:20528703

Calvo, R., Peters, D., Johnson, D., & Rogers, Y. (2014). Autonomy in Technology Design. In *CHI'14 Extended Abstracts on Human Factors in Computing Systems*. Toronto: ACM. doi:10.1145/2559206.2560468

Calvo, R. A., & Peters, D. (2014). *Positive Computing: Technology for Well-Being and Human Potential*. MIT Press.

Carbone, S., Rickwood, D., & Tanti, C. (2011, October). Workforce shortages and their impact on Australian youth mental health service reform. *Advances in Mental Health*, *10*(1), 92–97. doi:10.5172/jamh.2011.10.1.92

Christensen, H., & Hickie, I. B. (2010). E-mental health: A new era in delivery of mental health services. *The Medical Journal of Australia*, *192*(11), S2. PMID:20528702

Clarke, G., & Yarborough, B. J. (2013). Evaluating the promise of health IT to enhance/expand the reach of mental health services. *General Hospital Psychiatry*, *35*(4), 339–344. doi:10.1016/j.genhosppsych.2013.03.013 PMID:23701698

Clough, P. (2003). Old and new challenges in automatic plagiarism detection. *National Plagiarism Advisory Service, 2003.* Retrieved from http://ir.shef.ac.uk/cloughie/index.html

Collin, P. J., Metcalf, A. T., Stephens-Reicher, J. C., Blanchard, M. E., Herrman, H. E., Rahilly, K., & Burns, J. M. (2011, October). ReachOut.com: The role of an online service for promoting help-seeking in young people. *Advances in Mental Health*, *10*(1), 39–51. doi:10.5172/jamh.2011.10.1.39

Conrad, D., & Kellar-Guenther, Y. (2006). Compassion fatigue, burnout, and compassion satisfaction among Colorado child protection workers. *Child Abuse & Neglect*, *30*(10), 1071–1080. doi:10.1016/j.chiabu.2006.03.009 PMID:17014908

Currell, R., Urquhart, C., Wainwright, P., & Lewis, R. (2000). Telemedicine versus face to face patient care: Effects on professional practice and health care outcomes. *Cochrane Database of Systematic Reviews* Cd002098. doi:10.1002/14651858.cd002098 PMID:10796678

Davenport, T. H. (2013). *Process innovation: reengineering work through information technology*. Harvard Business Press.

DiMarco, C., Covvey, H. D., Bray, P., Cowan, D., DiCiccio, V., Hovy, E.,... Mulholland, D. (2007). The development of a natural language generation system for personalized e-health information. *Paper presented at the Medinfo 2007: the 12th World Congress on Health (Medical) Informatics; Building Sustainable Health Systems*.

Doherty, G., Coyle, D., & Sharry, J. (2012, May 5–10). Engagement with online mental health interventions: an exploratory clinical study of a treatment for depression. *Paper presented at the SIGCHI Conference on Human Factors in Computing Systems*, Austin, Texas, USA. doi:10.1145/2207676.2208602

Eysenbach, G., Powell, J., Englesakis, M., Rizo, C., & Stern, A. (2004). Health related virtual communities and electronic support groups: Systematic review of the effects of online peer to peer interactions. *BMJ (Clinical Research Ed.), 328*(7449), 1166. doi:10.1136/bmj.328.7449.1166 PMID:15142921

Ford, M., Wyeth, P., & Johnson, D. (2012, November). Self-determination theory as applied to the design of a software learning system using whole-body controls. *Proceedings of the 24th Australian Computer-Human Interaction Conference* (pp. 146-149). ACM. doi:10.1145/2414536.2414562

Friedman, B., Kahn, P. H., Jr., & Borning, A. (2006). Value sensitive design and information systems. In Human-computer interaction in management information systems: Foundations (Vol. 4). ME Sharpe.

Gagné. (2014). *Marylene. The Oxford handbook of work engagement, motivation, and self-determination theory*. Oxford University Press.

Gagné, M. (2003). The role of autonomy support and autonomy orientation in prosocial behavior engagement. *Motivation and Emotion, 27*(3), 199–223. doi:10.1023/A:1025007614869

Griffiths, K., Farrer, L., & Christensen, H. (2010). The efficacy of internet interventions for depres- sion and anxiety disorders: A review of randomised controlled trials. *The Medical Journal of Australia, 192*, S4–S11. PMID:20528707

Grohol, J. M., Anthony, K., Nagel, D. A. N., & Goss, S. (2010). Using Websites, blogs and wikis in mental health. In *The use of technology in mental health applications ethics and practice* (pp. 68-75).

Hoyt, T., & Pasupathi, M. (2008). Blogging about trauma: Linguistic measures of apparent recovery. *Relaunching soon, 4*(2), 56.

Hussain, M. S., Calvo, R. A., Ellis, L., Li, J., Ospina-Pinillos, L., Davenport, T., & Hickie, I. (2015). NLG-Based Moderator Response Generator to Support Mental Health. *Paper presented at the 33rd Annual ACM Conference Extended Abstracts on Human Factors in Computing Systems*. doi:10.1145/2702613.2732758

Littlewood, W. (1996). Autonomy: An Anatomy and a Framework. *System, 24*(4), 427–435. doi:10.1016/S0346-251X(96)00039-5

Liu, M., Calvo, R. A., Davenport, T., & Hickie, I. (2013, Nov 26). Moderator Assistant: helping those who help via online mental health support groups. *Paper presented at the Joint Workshop on Smart Health and Social Therapies, OzChi2013*, Adelaide, Australia.

National Survey of Mental Health and Wellbeing Summary of results. (2007). Australian Bureau of Statistics: Australian Bureau of Statistics, Canberra.

Pennebaker, J. W., Francis, M. E., & Booth, R. J. (2001). Linguistic Inquiry and Word Count (LIWC): A computerized text analysis program. Mahwah (NJ), 7.

Peters, D., & Calvo, R. (2014). Compassion vs. empathy: designing for resilience. *interactions, 21*(5), 48-53.

Piette, J. D. (2000). Interactive voice response systems in the diagnosis and management of chronic disease. *The American Journal of Managed Care*, *6*(7), 817–827. PMID:11067378

Reiter, E. (1999). Natural Language Generation in STOP. Retrieved from http://inf.abdn.ac.uk/research/stop/stop-nlg.htm

Reiter, E., Dale, R., & Feng, Z. (2000). *Building natural language generation systems* (Vol. 33). MIT Press. doi:10.1017/CBO9780511519857

Resnick, P., & Varian, H. R. (1997). Recommender systems. *Communications of the ACM*, *40*(3), 56–58. doi:10.1145/245108.245121

Riva, G., Banos, R. M., Botella, C., Wiederhold, B. K., & Gaggioli, A. (2012). Positive technology: Using interactive technologies to promote positive functioning. *Cyberpsychology, Behavior, and Social Networking*, *15*(2), 69–77. doi:10.1089/cyber.2011.0139 PMID:22149077

Riva, G., Calvo, R. A., & Lisetti, C. (2015). Cyberpsychology Applications of Affective Computing. In R. A. Calvo, S. K. D'Mello, J. Gratch, & A. Kappas (Eds.), *Handbook of Affective Computing*. New York: Oxford University Press.

Ryan, R., & Deci, E. (2000). Intrinsic and Extrinsic Motivations: Classic Definitions and New Directions. *Contemporary Educational Psychology*, *25*(1), 54–67. doi:10.1006/ceps.1999.1020 PMID:10620381

Ryan, R. M., & Deci, E. L. (2001). On Happiness and Human Potentials: A Review of Research on Hedonic and Eudaimonic Well-Being. *Annual Review of Psychology*, *52*(1), 141–166. doi:10.1146/annurev.psych.52.1.141 PMID:11148302

Ryan, R. M., Rigby, C. S., & Przybylski, A. (2006). The motivational pull of video games: A self-determination theory approach. *Motivation and Emotion*, *30*(4), 344–360. doi:10.1007/s11031-006-9051-8

Schueller, S. M., & Parks, A. C. (2012). Disseminating self-help: Positive psychology exercises in an online trial. *Journal of Medical Internet Research*, *14*(3), e63. doi:10.2196/jmir.1850 PMID:22732765

Slade, T., Johnston, A., Oakley Browne, M. A., Andrews, G., & Whiteford, H. (2009). 2007 National Survey of Mental Health and Wellbeing: Methods and key findings. *Australasian Psychiatry*, *43*(7), 594–605. PMID:19530016

Spear, H. J., & Kulbok, P. (2001). Autonomy and adolescence: A concept analysis. *Public Health Nursing (Boston, Mass.)*, *21*(2), 144–152. doi:10.1111/j.0737-1209.2004.021208.x PMID:14987214

Strecher, V. (2007). Internet methods for delivering behavioral and health-related interventions (eHealth). *Annual Review of Clinical Psychology*, *3*(1), 53–76. doi:10.1146/annurev.clinpsy.3.022806.091428 PMID:17716048

The World health report: 2001: Mental health: new understanding, new hope. (2001). *World Health Organization*.

Van Bilsen, H. (2013). *Cognitive behaviour therapy in the real world: Back to basics*. Karnac Books.

Varges, S., Bieler, H., Stede, M., Faulstich, L. C., Irsig, K., & Atalla, M. (2012, May 23-25). SemScribe: Natural Language Generation for Medical Reports. *Paper presented at the Eighth International Conference on Language Resources and Evaluation (LREC)*, Istanbul, Turkey.

Webb, M., Burns, J., & Collin, P. (2008). Providing online support for young people with mental health difficulties: Challenges and opportunities explored. *Early Intervention in Psychiatry*, *2*(2), 108–113. doi:10.1111/j.1751-7893.2008.00066.x PMID:21352141

Wiemer-Hastings, K., Janit, A. S., Wiemer-Hastings, P. M., Cromer, S., & Kinser, J. (2004). Automatic classification of dysfunctional thoughts: A feasibility test. *Behavior Research Methods, Instruments, & Computers*, *36*(2), 203–212. doi:10.3758/BF03195565 PMID:15354685

Ybarra, M., & Eaton, W. (2005). Internet-Based Mental Health Interventions. *Mental Health Services Research*, *7*(2), 75–87. doi:10.1007/s11020-005-3779-8 PMID:15974154

## KEY TERMS AND DEFINITIONS

**Augmentation:** The process of using computer programs to extend the human capabilities (e.g. moderation in forums), such as identifying members at risk of mental health issues, generating template responses, etc., in order to scale up the number of people they can support.

**Automation:** The process of using computer programs to automatically reduce or eliminate the need for human effort in a specific task.

**Intervention:** What is done to help a client/user, for example comments that contain suggestions, encouragements and online resources (i.e. links) posted by moderators or peer-supporters in response to a post in a mental health forum.

**Moderator:** A trained person who is responsible for reviewing posts in forums in order to identify members at risk of mental health issues and provide them with support through discussions and online resources.

**Natural Language Generation (NLG):** The process of producing text in natural language form (i.e. human-like) using artificial intelligence and computational linguistics.

**Natural Language Processing (NLP):** The use of artificial intelligence, machine learning and computational linguistics for computer applications to understand human speech/text.

**Online Peer-Support:** The process of providing and receiving support for a particular problem (e.g. mental health) through the members (i.e. community) of online forums with similar experience and knowledge.

**Positive Computing:** The design and development of technology to support wellbeing and human potential.

**Triage:** The process of prioritising posts/members based on the severity of the identified mental health issue (e.g. self harm).

# Chapter 5
# What Do Elderly Users Want and Need from Fitness Technologies?
## Findings from the ELF@Home Project

**John Waterworth**
*Umeå University, Sweden*

**Eva Waterworth**
*Umeå University, Sweden*

**Paula Álvarez**
*SGGPA, Spain*

**José Gutiérrez**
*SGGPA, Spain*

**Juan Luis Carús**
*CTIC Technology Centre, Spain*

**Sonia Garcia**
*CTIC Technology Centre, Spain*

## ABSTRACT

*It is well known that physical exercise has a significant beneficial effect on mental and physical health, and elderly fitness programs are a good and widely accepted approach to prevent frailty. In this chapter, we examine what elderly people actually want and need when it comes to technologies designed to support and encourage their physical fitness. We present the ELF@Home project as a case study, and report design insights and other results from user involvement in the project. User involvement is a key component of the approach and uses methods such as interviews, focus group meetings, early component and prototype tests with users, as well as inputs from medical experts. ELF@Home is a clear example of a "Positive Technology" approach. The project proposes the adoption of new technology in everyday life from the perspective of positive psychology, approaching this aim by designing devices and systems that are actually usable and desirable in supporting extended healthy living for this target population.*

## INTRODUCTION

According to the Constitution of the World Health Authority: "Health is a state of complete physical, mental and social well-being and not merely the absence of disease or infirmity" (WHO, 1948). Physical and mental wellbeing cannot be completely separated, and indeed go together in most current conceptions of health and, in particular, in successful ageing. Thanks to increasing computing power, reduced size

DOI: 10.4018/978-1-4666-9986-1.ch005

and costs of electronic components such as sensors and displays, it is now both possible and affordable for individual elderly people to be supported by technology that encourages them to exercise to maintain fitness and also allows them to check their own health status regularly. Sensor-based devices and popular interaction technologies developed for computer games make it feasible to design health- and fitness-supporting devices for use by the elderly at home and even when out of doors.

In this chapter, we examine the question of what elderly people – in the age range from 75 years and upwards – actually want and need when it comes to such technologies. How can we design devices and systems that are actually usable and desirable to support extended healthy living for this target population? Unless we can do that, the potential of technology to provide this kind of support for successful ageing will not be fulfilled. And how do we know whether or not we have succeeded in that aim? To address these questions, we report on findings from an ongoing project funded by the Ambient Assisted Living Joint Programme – ELF@Home: elderly sELF-care based on sELF-check of health conditions and sELF-fitness at home (ELF@Home, 2015).

## BACKGROUND

### Physical Exercise and the Elderly

Frailty syndrome (Fried et al., 2001) has emerged in recent years as an explanation for age disability when no other relevant pathology exists. Frailty is an important cause of loss of autonomy, conferring a high risk of falls, disability for activities of daily living (ADL disability), cognitive disease, hospitalization and mortality. Frailty is considered highly prevalent in old age and according to the SHARE study (Santos-Eggimann, 2009) in ten European countries, more than 42% of the elderly aged over 65 years are pre-frail and 17% are frail.

It is well known that physical exercise has a significant beneficial effect on health, and elderly fitness programs are a good and widely accepted approach to prevent frailty (Cadore et al., 2013) (Liu et al., 2009). Furthermore, in recent years there have been many investigations that conclude that the absence of this exercise is related to the development and worsening of many chronic diseases, such as cardiovascular disease, type 2 diabetes mellitus, colon and breast cancer, and cognitive decline in the elderly (Nascimento et al., 2014).

Ischemic heart disease, along with stroke and other cardiovascular diseases is one of the main causes of death in industrialized countries, and it has been observed that regular physical activity is associated with a lower risk of developing such diseases (Do Lee et al., 2003; Kesaniemi et al., 2001; Liu-Ambrose et al., 2010). In order to establish what kind of exercise would have most benefits for the elderly, it would be wise to consider the following:

- **The Correlation between the Amount of Physical Activity and Health Benefit:** You can get great health benefits by practicing small amounts of exercise and this benefit does not necessarily scale up by increasing the amount of the same, as in the case of ischemic heart disease.
- **The Intensity of Physical Activity:** We know that moderate and high intensity physical activity have a positive effect on cardiovascular health. Although there is no evidence about low intensity exercises, we do know that for people over 65 years of age there is a correlation between walking and a lower risk of ischemic heart disease.

- **Frequency of Physical Activity:** Since it has been shown that in people with cardiovascular risk factors training once a week does not reduce mortality, and practicing sporadic intense exercise even increases the risk of cardiovascular events, experts conclude that practicing exercise 3 times a week, and if possible, every day would be the best option.

Physical activity is also recognized as a highly protective factor in cognitive functions of the elderly, both in normal brain aging and in different stages of cognitive impairment. Many studies on healthy populations have shown how physical exercise is associated with less deterioration of cognitive function, highlighting the improvement in memory and attention. Reviews of the different studies on this topic (García et al., 2007; Kelaiditi et al., 2013), concluded that there is a high probability that exercise would have an impact on cognitive functions, preventing age relating cognitive decline and improving cognitive functions in mild cognitive impairment. Resistance or aerobic activities would be associated with improvements in cognitive performance, while non-aerobic exercises, such as stretching or relaxation, would not offer the same results.

From the point of view of public health, both cardiovascular disease and cognitive impairment are major problems, both for their prevalence and for the economic costs involved. There is an increased dependence on drugs in the prevention of cardiovascular disease, while we can observe a lack of effective pharmacological treatments for cognitive impairment. Therefore an increased emphasis on the value of physical exercise is of high importance, especially in the elderly, who are not always familiar with the need for physical activity and particularly not with organized health-maintenance and fitness-training programmes.

In terms of quality of life, and in particular psychological wellbeing, the amount and type of regular exercise undertaken by elderly persons has been correlated reliably with positive mental states. A large Swedish study (Lindwall et al., 2007) involving 860 persons aged 60-95 found that persons of both genders had lower depression scores if exercising regularly than if generally inactive. Similar findings were reported in several more recent studies, for example Mammen and Faulkner (2013), who stress the role of moderate regular exercise in preventing depression in the elderly.

## ELF@Home: Elderly Self-Care Based on Self-Check of Health Conditions and Self-Fitness at Home

To address these issues the ELF@Home research and innovation project was initiated in June 2013 and is scheduled to run until May 31st 2016. It is co-funded by the Ambient Assisted Living Joint Programme (AAL JP) and National Authorities in Spain, Sweden and Germany. The project approach capitalizes on the proven advantages of elderly fitness maintenance in developing a self-care solution based on self-check of health conditions and self-fitness maintenance at home and out of doors.

The ELF@Home system provides a personalized fitness plan to persuade and motivate elderly users by facilitating and simplifying their access to fitness programmes at home. A self-check system based on the use of various customized sensor devices is used to monitor health status and the activity lifestyle of the user. The system works as a personal trainer, generating for each individual user a personalized fitness plan based on his or her activity performance and health status. To achieve these goals the system is composed of biomedical sensors, a wearable physical activity sensor primarily for outdoor use, a simple TV interface for fitness sessions and a computer vision system used to analyse fitness exercise execution so that feedback and encouragement can be provided during fitness training sessions. These

*Figure 1. The ELF@Home technological vision*

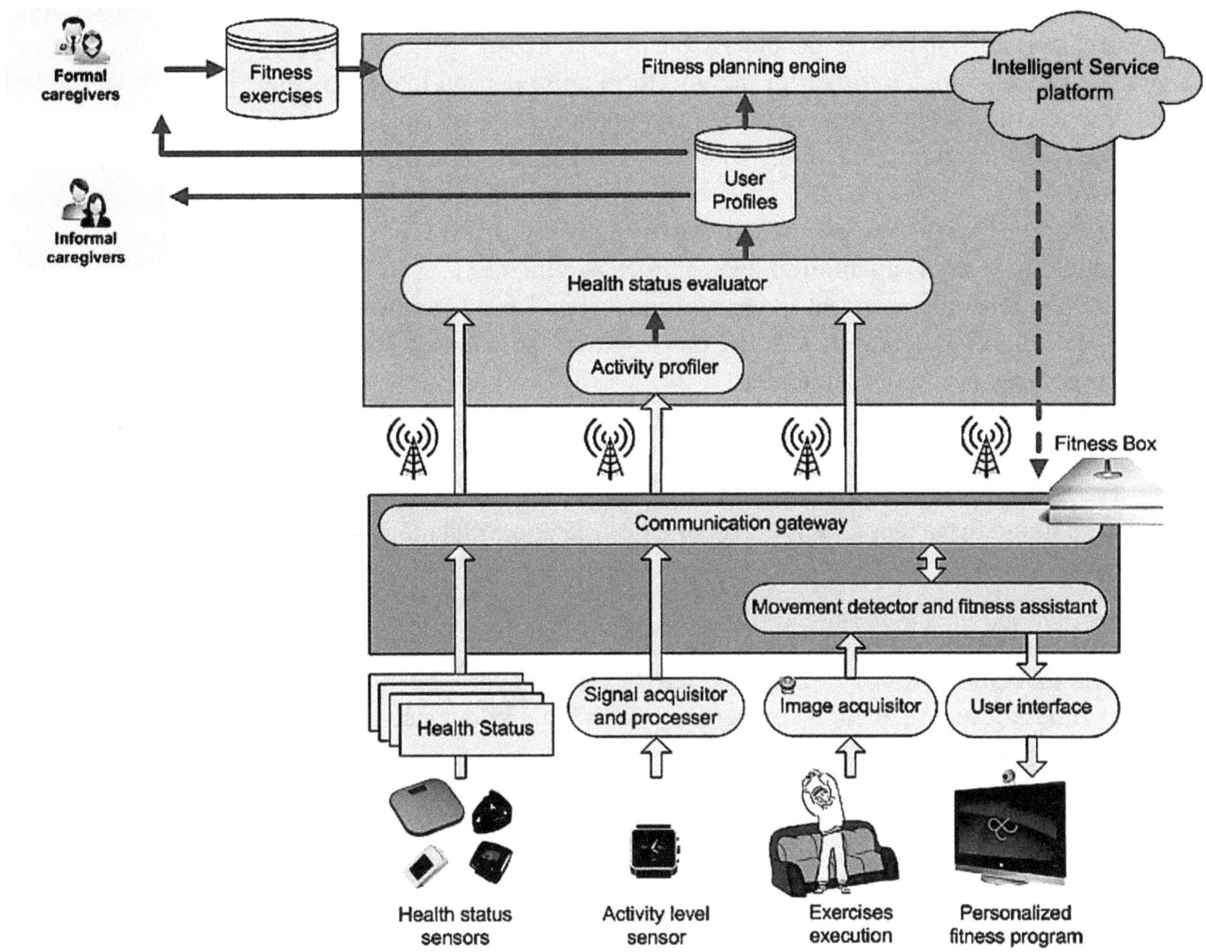


components are connected to the intelligent service platform, which provides customized exercise programmes (see Figure 1).

ELF@Home is a clear example of a "Positive Technology" approach exemplifying the scientific and applied use of technology for improving the quality of personal experience through its structuring (by using a goal, rules, and a feedback system) and personal augmentation (to achieve multimodal and mixed experiences). Based on the known link between mental wellbeing and regular exercise, the project proposes the adoption of new technology in everyday life from the perspective of positive psychology. It approaches this aim by designing devices and systems that are actually usable and desirable in supporting extended healthy living for this target population.

## USER INVOLVEMENT IN THE ELF@HOME PROJECT

The overall aim of user involvement in ELF@Home is to conduct a truly user-driven project, in which the users participate as part of the project team and on their own terms. In this way, the project has a better chance of developing a product or range of products that target users are likely to want to use, and will be able to use. We are working according to the e-Inclusion approach (Waterworth & Waterworth, 2009, 2012), which emphasises the elderly person's full participation in a project by building up their experience of technology in order for them to form opinions and to express their views about the proposed products during the process of design and implementation. This approach was motivated by prior experience with innovating technology with and for elderly users, and in particular the following insights:

- The elderly, like all "age groups" are not homogenous in terms of prior experience with interactive technology, overall capabilities, personalities and interests.
- They are generally reluctant to express their views, needs and priorities as regards new or proposed technology – they tend to be more "polite" than much younger people, less confident of their competence (at least initially).
- Due to their relative lack of exposure to current technologies, it is generally difficult for them to imagine the overall project vision or possibilities of technology.

We have found that to get a useful level of elderly user participation it is necessary to take the above factors into account by

1. Discussing individual needs, preferences and priorities as they relate to the project goals;
2. Forming focus groups of users to broaden the range of characteristics in terms of, for example, age and fitness levels, as well as to overcome individual reluctance to express views, and especially negative views of proposed innovations;
3. Holding regular meetings, with some "added value" for participants beyond the project goals, to maintain interest, keep the target users informed and involved in the innovation process.

This last activity might be something as simple as organizing coffee and cake for the group, or some other social activity such as a meal out or a visit to a place of interest. It is important to establish a social focus group of users, and to get to know individual users, their lifestyles, interests, hobbies, likes and dislikes. In the case of elderly fitness programmes, it is also necessary to obtain detailed guidance from medical experts.

## Who Are the Users?

The target group of the ELF@Home project is older people (aged over 65 years) who are living independently at home and not exhibiting frailty or pre-frailty symptoms. The aim is to empower end-users by allowing them to prevent frailty, dependency and functional decline by maintaining fitness at home. As a result, the use of this solution will help the elderly to stay independently at home and to deal autonomously with the activities of daily living. During the project design, we have involved four groups of users: two Spanish groups and two Swedish groups.

The Spanish primary user test population consisted of two groups. One group lives in a residential facility and consists of 10-15 users, with a 2:1 ratio of female:male, and an average age 80. They have chronic health conditions but no cognitive impairment. The other group consists of 23 females and 1 male, with an average age 85, living in a rural, sparsely-populated area. Both groups are characterised as currently physically inactive.

The Swedish primary users were also composed of two groups, one consisting of 12 users, 8 females and 4 males, with an age range of 70-85 years. They live independently, in the town of Skellefteå or the surrounding areas. The other group consists of 15 users, 10 females and 5 males, with an age range of 65-87 years. They live independently, mostly in the small town of Åsele or the surrounding rural areas. Both Swedish groups are characterized as physically active in general, though most have some health issues.

In both countries, potential users were identified by providers of social and health care, who verified that they met the project criteria of age and absence of cognitive impairment. From these, participants were self-selected into the project by indicating their willingness to take part and to try the technology and associated exercise programmes. None of the users had measured their own fitness or performance on any physical activities prior to their involvement in the project.

The Barthel Scale (Mahoney & Barthel, 1965) was used for selecting users to take part in the field trials. It is used to measure users' performance in activities of daily living (personal hygiene, dressing, eating, etc.). Fitness of users was assessed using the Short Physical Performance Battery (SPPB) (Guralnik et al., 1994) for evaluating lower extremity functioning in older persons. The result of this test is highly related to frailty, mortality and cognitive impairment. The SPPB test was used for evaluating performance in balance and in gait speed. Users carry out this test before the beginning of the field trials, half way through, and at the end, to determine whether their performance has improved.

Users are involved in the following project activities:

- Design of exercises, exercise programmes and fitness plans.
- Specification of fitness measures.
- Gathering users' functional and interface/interaction requirements:
  - Guided interviews with individual users.
  - Brainstorming with focus groups of elderly people.
  - Health/exercise information from medical experts.
  - Feedback and suggestions on specific design questions from users.
- Evaluating approach, components and overall system:
  - Conceptual evaluation.
  - Component tests and early prototype tests.
  - System prototype tests.
- Field trials.

## FITNESS ACTIVITIES AND MEASURES

The ELF@Home system will be able to collect a set of health indicators in order to track the health status of elderly users and to provide them with a personalized fitness program. The sensor-based measures collection is crucial to guarantee the effectiveness of the fitness activities and to prevent health-related problems. The choice of sensors to be used is based on user requirements (health status and/or problems).

Table 1 shows the measures proposed to define the user health status. For each proposed measure the measurement method and the acquisition frequency are described. The cardiovascular measures are the most important and they will be collected by the user using electronic sensors. The ELF@Home solution will evaluate the cardiovascular measures to decide if the user is in healthy conditions to do fitness activities and to evaluate the fitness plan execution. Anthropometric and functional ability measurements

*Table 1. Measures used to define user health status*

| | Measure | Method | Frequency |
|---|---|---|---|
| Cardiovascular measures | Blood pressure | Measured by the user using biomedical electronic sensors | Before, immediately after and one minute after exercising |
| | Heart frequency | | |
| | Oxygen saturation | | |
| Anthropometric measures | Weight | Measured by medical experts | Weekly |
| | Height | | |
| | Waist circumference | | |
| | Brachial perimeter | | |
| | Body mass index | | |
| Functional measures | Balance (standing on each foot) | Measured by medical experts | Monthly |
| | Walking speed | | |
| | Grip strength | | |

will be carried out by experts, and they will be used to evaluate the effectiveness of the fitness plan and to track the evolution of users' health and fitness status.

Healthy conditions to do exercises are defined using the following thresholds. If a user has medical values outside of the healthy thresholds, he or she should be advised to see a doctor.

- **Maximum Heart Rate:** 60% of $HR_{max}$.
  - $HR_{max}$ = 220 bpm – age (for males).
  - $HR_{max}$ = 210 bpm – age (for females).
- **Maximum Blood Pressure:** 160/90 mmHg.
- **Minimum Oxygen Saturation:** 92%.

Depending on the user profile, the fitness exercises suggested to the user will be different. The fitness plan is divided into 16 levels as can be seen in the Table 2. Each level is characterized by a number of series, repetitions and resting time between exercises. All users will start at level 1 and they will progress depending on their health status and their activity performance.

*Table 2. Fitness plans*

| Level | 1 | 2 | 3 | 4 | 5 | 6 | 7 | 8 | 9 | 10 | 11 | 12 | 13 | 14 | 15 |
|---|---|---|---|---|---|---|---|---|---|---|---|---|---|---|---|
| # Series | 2 | 2 | 3 | 3 | 3 | 3 | 3 | 3 | 3 | 3 | 3 | 3 | 3 | 3 | 3 |
| # Repetitions | 8 | 10 | 10 | 12 | 12 | 12 | 15 | 15 | 15 | 20 | 20 | 20 | 25 | 25 | 25 |
| # Resistance Exercises | 2 | | | | | | | | | | | | | | |
| # Strength Exercises | 2 | | | | | | | | | | | | | | |
| Resting Time | 45" | | | | | | | | | | | | | | |

*Table 3. The exercises*

| Type | Name | Objective |
|---|---|---|
| Resistance | Knee lifts | Gait and balance improvement |
| | Balance with a chair | Static balance |
| | Balance without a chair | Static balance |
| | Tandem gait | Dynamic balance |
| | Lateral walking | Dynamic balance |
| | Leg extension in a chair | Leg resistance |
| | Curl | Arm resistance |
| | Shoulder press | Shoulder resistance |
| Strength | Standing from a chair | Strength endurance |
| | Arms extension | Strength endurance |
| | Squat | Strength endurance |
| | Forward lunge | Strength endurance |
| | Backward lunge | Strength endurance |
| | Hip adduction | Strength endurance |
| | Trunk twist | Strength endurance |

At the beginning of the activity program, depending on the anthropometric measures and the functional measures, a medical expert will decide which exercises are not adequate for the user.

The exercises planning for each day should be generated randomly to provide a specific number of exercises from the resistance group and from the strength group. The exercise planning should be generated to last about 20 minutes including a warm-up stage. Table 3 shows the proposed exercises designed by medical experts and specifically for elderly people. For each exercise, its type and objective are described.

## USER FUNCTIONAL AND INTERFACE REQUIREMENTS

We tested the home-fitness idea and some approaches to motion-based interfaces in order to gather the users' functional and interface requirements and provide recommendations for the designers. In turn the designers proposed different approaches for each part of the interface to the elderly, in order to get their advice and feedback.

### Functional Requirements

The initial aim was to establish the functionalities of the complete service by taking into account end users opinions, as well as medical and enterprises expertise. Functional requirements are listed in Table 4.

The activity sensor is one of the main components of the ELF@Home solution and its functionality was widely discussed during the design stage. For a meaningful analysis of user activities, the activity sensor has to be able to measure movement in all axes, and heart rate. The minimum requirement for tracking the user's movement is to measure relative movement of the user. This could be done using

*Table 4. Functional requirements for ELF@Home*

| No. | Requirement | Importance | Description |
|---|---|---|---|
| FR1 | Sensor devices easy interaction | High | Sensors must be easy-to-use and unobtrusive |
| FF2 | Fitness exercises support | High | It must be a Combination of resistance and strength exercises |
| FR3 | Caregiver health status evaluation | Medium | At the start of the program, a formal caregiver must evaluate the user health status deciding which exercises are not adequate for him |
| FR4 | Medical variables acquisition | High | The system should indicate users the variables to be acquired according to the frequency acquisition. |
| FR5 | Check health conditions to do exercises | High | The health status must be analysed to detect if the user has healthy conditions to do the exercises. |
| FR6 | Warm up exercises support | High | Users must warm up before doing physical exercises |
| FR7 | Fitness exercises personalization support | High | Fitness exercises must be personalized for each user according to its health status.<br>The fitness exercises must be divided into levels and users will change the level according to its improvements. |
| FR8 | Fitness exercise sessions generation | Medium | Fitness exercise sessions must last around 20 minutes. They must be dynamic to improve the user motivation and combining equitably resistance and strength exercises. |
| FR9 | Fitness exercise assistance support | High | The system must assist elderly doing the exercises. It must encourage elderly and detect if they are not doing the exercise rightly. |
| FR10 | Outdoor exercises support | Low | The system should suggest outdoor exercises to users. |
| FR11 | Exercises motivation support | High | The exercises motivation is crucial to the system to ensure user involvement |

three accelerometers and three gyroscopes. For an absolute reference of the movement three magnetometer sensors should be used. Based on this sensor data it will be possible to determine the position of the user while moving (angled, upside-down, etc.). For measuring heart rates the sensor element has to be attached to specific areas of a body (e.g. a chest belt). There are a number of stand-alone sensors available on the market. They could send the measured data via a wireless protocol (e.g. Bluetooth or ANT+) to the activity sensor. The internal battery of the activity sensor must have a big capacity to enable a long-enough measurement session (e.g. a long walking session of about 4-5h). For uncomplicated handling by the user, charging the battery will be done via contactless charging (Qi-technology). One of the key requirements coming out of the user interviews regarding the activity sensor is about "wearability". The activity sensor has to be small, lightweight, easy to attach/mount and unobtrusive for normal body movements. One consequence of this is that the heart-rate sensor should be de-coupled from the activity sensor.

## User Interface Requirements

User interface requirements were gathered by interviewing end-users and by holding user focus group meetings. In this task we started by testing the home-fitness idea and motion based interfaces to gather the requirements and recommendations for the designers. This work continued during the later design phases of the project (see section on Early User Tests). The approach taken involved three main aspects:

1. Interviews with individuals,
2. Brainstorming with representative elderly users in focus groups, and
3. Study of similar available approaches.

To identify relevant views from interviews and focus groups, a set of open-ended questions was used to prompt discussions with users. Although most of the Swedish users are physically active to some extent, they all said that it is not enough and want their physical activities to be more frequent, more fun and more regular. Examples of the activities they do today are: walking (some with a dog), cycling, shoveling snow, morning workout (only one person did this), Nordic (cross-country) skiing, choir singing, and gardening. Most of the users regard music as helpful during exercise. None of the users were familiar with measuring their fitness or performance on activities.

From interviews, it was found that most of the users think that physical activities should be a regular routine in their daily lives. They want to do their physical activity both in their home and outside the home, but in Sweden they prefer to do most of it outdoors. All of the Swedish users liked the project idea, and think it is very important for elderly people to keep both physically and mentally active and fit. They are very interested in their own fitness and wellbeing. Users are willing to try different sensor devices, but they must see the benefit from using them and it must be unobtrusive and possible to wear both indoors and outdoors. All of the users would consider doing exercises in front of a TV if they can see the benefit of the exercises - if it is fun and motivating. They also see an advantage from being able to see their results in terms of fitness. There were different opinions about whether physical activities should be carried out individually or in groups. Some of the users want to exercise socially in groups but others would rather do it mostly by themselves. The most preferable would be to be able to do both. One idea was to include a social event into some of the exercise programmes, for example during a structured walk with others.

In focus group meetings, the following key points were raised:

- One of the most important tasks of designing a usable home-fitness system for the elderly is to design it so the users overcome the threshold of starting to do exercises, and to make the exercises fun so that they see the advantages of exercising.
- How the results are shown is also important and how this can help the elderly feel motivated to exercise.
- Ethical issues are important to them, mostly as regards their privacy. They want to know who is going to have access to their personal data apart from themselves. The ideal situation for them would be that doctors, nurses and their physiotherapist have access and can if necessary advise or take care of an acute situation. The physiotherapist could evaluate their exercises and correct them.

During this discussion it was also suggested that it would be advantageous to involve a healthcare centre that is only for the elderly and that could be connected to the ELF@Home system.

The visualisation of the results must be easy and quick to understand, with the user getting useful information from the displays Another important point that was raised during the focus group meetings was that it must be possible to use some of the project equipment naturally outdoors. It could, for example, be like a watch attached to the arm that can give the user information and measure physical status. Another example that was suggested was a T-shirt, but that solution also had some negative aspects such as needing cleaning, having to remember to put it on, you have to wear the same one every day, etc.

In the focus groups we have also discussed how the results could be used. It was felt that the results should be used to create awareness of what you do during the day (in the form of physical activity) and to become more aware of your physical condition and how it is affected by your activities. As one user expressed it "I will get to know my body, how it works and what is best for it". The results could also be used to discuss health status with friends and family, but not as a competition with other users. It is important that the results are presented in a positive way even though a value is outside normal values.

The Swedish users were asked if they were willing to wear a chest band that holds the sensors when outdoors, and they were willing to try it. They suggested that the best way to present the result in this case would be with vibrations. A voice that presented the result was also suggested but the drawback with that is that if you are walking with someone when you get some information from the chest band it could be embarrassing. The idea of a sound signal was also raised and discussed. The weakness with that was seen to be that you might not hear it if you listen to music through your earphones.

The overall preferred solution would be for the user to wear a watch that can both measure and display the information. That would also be the most unobtrusive solution. It should be possible to see the results both on the TV, when in the home, and on the watch when outside.

The following were initially identified as requirements for biomedical sensor use:

- Simple to use.
- Secure and private.
- More than one user able to share the same equipment.
- Little or no maintenance for the end user.
- Long battery life with charging as infrequent as possible.
- Easy to recharge when needed.

We also interviewed eleven healthcare experts (2 Swedish, 2 British and 7 Spanish) on their views of using existing commercial platforms when developing equipment for rehabilitation of the elderly. They most often answered that the hardware was good enough but that clinically tested software that really could be used as a stand-in for traditional rehabilitation training was not available. The platforms today are developed and used for entertainment and not for fitness, activity or health screening/monitoring on a level that was acceptable for the experts who were interviewed. All agreed about the potential usefulness of the ELF@Home solution and indicated that they would recommend it to their patients. The Spanish healthcare experts stated that they already recommend physical activity to their patients but that only a 50% of their patients actually do it.

## EARLY COMPONENT AND PROTOTYPE TESTS

It is an important part of our used-driven approach to expose the users to components of the system and prototypes as they are developed, to ensure that needs are met and to steer the course of design and implementation. The main focus of these early user tests was on the following aspects:

- Use and acceptability of using the sensors to measure health status.
- Design of the GUI (Graphical User Interface) for clarity and ease of interaction.
- Ease of use and acceptability of navigation with input by simple gesture and speech.
- Success of activity detection, and display of feedback on activities, in terms of usefulness, ease of use and understanding.
- Perceived usefulness and acceptability of individual indoor exercises.

The methods used were as follows:

- Focus groups and individual discussions were again carried out, this time around design concepts and sketches, using semi-structured interviews.
- Preliminary usage tests of the Kinect interface for games were carried out in a group context (one user at a time testing the system).
- Usage tests of successive versions of the system prototype combining the above components, carried out in a group context (one user at a time testing the system). Data included users' expressed opinions on individual exercises and view of self as shown by system.
- Ratings were also obtained by system from users after each exercise completed during above usage tests of prototype versions.

The results are structured below according to the different stages of using the ELF@Home indoor system.

### On Starting the System

Information from the sensors and from the fitness box is displayed to the user on the TV screen via the Graphical User Interface. The fitness box is the central device that users will have in their home, connected to the TV and to the Internet to provide the ELF@Home solution to them. Below we present versions of the GUI display screen designs, designed to guide the users through the ELF@Home self-check health and exercising programme. Once the users presence has been recognised by the system the first interactive screen offers a choice of seeing the "plan for today" or looking at displayed progress from earlier encounters with the system (if any), as shown in Figure 2.

The first comment from users on this version was that it looks a rather grey and like a typical "elderly product". User felt that the use of colour could improve the appearance. It was also mentioned that the exclamation sign "!" did not mean anything to the seniors. They wanted something that is easy to understand and obvious. In the light of these comments, the screen was redesigned, as shown in Figure 3.

When the user selects "plan for today", the initial design for the next screen was as shown in Figure 4.

This was felt to be confusing in terms of what the user can choose. The health measures should be done before performing an exercise, but it is not clear if she can then choose the indoor or outdoor ex-

*Figure 2. Initial screen of the ELF@Home application*

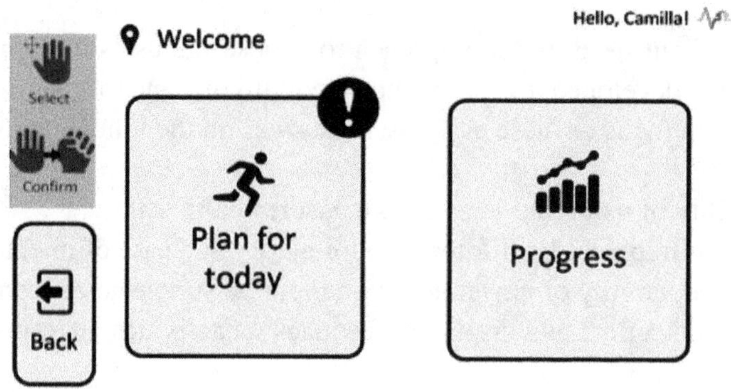


*Figure 3. Initial screen of the ELF@Home application, revised*

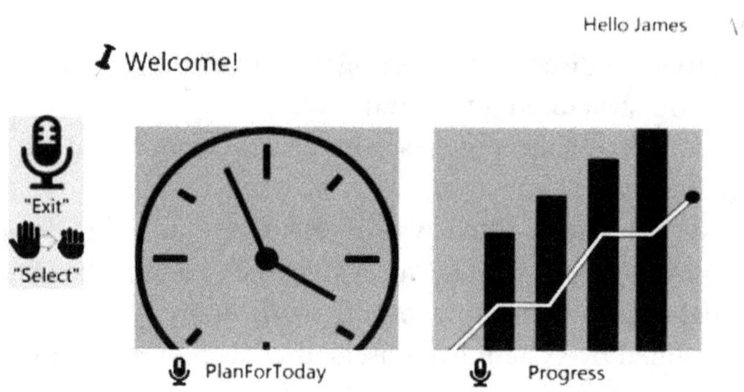


*Figure 4. Initial screen for showing "tasks for today"*

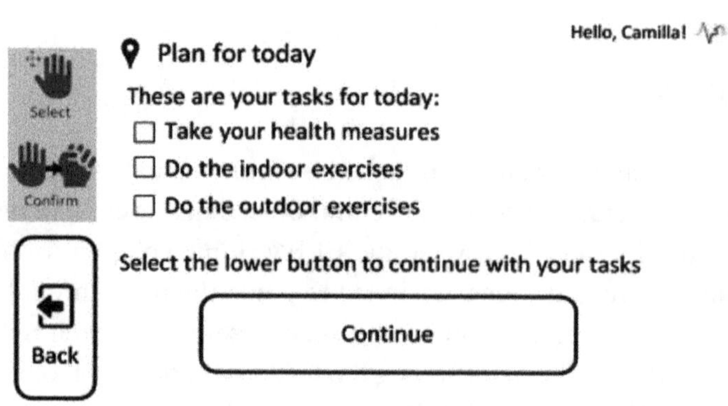

*Figure 5. Revised screen showing "tasks for today"*

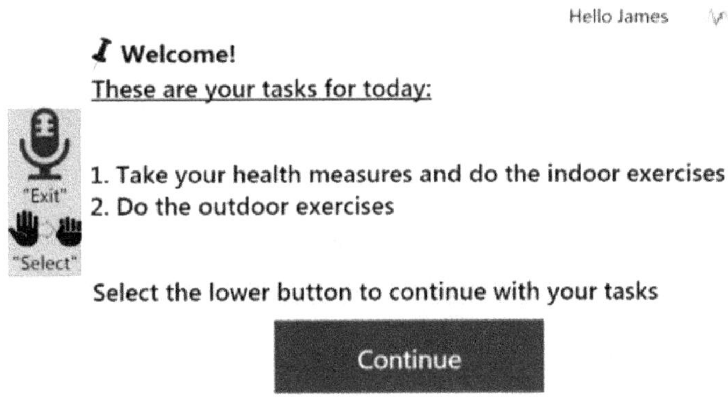


ercises. In fact, the boxes are not selectable. In this screen the user can only press "continue". This was made clearer in a revised version of the screen, shown in Figure 5.

## Taking Own Health Measures

In normal use, the first of the measures to be taken are heart rate and oxygen saturation. An improved version of this screen was designed to ensure that the way the device fits on the finger is clear, as shown in Figure 6.

Users found the initial version of a screen explaining how to take blood pressure readings unclear as regards to the exact use of the sensing device. A modified picture was provided in a revised version of the screen, with reference made to the image shown on the bracelet itself (see Figure 7).

Users also expressed a wish to be able to choose between an image of using a sensing device and an animation of how to put it on properly, especially in the case of measuring the blood pressure. It was also suggested that when showing the image of the blood pressure cuff it should be an image of a real person's arm with the cuff correctly positioned on it.

Sometimes there were communication problems between the sensors and the system. Users were clear that status information about the sensing devices is needed to give the user clearer feedback on what is

*Figure 6. Revised screen showing how to use the pulse oximeter.*

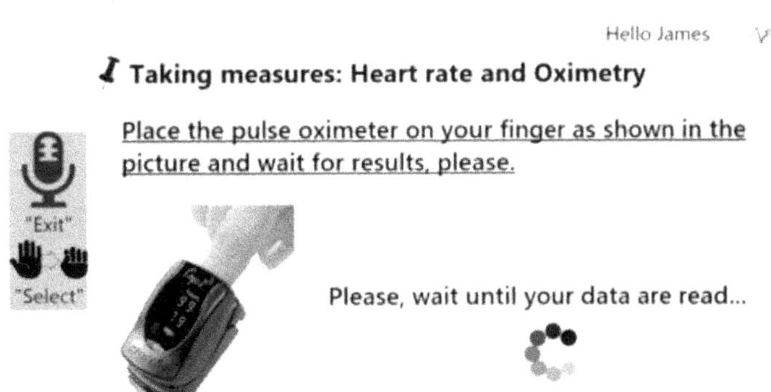

*Figure 7. Revised screen to explain taking blood pressure*

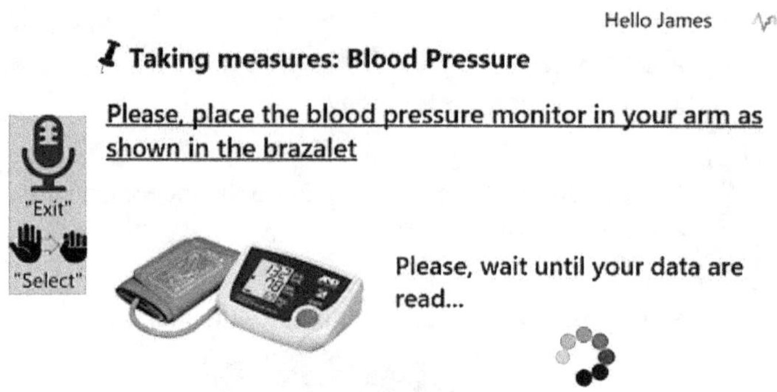


happening. In the light of this reaction from users, technical enhancements are being made to support a richer communication protocol so that more information can be shared with the users.

## When the Values Are Out of Range

In some cases, users will find that their measurements return values that are out of the healthy range as recognised by the system. The initial designs for screens presenting this information are shown as in Figure 8.

*Figure 8. Screenshots of initial design for values out of range*

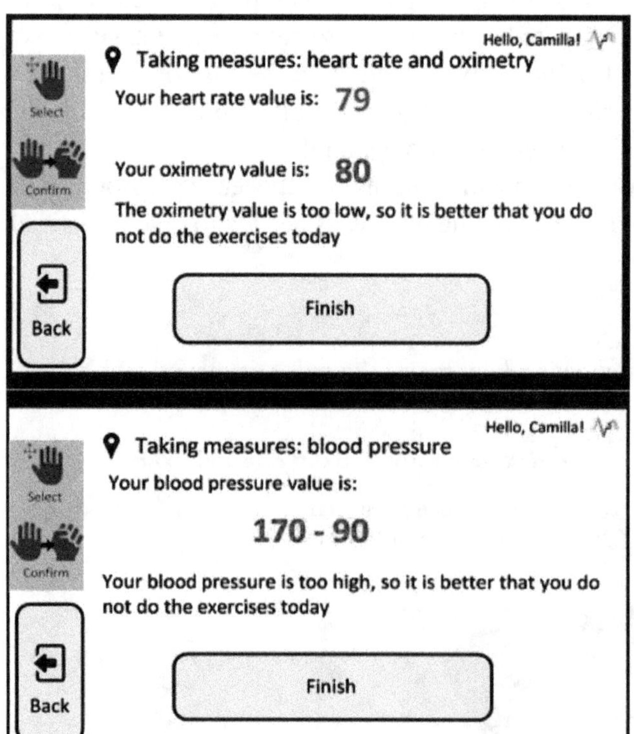

The main comment about these was that it would be helpful if more detailed advice could be given about what the user should do, for example "consult the healthcare centre" or "try again after you have had a rest".

## Interacting with the Camera Interface and using Speech Recognition

Initial trials of the idea of using a camera-based interaction technique were carried out with our users interacting with a Kinect, to establish the viability of this approach. In particular, we tested how well the groups of Swedish users could succeed in selecting chosen items from game-related visual menus, as shown in Figure 9.

In general, the approach worked well, although several users had problems with holding their hand in a fixed place for long enough to make their chosen selection.

The Spanish users tested a simple demo application that was based on pressing buttons that were the similar size and that were distributed in the screen in the same way as the application that was being designed for the fitness box. The users were shown a screen with two buttons and there were instructions in the screen that told them which button to press. Figure 10 shows the interaction map of the demo application.

*Figure 9. A user in Skellefteå trying out Kinect-based selection from a visual menu screen*

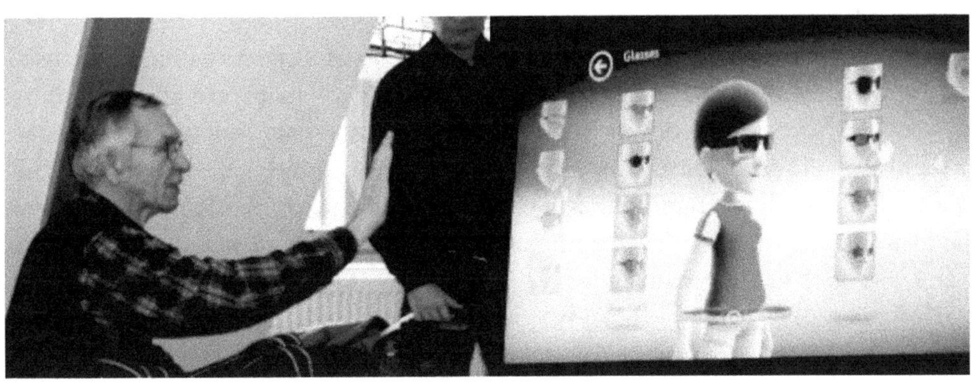

*Figure 10. User interaction basic demo application*

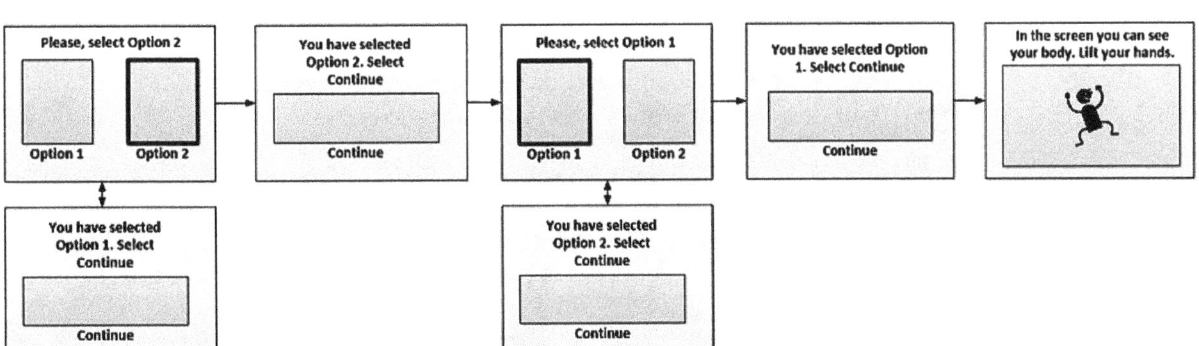

The users usually needed 3 or 4 iterations to succeed completely in navigating through all the screens on their own.

Before carrying out the indoor exercises, the position of the user's body must be detected by the Kinect sensor system and then an image of this is displayed on the TV interface. Various representations of the user's body were considered during early user trials. In discussions, users indicated that they preferred the option of a skeleton representing the user, as compared to other possibilities, including an animated generalised man or woman, a camera image of self, and a shadow figure. They preferred not to see themselves portrayed realistically but to see themselves as a skeleton. Eventually a green stick figure, with red markings indicating poorly detected portions, was selected by the users as the clearest and easiest representation to understand (see Figure 11).

As shown in Figure 11, to continue the user must select "continue" by allowing the hand cursor to hover over the purple button. The hand is then closed and, when opened, "continue" is selected. As this kind of interaction is usually new to the users, they need some training time to be able to do it right. The users will often have problems selecting the buttons, so the GUI tries to maximize the button size, so it is easier for them to select the buttons.

This mode of interaction causes some problems for users. They find the "hand open" gesture difficult and unintuitive, and have expressed the view that only a "hand closed", when over the purple button, should be used instead. The complete operation of moving the hand over the button, closing the hand, and then opening the hand again to complete the gesture, takes some time. Several users find it difficult to hold the hand in place over the target for this amount of time. This problem seems to be exacerbated by the positioning of the "continue" button at the bottom of the screen, since it is generally less tiring to hold the hand still at shoulder height.

In order to design and validate possible speech recognition aspects of the interface (used for simple commands), the Swedish users were asked to record some words that were going to be used as voice commands. They recorded them both in English and in Swedish and they used the Kinect recording functionality and an audio recorder (Olympus LS10). These recordings were analysed and no significant differences were found in the recognition results, validating the use of the Kinect as a microphone. Users liked the idea of using simple speech commands for some common functions, as long as it worked effectively and was done in their own language.

*Figure 11. Representation of user's body on the TV interface*

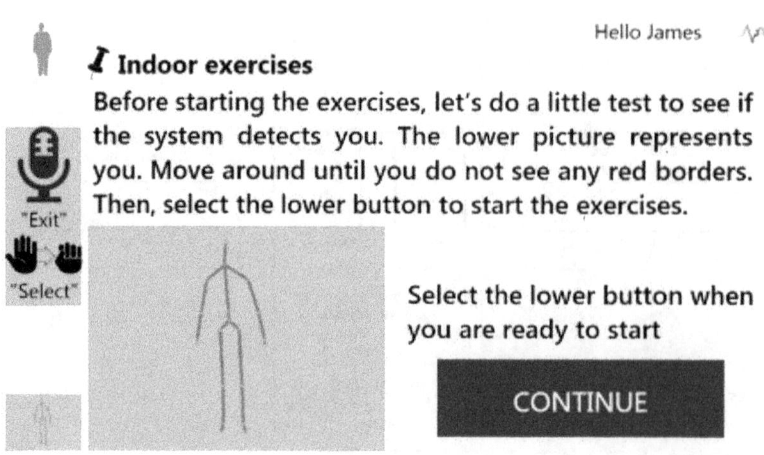

In use with the prototype, the users appreciated the speech interaction and most of the time it works more effectively than using the hand gesture. Speech recognition is not implemented for all commands yet, but the users would prefer it to be. However, the Spanish tests found problems with speech recognition in the larger rooms used for their groups. This may be the result of echo (although not perceptible by people) negatively affecting the speech recognition.

## Doing the Indoor Exercises

Before starting the exercises, it is vital that the users warm up. For this, a short videos is shown in the system TV interface. Similarly, a demo video of each exercise is offered before the user selects to carry it out, as shown in Figure 12.

It was done this way because most of the users thought that the video should not be played at the same time as they are doing their exercise. They felt that it would better if it were shown before, with the possibility to look at it again if one does not remember how to do the exercise. If the video were shown at the same time as the user was performing her exercise she would feel stressed that the exercise was being performed too slowly and that the exercise was not done well enough. This would make them feel not good enough and then they would tend not do the exercises.

The Swedish user group in Skellefteå would prefer that an elderly person was shown doing the exercises, but the group in Åsele thought it was OK with a younger user. The Spanish care staff expected their users to prefer a younger person doing the exercises, as in their experience older patients usually respond better to younger health professionals than to older ones. Generally users liked the demos video but felt that it should be possible to see it again after starting an exercise. The view was also expressed that the video should include a voice giving more detailed instructions. Also, some of the exercises should show the person from the side in order to see more clearly how the exercise should be performed. Many of these improvements will be included in later versions of the prototype.

At the end of an exercising session, the user is shown another "warm up" video to wind down well after the training. Several users found this confusing, since the term "warm up" suggests that the session is just starting. Instead, it was suggested that the screen should refer to "cool down" or "finishing off". This text will therefore be changed in the next version of the prototype. Both the warm up exercises (at the beginning and end of a training session) were very confusing, the users did not understand or remember what to do. The warm up exercise at the end they thought should in their opinion only be stretching. Another comment about the video was that the performer should not look so serious. It would be nicer with a performer who smiled and looked like she enjoyed doing the exercises.

*Figure 12. The demonstration videos*

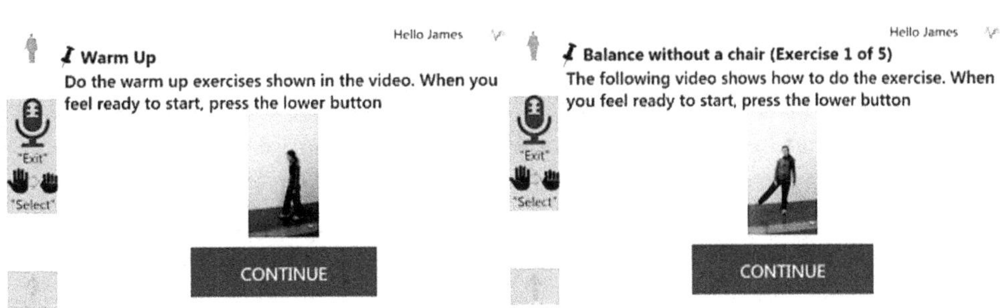

The sequence of images below (Figure 13) shows how the system provides feedback on the way users are carrying out each exercise. Until each criterion is met (as indicated by the buttons to the right of the figure), the user cannot move on to complete the exercise.

There have been a lot of discussions about how to show the steps of the exercise. The version shown above is a middle way that has been agreed upon. During the tests we have also discussed the text of the different steps, how to describe the steps in words. The users also want to add a voice in the demo video that describes the steps in detail.

## FUTURE RESEARCH

User involvement has played a key part in the continuing design and development of the system, resulting in concrete changes. Some technical problems were also identified from our completed user studies and these have been rectified and in some cases led to overall improvement of the implementation approach. Many other comments and opinions were gathered from the early user trials, and these are under active consideration and discussion amongst the project team. This work will continue with the activity sensor and related developments for the outdoor parts of the system.

Limitations of the work done within the project include the sampling of participants. As described in the section "Who are the Users?" above, our two user groups (in Spain and Sweden) are rather different in profile, especially in terms of level of prior physical activity and the male:female ratio. In both countries, users self-selected their involvement in the project and so may be more motivated than the average elderly person to adopt new technology. Also, although we have developed a working prototype ready for testing, this is not yet finalised in terms of design and its efficacy has not yet been verified. The final version of the ELF@Home system will be ready for piloting in users' everyday environments towards the end of 2015.

The key features that will differentiate the final ELF@Home system from products available in the market for the maintenance health and fitness are, as follows:

- Close involvement of actual users with health issues over a long term and including realistic trials of use is novel for this type of product.
- The availability of continuous monitoring of user's activity and the automatic personalization of fitness exercises according to the monitored life style, made possible by the technical advances embodied in the project, are also unique.
- The close involvement of medical experts in the design of the exercises and testing procedures is also unusual.

All of these features contribute to the customisability of the approach, which has a huge potential for further development to deal with specific types of fitness problem and specific types of users.

In the work so far, we have focused on particular types of elderly users. Future research and development will be needed to address the needs of other groups, for example young and middle aged users, users with specific conditions or disabilities needing rehabilitation, very old users, amongst many other possible target groups. The trend towards the development of positive technology for the maintenance and improvement of health seems irresistible. Individual citizens and society in general benefits from the availability of individualised health and fitness support, including both assessment and intervention plans.

*Figure 13. Feedback on performance of an exercise*

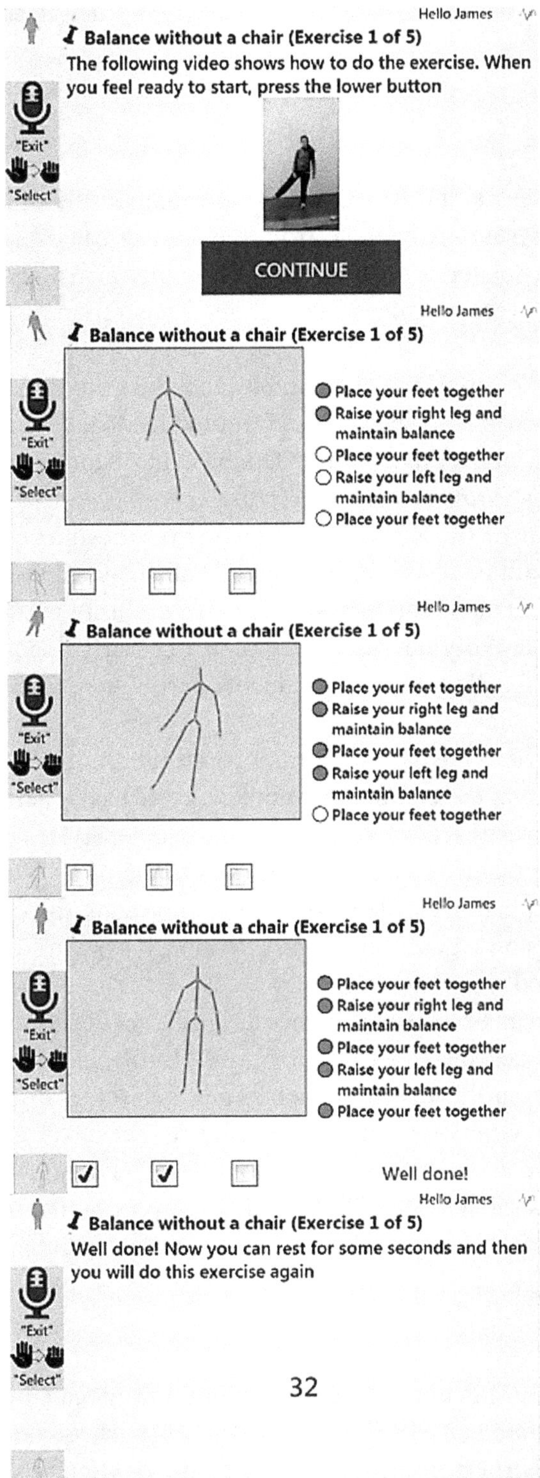

In the future, this need will increasingly be met by technical means – and in this respect ELF@Home is a piöneering example. A great deal of further research will be needed to achieve this on a broader scale.

## CONCLUSION

Elderly users' opinions on design and functionality have guided the development of relevant ELF@ Home components and the system as a whole from the start of the project. In the early user tests reported in this document, user-related aspects of the sensing platform and of the GUI and interaction for indoor exercise programmes were examined. This chapter has reported the results from both Spanish and Swedish user groups.

Generally speaking, user reaction was favourable and the components and early versions of the prototype were found to be acceptable and usable. Detailed feedback was provided on some aspects of the user interface and way of interacting, and this feedback has been – or will be – taken account of in further iterations of the ELF@Home prototype system.

The main innovations of the ELF@Home service relate to the design of a solution specifically adapted to elderly people, through continuous user involvement at all stages of the project. The system has been designed to minimize end user intervention and maximize usability and pleasure. User interfaces and fitness exercises have been carefully designed according to elderly needs and abilities, and with their ongoing feedback. The users feel that they are a valuable part of the project team and take this role very seriously.

From a technical point of view, the most important contributions of ELF@Home to advance the state of the art in elderly fitness lie in the continuous monitoring of user's activity levels and the automatic personalization of fitness exercises according to the monitored life style. This distinguishes ELF@Home from what is available in the marketplace. It is a clear example of a ''Positive Technology'' approach through the scientific and applied use of technology for improving the quality of personal experience through its structuring (by using a goal, rules, and a feedback system) and personal augmentation (to achieve multimodal and mixed experiences).

Regular physical exercise can be expected to have a significant beneficial effect on health, and elderly fitness programs are a widely accepted approach to prevent frailty and minimize or prevent the development and worsening of many chronic diseases, such as cardiovascular disease, type 2 diabetes mellitus, colon and breast cancer, and cognitive decline in the elderly. Because we test the health and wellbeing status of our trial users before and after extensive use of ELF@Home, we will be able to evaluate the extent to which the service as implemented has a positive impact on the lives of the target users.

## ACKNOWLEDGMENT

ELF@Home (AAL-2012-5-123) is a project co-funded by European Commission under the Ambient Assisted Living Joint Programme (AAL JP, Call 5, 2012), Ministerio de Industria Energía y Turismo in Spain (MINETUR), Swedish Governmental Agency for Innovation Systems in Sweden (VINNOVA) and Federal Ministry of Education and Research in Germany (BMBF).

## REFERENCES

Cadore, E. L., Rodríguez-Mañas, L., Sinclair, A., & Izquierdo, M. (2013). Effects of different exercise interventions on risk of falls, gait ability, and balance in physically frail older adults: A systematic review. *Rejuvenation Research*, *16*(2), 105–114. doi:10.1089/rej.2012.1397 PMID:23327448

Do Lee, C., Folsom, A. R., & Blair, S. N. (2003). Physical activity and stroke risk a meta-analysis. *Stroke*, *34*(10), 2475–2481. doi:10.1161/01.STR.0000091843.02517.9D PMID:14500932

Elderly self-care based on self-check of health conditions and self-fitness at home. (2015). ELF@Home. Retrieved from http://www.elfathome.eu

Fried, L. P., Tangen, C. M., Walston, J., Newman, A. B., Hirsch, C., Gottdiener, J., & McBurnie, M. A. et al. (2001). Frailty in older adults: Evidence for a phenotype. *Journal of Gerontology*, *56A*, M146–M156. PMID:11253156

García García, J., & Larrión Zugasti, J. L. (2007). *Deterioro cognitivo y fragilidad. In J.M.L. Arrieta, & F.J.G. Garcia (Eds.), El anciano con demencia* (pp. 59–83). Madrid: Sociedad Española de Medicina Geriátrica.

Guralnik, J. M., Simonsick, E. M., Ferrucci, L., Glynn, R. J., Berkman, L. F., Blazer, D. G., & Wallace, R. B. et al. (1994). A short physical performance battery assessing lower extremity function: Association with self-reported disability and prediction of mortality and nursing home admission. *Journal of Gerontology*, *49*(2), M85–M94. doi:10.1093/geronj/49.2.M85 PMID:8126356

Kelaiditi, E., Cesari, M., Canevelli, M., Van Kan, G. A., Ousset, P. J., Gillette-Guyonnet, S., & Vellas, B. et al. (2013). Cognitive frailty: Rational and definition from an (IANA/IAGG) international consensus group. *The Journal of Nutrition, Health & Aging*, *17*(9), 726–734. doi:10.1007/s12603-013-0367-2 PMID:24154642

Kesaniemi, Y. K., Danforth, E. Jr, Jensen, M. D., Kopelman, P. G., Lefèbvre, P., & Reeder, B. A. (2001). Dose-response issues concerning physical activity and health: An evidence-based symposium. *Medicine and Science in Sports and Exercise*, *33*(Suppl. 6), S351. PMID:11427759

Linwall, M., Rennemark, M., Halling, A., Berglund, J., & Hassmén, P. (2006). Depression and exercise in elderly men and women: Findings from the Swedish national study on aging and care. *Journal of Aging and Physical Activity*, *15*, 41–55. PMID:17387228

Liu, C. J., & Latham, N. K. (2009). Progressive resistance strength training for improving physical function in older adults. *Cochrane Database of Systematic Reviews*, CD002759. PMID:19588334

Liu-Ambrose, T., Nagamatsu, L. S., Graf, P., Beattie, B. L., Ashe, M. C., & Handy, T. C. (2010). Resistance training and executive functions: A 12-month randomized controlled trial. *Archives of Internal Medicine*, *170*(2), 170–178. doi:10.1001/archinternmed.2009.494 PMID:20101012

Mahoney, F. I., & Barthel, D. (1965). Functional evaluation: The Barthel Index. *Maryland State Medical Journal*, *14*, 56–61. PMID:14258950

Mammen, G., & Faulkner, G. (2013). Physical Activity and the Prevention of Depression. *American Journal of Preventive Medicine*, *45*(5), 649–657. doi:10.1016/j.amepre.2013.08.001 PMID:24139780

Nascimento, B. R., Brant, L. C., Moraes, D. N., & Ribeiro, A. L. (2014). Global health and cardiovascular disease. *Heart (British Cardiac Society)*, *100*(22), 1743–1749. doi:10.1136/heartjnl-2014-306026 PMID:25327515

Nielsen, J. (1994a, April 24-28). Enhancing the explanatory power of usability heuristics. *Proc. ACM CHI'94 Conf.*, Boston, MA (pp. 152-158).

Santos-Eggimann, B., Cuénoud, P., Spagnoli, J., & Junod, J. (2009). Prevalence of frailty in middle-aged and older community-dwelling Europeans living in 10 countries. *Journal of Gerontology*, *64*, 675–681. PMID:19276189

Waterworth, E. L., & Waterworth, J. A. (2009). Designing ICT for the over 80s. In *Topo, P. & Östlund, B. (2009), Dementia, Design and Technology: Time to Get Involved*. Amsterdam: IOS Press.

Waterworth, E. L., Waterworth, J. A., Peter, C., & Ballesteros, S. (2012, June 6-8). Seniors in charge of ICT innovation. *Proceedings of the 5th Workshop on Affect and Behaviour Related Assistance PETRA 2012*, Crete.

WHO. (1948). Preamble to the Constitution of the World Health Organization as adopted by the International Health Conference, New York, 19-22 June, 1946; signed on 22 July 1946 by the representatives of 61 States (*Official Records of the World Health Organization*, no. 2, p. 100) and entered into force on 7 April 1948.

## KEY TERMS AND DEFINITIONS

**Aerobic:** Aerobic exercises are of low to moderate intensity, usually sustainable for prolonged periods of time and not requiring lactate formation in the body.

**Ambient Assisted Living:** Information and communication technology designed and applied to improve the quality of life of old and vulnerable people.

**Cardiovascular:** Cardiovascular disease affects the blood circulation of the body, often the heart itself.

**Frailty Syndrome:** The tendency in ageing adults to be increasingly vulnerable to falls, mechanical disabilities, infection, and so on, raising the probability of their hospitalization and eventual death.

**Health:** A person's health status is their level of physical, mental and social well-being.

**Ischemic Heart Disease:** A disease characterized by reduced blood supply to the heart, and which is the most common cause of death in many developed countries.

**Type 2 Diabetes Mellitus:** A chronic condition in which there are high levels of sugar in the blood and a range of possible symptoms including fatigue, reduced libido, susceptibility to infections, hunger and increased thirst.

# Chapter 6
# Tools for eMental-Health:
## A Coping Processor for Adaptive and Interactive Mobile Systems for Stress Management

**Manolya Kavakli**
*Macquarie University, Australia*

**Amir Maddah**
*Macquarie University, Australia*

**Heidi Ranjbartabar**
*Macquarie University, Australia*

**Kiumars Ranjbartabar**
*Macquarie University, Australia*

## ABSTRACT

*This chapter focuses on how to develop tools for positive technology and more specifically, mobile e-mental health systems using a virtual stress counselor. The main objective is to develop a framework for mobile e-mental health systems reviewing existing e-mental health apps and discussing necessary system requirements. The chapter states that current e-mental health apps do not offer any facilities to promote social interaction between the counselor and the user. The proposed framework requires personalized interactions between a virtual counselor and a student. It provides personalized feedback to reduce stress level and enhances personal stress management strategies. This requires integration of technologies for facial expression detection, speech and emotion recognition as well as other psycho-physiological feedback. A prototype system for e-mental health has been developed and the components of the system architecture have been widely discussed including the need for a coping processor. Finally, conclusions are drawn regarding the tools for positive technology.*

## INTRODUCTION

Virtual Reality (VR) has resulted in creative solutions offering entirely new options for human computer interaction (HCI). VR technologies combined with social networking and mobile phone technology present a new cyber-landscape that have potential to supplement or complement traditional professional practices; producing new learning processes, environments, and tools; and expanding borders of science beyond anything this world has ever seen. VR applications have demonstrated that they can reduce fear (Malbos et al., 2013), acute pain in burn patients (Hoffmann et al., 2000), eating disorders (Riva et al, 1999), post-traumatic stress disorder (Rothbaum et al., 1999), and stress in cancer patients (Scheider

DOI: 10.4018/978-1-4666-9986-1.ch006

and Workman, 1999). Therefore, VR applications deserve to be considered as positive technology tools and may be used to improve physical and mental health.

There is a significant need to promote mental health and wellbeing by the development of e-mental health applications that link mobile tools with traditional forms of counselling. Today, almost three-quarters of Australians report that stress has an impact on their physical health. High demand for mental health services and limitations of online facilities available add pressure on service providers. As a result, online mental health services that use health promotion technologies in Australia have been going through rapid changes in models of service delivery to address the demand. A virtual advisor always accessible on a smart phone is a promising way to address the aforementioned problem.

The main objective of this chapter is to review e-mental health systems, to present a debate on the development of e-mental health systems using VR as a tool for positive technology, and to evaluate their use discussing relevant ethical issues. To be able to evaluate potentials of VR-based mobile e-mental health systems we present a framework after reviewing existing e-mental health apps and discussing necessary system requirements. The proposed framework is based on personalized interactions between a virtual counselor and a student requiring help to manage their stress levels during exams and expected to provide personalized feedback to reduce stress level and enhance personal stress management strategies of students. In this chapter, we explore the use of virtual stress counsellors investigating a number of research questions such as:

Is the use of avatars meaningful in e-mental health applications as virtual stress counselors?

- Is it possible to improve the stress management skills of a person by interacting with an avatar?
- How can we use avatars and animation technology to improve coping processes?

The remaining section of this chapter focuses on how to develop tools for positive technology and more specifically, a mobile application presenting a virtual exam-stress counselor. First e-mental health systems are reviewed, and system requirements are defined, then, a generic framework is proposed. Finally, the components of the system architecture are discussed and conclusions regarding the tools for positive technology are drawn and associated ethical concerns are discussed in the evaluation of solution.

## E-Mental Health Systems as Positive Technology Tools

Technology has been pushing fundamental changes in social life. As stated by Psotka (2013), more than two billion people were using the Internet globally in 2010 including three quarters of the American population more than a doubling increase since 2000, and online learning increased from 45,000 enrollments in 2000 to roughly one million in 2007 showing signs of continuing to grow at more rapid pace, a power function expansion. This is expected to increase with the adoption of augmented reality technology that may allow to present scenarios that include features not available in reality. This would be the case when cueing stimuli are presented to determine what level of augmented information can be used by patients to provide insight for the development of compensatory strategies aimed at improving day to day functional behavior (Rizzo et al, 2003).

Although VR, computer games, and social media may be seen as disruptive technologies by some researchers (e.g., Psotka, 2013) due to the public's enthusiastic adoption of these new technologies, we refer them as positive technology tools due to their potential to change the quality of life for the people using them. The most popular social networks, such as Facebook™, the virtual world Second Life™, and massively multiplayer online games (MMOGs), such as World of Warcraft and the SIMs have inspired the public's imagination and their motivation to learn. World of Warcraft and Second Life have reported participation of 8.5 and 6.5 million users, respectively (Bainbridge, 2012; Squire & Steinkuehler, 2006). With such expansive participation in social media, informal learning has been "virtually" transformed by these emergent settings (Psotka, 2013). Another type of expansive participation has been the use of mobile applications. As smartphones and tablets' popularity increases, so does the number of mobile applications to support the users. For example, driven by these applications, Australia's enthusiasm for touch-screen phones rapidly increased in 2012. In its report, the Australian Communication and Media Authority (ACMA) has estimated that 49% (8.67 million) Australian adults would have used a smartphone in 2012, compared with 25% (4.25 million) in 2011, representing a 104% increase as stated by the Australian Financial Review in 2013. There is a growing demand for mobile applications. Australia's telephony market was estimated to be worth over $15 billion per annum in 2013 by the Australian Financial Review. In 2010, 300,000+ mobile applications were downloaded 10.9 billion times. Global downloads was expected to reach 76.9 billion in 2014 and to be worth US$35 billion (Mobithinking, 2012).

While these statistics demonstrate the potential usability of mobile apps in e-mental health by Australian adults, the demand is even greater for the young generations due to their greater use of mobile technology. In 2013, 89% of young Australians owned a smartphone and 83% downloaded an app for seeking help. There is a general need to promote mental health and wellbeing of young generations in Australia by the development of e-mental health applications that link mobile tools with traditional forms of counselling.

There is a high demand for mental health services. However, access to online facilities available are limited. As a result, online mental health services that use health promotion technologies to promote youth wellbeing in Australia have been going through rapid changes in models of service delivery to address the demand. There are self-help resources available, however, the impact of these on young people's wellbeing is unknown.

The traditional ways of providing face-to-face counseling services have been proven to be effective in helping students to get over stressful periods. However, given the high demand of such services, especially during the exam period, it is very unlikely that those issues be addressed timely for every student. Some people fear social stigmatization and worry about being witnessed by acquaintances while visiting psychologists. These factors make it challenging to reveal a student's emotional problems related to exam stress. Consequently, the availability of an intelligent and human-like virtual advisor would allow students to have easy access via computers and smart phones to exam-stress related confidential advice and timely support (Li et al., 2012).

## Coping Theory in Stress Management

Stress is defined as a relationship between the person and the environment that is perceived as relevant to the person's well-being and in which the person's resources failed to meet the demand (Coyne et al. 1980). Stress arises when individuals perceive a discrepancy between the physical or psychological demands of a situation and the resources of his or her biological, psychological or social systems (Sarafino, 2012). An appropriate level of stress can help students to concentrate on preparing for their assessment tasks by triggering the secretion of a charged chemical called "adrenaline" in the central nervous system thus boosting our capability to cope with stress, anger or fear through increased heart rate, blood pressure, cardiac output and carbohydrate metabolism (Karavolos et al. 2008). However, too much stress will result in negative impacts on memory, exam performance, mental health and physical well-being (Lee 2010; Yang and Shin 2008). One common consequence of exam stress is distress or depression. To proactively prevent these negative impacts from happening, stress management and its optimization is essential.

Stress has significant effects on the mental health of students from diverse age groups and educational levels (Kernan, Wheat & Lerner 2008; Vaez & Laflamme 2008). Although appropriate level of stress boosts concentration and self-discipline of students, the excessive stress and related symptoms such as anxiety, worry and fear of failure can potentially result in poor exam performance and have negative impact on student's mental and psychical health (Li et al., 2012). Exam stress has been reported to lead to depression, anxiety, substance abuse, delinquency and suicide (Lee 2010; Yang and Shin 2008). Improved accessibility to counseling services for at-risk students is found to be among the best intervention strategies to improve such situations (Washburn & Mandrusiak 2010).

Exam stress is common for students of all ages, regardless of their socio-economic, cultural and educational background. Stress is an inevitable aspect of college student's life (Baghurst, 2013). There are many students worldwide suffering from stress and anxiety every day. There are various reasons for experiencing stress. If chronic stress is not addressed timely, it may result in serious debilitating consequences including insomnia, depression and even suicide (Ross et al, 1999, Krantz & Kiecolt-Glaser, 2014). Stress has negative effects on students' academic performance and impairs efforts to be physically active (Stults-Kolehmainen, 2013). During exam time, face to face counselling has been proven to be effective in helping students to overcome a stressful period, however many students hesitate to talk to counsellors when such need arise. There are research studies claiming that the availability of an intelligent and human-like virtual advisor, such as a virtual counselor on their mobile phone, would allow students to have an easy access to exam-stress-related confidential advice and timely support (Li et al, 2012).

Coping (Stress management) involves constantly changing cognitive or behavioral efforts to manage situations appraised as taxing or exceeding a person's resources (Amirkhan & Auyeung 2007). Lazarus and Folkman (1984) suggested that there are two types of coping responses emotion focused and problem focused: Emotion-focused coping involves trying to reduce the negative emotional responses associated with stress such as embarrassment, fear, anxiety, depression, excitement and frustration. Emotion-focused coping does not provide a long term solution and may have negative side effects as it delays the person dealing with the problem (McLeod, 2009). Women tend to use more emotion-focused strategies than men (Billings & Moos, 1981). However, this may be the only realistic option when the source of stress is outside the person's control. Problem-focused coping targets the causes of stress in practical ways which tackles the problem or stressful situation that is causing stress, consequently directly reducing the stress (McLeod, 2009). Problem focused strategies aim to remove or reduce the cause of the stressor, including problem-solving, time-management, and obtaining instrumental social support.

In addition to Lazarus and Folkman's (1984) classiffication on coping modes by function (as either problem focused or emotion focused), delineating coping as dealing mainly with the problem or with its emotional and physiological outcomes, respectively, another distinction between coping modes refers to the approach–avoidance classification and encompasses two major forms of techniques: active coping (approach) and passive coping (avoidant). Active coping involves a person taking active initiatives to change the situation through actions and/or cognition. It has been found to be more effective in mitigating stress compared to passive coping. Passive coping involves a person trying to ignore the stressful problem (Compas et al. 2001).

Previous studies empirically show that students can be trained to handle stress better (Monkong et al. 2009). Therefore, it is possible to assume that a virtual counsellor helping students enhance their coping strategy and convert stress into efficient work will be beneficial for mental health. Coping theory states that coping with stress can be considered as either a personal problem solving style, or as a problem solving process (Monkong et al. 2009). There are three general coping processes in stress management: avoidance, seeking support and problem-solving. One must explore whether and to what extent a virtual counselor can inspire the two relatively more positive, effective and healthier coping processes, namely seeking support and problem-solving. As discussed by Kavakli et al. (2012), two corresponding constructs namely "perceived social support" (i.e., corresponding to the acquisition of social support) and "perceived exam control" (i.e., corresponding to the feeling of having the capacity to handle the problem) become variables of interest. These variables should be examined as they relate to final coping outcomes. One must find out whether student's interactions with a virtual counselor directly impact coping outcomes and if so, how this interaction can be optimized. To achieve this, authors present an integrated system architecture.

## BACKGROUND

While the significance of the need for mobile tools for e-mental health apps has been discussed in the previous section, in this section it would be beneficial to discuss if there is actually any value in working on the development of virtual stress counselors. Existing virtual stress counselors are either text-based or offer limited intelligence. Exceptions include "Ellie," a virtual psychologist developed at Institute for Creative Technologies helps psychologists by analyzing a person's words and their mannerisms to determine their emotional state (USC, 2014). Users respond to a series of questions from Ellie that tracks the user's eye gaze, how often they smile, if they lean back or forward, inflections in their voice, and other signals, recording 30 measurements per second and monitoring about 60 different features, using an Xbox Kinect sensor. Although Ellie may help psychologists view each patient objectively, she cannot diagnose health problems of individuals. There are also voice-based artificial intelligence (AI) systems to support healthcare professionals in their diagnosis. However, like Ellie, most of these require the presence of human psychologists on telephone or online or offer limited interactive capabilities such as the virtual doctor (KCCI, 2011) who greets users online just like a real doctor, but leaves the examination and diagnosis to the actual doctors.

*Is using avatars meaningful in e-mental health applications as virtual stress counselors?* This question can be answered by a number of important references. These references show that people tend to react to avatars as if reacting to real human beings. Slater and colleagues (2006) replicated a famous yet controversial experiment (Milgram 1963) in a virtual environment. They found that in spite of the fact that all participants know that they were interacting with virtual characters and a virtual environment, they responded to the situation at the subjective, behavioural and physiological levels as if it were real. This is also evidenced by psycho-physiological measures such as an increase in the participant's heart rate (Slater et al. 2006). Other researchers took this fact even a step further and suggested that people feel more comfortable when interviewed by media-mediated electronic doctors and are more likely to release their flinched mind during the consultation process in contrast to human doctors Yoshida et al. (2002).

There is a consensus on that the experience of presence is a complex, multidimensional perception, formed through an interplay of raw multi- sensory data and various cognitive processes (e.g., Ijsselsteijn

& Riva, 2003, Riva, 2004, Sanchez-Vives & Slater, 2005, Baumgartner et al., 2006) and VR can supplement certain aspects of presence. For example, Riva et al. (2007) analyzed the relationship between presence and emotions. The results confirmed the efficacy of VR as affective medium: the interaction with "anxious" and "relaxing" virtual environments produced anxiety and relaxation.

*Is it possible to use avatars and animation technology to improve human skills on coping processes?* There is theoretical evidence that taking another person's perspective of events recruit some of the same mental processing and activate some of the same neural networks as would be activated if the person really was experiencing the imagined situation (Smith & Kosslyn, 2006). Such thinking relies on motor cognition. Motor cognition is mental processing in which the motor system draws on stored information to plan and produce our own actions, as well as to anticipate, predict, and interpret the actions of others (Smith & Kosslyn, 2006). These studies highlight the importance of watching another person to replicate the motor actions, and provide a good basis to cope with unfamiliar situations. In the concept of motor cognition, shared motor representations refer to the person's ability to represent actions made by other people, mentally. Same types of motor representations are formed when the person observes someone else act as when they themselves perform the same action (Smith & Kosslyn, 2006). Such shared representations of the meaning of words and social interactions become internalized and represented so that they can be used in mental processing even in the absence of an on-going social interaction. Theoretically, if these shared motor representations can be identified and addressed in a computer code, it should be possible to use an avatar as a positive technology tool to simulate social interaction between humans and avatars.

There are an impressive number of behavioral and neurophysiological studies demonstrating that perception and action have a common neuronal coding in shared representations between self and others. While the concept of motor cognition relies on the fact that cognition is embodied in action, and motor priming states that watching a movement or an action facilitates making a similar motor response oneself,

how human or machine like this avatar should be? There is no consensus on this research question. Castiello and colleagues (2002) explored motor priming studying behavioral responses to actions by a robot arm and a human arm. They found that the participants' responses were faster when the model used was human. There is neurophysiological evidence that certain brain regions involved in executing actions are activated by the mere observation of action (the so-called "mirror system" as described by Rizzolatti et al, 1996, Gallesse et al, 1996). However, it is unknown whether this mirror system causes interference between observed and simultaneously executed movements. Kilner et al. (2003) found that observing another human make incongruent movements interferes with movement execution but observing a robotic arm making incongruent movements does not.

*Is it possible to improve the stress management skills of a person by asking them to watch and interact with an avatar demonstrating how to cope with pressure?* Should this be seen as a human or machine demonstration? These are interesting research questions yet to be answered. However, it is clear that one should take into account the effect of motor priming when developing e-mental health apps. Although the idea sounds promising, there are major challenges in the development of virtual counselors, especially if they are expected to convey a feeling of social interaction. Some of these challenges have been successfully addressed. For example, Rickel et al. (2002) managed to create virtual humans that can exhibit non-verbal human behaviours such as emotions and gestures. While this addresses behavioral realism challenge, the advancements in "Chatbot" technology address the conversational realism. For example, virtual advisors such as "Franco" can simulate conversations of a human and answer questions related to military aircraft, ships and geographic information (Broughton et al. 2002). This complements the features of a virtual human developed by Rickel et al. (2002) and makes the idea of a highly-realistic virtual counselor possible. Such an integrated system would give an opportunity to test if there is value in using highly realistic avatars for motor priming and developing shared presentations in motor cognition and control.

## AN E-MENTAL HEALTH FRAMEWORK

This section discusses the requirements for an e-mental health system, after reviewing e-mental health applications.

### E-Mental Health Apps

Current e-mental health apps do not offer any facilities to promote social interaction between the counselor and the user. For example, Smedberg and Sandmark (2012) designed a prototype of a mobile phone app for self-reflection. This app is integrated in a larger web based stress management system. The user input is sent to the web based system. Based on the documented stress situation, an expert in the web based stress management system recommends relevant stress exercises to work on. The goal of the mobile app is to help people become more aware of patterns of stressful events. The application has two main parts: First part is registration and management of stressful situations. The other part is to display statistical data about the situations. It logs and displays basic information about self-perceived stress situations, such as location and time. The mobile phone app is used only for monitoring. The main problem with this app is the lack of interaction between the user and the counselor.

Another interesting example is an e-health game developed by Dennis and O-Toole (2014). The game makes use of attention-bias modification training (ABMT), an emerging cognitive treatment for anxiety. In this treatment, patients are expected to ignore a threatening stimulus (such as an angry face) and instead they focus on a non-threatening stimulus (such as a neutral or happy face). This type of training has been shown to reduce anxiety and stress among people suffering from high anxiety. The study involved 75 participants who all scored relatively high on an anxiety survey. They were required to follow two characters around on the screen, tracing their paths as quickly and accurately as possible. After playing the game for 25 to 45 minutes, the participants were asked to give a short speech to the researchers while being recorded on video. Public speaking was an especially stressful situation specifically for these participants. The videos revealed that participants who played the ABMT-based version of the game showed less nervous behavior and speech during their talk and reported less negative feelings afterward.

Ranjbartabar et al. (2015b) developed a mobile stress management system prototype for students with mental health problems. The app allows registered doctors to upload their customized questionnaires. There is no interaction between the doctor/counsellor and the user. The goal of this app is to measure student's excessive stress and anxiety by a questionnaire and based on this qualitative measurement to return feedback to the student about appropriate treatment options for reducing the stress level. They tested the prototype with 10 students who participated the study for two months. Participants were university students in the age range of 18 to 25. They were asked to use the application for one month during their exams and one month after their exams at least twice per week. The results show that although 80% of the students had high and 20% had mild levels of stress during the first month, 90% had a lower level of stress in the second month. After the testing period, they drew the comparisons between the diagnostics

*Table 1. Functionalities of top eMental health apps*

| Functions of the Apps | Counseling | | | | Relaxation Feedback | | | | Score |
|---|---|---|---|---|---|---|---|---|---|
| | Video | Audio | Text | Questionnaire | Physiological | Personal | Multilingual | Musical | |
| Take a break | | 1 | | 1 | | | | 1 | 3 |
| End Anxiety | | 1 | | | | | | | 1 |
| Stress Test | | | | 1 | | 1 | | 1 | 3 |
| I can be free | 1 | 1 | | | | | | 1 | 3 |
| Stress Check | | | 1 | | 1 | 1 | | | 3 |
| Stress quotes | | | 1 | | | | | | 1 |
| Sleep Easily | | 1 | | | | | | 1 | 2 |
| eMentalHelp | 1 | | 1 | | 1 | | 1 | 1 | 5 |
| | 25% | 50% | 38% | 25% | 25% | 25% | 13% | 63% | |

of the prototype and the opinion of a certified practitioner. The results indicate that the application was able to correctly diagnose mental health problems of the participants. The questionnaire was designed by consulting a medical practitioner.

Prior to the app development, Ranjbartabar et al. (2015a) reviewed e-health mobile applications on both iPhone and Android platforms. They listed the functionalities of e-health apps. The selection of these mobile apps was based on overall user rating, as these are free apps that come in the top seven in the search result. In Table 1, authors present a comparative analysis based on this review, including the app developed by Ranjbartabar et al (2015b):

- "Take a break" app is one of the highly rated applications that allow users to listen to audio records of meditation with sounds of nature or music in the background. While listening to the audio, the speaker gives instructions and requests the user to follow a number of movements. The suggested positions are useful and users can select comforting background sounds of ocean, rain, etc. However, the application is not personalized and does not consider users' circumstances. It is voice based, monolingual, and its use is limited by people who have no hearing problems.
- 'End Anxiety Hypnosis' app teaches self-hypnosis to its users. Hypnosis may not alleviate the stress level of all users, if not practiced properly. It is not guaranteed to be performed correctly by all either; therefore, it might have negative effects on users.
- "Stress Test App" is used to examine severity of the stress. It provides a questionnaire made up of 30 questions to measure users' stress level. To help users to relax, it provides a number of stress relief audio records and helps them to monitor their stress using graphs. Its core weakness is the rigid questionnaire and the suggestion of only a limited number of solutions.
- "I can be free" helps users to overcome their fears by talking and playing music.
- "Stress Check by Azumio - Lite" assesses the level of psychological or physical stress and measures users' stress by monitoring heart rate after touching the camera lens. Its main problem is the accuracy of the sensors.
- "Anti-stress quotes" provides different quotes to stressful people. Its weakness is not customizing the quotes, and not providing any solutions based on users' personal situation.
- "Sleep Easily by Shazzie" provides various meditation methods to help users to sleep at ease.

- "eMental Health" In addition to relaxation music and watching videos, the application provides features such as, access to Facebook, a questionnaire for better mental diagnostic, emergency alert to locate family and friends, a facility to locate and rate doctors, user's status for following-up, data and statistics to research centres, facility to customize the questionnaire by doctors, text-based and multilingual support, coverage of a wide range of mental health problems.

As seen in Table 1, none of these eMental Health apps provides a virtual stress counselor that is available for social interaction. 63% rely on musical feedback and 50% make use of audio records. 38% is text-based. Only 25% provides personal feedback, make use of questionnaires and video records, and measures psycho-physiological feedback. This comparative analysis demonstrates the fact that the top rated e-mental health apps do not facilitate social interaction with a virtual counselor in the current state.

## Requirements for an E-Mental Health System

Requirements analysis is critical to the success of an application development, similar to any software project. The requirements should be documented, measurable, and verifiable. System Analysts can employ several techniques or a combination of these to elicit the requirements from the user. These may include the development of scenarios, the identification of use cases, the use of observation, holding interviews, or focus groups and creating requirements lists. Prototyping may be used to develop a sample system that can be demonstrated to users. Author has specified the requirements for an e-mental health system including four different types of feedback: affective, personalized, agent-based, gender-adaptive, and stress-related coping feedback.

**Requirement 1:** Affective feedback. Affective feedback is an attribute to emotionally responsive user interfaces. Computers cannot respond properly to the users, since they have limitations in the interpretation and evaluation of the users' social signals. If computers are expected to be genuinely intelligent and to interact naturally, they must have the ability to recognize, understand, even to have and express emotions. In literature, there are attempts to develop affective agents. For example, (Cassell et al. 1999) developed technologies for sensing user affects through a variety of physiological, nonverbal and verbal channels (e.g., facial expression, postures, galvanic skin response, muscle contraction and speech.) Others developed systems for displaying affective signals using a variety of modalities (e.g., speech and facial expression (Tosa 1994)). Ball and Breese (2000), Allbeck and Badler (2002), and Rosis et al. (2003) generated affect and personality using a variety of behavioural cues including vocal cues, verbal cues, facial expressions, gestures and postural information. Vanhala and Surakka (2005) developed an affective system reading various physiological signals from the user's facial muscles and heart rate. They used a special chair to analyse users' emotion-related behavior in the production of electronic social-emotional cues for the user while interacting with digital media. They combined this feedback with Finnish speech synthesizers. These studies demonstrate the feasibility of using psycho-physiological feedback for sensing the affective response.

**Requirement 2:** Personalised feedback. Kavakli et al (2012) stated that *personalization* is highly important for a virtual counsellor, as students wish to get relevant and tailored advice for themselves; and the agency and/or empathy has to be established between the user and the virtual counsellor. Empathy is the capacity to understand what another person is experiencing from within the other person's frame of reference, i.e., the capacity to place oneself in another's place. Watching another person or an avatar may provide a means whereby people can determine agency. The similarity between the avatar and the user is an important factor to establish agency. Kavakli et al (2012) designed a prototype e-mental health system and elicited the requirements for this conducting a pilot study with students. They found that students require the virtual counsellor to exhibit humane features that they can relate to. If appropriately built, such a system would give students a better sense of control over their exams and a sense of social support that they otherwise might find difficult to obtain. Students in their experiments stated that such a system would significantly reduce the stress level and provide effective strategies in managing exam stress. Desktop computers are no longer sufficient for providing timely support for mental health problems. Especially, young people and females prefer to use more contemporary and personalized mobile tools.

**Requirement 3:** Agent-based feedback. The agent-based feedback presented by the avatar has implications in the acceptance of technology. As reflected by students during the interview process (Kavakli et al., 2012), the use of avatar "has a good call" and "students really need this". Kavakli et al. (2012) proposed an avatar-based interface between the user and the system. The social interaction is achieved through a *personalised* avatar using an embodied conversational agent. There is a need to study how personalized avatars could influence people's coping processes. They suggested that one must examine how to effectively mimic the knowledge, diagnosis and behaviour of counsellors through an intelligent embodied agent, to help students better cope with exam stress.

**Requirement 4:** Gender-adaptive feedback. Kavakli and Chen (2014) conducted a survey regarding the perception of Information Technology (IT) with 20 male and 20 female participants. They asked participants to identify the gender of their IT device and compared the responses of females to males. They found gender differences in the perception of IT, as well as the user interaction with the technology using gestures (specifically, gesture types, frequency and occurrences.) Their findings state that in general including male and female participants' responses, desktop computers seem to be perceived as a more masculine technology (43.3%), mobile phones are perceived more feminine (50%), laptops have no gender (68%), neither does the Internet (73%). However, when comparisons are drawn between males and females, Kavakli and Chen (2014) found that there are gender differences in the perception of the gender of technology. Majority of males think that their IT device has no gender. All males consider the internet with no gender at all. If there is a gender associated with it, desktop is masculine (40%), mobile phone (20%) and laptop are feminine technologies (14.2%). More interestingly, Kavakli and Chen (2014) stated that more than 86.6% of females think that their desktop has a gender (while more than half of females think that their desktop is masculine, the other half think that it is feminine). Their perception of mobile technology is primarily feminine (80%), but their laptop (36.3%) and Internet (33.3%) are partially feminine, while majority of them think that their laptop and internet has no gender. These findings imply that while males show a tendency to objectify the technology, they do not seem to associate with the personality or gender behind their IT device. For them, an IT device is an object, whereas a large proportion of females seem to perceive personality and gender associated with their IT device. They suggested that these differences between males and females may be the driving force behind their use of technology.

**Requirement 5:** Stress-related Coping feedback. Kavakli et al. (2012) conducted semi-structured and in-depth interviews demonstrating a preliminary prototype to potential users. Interviews with

14 undergraduate students were recorded and then transcribed. Open, axial and selective coding methods were used to analyze the data (Glaser and Strauss 1967). A tranquil environment of a counselling clinic was simulated in the Virtual Reality Lab to capture genuine reactions of students in dialogue with the prototype of the Virtual Counsellor (ESCAP). The results (Kavakli et al, 2012) indicate that a Virtual Counsellor is potentially a very promising tool. In the interviews, 21% of the respondents admitted that they have issues with exam stress. However, the common stress symptom indicators (UOM 2010) failed to detect the students' exam stress. Measurement of stress and providing proper Stress Management feedback is very important for an e-Mental Health app. There are good examples of questionnaires that can be used for this purpose. For example, Ranjbartabar (2015) investigated whether a single questionnaire developed by a medical practitioner is enough to detect mental health problems and found that it is sufficient. Shibli et al. (2014) used Dr. OZ's Anxiety Scale Test to assess examination/test anxiety among 60 college students and found that it successfully depicts examination anxiety among subjects. Their results also reflected gender based examination anxiety among subjects. They stated that females are more prone to anxiety. This also stresses the necessity of gender adaptive feedback.

## AN AFFECTIVE VIRTUAL STRESS COUNSELOR SYSTEM

This section discusses the development of a framework for an e-mental health system handling *personalized* interactions between a virtual counselor and a student requiring help to manage their stress levels during exams. Authors propose an affective system integrating technologies for facial expression detection, speech recognition, emotion recognition from speech and other psycho-physiological readings such as heart rate and skin conductivity. To give a personality to the system, authors call this affective system Dr McQuerry.

The proposed framework is underpinned by coping theory. Coping is considered as a problem solving process. The framework highlights constructs of interest that emerged from qualitative data analysis stage conducted by Kavakli et al. (2012). They identified moderating variables for coping processes as personality, gender, attribution style in their pilot studies regarding the credibility, competence, and attractiveness of the gender of a virtual counselor. In the proposed framework, students verbally interact with the highly personalized and animated virtual counsellor avatar, Dr McQuerry. Dr McQuerry is an embodied conversational agent with the behavioral traits of facial expressions and gestures to make the conversation more immersive.

The benefits of this affective system for the community have been largely discussed before, but the benefits to the research domain would be as follows:

- To find thresholds for the measures of psycho-physiological feedback for sensing the affective response.
- To explore correlations between students' stress level, "perceived social support", "perceived exam control", "speech rate", "perceived personality", and "gender" of the avatar.
- To develop evaluation methods to test the effectiveness of a virtual counselor in providing personalized feedback to reduce student's stress level and enhance their exam stress management strategies.

## System Architecture

As raised by users in the interviews by Kavakli et al. (2012), the central focus in an e-mental health system should be personalization and anthropomorphism. Personalization refers to providing tailored exam management advice to accommodate individual differences. Anthropomorphism (Zanbaka et al., 2006) refers to the extent a virtual agent resembles the appearance or behavioral attributes of a human counselor. This aligns well with afore-mentioned design goals for a virtual counselor, "behavioral and conversational realism".

Figure 2 illustrates the interaction between the various components of the system and demonstrates the system architecture that maximizes personalization and anthropomorphism. Dr McQuerry interacts with students, using the following components: the Behavioral Module (via animation and conversation processor), User Module (via emotion processor), Learning Module (via a coping processor) and an Expert System (via a decision support and knowledge processor). Interactive Drama Engine mediates the relations between these modules. Although the integration of these components in Dr McQuerry is novel, the components have been developed step by step in various previous projects. Learning Module and Expert System have been explained in detail in Kavakli et al (2012). The project contributes to the research domain not only with the integrated system development, but also with the concept development, especially regarding our approach to the coping processes. The mechanics of Coping Processor is original to this chapter and therefore requires further discussion in the remaining parts of the chapter.

The interface between the user and the system is an avatar (Dr McQuerry) that exhibits both facial and upper body animations, such as hand gestures. The system automatically evaluates users' speech and emotions. The User Module contains user data for more personalized diagnosis. Associated diag-

*Figure 1. Main screen, questionnaire screen for diagnosing depression*
*Ranjbartabar et al, 2015.*

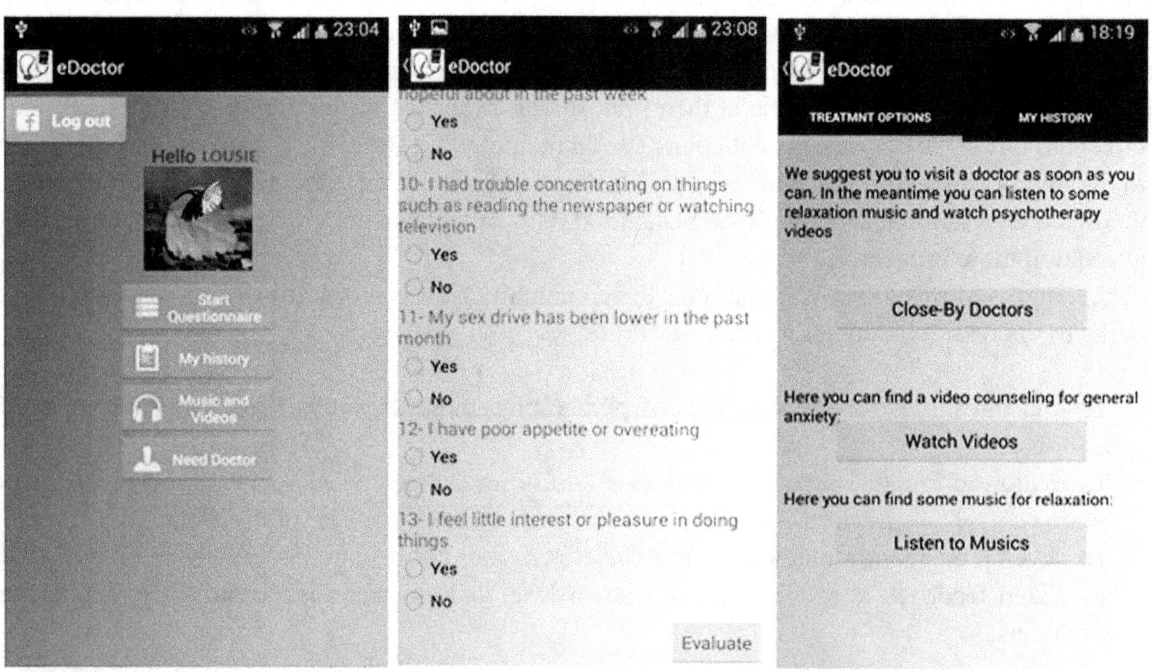

*Figure 2. System architecture for a eMental health system*

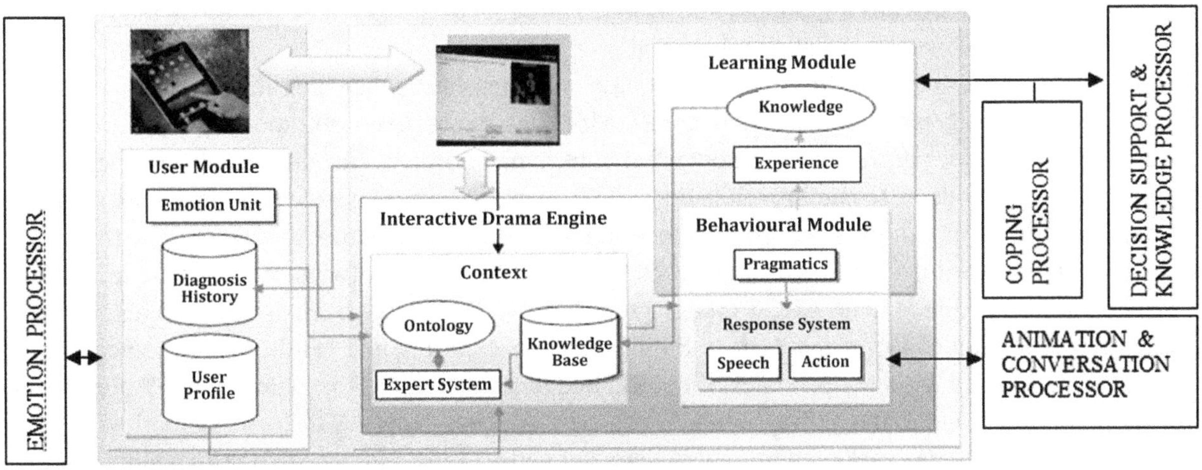


nosis captured in previous or current counseling sessions is stored in the user module. The Emotion Unit captures the emotion of the user. Fine tuning is conducted by the inference engine of the expert system to give a human touch to the avatar by facilitating and generating an appropriate non-verbal expression (both facial and hand gestures). The diagnosis history stores the diagnosis and interactions of current and previous counseling sessions of the user with the system. It is updated by the experience unit of the Learning Module. The information from the diagnosis history may serve as an acquaintance of Dr McQuerry with the user and begin the process of initial dialog with reference to earlier counseling sessions. The Learning Module stores vital conversational details between the user and the system for reference in current and future consultation sessions. For further descriptions on technical details of system design, please refer to (Rudra et al. 2012). The user profile stores the data about individual characteristics for better understanding of socio-economic and cultural background of the user to assist in diagnosis. The intelligence and behavior of the avatar is controlled by the context and behavioral modules of the interactive drama engine respectively. The Context Module implements the generation of advice in the coping process outlined in our research model and consists of an expert system. The decisions made by the expert system during the course of the conversation is drawn from the application of inference rules on the knowledge base developed by consulting existing literature, clinical documents and experts in student psychology. The knowledge base for the virtual counselor needs to be rigorously verified by domain experts. Compiling a counseling knowledge base will be an ongoing process even after implementation of the system. Therefore, it requires regular updates by knowledge experts in the domain of student psychology.

Customization of the system remains a challenge, since we need to cater for students from different cultural, social and ethnic backgrounds. The ontology provides a persona to the avatar, Dr McQuerry and guides the reasoning process by cross checking the diagnosis history, experience from the current session and current emotional state of the user. It governs the behavior of the avatar during its conversation with the user. Post diagnosis, data from the Experience Unit is documented in the diagnosis history database for future consultation with the same user. Pragmatics governs how the avatar comprehends a situation and produces conversation with the user. Any new experience of the agent is stored as knowledge for updating the expert system's knowledge base after consultation with a psychologist. The Context Module sends diagnosis related questions and decisions to the behavioral module which codes the speech and gesture (action) mark-up files for emoting the avatar. The behavioral module is the core to the realization of one of our research goals - believability to the user of the system.

Creating character believability involves not only creating intelligence or realism but also providing affective connection between humans and agents. Modeling expressive agent motions that can embody distinctive personalities and engage in nonverbal communication is a current topic in Artificial Intelligence (AI). With today's technology, it is possible to sense the emotions of a user from the statistical prosodic feature of speech by an emotion detection software. Such an emotion detection software was developed at Vox Institute, Geneva by (Zei, 2010) using PRAAT (Dutch for 'talk') software technology. This software was utilized in an ARC Linkage grant LP0216837 (Kavakli, Bossomaier, Tien, Cooper), "Cognitive Modeling of Computer Games Pidgins". Their experimental results show the accuracy of the system to classify the emotion states of neutral and anger with 94% for males and 95% for females (Rudra et al., 2007 and 2007b). Pidgin words can be classified using SVM for the emotion states of neutral and anger and can make a non-player-character (NPC) react not only by the meaning of the utterance of the user but also their emotional state. Collecting data about skin conductivity and heartbeat, based on the context and the sensed emotion of the student, the avatar of Dr McQuerry (Figure 3) can be emoted in real-time through dynamically generated XML from the system database using a behavioral markup language (BML). This technique is similar to the one in GRETA (Pelachaud, 2009) which is a multi-lingual embodied conversational agent.

## System Implementation

An e-mental health system has been developed as a prototype using a Content Management System to publish web pages so that a psychologist can design as many interactive sessions as required. The tool is accessible using an Iphone. A number of animations have been completed for the pilot study. Three prototypes as an avatar for Dr McQuerry have been developed at various levels of realism for testing as seen in Figure 4, using various technologies, such as Xist Face Tracking and Motion Builder, Mascarad and 3D Max, and Crazy Talk.

- **Code:** A server based design approach was used for the application for ease in publishing to many platforms at once and centralizing for immediate deployment of updates. Code encapsulates Information and Media. A Model View Controller paradigm provided by the Django 1.6 frame-

*Figure 3. Creating an emoted avatar using Face tracking technology*
*Kavakli et al., 2012.*

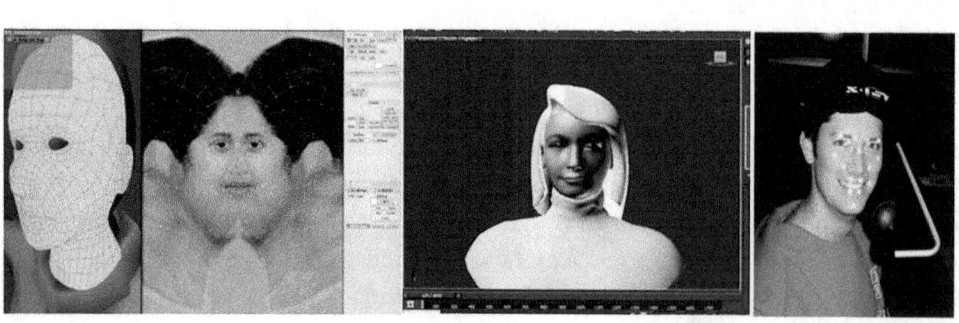

*Figure 4. Prototype of Dr McQuerry*

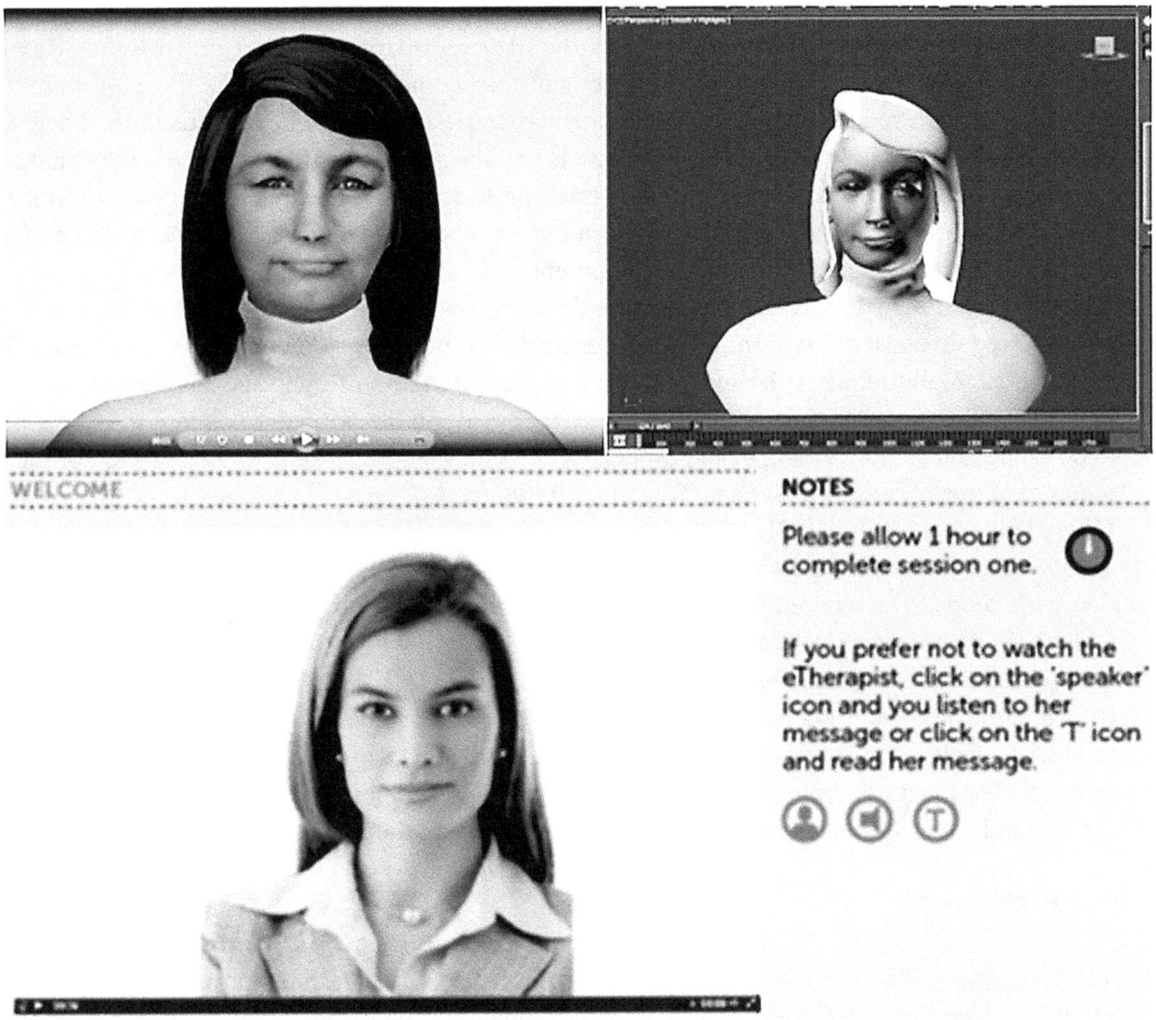


work was implemented. Django uses the python scripting language to quickly provide a web/database interface that is well supported, scalable, and easy to maintain. The application interfaces with a MySQL database at the moment, which was chosen for ease and speed of setup for the pilot. Through the use of Python, javascript and libraries such as JQuery Mobile, it is possible to access the smartphone to crowdsource information and media. Conversion tools such as phone gap can allow compilation of the application to run natively on the application if this is needed. PhoneGap is a free and open source framework that allows you to create mobile apps using standardized web APIs for various platforms such as iOS, Android, Blackberry 10, Firefox, and Windows 8.

- **Xist Face Tracking and Motion Builder:** As seen in Top Left in Figure 4, Face tracking technology can help build an avatar with realistic facial expressions using Xist Infrared Face Tracking device and Motion Builder software. 3D Studio Max and Softimage|XSI with FBX plug-ins have been used for 3D modelling of the avatar, similar to the methods used in Kavakli and Kartiko (2009). 3D Studio Max has a built in exporter for.FBX format which MotionBuilder reads. In

MotionBuilder, it is possible to set up the rig of the character and apply the Motion-Capture (mo-cap) animation onto the character's skeleton, see Figure 1. There are a number of problems that have to be addressed. In the implementation, the file export from Motion Builder to 3D Max has been found problematic. Facial muscle movements can be jammed during the file export process. This may require re-capturing the animations and cause repetitions in face tracking. There is a trade off in between how realistic the animations and the model should be to assess the benefits of using this laborious3D modelling and face tracking technology. It may be seen too complicated since it requires a real professional actor, or a real psychologist, as well as a face tracking expert and an animator, as well as software development and content development teams.

- **Mascarad and 3D Max:** Mascarad is a simple video tracking software. However, the use of the software requires extensive training and the end result is not successful due to its complexity. The software generally requires the manipulation of each animation to get reasonable results which may be much more complex than expected. After tweaking the animations, there may be a need to do video and audio tracking again, especially if the new audio records to be collected or the 3D model requires revisions, as seen in Top Right in Figure 4.
- **CrazyTalk:** CrazyTalk is a 2D animation program, easy and quick to use. CrazyTalk Animator is suitable for beginners, educators, video editors and all users that need a total 2D Animation solution with deep character creation and performance animation tools (see Figure 4 Bottom model). CrazyTalk Animator focuses on total animation production with actors, props, scenes, camera & a complete time-line for precision animation. With CrazyTalk Animator it is possible to choose from a number of pre-modelled characters. The avatars are primarily talking heads with full-body motion. However, the characters are actual models and generally look too good looking to represent a professional psychologist in practice. It is simple to implement as it requires only mapping the lip model and animation to the actual video stream, and therefore easier to produce.

## Coping Processor

What differentiates this affective e-mental health system from any other expert system development is the idea of development of a Coping Processor which can act as an extension to human mind informing the person about the coping strategies for stress management. Coping Processor requires a 3-stage development as discussed below:

1. **Identification of Moderator Variables (Individual Characteristics):** Due to disparity in coping taxonomies, people with different characteristics handle stress in different ways. This requires the use of different coping strategies depending on the user profile. Individual characteristics that potentially modulate the effectiveness of strategy include personality, age, gender, the level of maturity and attribution styles (Amirkhan and Auyeung, 2007). Understanding the influence of individual characteristics on coping processes provides the developers with the ability to explore how to maximize the effectiveness of a virtual counsellor in counseling a student under stress. Kavakli et al. (2012) state that tailored exam stress management strategies based on individual characteristics are deemed more effective for students and suggested to use the Guilford-Zimmerman Temperament personality scale (Guilford 1976), which had been widely used in literature and demonstrated to have good psychometric properties (Wang and Gan, 2010), to assess individual characteristics.

There is evidence that the acceptance of the avatar of a virtual counsellor highly depends on its characteristics. Kavakli et al. (2012) conducted pilot tests with potential system users (25 university students). They gave the listeners 4 different states of the same speech spoken by males and females (e.g., 10Hz, 30 Hz, fast, slow) and asked them to assess the credibility, pleasantness, dynamism, and clarity of the speech in 8 samples given on an evaluation sheet. In 200 samples, Kavakli et al (2012) found that in general the voices of male advisors are considered more pleasant and credible than female advisors. On the other hand, the voices of female advisors are considered more clear, dynamic and competent than male advisors' by most users. This gives interesting implications regarding the design of virtual psychologists, stating that one should consider the gender of the virtual advisor carefully to maximize its effect on users. Further investigations should be carried out in this aspect.

2. **Establishment of Association with the Virtual Counselor:** Kenton (1989) stated that "Even when men and women are objectively equal on these dimensions, receivers perceive men as being more persuasive as speakers." Feldstein et al. (2001) conducted a set of experiments assuming that listeners regard speakers whose global speech rates they judge to be similar to their own as more competent and more socially attractive than speakers whose rates are different from their own. They also investigated gender influences on those perceptions. Their participants were 17 male and 28 female listeners. They judged each of 3 male and 3 female speakers in terms of 10 unipolar adjective scales. They used 8 of the scales to derive 2 scores describing the extent to which the listener viewed a speaker as *competent* and *socially attractive*. The 2 scores were related by trend analyses. They examined trend components of the data by split-plot multiple regression analyses. In general, the results supported both hypotheses. Their findings state that the participants judged speakers with speech rates similar to their own as more competent and socially attractive than speakers with speech rates slower or faster than their own. However, the ratings of competence were significantly influenced by the gender of the listeners, and those of social attractiveness were influenced by the gender of the listeners and the speakers. The profile, gender, and speech rate of the user to display an avatar should be taken into account so that the user can associate with the avatar as persuasive and competent. Two important measures have to be taken into account in terms of speech rates and gender:
    a. Listeners' perceptions of the speakers' speech rates as compared with their own and
    b. Comparisons of the actual speech rates of the speakers and listeners.
3. **Designing a Coping Processor using Questionnaires:** Another important component of the Coping processor is the choice of the questionnaires to be used to measure the level of stress. Macquarie University has a Counselling service called UniWellBeing (http://students.mq.edu.au/support/health_and_wellbeing/counselling_service/). The UniWellbeing Course is a free, online and internet-delivered treatment Course for Macquarie University students. The UniWellbeing Course is designed to teach practical, proven, skills for managing symptoms of stress, anxiety, worry, low mood and depression. Many young adults have difficulties with stress but, few people seek and have access to treatment. The site states that as many as 50% of students experience stress, anxiety, worry, low mood and depression. The UniWellbeing Course is designed to help students learn practical strategies to stay emotionally healthy. Students can apply to participate in the Course by completing the CAPS Self-Referral Questionnaire that can be seen in Figure 5, Figure 6, and Figure 7. Two important measures have to be taken into account to design Questionnaires:

*Figure 5. Macquarie University exam stress questionnaire (page1)*

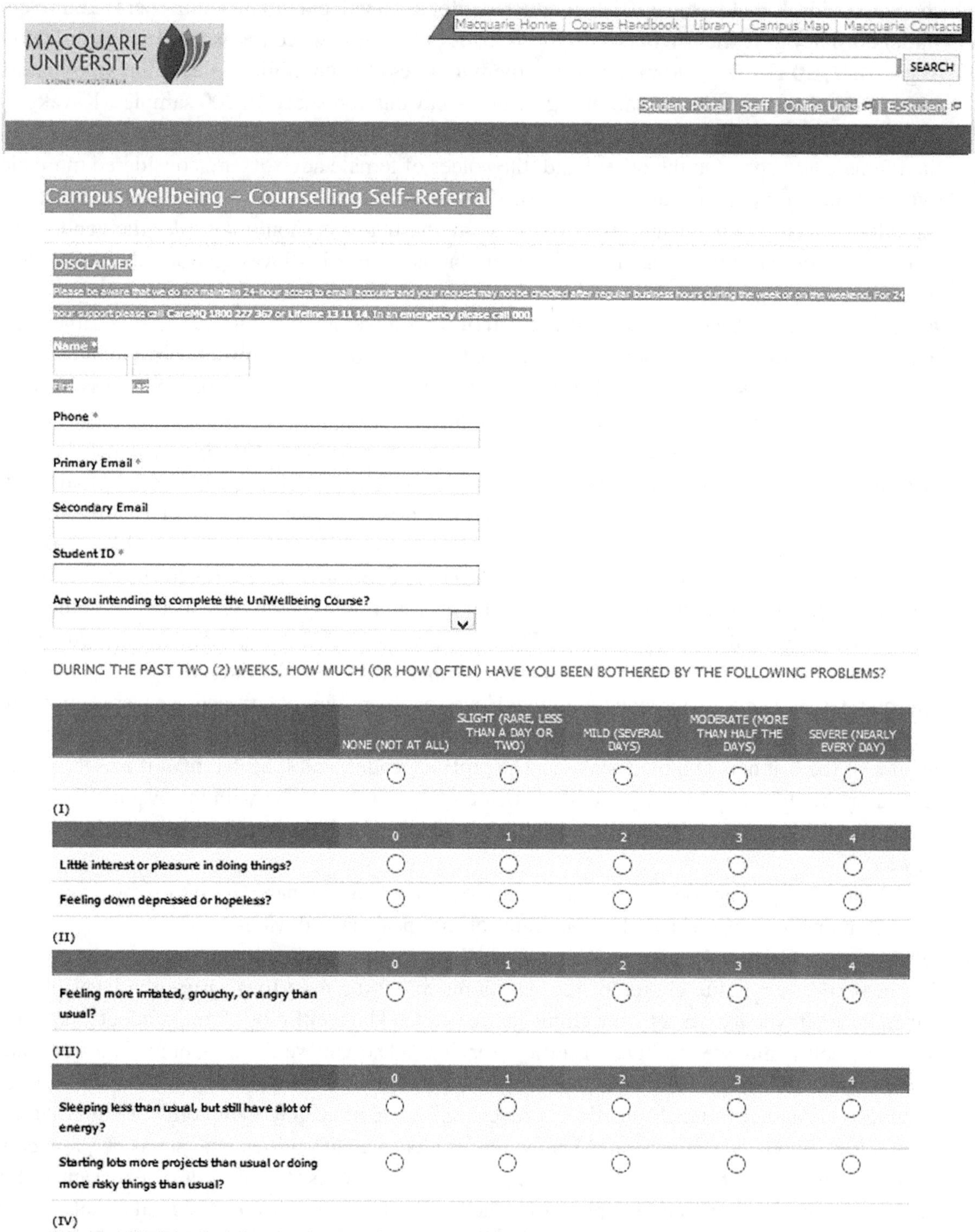

Macquarie Home | Course Handbook | Library | Campus Map | Macquarie Contacts

MACQUARIE UNIVERSITY

SEARCH

Student Portal | Staff | Online Units | E-Student

Campus Wellbeing – Counselling Self-Referral

DISCLAIMER

Please be aware that we do not maintain 24-hour access to email accounts and your request may not be checked after regular business hours during the week or on the weekend. For 24 hour support please call CareMQ 1800 227 367 or Lifeline 13 11 14. In an emergency please call 000.

Name *

First Last

Phone *

Primary Email *

Secondary Email

Student ID *

Are you intending to complete the UniWellbeing Course?

DURING THE PAST TWO (2) WEEKS, HOW MUCH (OR HOW OFTEN) HAVE YOU BEEN BOTHERED BY THE FOLLOWING PROBLEMS?

| | NONE (NOT AT ALL) | SLIGHT (RARE, LESS THAN A DAY OR TWO) | MILD (SEVERAL DAYS) | MODERATE (MORE THAN HALF THE DAYS) | SEVERE (NEARLY EVERY DAY) |
|---|---|---|---|---|---|
| | ○ | ○ | ○ | ○ | ○ |
| (I) | | | | | |
| | 0 | 1 | 2 | 3 | 4 |
| Little interest or pleasure in doing things? | ○ | ○ | ○ | ○ | ○ |
| Feeling down depressed or hopeless? | ○ | ○ | ○ | ○ | ○ |
| (II) | | | | | |
| | 0 | 1 | 2 | 3 | 4 |
| Feeling more irritated, grouchy, or angry than usual? | ○ | ○ | ○ | ○ | ○ |
| (III) | | | | | |
| | 0 | 1 | 2 | 3 | 4 |
| Sleeping less than usual, but still have alot of energy? | ○ | ○ | ○ | ○ | ○ |
| Starting lots more projects than usual or doing more risky things than usual? | ○ | ○ | ○ | ○ | ○ |
| (IV) | | | | | |

*Figure 6. Macquarie University exam stress questionnaire (page2)*

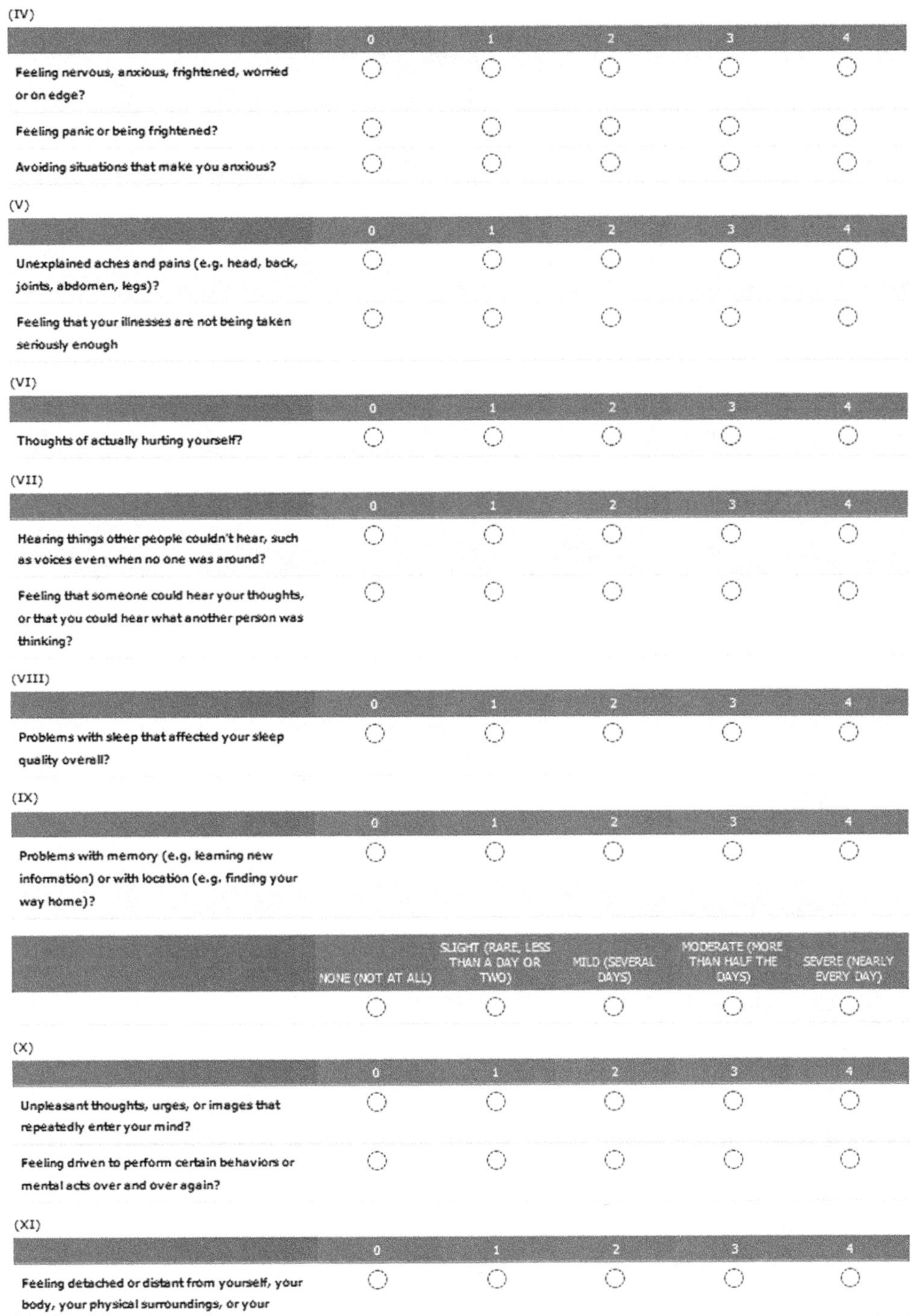

(IV)

| | 0 | 1 | 2 | 3 | 4 |
|---|---|---|---|---|---|
| Feeling nervous, anxious, frightened, worried or on edge? | ○ | ○ | ○ | ○ | ○ |
| Feeling panic or being frightened? | ○ | ○ | ○ | ○ | ○ |
| Avoiding situations that make you anxious? | ○ | ○ | ○ | ○ | ○ |

(V)

| | 0 | 1 | 2 | 3 | 4 |
|---|---|---|---|---|---|
| Unexplained aches and pains (e.g. head, back, joints, abdomen, legs)? | ○ | ○ | ○ | ○ | ○ |
| Feeling that your illnesses are not being taken seriously enough | ○ | ○ | ○ | ○ | ○ |

(VI)

| | 0 | 1 | 2 | 3 | 4 |
|---|---|---|---|---|---|
| Thoughts of actually hurting yourself? | ○ | ○ | ○ | ○ | ○ |

(VII)

| | 0 | 1 | 2 | 3 | 4 |
|---|---|---|---|---|---|
| Hearing things other people couldn't hear, such as voices even when no one was around? | ○ | ○ | ○ | ○ | ○ |
| Feeling that someone could hear your thoughts, or that you could hear what another person was thinking? | ○ | ○ | ○ | ○ | ○ |

(VIII)

| | 0 | 1 | 2 | 3 | 4 |
|---|---|---|---|---|---|
| Problems with sleep that affected your sleep quality overall? | ○ | ○ | ○ | ○ | ○ |

(IX)

| | 0 | 1 | 2 | 3 | 4 |
|---|---|---|---|---|---|
| Problems with memory (e.g. learning new information) or with location (e.g. finding your way home)? | ○ | ○ | ○ | ○ | ○ |

| | NONE (NOT AT ALL) | SLIGHT (RARE, LESS THAN A DAY OR TWO) | MILD (SEVERAL DAYS) | MODERATE (MORE THAN HALF THE DAYS) | SEVERE (NEARLY EVERY DAY) |
|---|---|---|---|---|---|
| | ○ | ○ | ○ | ○ | ○ |

(X)

| | 0 | 1 | 2 | 3 | 4 |
|---|---|---|---|---|---|
| Unpleasant thoughts, urges, or images that repeatedly enter your mind? | ○ | ○ | ○ | ○ | ○ |
| Feeling driven to perform certain behaviors or mental acts over and over again? | ○ | ○ | ○ | ○ | ○ |

(XI)

| | 0 | 1 | 2 | 3 | 4 |
|---|---|---|---|---|---|
| Feeling detached or distant from yourself, your body, your physical surroundings, or your | ○ | ○ | ○ | ○ | ○ |

*Figure 7. Macquarie University exam stress questionnaire (page3)*

| | NONE (NOT AT ALL) | SLIGHT (RARE, LESS THAN A DAY OR TWO) | MILD (SEVERAL DAYS) | MODERATE (MORE THAN HALF THE DAYS) | SEVERE (NEARLY EVERY DAY) |
|---|---|---|---|---|---|
| | ○ | ○ | ○ | ○ | ○ |

(X)

| | 0 | 1 | 2 | 3 | 4 |
|---|---|---|---|---|---|
| Unpleasant thoughts, urges, or images that repeatedly enter your mind? | ○ | ○ | ○ | ○ | ○ |
| Feeling driven to perform certain behaviors or mental acts over and over again? | ○ | ○ | ○ | ○ | ○ |

(XI)

| | 0 | 1 | 2 | 3 | 4 |
|---|---|---|---|---|---|
| Feeling detached or distant from yourself, your body, your physical surroundings, or your memories? | ○ | ○ | ○ | ○ | ○ |

(XII)

| | 0 | 1 | 2 | 3 | 4 |
|---|---|---|---|---|---|
| Not knowing who you really are or what you want out of life? | ○ | ○ | ○ | ○ | ○ |
| Not feeling close to other people or enjoying your relationships with them? | ○ | ○ | ○ | ○ | ○ |

(XIII)

| | 0 | 1 | 2 | 3 | 4 |
|---|---|---|---|---|---|
| Drinking at least 4 drinks of any kind of alcohol in a single day? | ○ | ○ | ○ | ○ | ○ |
| Smoking any cigarettes, a cigar, or pipe or using snuff or chewing tobacco? | ○ | ○ | ○ | ○ | ○ |
| Using any of the following medicines ON YOUR OWN, that is, without a doctor's prescription, in greater amounts or longer than prescribed [e.g., painkillers (like Vicodin), stimulants (like Ritalin or Adderall), sedatives or tranquilisers (like sleeping pills or Valium), or drugs like marijuana, cocaine or crack, club drugs (like ecstasy), hallucinogens (like LSD), heroin, inhalants ir solvents (like glue), or methamphetamine (like speed)]? | ○ | ○ | ○ | ○ | ○ |

Continue

a. **Perceived Exam Control (PEC):** Prior research on college students used the perceived academic control construct to assess students' sense of control over their academic achievements (Perry et al. 2005; Ruthig et al. 2007). Kavakli et al. (2012) propose to adapt the Perceived Academic Control Scale (Perry et al. 2001) to measure and assess PEC (Perceived Exam Control).
b. **Perceived Social Support (PSS):** Perceived social support refers to the provision of various resources including psychological and material resources that serve as a buffer against stressful events. Such resources can be provided by 4 strategies:
    i. Preventing the situation being perceived as stressful, for example through introducing continuous assessment methods or reducing the weight of exams,
    ii. By providing a solution to a stressful problem,
    iii. By minimizing its perceived importance, or
    iv. Facilitating healthy behavioral responses to the event (Crockett et al., 2007).

It is assumed that Dr McQuerry as an embodied conversational agent with highly intelligent, interactive and personalized advice should enhance user's perceived social support. This is achieved through providing tailored advice to manage stress (2nd strategy mentioned above), forming an appropriate attitude towards the exam (3rd strategy) and facilitating healthy behavioural responses to better handle stress (4th strategy).

4. **Measurement of Coping Outcomes:** Kavakli et al. (2012) propose to measure the stress level of students before and after their interview with Dr McQuerry who asks students questions about their mental state. Dr McQuerry may capture user's speech and facial expressions using built in cameras and motion tracking sensors. Both objective measures including participants' heart rate and skin conductivity, and self-reported stress level measures must be used. Further investigation has to be carried out to find out whether the use of the system has enhanced their stress management skills, as discussed below:
    a. **Objective Measures:** Heart rate and skin conductivity. Andreassi (2006) states that psychophysiology is the study of relations between psychological manipulations and resulting physiological responses. Psycho-physiological feedback is measuring subject's quantifiable physiological processes, such as heart rate, sweat, skin temperature and blood pressure. Anttonen and Surakka (2005) state that emotions can be conceptualised by valence (level of excitement) and arousal (level of pleasure). Scientists have used heart rate for measuring valence, while heart rate variability and galvanised skin response (skin conductivity level) have been used in measuring arousal (Anttonen and Surakka 2005; Ganglbauer et al. 2009). Examples include, NASA measuring the stress level in astronauts using psycho-physiological feedback, the Wild Divine games for relaxation, medical games for detecting and treating medical disorders (e.g., Dzhafarova et al. 2007). Among these, a relaxation game developed by Bersak et al. (2001) involves players racing against each other. Each player is connected to a device measuring their galvanized skin response, which is used to calculate their levels of relaxation and subsequently to control their speed levels. Based on these insights, Kavakli et al (2012) propose to use psycho-physiological feedback to measure the heart rate and skin conductivity of students to reveal their stress level.

b. **Subjective Measures:** Perceived stress. As suggested by Kavakli et al. (2012), the perceived stress construct can be measured through students' self-reported stress level using questionnaires with seven scales to rank (Cohen et al., 1983). In the Perceived Stress Scale (PSS), typical questions include: "During the last month, how often have you:...been upset because of something that happened unexpectedly;...felt that you were unable to control the important things in your life;...?" Responses (1=Never;7=Very often) are summed so that higher scores indicate greater perceived stress. Internal reliability of this shortened measure has been reported to be similar to PSS (Cohen et al., 1983; Shiovitz-Ezra et al. 2009).

5. **Identification of an Exam Stress Management Strategy:** Another important factor on student's coping process is the identification of more active exam stress management strategies. Kavakli et al. (2012) propose to use the items in Amirkhan and Auyeung (2007), which captures people's intention to implement certain coping strategies, to assess if there are any improvements in students' coping strategy after being exposed to a session with Dr McQuerry.

## SOLUTION, EVALUATION, AND RECOMMENDATIONS

### Implementation of the Framework

This section focuses on the implementation of the proposed e-Mental Health framework for Virtual Stress Counseling. The main objective of this chapter was to develop a framework for mobile e-mental health systems reviewing existing e-mental health apps and discussing necessary system requirements. The chapter stated that current e-mental health apps do not offer any facilities to promote social interaction between the counselor and the user. The proposed framework, therefore, requires personalized interactions between a virtual counselor and a student. It provides personalized feedback to reduce stress level and enhances personal stress management strategies. The e-mental health framework integrates technologies for facial expression detection, speech and emotion recognition and other psycho-physiological feedback such as heart rate and skin conductivity. A prototype system was developed without the use of psycho-physiological feedback in the first iteration. The current prototype uses a Content Management System to publish web pages so that a psychologist can design as many interactive sessions as required. The tool is accessible using a smart phone. A number of animations have been completed for the pilot study. Three prototypes as an avatar for Dr McQuerry have been developed at various levels of realism for testing, using various technologies, such as Xist Face Tracking and Motion Builder, Mascarad and 3D Max, and Crazy Talk. Further empirical studies are planned to conduct a comparative analysis on the usability of psycho-physiological feedback for sensing the affective response in immersive virtual reality versus mobile devices. The proposed system has been divided into 4 modules associated with 4 processors: the Behavioral Module (via animation and conversation processor), User Module (via emotion processor), Learning Module (via a coping processor) and an Expert System (via a decision support and knowledge processor). The stages of implementation can be listed as follows:

For the first stage of implementation, the correlations between student's stress level, exam control and perceived social support, speech rate, personality, and gender of the avatar must be investigated. It is proposed to test the usability of the e-mental health system Dr McQuerry in immersive virtual reality (VR), mobile, and online platforms to evaluate the efficiency of the framework for mobile e-mental health systems, conducting surveys with a large number of undergraduate students to assess the acceptance of the avatar. The surveys can then be analysed and conclusions be drawn for the first concept to start an iterative system design process.

Second stage of implementation involves conducting large scale experiments with undergraduate students during the exam period to empirically verify the impact of the prototype on students, displaying the avatar using an immersive VR system to maximize the user experience of anthropomorphism and personalization. Qualitative data using questionnaires (Guilford-Zimmerman Temperament personality scale, PEC, PSS and Dr. OZ's Anxiety Scale Test) can be collected during the experiments as previously discussed. In these experiments, the stress level of students monitoring qualitative and quantitative measures such as heart beat and skin conductivity, before and after their interactions are measured. The ECG, EMG, GSR and other quantitative measures are recorded. The results can be compared to moderator variables explained previously and the conclusions are drawn for fine-tuning the system.

Third stage of implementation involves conducting large scale experiments with undergraduate students during the exam period to empirically verify the impact of the prototype on students, displaying the avatar using smart phones. In these experiments, the stress level of students using a sensor based mobile application tracking qualitative and quantitative measures such as heart beat and skin conductivity are measured before and after their interactions. Continuous real time monitoring can be achieved using wireless network sensors. The ECG, EMG, GSR, heart-rate, optical pulse and other quantitative measures are recorded. The results can be compared to moderator variables explained previously and the conclusions are drawn for fine-tuning the system.

Fourth stage of implementation involves evaluation of the data collected in both experiments. The system developed for VR and mobile applications are refined and an online prototype is produced for mass distribution. For example, *Android*-based mobile devices enable a real-time calculation of heart rate and other quantitative measures for the two experimental studies. Thus, ECG, EMG, GSR data can be acquired in real time by *Shimmer*TM sensors and transmitted via *Bluetooth*, to be processed and evaluated on the mobile device. The aim here is to recognize emotions of the user by collecting and analyzing data from different types of sensors on the smartphones. To achieve this, a machine learning approach to gather, analyze and classify device usage patterns, and develop a social network service client for Android smartphones can be adopted. Shimmer3 IMU Evaluation Kit has Bluetooth streaming functionality. It is supported by a range of development software tools and applications including MatLAB and C# applications. Data can be analysed in MatLAB to find various behavioral patterns of the current emotional state and profile of the users using Bayesian Network classifier for emotion recognition. It is expected that the system can classify user emotions into 7 classes such as happiness, surprise, anger, disgust, sadness, fear, and neutral with high accuracy on a mobile platform. A mobile camera to detect facial expressions of the users and Support Vector Machines (SVMs) for classifying 7 basic emotions and neutral expression can be used. The facial expression features for emotion recognition can be extracted by Active Shape Model (ASM) fitting landmarks on a face and then dynamic features can be generated by the displacement between neutral and expression features.

Fifth stage of implementation involves conducting usability analysis after distributing the system to volunteers to test VR, mobile, and online versions of the system, evaluate the results and develop a framework for mobile e-mental health systems.

## EVALUATION AND ETHICAL CONCERNS

This section focuses on ethical issues in the use of VR and interactive computer simulations that might be critical in Virtual Stress Counseling. VR as a positive technology offers fresh and highly effective new approaches to creativity in the context of education, such as a more individual approach to learning and coping that creates opportunities for counsellors to engage users providing individual feedback. Thus, VR Technology may provide opportunities for individualized, automatic feedback, and promote collaboration and peer interaction in new powerful ways (Psotka, 2013). On the other hand, VR and interactive computer simulations can stretch and shape students' minds in ways that have not yet been explored by educators in large-scale implementations as disruptive technologies at its core (Psotka, 2013 and they may never fit into the existing framework of education unless current approaches to the use of educational technologies change. One of VR's assumed assets is its capacity to deliver high fidelity training or rehabilitation environments that are designed to promote transfer of VR-acquired learning or behavior to the real world; this asset is expected to support "positive" outcomes and to promote human welfare, but it is not hard to imagine the development of scenarios that could serve less "noble" purposes (Rizzo et al, 2003).

Ethical issues can be discussed under the following headings:

- **Borders of Reality and Addiction to Fantasy:** As users of simulations get habituated in a virtual world, the borders of reality may get blurred for them. Users may associate their poor performance in real world conditions with the characteristics of reality and might choose to escape to VR exposures. Rather than spending more time facing the physical reality, they may choose to spend more time in VR. This may result in individuals experiencing increased difficulties in accepting their conditions or status in reality, as well as addiction to fantasy.
- **Misrepresentations, Biased Representations, and Indecent Representations:** Even if virtuality and reality are not opposite concepts, simulation and reality, and representation and reality, certainly are (Brey, 2008). Brey (2008) argues that representations in VR or simulations of reality can become morally problematic for three reasons: failing to uphold standards of accuracy (misrepresentations), failing to uphold fairness and unfairly disadvantaging certain individuals or groups. (biased representations), and violation of standards of decency and public morality (indecent representations).
- **Altered Sense of Reality:** As VR technology becomes more accessible, individuals may seek to enter virtual environments in order to increase their own understanding of their psychological processes (Whalley, 1994). Such independent exploration, which lacks the therapeutic support and guidance, could prove to be detrimental to individuals with altered levels of reality-testing, experiencing hallucinations and delusions (Rizzo et al., 2003).
- **Avatars and Dependency:** In virtual environments, users assume control over a graphically realized character called an avatar. Avatars can be built after the likeness of the user, but more often, they are generic persons or fantasy characters. Engagement between Human and Computer Interaction may be perceived as Human to Human Interaction, leveraging human cognitive, perceptual and social attributes in a way that promotes interaction with technology in a social manner (Turk and Robertson, 2000), so much so that such engagement and bonding may enable users to build personal relationships with computers (Rizzo et al., 2003). According to the argument from a moral perspective, it is possible to establish a strong association with a virtual human that

may potentially create dependency, if the VR simulation is inhabited with very convincing and believable avatars. This argument has gained empirical support by Slater et al. (2006). The emotions appealed to in the treatment of virtual humans are the same emotions that are appealed to in the treatment of real humans, because these actions resemble each other so closely (Brey, 2008). Dependency on avatars may result in a threat to psychological well-being by way of providing an unhealthy substitute for physical proximity and real human to human interaction. It may promote social withdrawal and antisocial personality disorder.

- **Agency, Ownership, and Identity:** For any object or structure found in a virtual world, one may ask the question: Who has the ownership? Does the user or the company that developed the avatar assert intellectual property rights to the avatar? What kind of framework of rights and duties should be applied to virtual property? (Burk, 2005).
- **Depiction of Real Persons, Right to Privacy and Publicity:** Virtual reality and simulations may include characters that are modeled after the likeness of real persons, whether living or deceased, including manipulated or computer-generated images of real persons who are placed in fictional scenes or are made to perform behaviors that they have not performed in real life, often made without the person's consent (Brey, 2008).
- **Therapist/Client Relationship and De-Humanisation:** In any social interaction, nonverbal communication is of paramount importance in the therapist/patient relationship and the success of the treatment. Much of this nonverbal communication comes from facial expression, body posture, hand gestures, and intonations. The VR presentation of therapist is extremely important for the establishment of association with the therapist. If this association cannot be established successfully in VR due to weak representation of virtual humans or proceduralised interactive exposures, this may have negative consequences in the association of the client with therapist in reality and dehumanizing behavior and serves to diminish or habituate a person's sensitivity to human therapists.
- **Exposure Therapy:** Exposure therapy should be used to enhance therapy, rather than substitute for it. Therapists should only attempt to use VR for exposure therapy if they are qualified to provide exposure therapy. Likewise, clinicians should only use the VR applications for neuropsychological testing if these are areas of expertise (Rizzo et al., 2003).
- **Mistakes in Diagnosis and Treatment:** As predicted by Rizzo et al. (2003), although the current therapeutic uses of VR still require a clinician to be present, future uses will probably not have this requirement. Individuals will be able to download or purchase locally VR assessment and therapeutic tools. This may contribute to faulty self-diagnosis and inadequate self-treatment.
- **Access to Exposure Therapy:** Universal and fair access to services will need to be addressed not to cause a digital divide to occur in the access to sophisticated VR scenarios for assessment/diagnosis, therapy, stress management, and personal growth promoting applications, so that community-based mental health clinics or educational institutions serving lower socioeconomic communities or people living in lower socioeconomic conditions and more disadvantaged locations in terms of broadband access may have a fair access to VR technology, and these services are not limited to a more exclusive group of people.

## FUTURE RESEARCH DIRECTIONS

The e-mental health apps must provide personalized feedback to reduce stress level and enhance personal stress management strategies. This requires the development of an affective system integrating technologies for facial expression detection, speech recognition, emotion recognition from speech and other psycho-physiological readings such as heart rate and skin conductivity. Currently, a prototype system has been developed without the use of psycho-physiological feedback at this stage. Further studies are required to conduct a comparative analysis on the usability of psycho-physiological feedback for sensing the affective response in immersive virtual reality versus mobile devices.

The current scope of the research in the proposed framework is limited to student psychology but it can be further extended to the application areas of employee stress diagnosis and management, and intelligent virtual companion for people who are in need of close support. The system can support people who are going through breakups or survived domestic violence, victims of post-traumatic stress disorders and people suffering from depression. The proposed framework can be applied to these areas with modifications to the database and behavioral modeling of the avatar.

## CONCLUSION

In this chapter, we reviewed e-mental health systems, presented a debate on the development of e-mental health systems using VR as a tool for positive technology, and evaluated their use discussing relevant ethical issues. To be able to evaluate potentials of VR-based mobile e-mental health systems we presented a framework after reviewing existing e-mental health apps and discussing necessary system requirements. The proposed framework is based on personalized interactions between a virtual counselor and a student requiring help to manage their stress levels during exams. There is a significant need to promote mental health and wellbeing of young generations by the development of e-mental health applications that link mobile tools with traditional forms of counselling. Almost three-quarters of Australians report that stress has an impact on their physical health. As smartphones and tablets' popularity increases, so does the number of mobile applications to support the users. As demonstrated in the beginning of this chapter, driven by mobile apps, Australia's enthusiasm for touch-screen phones has rapidly increased. While the statistics demonstrate the potential usability of mobile apps in e-mental health by Australian adults, the demand is even greater for the young generations due to their greater use of mobile technology. High demand for mental health services and limitations of online facilities available add pressure on service providers. As a result, online mental health services that use health promotion technologies to promote youth wellbeing in Australia have been going through rapid changes in models of service delivery to address the demand. The traditional ways of providing face-to-face counseling services have been proven to be effective in helping students to get over stressful periods. However, given the high demand of such services, especially during the exam period, it is very unlikely that those issues be addressed timely for every student. A virtual advisor always accessible on a smart phone is a promising way to address the aforementioned problem.

In this chapter, we focused on how to develop tools for positive technology and more specifically, mobile e-mental health systems using a virtual stress counsellor. We stated the significance of the need for mobile tools for e-mental health apps and discussed whether there is actually any value in working on the development of virtual stress counselors. Then, we addressed a number of research questions such as:

- Is the use of avatars meaningful in e-mental health applications as virtual stress counselors?
- Is it possible to improve the stress management skills of a person by interacting with an avatar?
- How can we use avatars and animation technology to improve coping processes?

To answer these questions, the chapter reviewed e-mental health tools to identify system requirements, proposed a framework, and discussed the components of the system architecture as well as its implementation to draw conclusions regarding the tools for positive technology. The chapter provided evidence that people tend to react to avatars as if reacting to real human beings as well as that taking another person's perspective of events activates some of the same neural networks as would be activated if the person really was experiencing the imagined situation. Therefore, our conclusion is it is possible to use avatars as virtual stress counselors to improve stress management skills of people interacting with them. The proposed framework demonstrates the requirements and components of system architecture to achieve this.

There are major challenges in the development of virtual counselors, especially if they are expected to convey a feeling of social interaction. In this chapter, leveraging the feasibility of systems like Ellie (KCCI, 2011), we have proposed a framework for the development of eMental-Health tools, making use of an avatar (Dr McQuerry) simulating a stress counsellor with facial expressions and conversational intelligence. It has been demonstrated that the design and evaluation of a mobile system that acts as a virtual counselor and helps students with exam stress management may address the current problems of student's mental and physical well-being through the suggestion of effective stress management techniques. Coping theories in stress management and how virtual counselors can be designed to help students to positively cope with the exam stress are discussed given the context of a coping processor. The proposed framework requires integration of various technologies which are available today and the feasibility of the approach has been discussed with various examples. The outcome is an affective system integrating technologies for facial expression detection, speech recognition, emotion recognition from speech and other psycho-physiological readings such as heart rate and skin conductivity. Finally, we have drawn attention to a number of ethical considerations associated with the development of virtual counsellors.

## REFERENCES

Andreassi, J. L. (2006). *Psychophysiology: Human behavior and physiological response*. Lawrence Erlbaum Assoc Inc.

Allbeck, J., & Badler, N. (2002). Embodied Autonomous Agents. In K. Stanney (Ed.), *Handbook of Virtual Environments* (pp. 313–332). Lawrence Erlbaum Associates.

Amirkhan, J., & Auyeung, B. (2007). Coping with stress across the lifespan: Absolute vs. relative changes in strategy. *Journal of Applied Developmental Psychology*, *28*(4), 298–317. doi:10.1016/j.appdev.2007.04.002

Anttonen, J., & Surakka, V. (2005). *Emotions and heart rate while sitting on a chair* (pp. 491–499). ACM. doi:10.1145/1054972.1055040

Aldwin, C. (2007). *Stress, coping, and development: An integrative perspective*. NY: The Guilford Press.

ADDA. (2013). Anxiety and Depression Association of America. Screening for Depression. Retrieved from http://www.adaa.org/iving-with-anxiety/ask-and-learn/screenings/screening-depression

Baghurst, T., & Kelley, B. C. (2013). An Examination of Stress in College Students Over the Course of a Semester.

Ball, G., & Breese, J. (2000). Emotion and personality in a conversational agent. In *Embodied Conversational Characters. (pp.xx)*. Cambridge, MA: MIT Press.

Baumgartner, T., Valko, L., Esslen, M., et al. (2006). Neural correlate of spatial presence in an arousing and noninteractive virtual reality: an EEG and psychophysiology study. *Cyberpsychology & behavior*, *9*, 30–45.

Bersak, D., McDarby, G., Augenblick, N., McDarby, P., McDonnell, D., McDonald, B., & Karkun, R. (2001). Intelligent biofeedback using an immersive competitive environment. *Proceedings of Designing Ubiquitous Computing Games Workshop at UbiComp.*

Billings, A. G., & Moos, R. H. (1981). The role of coping responses and social resources in attenuating the stress of life events. *Journal of Behavioral Medicine*, *4*(2), 139–157. doi:10.1007/BF00844267 PMID:7321033

Brey, P. (2008). Virtual Reality and Computer Simulation. In K. Himma & H. Tavani (Ed.), Handbook of Information and Computer Ethics. John Wiley & Sons. doi:10.1002/9780470281819.ch15

Botella, C., Garcia-Palacios, A., Baños, R. M., & Quero, S. (2009). Cybertherapy: Advantages, Limitations, and Ethical Issues. *PsychNology Journal*, *7*(1), 77–100.

Broughton, M., Carr, O., Taplin, P., Estival, D., Wark, S., & Lambert, D. (2002). *Conversing with Franco, FOCAL's virtual adviser.* Retrieved from http://www.dominique-estival.net/ConversingWith-Franco_final.pdf

Burk, D. (2005). Electronic Gaming and the Ethics of Information Ownership. *International Review of Information Ethics*, *4*, 39–45.

Cassell, J., Bickmore, T., Campbell, L., Chang, K., Vilhjàlmsson, H., & Yan, H. (1999). Embodiment in Conversational Interfaces: Rea. *Proceedings ACM SIGCHI* (pp. 520-527). ACM Press.

Castiello, U., Lusher, D., Mari, M., Edwards, M. G., & Humphreys, G. W. (2002). Observing a human or a robotic hand grasping an object: Differential motor priming effects. In W. Prinz & B. Hommel (Eds.), *Attention and performance XIX* (pp. 314–334). Cambridge, MA: MIT Press.

Cohen, S., Kamarck, T., & Mermelstein, R. (1983). A global measure of perceived stress. *Journal of Health and Social Behavior*, *24*(4), 385–396. doi:10.2307/2136404 PMID:6668417

Coyne, J. C., Lazarus, R. S., Kutash, I. L., & Schlesinger, L. B. (1980). *Handbook on stress and anxiety.* San Francisco: Jossey-Bass.

Compas, B. E., Connor-Smith, J. K., Saltzman, H., Thomsen, A. H., & Wadsworth, M. E. (2001). Coping with stress during childhood and adolescence: Problems, progress, and potential in theory and research. *Psychological Bulletin*, *127*(1), 87–127. doi:10.1037/0033-2909.127.1.87 PMID:11271757

Crockett, L. J., Iturbide, M. I., Stone, R. A. T., McGinley, M., Raffaelli, M., & Carlo, G. (2007). Acculturative stress, social support, and coping: Relations to psychological adjustment. *Cultural Diversity & Ethnic Minority Psychology*, *13*(4), 347–355. doi:10.1037/1099-9809.13.4.347 PMID:17967103

David, S., Krantz, B. T., & Kiecolt-Glaser, J. (2014). *How stress affects your health*. American Psychological Association.

Dennis, T. A., & O'Toole, L. J. (2014). Mental Health on the Go: Effects of a Gamified Attention-Bias Modification Mobile Application in Trait-Anxious Adults. *Clinical Psychological Science*.

Dzhafarova, O. A., Donskaya, O. G., & Zubkov, A. A. (2007). Biofeedback computer games. *Biomedical Engineering*, *41*(4), 186–190. doi:10.1007/s10527-007-0040-3

Feldstein, S., Dohm, F., & Crown, C. L. (2001). Gender and speech rate in the perception of competence and social attractiveness. *The Journal of Social Psychology*, *141*(6), 785–806. doi:10.1080/00224540109600588 PMID:11827225

Gallese, V., Fadiga, L., Fogassi, L., & Rizzolatti, G. (1996). Action recognition in the premotor cortex. *Brain*, *119*(2), 593–609. doi:10.1093/brain/119.2.593 PMID:8800951

Ganglbauer, E., Schrammel, J., Deutsch, S., & Tscheligi, M. (2009). Applying psychophysiological methods for measuring user experience: possibilities, challenges and feasibility. *Proceedings of the Workshop on user experience evaluation methods in product development.*

Glaser, B., & Strauss, A. (1967). *Grounded Theory: The Discovery of Grounded Theory*. New York: de Gruyter.

Guilford, J. S. (1976). *The Guilford-Zimmerman Temperament Survey handbook*. San Diego, CA: EdITS.

Hoffman, H. G., Doctor, J. N., Patterson, D. R., Carrougher, G. J., & Furness, T. A. III. (2000). Virtual reality as an adjunctive pain control during burn wound care in adolescent patients. *Pain*, *85*(1), 305–309. doi:10.1016/S0304-3959(99)00275-4 PMID:10692634

Ijsselsteijn, W. A., & Riva, G. (2003). being there: the experience of presence in mediated environments. In: G. Riva, F. Davide, & W.A. Ijsselsteijn (Eds.), Being there: concepts, effects and measurements of user presence in synthetic environments (pp. 3–16). Amsterdam: Ios press. Retrieved from www.emergingcommunication.com/volume5.html

Virtual Doctor can advise on when to go to the ER. (2011). *KCCI*. Retrieved from http://www.kcci.com/Virtual-doctor-can-advise-on-when-to-go-to-ER/3903134

Karavolos, M. H., Spencer, H., Bulmer, D. M., Thompson, A., Winzer, K., Williams, P., & Khan, C. M. et al. (2008). Adrenaline modulates the global transcriptional profile of Salmonella revealing a role in the antimicrobial peptide. *BMC Genomics*, *9*(1), 458. doi:10.1186/1471-2164-9-458 PMID:18837991

Kartiko, I., Kavakli, M., & Cheng, K. (2009, August 11-14). The impacts of animated - virtual actors' visual complexity and simulator sickness in virtual reality applications. In B. Werner (Ed.), *Proceedings of the 2009 6th International Conference Computer Graphics, Imaging and Visualization* (pp. 147-152). IEEE Computer Society. doi:10.1109/CGIV.2009.66

Kavakli, M., & Chen, Y. L. (2014, October 12-16). Gender Differences in Gesture-based Interaction. *Proceedings of the Seventh International Conference on Advances in Human-oriented and Personalized Mechanisms, Technologies, and Services CENTRIC '14*, Nice, France (pp. 1-7).

Kavakli, M., & Kartiko, I. (2007, May 30 - 31). Avatar Construction for Believable Agents. *Proceedings of the tenth international conference on computer graphics and artificial intelligence 3IA '07*, Athens, GREECE (pp. 1-6).

Kavakli, M., Li, M., & Rudra, T. (2012). Towards the development of a virtual counselor to tackle students' exam stress, Transactions of the SDPS. *Journal of Integrated Design and Process Science*, *16*(1), 5–26.

Kavakli, M. (2012, July 17-20). Interacting with virtual humans and detection of facial expressions: What makes an avatar more real than real? Proceedings of the IADIS Conference on Game and Entertainment Technologies GET '12, Lisbon, Portugal (pp.1-8).

Kilner, J. M., Paulignan, Y., & Blakemore, S. J. (2003). An interference effect of observed biological movement on action. *Current Biology*, *13*(6), 522–525. doi:10.1016/S0960-9822(03)00165-9 PMID:12646137

Lazarus, R. S., & Folkman, S. (1984). *Stress, appraisal, and coping*. New York: Springer.

Lee, S., & Espelage, D. L.Jun Sung Hong. (2010). An ecological understanding of youth suicide in South Korea. *School Psychology International*, *31*(5), 531–546. doi:10.1177/0143034310382724

Li, M., Rudra, T., & Kavakli, M. (2012, April 16-17). E-counsellor - An Avatar for Student Exam Stress Management. *Proceedings of the 3rd International Conference on Information Management and Evaluation ICIME '12*, Atilim University, Ankara, Turkey (pp.185-193).

Malbos, E., Rapee, R. M., & Kavakli, M. (2013). A Controlled Study of Agoraphobia and the Independent Effect of Virtual Reality Exposure Therapy. *The Australian and New Zealand Journal of Psychiatry*, *47*(12), 160–168. doi:10.1177/0004867412453626 PMID:22790176

Matthew, A., & Stults-Kolehmainen, R. S. (2013). *The Effects of Stress on Physical Activity and Exercise*. Springer.

McLeod, S. A. (2009). Emotion Focused Coping. *Simply Psychology*. Retrieved from www.simplypsychology.org/stress-management.html#em

Milgram, S. (1963). Behavioral study of obedience. *Psycho J*, *67*, 371–378. PMID:14049516

Monkong, L., Pongpanich, S., Viwatwongkasem, C., Chantavanich, S., Wongpiromsarn, Y., & Katz, L. S. (2009). The effectiveness of program developed from cognitive experiential self-theory and life skills technique on adolescent coping with stress. *Nepal Medical College Journal*, *11*(4), 225–228. PMID:20635598

Pelachaud, C. 2009. Modelling Multimodal Expression of Emotion in a Virtual Agent, *Philosophical Trans. B,* 364, 3539-3548.

Perry, R. P., Hladkyj, S., Pekrun, R. H., Clifton, R. A., & Chipperfield, J. G. (2005). Perceived academic control and failure in college students: A three-year study of scholastic attainment. *Research in Higher Education*, *46*(5), 535–569. doi:10.1007/s11162-005-3364-4

Psotka, J. (2013). Educational Games and Virtual Reality as Disruptive Technologies. *Journal of Educational Technology & Society*, *16*(2), 69–80.

Ranjbartabar, H., Maddah, A., & Kavakli, M. (2015a, June 28-July 1). eMedicalHelp: A Customized Medical Diagnostic Application: Is a single questionnaire enough to measure stress? *Proceedings of the 2015 IEEE/ACIS 14th International Conference on Computer and Information Science (ICIS)*, Las Vegas, USA. IEEE.

Ranjbartabar, H., Maddah, A., & Kavakli, M. (2015b). An eMental-Health Application and Customised Questionnaires for Stress Measurement. *International Journal of Computer & Information Science*, 16(2), 1-7.

Rickel, J., Marcella, S., Gratch, J., Hill, R., Traum, D., & Swartout, W. (2002). Toward a new generation of virtual humans for interactive experiences. *IEEE Intelligent Systems*, *17*(4), 32–38. doi:10.1109/MIS.2002.1024750

Rizzolatti, G., Fadiga, L., Fogassi, L., & Gallese, V. (1996). Premotor cortex and the recognition of motor actions. *Brain Research. Cognitive Brain Research*, *3*(2), 131–141. doi:10.1016/0926-6410(95)00038-0 PMID:8713554

Riva, G. (2004). The psychology of ambient intelligence: activity, situation and presence. In G. Riva, F. Davide, F. Vatalaro, & M. Alcañiz (Eds.), *Ambient intelligence: the evolution of technology, communication and cognition towards the future of the human-computer interaction* (pp. 19–34). Amsterdam: Ios Press. Retrieved from www.emergingcommunication.com/volume6.html

Riva, G., Bacchetta, M., Baruffi, M., Rinaldi, S., & Molinari, E. (1999). Virtual reality based experiential cognitive treatment of anorexia nervosa. *Journal of Behavior Therapy and Experimental Psychiatry*, *30*(3), 221–230. doi:10.1016/S0005-7916(99)00018-X PMID:10619546

Riva, G., Botella, C., Légeron, P., & Optale, G. (Eds.), (2004). Cybertherapy: Internet and Virtual Reality as Assessment and Rehabilitation Tools for Clinical Psychology and Neuroscience (Vol. 99). Amsterdam: IOS Press.

Riva, G., Mantovani, F., Capideville, C. S., Preziosa, A., Morganti, F., Villani, D., & Alcaniz, M. et al. (2007). Affective Interactions Using Virtual Reality: The Link between Presence and Emotions. *Cyberpsychology & Behavior*, *10*(1).

Rizzo, A. S., Schultheis, M. T., & Rothbaum, B. O. (2003). Ethical Issues for the Use of Virtual Reality in the Psychological Sciences. In S. Bush & M. Drexler (Eds.), *Ethical Issues in Clinical Neuropsychology* (pp. 243–280). Lisse, Netherlands: Swets & Zeitlinger Publishers.

Rosis, F. D., Pelachaud, C., Poggi, I., Carofiglio, V., & Carolis, B. D. (2003). From Greta's mind to her face: Modelling the dynamics of affective states. *Int. Journal of Human-Computer*, *Studies in Health Technology and Informatics*, *59*(1-2), 81–118.

Ross, S. E., Bradley, N., Heckert, C., & Teresa, M. (1999). Sources of stress among college students.

Rudra, T., Li, M., & Kavakli, M. (2012, January5-7). ESCAP: Towards the Design of an AI Architecture for a Virtual Counselor to Tackle Students' Exam Stress. *Proceedings of the Hawaiian International Conference on System Sciences (HICSS)*, Hawaii (pp. 1-10). doi:10.1109/HICSS.2012.249

Rudra, T., Kavakli, M., & Tien, D. (2007a, Oct 30–Nov 2). Emotion Detection from Male Speech in Computer Games. *Proceedings of the IEEE TENCON '07*, Taipei International Convention Center, Taiwan (pp. 1-4).

Rudra, T., Kavakli, M., & Tien, D. (2007b, January 15-18). Emotion Detection from Female Speech in Computer Games. *Proceedings of the 4th International Conference on IT and Application ICITA '07*, Harbin, China (pp. 712-716). IEEE.

Sanchez-Vives, M.V., & Slater, M. (2005). From presence to consciousness through virtual reality. nature review neuroscience, 6, 332–339.

Sarafino, E. P. (2012). Health Psychology: Biopsychosocial Interactions (7th ed). Asia: Wiley.

Mental Health on the go: Reducing anxiety with smartphone app. (2014, March 18). Association for Psychological Science. *ScienceDaily*. Retrieved from www.sciencedaily.com/releases/2014/03/140318111900.htm

Shibli, N., Hasan, I., Shakeel, A., Shakeel, S., Yousaf, S., & Iqbal, M. (2014). Dr. Oz's Anxiety Scale as an Indicator of Test/Examination Anxiety among Male/Female College Students, *Int. Journal of Scientific and Research Publications*, *4*(12).

Shiovitz-Ezra, S., Leitsch, S., Graber, J., & Karraker, A. (2009). Quality of Life and Psychological Health Indicators in the National Social Life, Health, and Aging Project. *The Journals of Gerontology: Series B*, *64*(Suppl. 1), i30–i37. doi:10.1093/geronb/gbn020 PMID:19204071

Slater, M., Antley, A., Davison, A., Swapp, D., Guger, C., Barker, C., & Sanchez-Vives, M. V. et al. (2006). A virtual reprise of the Stanley Milgram obedience experiments. *PLoS ONE*, *1*(1), e39. doi:10.1371/journal.pone.0000039 PMID:17183667

Smith E.E., & Kosslyn, S.M. (2007). *Cognitive Psychology: Mind and Brain, Chapter11 Motor Cognition and Mental Simulation.* USA: PHI Pearson Higher education.

Smedberg, A., & Sandmark, H. S. (2012). Design of a Mobile Phone App Prototype for Reflections on Perceived Stress. *Proceedings of the Fourth International Conference on eHealth, Telemedicine and Social Medicine TELEMED '12*, Valencia, Spain. IARIA.

Schneider, S. M., & Workman, M. L. (1999). Effects of virtual reality on symptom distress in children receiving chemotherapy. *Cyberpsychology & Behavior*, *2*(2), 125–134. doi:10.1089/cpb.1999.2.125 PMID:19178248

Tosa, N., Murakami, K., Kakimoto, M., & Sato, S. (1994). Neuro-Character. *Proceedings of the AAAI '94 Workshop, AI and A-Life and Entertainment*.

Turk, M., & Robertson, G. (2000). Perceptual user interfaces. *Communications of the ACM*, *43*(3), 33–34. doi:10.1145/330534.330535

Stress Management Flyer. (2010). University of Melbourne. Retrieved from http://www.services.unimelb.edu.au/asu/download/Study-StressManagement-Flyer.pdf

White, S. (2013). Meet Ellie, The Virtual Psychologist. *Technology Guide*. Retrieved from http://www.technologyguide.com/news/virtual-psychologist-could-change-the-future-of-mental-health/

Vaez, M., & Laflamme, L. (2008). Experienced stress, psychological symptoms, self-rated health and academic achievement: A longitudinal study of Swedish university students. *Social Behavior and Personality*, *36*(2), 183–196. doi:10.2224/sbp.2008.36.2.183

Wang, Z., & Gan, Y. (2010). Coping mediates between social support, neuroticism, and depression after earthquake and examination stress among adolescents. *Anxiety, Stress, and Coping*, 24(3), 343-358. PMID:20865589

Washburn, C. A., & Mandrusiak, M. (2010). Campus suicide prevention and intervention: Putting best practice policy into action. *Canadian Journal of Higher Education*, *40*(1), 101–119.

Yang, S., & Shin, C. S. (2008). Parental attitudes towards education: What matters for children's well-being? *Children and Youth Services Review*, *30*(30), 1328–1335. doi:10.1016/j.childyouth.2008.03.015

Vanhala, T., & Surakka, V. (2005). An agent framework for the development of psycho- physiologically interactive systems. *Proceedings of HCI International 2005*, Las Vegas, Nevada, USA.

Yoshida, A., Hagita, Y., Yamazaki, K., & Yamaguchi, T. (1993). Which do you feel comfortable, interview by a real doctor or by a virtual doctor? A comparative study. *Proceedings of the 2nd IEEE International Workshop on Robot and Human Communication* (pp. 370-374)

Zanbaka, C., Goolkasian, P., & Hodges, L. F. (2006). Can a virtual cat persuade you? The role of gender and realism in speaker persuasiveness. In CHI 2006 proceedings. Montreal Quebec Canada.

Zei Pollerman, B. (2010, March 10-13). Karasek's Demand/Control model, emotions and Health (Poster). *Proceedings of the 68th Annual scientific meeting* (pp. 72).

## KEY TERMS AND DEFINITIONS

**Avatar:** An embodiment or manifestation of a person or idea. It is generally an icon, model, or image representing a particular person in a computer game or in a virtual world.

**Coping Processes:** There are three general coping processes in stress management: avoidance, seeking support and problem-solving.

**Coping:** Stress management that involves constantly changing cognitive or behavioral efforts to manage situations appraised as taxing or exceeding a person's resources.

**Embodied Conversational Agent:** Computer generated characters that demonstrate same properties as humans in face-to-face conversation, including verbal and nonverbal communication. An embodied conversational agent constitutes a type of multimodal interface where the modalities are those natural to human conversation such as speech, facial expressions, hand gestures, and body posture. It may refer to a software agent in an interaction with a human or represent humans in a virtual environment using avatars.

**Empathy:** The capacity to understand what another person is experiencing from within the other person's frame of reference, i.e., the capacity to place oneself in another's place.

**Motor Cognition:** Mental processing in which the motor system draws on stored information to plan and produce our own actions, as well as to anticipate, predict, and interpret the actions of others.

**Perceived Exam Control:** The feeling of having the capacity to handle the problem.

**Perceived Social Support:** The acquisition of social support.

**Stress:** A relationship between the person and the environment that is perceived as relevant to the person's well-being and in which the person's resources failed to meet the demand.

# Section 3

# Positive Interventions:

## Health Care

# Chapter 7
# An Emerging Model of Pregnancy Care:
## The Introduction of New Technologies in Maternal Wellbeing

**Claudia Carissoli**
*Università Cattolica del Sacro Cuore, Italy*

**Daniela Villani**
*Università Cattolica del Sacro Cuore, Italy*

**Giuseppe Riva**
*Università Cattolica del Sacro Cuore, Italy & I.R.C.C.S. Istituto Auxologico Italiano, Italy*

## ABSTRACT

*Pregnancy is a very special time in a woman's life, a time of important and complex step that can lead to the fall the previous personal balances and looking for new. This phase potentially critical, is often accompanied by anxiety, negative emotions, worries and stress about themselves, the couple's life, the baby. Among the many interventions available for the welfare of pregnant women, new technologies are playing an increasingly important role, thanks to its spread, the lower costs and its peculiar characteristics (interactivity, sociality, customizability, ubiquity, multimediality, velocity, etc). Smartphones and tablets in particular are proving excellent tools to accompany women on this journey toward a healthy motherhood.*

## INTRODUCTION

Pregnancy is a complex phase in a woman's life, a period in which she changes her status from daughter to mother in just a few months. Becoming a mother requires a profound reconstruction of self (Barclay et al., 1997). This process of change is not bounded by a particular time frame, and it can even happen before the end of the neo-maternal month (Rubin, 1984).

In addition to biological changes, pregnancy leads to a search for a new identity that has to be positioned at the individual, couple and social levels (Stern et al., 1998; Bibring, 1959; Ammaniti et al., 1996; Monti et al. 2006).

DOI: 10.4018/978-1-4666-9986-1.ch007

In this sense pregnancy is a psychologically complex period in a woman's life, and every pregnancy could be seen as a phase of potential vulnerability. Indeed, this metamorphosis is characterized by physiological and psychological changes that can enhance anxiety or other negative emotional states and favor risky behaviors, such as the lack of attention to personal hygiene and prenatal screening, poor diet, alcohol consumption, smoking and drug use (Lindgren, 2001).

A wide consensus exists about the role of maternal psychological state in influencing the development of the child and the course of the pregnancy: negative emotions, such as anxiety and stress, are often associated with a redoubt variability in the fetal cardiac frequency, greater motor activity (which can cause spontaneous abortion), various pregnancy complications, pre-term birth and low birth weight (Hoffman & Hatch, 2000; Dunkel-Schetter, 1998; Dayan et al., 2002). Davies and colleagues showed that the level of maternal cortisol, measured between 30-32 weeks of gestation, is a predictor of a difficult temperament in children at two months of age (Davis et al., 2007); it is also inversely related to scores of cognitive and motor development in children at both three and eight months (Buitelaar et al., 2003). Anxiety detected at 32 weeks gestation was predictive of severe behavioral problems in children at 4 years of age (O'Connor et al., 2002).

This situation appears even more critical in cases of anxiety or depression disorders during pregnancy that are related to postpartum depression (Grant et al., 2008; Austin et al., 2007) and to negative effects on infant mental development (Tronick, 1999). Postnatal depression has been clearly associated with negative health consequences for both women and their babies (O'Hara and Swain, 1996).

Specifically, impaired maternal-infant interactions have been linked to vulnerability in infants and children (Murray et al., 1996), to attachment insecurity and delay in cognitive and emotional development (Hipwell et al., 2000; Murray et al., 1992; Cogill et al., 1986; Cummings & Davies, 1994), and to social and interaction difficulties (Murray et al., 1999).

As well-being of the mother is critical for optimal pregnancy outcomes, it is important to regulate maternal stress and provide expecting mothers with coping strategies to increase their quality of life and to maximize infant health and development.

This chapter pursues a threefold objective. First, it aims to investigate how it is possible to enhance women's well-being during pregnancy by taking into consideration the three levels of well-being identified by positive psychology. Second, it aims to analyze how actual mothers-to-be use new technologies to meet several needs. Finally, it aims to describe the Italian mobile app "BenEssere Mamma," which was developed by the chapter's authors to support mothers' well-being during pregnancy.

## HOW TO ENHANCE WOMEN'S WELL-BEING DURING PREGNANCY

Pregnancy, evoking a range of emotions from great joy and anticipation to crippling anxiety, is likely to increase several needs, including the needs for information, to share experiences with others or to be instantly connected, and to consult professionals (Tripp et al., 2014). There are several ways to meet these needs, including self-soothing techniques, psycho-education and relaxation, that are particularly important in this transitional and meaningful time (Beddoe & Lee, 2008).

According to the positive psychology perspective – which emerged as the scientific study of positive personal experience, positive individual traits, and positive institutions (Seligman, 2003; Seligman and Csikszentmihalyi, 2000) - it is critical to focus on human strengths, healthy processes, and fulfillment in order to improve quality of life, as well as to increase wellness and resilience in individuals, organizations, and societies. This is also true for pregnant women.

Keyes and Lopez (Keyes & Lopez, 2002) suggested that positive functioning could be achieved by working on three levels of well-being: (a) high emotional well-being, (b) high psychological well-being, and (c) high social well-being. This means that positive psychology identifies three characteristics of our personal experience—affective quality, engagement/actualization, and connectedness—that serve to promote personal well-being.

By following this categorization it is possible to identify three critical perspectives to take into consideration in order to improve quality of life and well-being during pregnancy.

## Fostering Maternal Positive Emotional States (Hedonic Perspective)

Theoretical perspectives suggest that the experience of positive emotions may be important in helping individuals recover quickly from stress. According to the Broaden-and-Build Theory of positive emotions (Fredrickson, 2001), the form and function of positive and negative emotions are distinct and complementary. Negative emotions (e.g., fear, anger, and sadness) narrow momentary thoughts and actions to produce autonomic nervous system activation that prepares the body for specific actions that served the ancestral function of promoting survival. By contrast, positive emotions (e.g., joy, interest, and contentment) broaden an individual's momentary thought–action repertoire, which in turn can build that individual's enduring personal resources, resources that also served the ancestral function of

promoting survival. One implication of the Broaden–and–Build model is that positive emotions have an undoing effect on negative emotions. In this sense, experiences of positive emotions, in turn, should broaden habitual modes of thinking and build personal resources for coping with adversity. Positive emotions are likely to be the active ingredient that energizes this upward spiral that optimizes health and well-being.

Although studies have investigated the relationship between stress/negative emotional states and delivery and neonatal complications, up to now the association of positive emotional states with these variables has been less investigated. Nevertheless, some preliminary evidence underlines the importance and beneficial effects of maternal positive affect in the context of pregnancy and birth outcomes.

Concerning the motherhood period, positive appraisal has been associated with a high level of stability in coping and less distress throughout pregnancy (Yali & Lobel, 2002). A recent study demonstrated that positive life events predicted significantly lower third-trimester maternal morning cortisol levels across the cortisol awakening response (Pluess et al., 2012). These findings suggest that positive affect dampens endocrine and psychological responses to stress in pregnancy, which may be protective for the developing fetus. Furthermore, in healthy pregnant women, Costa and colleagues (2003) examined leisure-time physical activity (LTPA) patterns during pregnancy and the association with psychological well-being. Authors found a consistent association between enhanced psychological well-being, as measured by a variety of psychosocial inventories, and LTPA participation, particularly during the first and second trimesters of pregnancy. According to this study, even low-intensity regular exercise may be a potentially effective low-cost method of enhancing psychological well-being.

Concerning the relationship between positive affective states and delivery experience, a recent study described associations of positive state of mind and emotional stability in the immediate post-partum period with having experienced a normal delivery (Hernandez-Martinez et al., 2011). However, positive affect was assessed in the immediate post-partum period, so it was not possible to state in a definite way if the positive delivery experience may have caused the higher positive affect in these women or vice versa.

Voellmin and colleagues (2013) assessed the relationship between positive affect and length of gestation and suggested that higher levels of positive affect in pregnancy are associated with longer length of gestation and with a reduced risk of delivering preterm. Specifically, the level of positive affect in the early second trimester of pregnancy, as well as the rate of increase in positive affect over the course of pregnancy, were positively associated with a longer length of gestation.

These preliminary studies suggest the importance of orienting mothers towards the cultivation of positive experiences in their lives.

## Promoting Maternal Growth and Fulfillment (Eudamonic Perspective)

Supportive and educational care is provided for most women who give birth. In several countries offering health care, there are many standard interventions—both public and private—available to support women in this particular phase of life. The characteristics and duration of care vary according to the status and training of the persons providing it (Rush et al., 1991). For example, the typical intervention offered in Italy is a childbirth class designed to provide information about maternal and fetal health from pregnancy to childbirth. Although very useful and popular, these courses are begin during the sixth or seventh month of pregnancy, when a lot of changes and doubts have already happened. Furthermore, mothers-to-be often struggle to follow these courses because of inconvenient hours, lack of time or long journeys required to reach the course locations. In addition, only a few of these courses include training for developing personal skills like resilience or coping skills to deal with maternity and childbirth effectively. Thus, the psychological component is often less explored than the educational-informative one.

The focus on mind-body practices that cultivate general health, diminish distress, and increase self-awareness may be particularly effective in addressing both the physical and psycho-emotional aspects of pregnancy and labor (Beddoe and Lee, 2008). Indeed, regular and moderate physical exercise can be helpful in the management of stress and other associated conditions or symptoms accompanying pregnancy, such as gestational diabetes and hypertension (Melzer et al., 2010). As well as physical exercise during pregnancy, routine prenatal care also includes relaxation and meditation practices during, which have various notable effects (Dunn et al., 2012; Beddoe & Lee, 2008).

Both these interventions represent possible effective approaches to well-being and quality of life during pregnancy, and they can also offer good strategies to support women in labor pain management. Labor pain is a subjective and multidimensional experience that varies according to each woman's individual perceptions and reactions to nociceptive information during labor and is influenced by several psychosocial, cognitive, and physiological factors (Lowe, 2002). Relaxation and meditation interventions have become popular for pain management in labor. On one hand, women are seeking alternatives to traditional treatment approaches, including analgesics and anesthesia, which can be invasive and are sometimes associated with negative side effects for both mother and infant (Smith et al., 2011). On the other hand, it is suggested that practitioners use a multidisciplinary approach to pain management in labor and incorporate non-pharmacological approaches that can be tailored to individual preferences and needs (Jones, 2012). As maternal prenatal anxiety is negatively associated with pre-labor self-efficacy for childbirth and labor pain (Beebe and Lee, 2007), relaxation and meditation represent good practices to help women feel more competent in coping with this specific experience, to reduce complication rates, and to have an overall better experience (Dunn et al., 2012 ; Gedde-Dahl & Fors, 2012).

The effects of relaxation and meditation practices during pregnancy will be described in the following paragraphs.

## Relaxation Strategies for Pregnant Women

When combined with regular exercise, relaxation techniques contribute to a reduction in preterm birth, longer gestation, increase in birth weight, and reduced risks of Caesarean section and instrumental extraction. The immediate impact of relaxation on pregnant women indicates a reduction in experienced stress or anxiety (Nickel et al., 2006; Bastani et al., 2005, 2006; Teixeira et al., 2005; Field et al., 2004, 1999; Urizar et al., 2004). Furthermore, relaxation could improve fetal health by reducing the basal fetal heart rate and increasing the number of fetal heart accelerations (Akbarzade et al., 2015).

The studies typically included a wide range of interventions like applied relaxation, massage, hypnotherapy, yoga therapy, verbal instructions, breathing instructions, progressive muscular relaxation (PMR) and guided imagery (GI). All of these techniques have shown promising results regarding a reduction in perceived stress and various physical symptoms and promotion of positive affect and well-being (Urech et al., 2010; Beddoe & Lee, 2009; Vieten & Astin, 2008; Nickel et al., 2006; Bastani et al., 2005,2006; Naredran et al., 2005; Teixera et al., 2005).

Although a variety of interventions exists, so far only a few research groups have directly evaluated whether different relaxation techniques have different impacts during pregnancy with randomized controlled trials. Thus, results obtained are heterogeneous with respect to the pattern of variables that are affected by the interventions (Field et al., 2006a, 2004, 1999; Teixeira et al., 2005).

Among the interventions, yoga therapies (Satyapriya et al., 2009; Narendran et al., 2005) and PMR over a longer period (Nickel et al., 2006; Field et al., 1999, 2004) are more likely to enhance psycho-biological well-being (Field et al., 1999) compared to massage therapy and a PMR relaxation group over 5 weeks. The massaged pregnant women showed reduced anxiety levels and stress hormones, fewer sleep disturbances, and fewer incidences of back pain and obstetric and postnatal complications. Only women in the PMR group had decreased anxiety levels after their first session.

Teixeira et al. (2005) investigated active versus passive relaxation techniques in pregnant women. Active relaxation was based on hypnotherapeutic methods, whereas women in the passive relaxation group sat quietly and read women's fashion magazines. A reduction in anxiety and heart rate, but not in stress hormones, was found in the women who participated in active relaxation. The effects of passive relaxation were comparable to those evoked by active relaxation. The outcomes of these studies indicate that different relaxation techniques can have different impacts on psycho-biological well-being in pregnant women.

Urech et al. (2010) evaluated the effects of a brief PMR and GI relaxation exercise, as well as a passive relaxation control condition, on pregnant women's psychological, endocrine and cardiovascular activity. Results indicated specific beneficial effects of the active relaxation techniques on pregnant women's psychological and/or cardiovascular state. Specifically, the GI condition was more effective for inducing relaxation than PMR. In addition, the GI, but not the PMR condition, was more effective in increasing self-reported relaxation than a passive relaxation control condition. Moreover, participants were more comfortable with GI than PMR. By including both physiological level assessment and self-reported experience, a discrepancy emerged between the two approaches. Apparently, the muscle relaxation exercises were more effective on cardiovascular arousal, whereas guided imagery achieved better results in terms of subjective relaxation measures. The implication for clinical practice is related to the importance of choosing psychological interventions that can be easily perceived as effective. Since GI is a comfortable relaxation technique and appears to be especially suitable to participants, it is likely that this technique will enhance compliance in pregnant women in a longer-term exercise program. Tragea and colleagues (2014) have recently examined the effectiveness of two relaxation techniques (progressive muscle relaxation and diaphragmatic breathing) during pregnancy. The results of the study demonstrate significant benefits from the use of the techniques in the pregnant women's psychological state. The systematic implementation of the proposed relaxation techniques contributed to a reduction in perceived stress and anxiety and increased the women's sense of internal control. Authors also found changes in many lifestyle factors to be associated with stress.

### Mindfulness for Pregnant Women

Mindfulness constitutes another effective approach in symptom reduction and general health improvements in pregnancy, such as management of anxiety, depression, back pain, and stress (Kabat-Zinn, 1994). Preliminary data supporting the potential benefits of mindfulness in the perinatal period has been found by Dunn and colleagues (2012). Based on that and other recent pilot studies (Duncan and Bardacke, 2009; Vieten and Astin 2008), it is possible to suggest that women who learn mindfulness during pregnancy are likely to use those skills to manage stressful aspects of pregnancy, childbirth and parenting, resulting in reductions in psychological distress and improvements in psychological well-being. Specifically, Duncan and Bardacke (2010) found that a mindfulness-based childbirth and parenting education program led to reductions in anxiety and depression; also, positive affect increased in women during the third trimester of pregnancy (Duncan & Bardacke, 2010). Similarly, Vieten and Astin (2008) carried out a study evaluating a psychosocial mindfulness-based intervention administered in the second half of pregnancy, and they found reductions in anxiety and negative mood when compared to wait list control. Altogether these pioneer researches indicate the importance of teaching mindfulness in the perinatal period and the potential effect of improving the developmental trajectory of parents and infants by broadening women's personal repertoire of coping strategies (Dunn et al., 2012).

## Enhancing Maternal Integration and Connectedness (Social Perspective)

Abundant evidence suggests that social support from family, friends, co-workers, and other social ties is associated with physical health and psychological well-being in different phases of the lifespan (House et al., 1988).

Social support plays a critical role in reducing the risk of depression and stress susceptibility and improving overall maternal well-being (Stice et al., 2004; Israel et al., 2002; Mathiesen et al., 1999). For this reason, social support may be especially important to consider as a protective factor for mothers during pregnancy (Dunkel-Schetter, 2011). It is possible to identify several persons that could contribute to the psychological well-being of future mothers. Professionals at different levels can provide information about prenatal care and assistance with daily tasks that are burdensome, as well as caring about and understanding stressors. Emotional support can also come from a husband/partner and friends, and it can be an emotional buffer that shields individuals from the negative effects of stress and depression (Campbell et al., 2009; Cooper et al., 2009; Mulsow et al., 2002).

The role of social and marital support has been extensively studied concerning antenatal depression, as documented by a recent review (Lancaster et al. 2010), while just a few studies (Roos et al., 2013; Nasreen et al., 2011) have investigated the relationship between social and marital support and antenatal anxiety.

Social support is significantly associated with psychological well-being in pregnancy (Dunkel-Schetter et al., 1996; Dunkel-Schetter, 2011). Specifically, several studies underline the association between quality of support, support satisfaction, perceived availability of support and actual receipt of support and significantly less prenatal and postpartum depression, less anxiety, fewer stressors, and improved health (e.g., Oakley et al., 1996; Collins et al., 1993; Tietjen & Bradley, 1985; Oakley, 1990, 1992; Cutrona, 1984).

## INTEGRATING TECHNOLOGIES INTO MOTHER-TO-BE WELL-BEING: CURRENT SCENARIOS

E-health and m-health are becoming the new way to promote healthcare by using information and communication technologies worldwide (Watterson et al., 2015; Bert et al., 2013). The rapid expansion of web access and mobile technologies gives the opportunity to improve well-being by fostering healthy behavior, reducing risky behavior and extending prevention and care-seeking culture. Internet and mobile technologies may represent a low-cost solution to cope with some global health challenges like lack of health care providers, lack of information or limited training for health workers (Watterson et al., 2015;).

New technologies offer new strategies to achieve the United Nation Millennium Development Goals (MDGs). Mobile phones and smartphones may offer easy health information access and provide support and skills to face with a specific health condition; these devices can also be used by care providers to monitor health status, offer training, answer questions and stay in touch with their patients (Rotheram-Borus et al., 2012).

A key factor in achieving MDG5 and improving maternal health is a healthier pregnancy that implies less risk of pregnancy-related complications and lower fetal and infant mortality rates (MDG4).

Pregnancy, in fact, can be considered a unique "teachable moment" for health and wellness interventions: women in this phase of their life are willing to make significant behavioral changes to improve fetus and maternal health. According to Peyton (2014) and Rotheram-Borus et al. (2012), although pregnant women lack pregnancy-related information, they are interested in nutrition, diet, exercise, growth stages of the fetus, gestational diseases, emotional states and fluctuation and more general information on pregnancy from the very beginning.

Internet, smartphones and mobile services are more and more being considered the best information source by pregnant women (Lagan et al., 2011) because they are able to offer new and powerful instruments to promote positive emotional states and to develop coping skills in order to let women live an aware, informed and healthy pregnancy.

The current scenario includes several technologies that will be described in the next paragraphs. First, the Internet, which is used both as a source of information and a source of social support, as well as to support self-help psychological training. Second, mobile services and mobile applications are designed to suggest correct behaviors and to meet pregnant women's different needs.

## Internet as a Source of Information and Social Support

The Internet is changing our relationship with health: today we have easy access to information on diseases, treatments and healthy behavior, and we can find answers to all of our questions in a click.

Pregnancy-related websites are more and more available on the Internet and pregnancy e-health is now practiced worldwide. According to Lagan and colleagues, in 2011 there were almost 136 million websites containing pregnancy-related information online and these sites' usage by pregnant women is constantly growing (Lagan et al., 2011).

According to a recent survey, the usage rate of the Internet amongst pregnant women is massive: participants affirmed to have used the Internet at least 10 times during their pregnancy. They also stated that they were mainly interested in antenatal or intrapartum issues and complications of pregnancy (Lagan et al., 2010). The Internet is often used to obtain further information about things mentioned by health care providers, or for assistance in making conscious decisions related to pregnancy and childbirth (epidural, induction or cesarean, etc). Sixty-three percent of women are influenced by Internet content in thinking and managing their pregnancy and childbirth (Lagan et al., 2010).

E-health consultations may help women feel empowered and informed enough to become "expert patients," able to negotiate their health care in an active and proactive manner with careful research and self-education (Johnson, 2014).

According to some studies, pregnant women consider online resources one of the main sources of useful information (Hearn et al., 2014; O' Higgins et al., 2014): women regularly use the Internet to get information and consider it the third most useful source of information after family and friends (O'Higgins et al., 2014). In some cases, women stated that the Internet is the only source they used to seek information about pregnancy (Lagan et al., 2010), or that it was their second source of information after doctors (Lima-Pereira et al., 2013).

E-health represents a common practice worldwide: a U.S. survey affirms that more than 75% of pregnant women practiced pregnancy e-health (Declercq et al., 2007). In Italy, around 95% of the women in the sample were Internet users, and almost all of them used the Internet for pregnancy-related topics (Bert et al., 2013). In Spain, the 95.5% of women interviewed reported daily Internet access (Lima-Pereira et al., 2013). In Sweden, 91% of women have access to the Internet and 84% of women used the Internet as source of information on pregnancy (Larsson, 2009). In China, the data are similar to those of the Western world (Gao et al., 2013).

This new trend in managing health raises theoretical and practical issues, such as ensuring quality and trustworthiness of content and avoiding the risk of misunderstandings or incomplete comprehension by women.

Although women consider the information they retrieve online good and useful, sometimes they don't have the appropriate knowledge to evaluate the quality of online content. Nevertheless, they would like to be oriented in choosing reliable sites or online content from healthcare providers (Lagan et al., 2010; Hearn et al., 2014; Romano, 2007). Thus, healthcare professionals may play an important role in safeguarding well-being, guiding mothers in online searches and recommending high-quality websites (O'Higgins et al., 2014; Bert et al., 2013; Larsson, 2009).

The Internet doesn't just meet the need for information. The web, in fact, is becoming a new way of finding social support: pregnant women access the Internet to share information through online discussion forums and to find support from other pregnant women or new mothers. By belonging to groups, even virtual ones, women can reduce their anxiety and feelings of isolation, receive reassurances and feel helped and relieved in the decision-making process (Lagan et al., 2010).

One possible reason for seeking support online may be the decline of the extended family: in the past, extended family members accompanied women in this transition to motherhood, but now, because of frequent loss of proximity, women may feel isolated and lonely. Discussion forums, social media platforms and online communities provide places to exchange advice, information and support (Miyata, 2002, Sharf, 1997, Preece, 2001, Wellman and Frank, 2001). Generating a sense of community with other women going through similar experiences can reduce loneliness (O'Higgins et al, 2014). Thanks to online resources, mothers-to-be can find a sense of belonging to a social community and social support, both of which are so important for their psychological well-being (Dunkel-Schetter et al., 1996; 2001). Online forums can promote individual empowerment by the sharing of information, which furthers the demand for accurate data and challenges health professionals (Lima-Pereira et al., 2012)

Internet forums enable women to connect with people with the same interests or that are living the same experience. In this way virtual communities are able to offer support, comfort, answers and a space where women can vent and share their private emotions and fears (Romano, 2007).

Several advantages have contributed to make the Internet so popular in this specific phase of life: not only the anonymity and the asynchronous communication, but also the convenience and the effectiveness.

Anonymity is fundamental: women appreciate the opportunity to talk about their pregnancies and doubts anonymously before announcing their pregnancy to their families, and even after because anonymity reduces shame for sharing private matters (sex and sexuality, vaginal bleeding and discharge or emotional changes in pregnancy and early parenthood, discomfort of pregnancy, breast changes, etc.). Online it is possible to anonymously post questions and receive answers, comfort and support. Anonymity lets women feel free to ask and talk about every aspect of pregnancy or private life and enables them to receive support and suggestions for every topic. No "silly" demands exist online; everybody can feel free to ask any questions without fear of judgment.

Asynchronous communication allows mothers-to-be to get in touch with friends or other mothers when and how they prefer, especially at night in the last trimester when sleep becomes difficult.

On Facebook, one of the most famous social networks in the world, people can share information, photos and emoticons about their lives in every moment and keep in touch with friends and family members, allowing the creation of social capital, which is essential for well-being (Johnson, 2014). As Bartholomew pointed out, "Facebook serves an important function in the acquisition of social capital and social support resources, which are beneficial at the transition to parenthood" (Bartholomew et al., 2012: 464).

Immediacy, easiness, convenience, effectiveness, interactivity, clarity and control are other aspects that make surfing the Web so appealing (Lagan et al., 2010). Women can access the Internet instantly from home, the workplace or public spaces (thanks to wireless access and mobile phones) without going out, wasting time or waiting for a medical consultation (Romano, 2007).

## Web-Based Training Programs

More and more people are looking for self-help programs to enhance their well-being and health, which is consistent with the rapid growth of web-based interventions and smartphone apps in behavioral healthcare (Luxton et al., 2011). Self-help programs, such as interventions that people practice individually without contact with a professional in the field, have been demonstrated to be effective in helping people enhance their quality of life (Haug et al., 2012 ; Newman et al., 2011; Cuijpers et al., 2010; Sethi et al., 2010; Van Vliet and Andrews, 2009; Williams et al., 2001).

This type of intervention is supported by technologies that enable individuals to overcome limits related to traditional support, such as time, resources, flexibility, accessibility and availability (Taylor and Luce, 2003).

Internet-based interventions have been demonstrated to be effective in reducing depression, anxiety, phobias and addictions; Web-based programs are salutary for people suffering from these diseases and successful in reaching woman with lower socio-economic status (Haga et al., 2013)

Web-based applications consist of self-help programs that are able to enhance personal empowerment and support women during pregnancy or at the beginning of motherhood. These are nowadays becoming a new strategy to promote subjective well-being and deal with pregnancy concerns, such as the risks of post-partum depression. Table 1 is a selection of some promising web-based programs.

## Mobile Services

The Global Observatory for eHealth (GOe) of the World Health Organization (WHO) defines m-health or mobile health as the "medical and public health practice supported by mobile devices, such as mobile phones, patient monitoring devices, personal digital assistants (PDAs), and other wireless devices." According to the World Health Organization (WHO), m-health can play an important role in promoting healthier pregnancy not only in developing countries, but also in lower income populations in developed states.

M-health may represent a booster for healthier pregnancy management. As a part of the "continuum of care" of the modern clinic and community, it can be useful to encourage correct behavior (physical exercise and weight control), provide clear and focused health information and help women become competent and learn skills to cope with physical and emotional changes in pregnancy (Peyton et al., 2014; Tamrat et al, 2012).

Mobile communication makes quick, low-cost and widespread healthcare services feasible; text SMS, voice call or IVR (Interactive Voice Response) offer the opportunity to reach a big part of the target population (including those living in rural and poor areas).

Mobile devices enable efficient perinatal education campaigns. Thanks to advice and personalized "tips" sent by text or voice-recorded messages, it is possible to suggest correct behaviors and make mothers more aware of information pertaining to pregnancy, dangerous symptoms, proper nutrition and risky behavior. Free vouchers for healthcare providers are a further well-being booster (Lund et al., 2014).

The "text4baby" (Parker et al., 2012) program is an effective and successful example of mobile phone education training. In the United States, future moms can sign up for the "text4baby" service by sending a text message with their child's expected birth date and postal code. They will receive three messages a week offering evidence-based information relevant to the stage of pregnancy they are in; each message includes a toll-free telephone number linked to low-cost services related to the message topic that are consistent with the mother's location.

The IVR system (Interactive Voice Response) is an alternative tool to provide similar interventions for illiterate or less educated people. "Aponjon" is a Voice (IVR) and SMS mobile health service that provides weekly text and voice health messages to pregnant women, mothers with newborn babies and their family members in Bangladesh. Aponjon gives reliable and accurate messages about pregnancy

*Table 1. Examples of Web-based programs for the well-being of pregnant women and new mothers*

| Name and Location | Description | Technical Features | Clinical Approach/Results |
|---|---|---|---|
| Mamma Mia (Haga et al., 2013) Norway | This is a free, Web-based self-help intervention designed to reduce the risk of postpartum depression and to promote subjective well-being in pregnant women or new mothers with mild-to-moderate symptoms of depression.<br>The program consists of 44 sessions over a period of 11 months: for each session, the user receives an email with a hyperlink; by activating the link, the user gains access to Mamma Mia and proceeds in a predetermined sequence of Web pages. | • Free<br>• Self-help intervention<br>• Compatible with different operating systems<br>• English language<br>• Attractive content and interfaces<br>• Discussion forum | • Assessment of depressive symptoms, metacognitive therapy, positive psychology, couples therapy, breastfeeding, and psycho-education<br>• First trial feedback is positive both in terms of acceptability and effectiveness by women and their partners |
| MomMoodBooster (Danaher et al., 2013) Australia | This is a free web-based program to help new mothers deal with postpartum depression.<br>The program consists of sox sessions (Getting Started, Managing Mood, Increasing Pleasant Activities, Managing Negative Thoughts, Increasing Positive Thoughts and Planning for the Future) introduced by a video explaining the session goal. Participants can complete the program in 6-12 weeks (every session can be completed in 2 weeks) with 6-12 coach calls.<br>It proposes different interactive activities designed to encourage participant engagement and behavioral change. | • Free<br>• Self-help intervention<br>• Compatible with different operating systems<br>• English language<br>• Attractive and interactive content and interfaces<br>• Discussion forum<br>• Coach calls | • Based on Milgrom's adaptation of the Coping With Depression Course (CWDC) for postpartum depression as well as an adaptation of the CWDC for Web-based delivery<br>• A pilot study tested the efficacy with a clinical sample of 53 women recruited from the United States and Australia. Women were very engaged with the program and showed significant clinical improvements. |
| MODIAB-web (Adolfsson et al., 2014) Sweden | This is a web-based support for pregnant women and new mothers with type 1 diabetes mellitus that aims to promote well-being and diabetes management.<br>It consists of three parts: 1) evidence-based information (being pregnant, labor and childbirth, and life as a new mother); 2) a self-care diary for self-reported monitoring; and 3) a discussion forum for peer support moderated by the research group. | • Free<br>• Self-help intervention<br>• Compatible with different operating systems<br>• Swedish language<br>• Discussion forum | • Based on a holistic approach<br>• Provides person-centered support in addition to usual care<br>• The first trial is supposed to be completed in February 2016 |

symptoms, nutrition and obstetric danger signs congruent with the week of pregnancy or the age of the baby (Ahsan & Raihan, 2013).

## Mobile Apps

New intervention areas are continuously emerging thanks to smartphones and mobile applications. In 2012, according to global research and consulting firm Strategy Analytics (2014), the number of active smartphone users worldwide was 1 billion; another billion will become smartphone users by 2015.

Smartphones and apps have significantly expanded healthcare possibilities. According to research-2guidance reports, 500 million smartphone users worldwide will use at least one mHealth app by 2015. By 2018 it is forecasted that more than 50% of smartphone and tablet users will have downloaded m-health applications (Research2guidance 2014 and 2015 report).

According to the European Commission's Green Paper on mobile health (2014), mobile health covers medical and public health practice supported by mobile devices, such as mobile phones. It also includes applications (''apps'') that are primarily intended to maintain or improve healthy behaviors, quality of life and the well-being of individuals directly or indirectly. Mobile apps can encourage adherence to a healthy lifestyle, resulting in more personalized treatments.

These new media may be capable of providing educational and training content that can help future mothers satisfy their need of communication, information and connection with others (Tripp et al., 2014; Romano, 2007).

According to some researchers, smartphones are the most common devices used by pregnant women who are active Internet users. Further, the mobile versions of websites are preferred to static resources because of their ubiquitous accessibility (Hearn et al., 2014; Waring et al., 2014).

These new devices have features capable of enabling pregnant women to communicate, track the progress of their pregnancy and alleviate their anxiety thorough interactive professional and private consultation (Tripp et al., 2014).

According to Rotheram-Borus and colleagues, there are six foundational functions for m-health interventions for pregnant women (Rotheram-Borus et al., 2014):

1. Informing about health, behaviors and resources;
2. Training, sending text messages, calls, pictures, or even videos that recommend the desired behaviors;
3. Monitoring behavior in real time to help people in adopting new habits;
4. Shaping healthy behaviors thanks to feedback, prompts, alerts, reminders, encouragement, and rewards provided at the right moment;
5. Supporting development and maintenance by linking women to peers, friends, family, or healthcare workers for social support and instrumental support services;
6. Linking to hospitals, clinical or emergency services to better manage critical situations.

Jihye and Iftekahr (Jihye and Iftekhar, 2016) analyzed some international pregnancy apps according to the framework created by Rotheram-Borus and colleagues and pointed out that apps generally contain more than one function (e.g., informing, training, monitoring, shaping and linking).

According to Jihye and Iftekahr's study, the informing function is important for users but not critical to app adoption because of the availability of other information services and online materials.

It is well known that pregnancy increases the need for information and that women surf the Web to find rapid and complete answers to their questions (Lagan et al., 2010, Lagan et al., 2011). Additionally, as the months pass, women show different informational needs. At an early stage they want information about indicators of pregnancy or dietary concerns, food aversion, banned food and, advice for vomiting and nausea. Then in the second trimester they desire to know more about unusual symptoms, and during the last trimester they are more and more focused on childbirth events (premature birth, epidural, hospital quality) or newborn parenting questions (Peyton et al., 2014).

This deep need for information does not seem satisfied by printed material. Brochures and leaflets are perceived as too general and lacking details, and they are often lost or discarded; books are considered expensive, difficult to search in, and limited in view.

Pregnancy apps are able to provide an appropriate, positive and effective response to these problems. Informative apps are the most common and usually provide a large range of general information about pregnancy, fetus development, maternal nutrition, advice and information on diseases such as gestational diabetes.

Among informative apps, women show a clear preference for interactive ones, which allow women to enter their personal information and then get recommendations and suggestions "tailor-made".

The users receive advice and information related to their specific gestational week, which helps them experience a new level of awareness of the responsbilities of pregnancy (Johnson, 2014). These apps often show 3D images of a developing fetus, reminders for healthcare appointments, pregnancy milestones, timely advice about pregnancy symptomatology, info on foods and weight and exercises to engage in, all of which have the possibility to invoke behavioral change as a result (monitoring and shaping functions).

Monitoring and shaping functions are crucial in keeping people using apps. It has been demonstrated that mobile phones may be acceptable for monitoring or self-monitoring by much of the population. Their behaviors—reminders, alarms, warnings and supportive messages—effectively promote healthy behavior including cessation of smoking, managing diabetes, engaging in physical activities and weight control (Rotheram-Borus et al., 2014). Some apps, for example, include a "bump photos" section, a feature which allows women to create a gallery of images of their growing baby bump. This capability may be a way to develop more awareness of pregnancy and to promote healthy behaviors and bonding (Johnson, 2014).

Supporting functions include features that enable women to obtain social support thanks to mobile online communities.

An interesting example of peer-to-peer support promoted by SMS contact is the Diabetes Buddy project. The Diabetes Buddies program is a pilot project to promote a healthy lifestyle and better management of diabetes thanks to reciprocal support among women in South Africa. During the course of 12 weeks, women were able to contact each other outside of the group sessions by a mobile phone; this allowed ongoing support between buddies. Furthermore, one SMS (or probe) was sent daily to each participant with the goal of helping the women gather information to use in the management of their disease (Rotheram-Borus et al., 2012).

The linking function is the least developed feature at the moment, but it is the one that can become the real "killer" capability. This function allows the app to be integrated into the overall system of healthcare and make a quick connection between women and health professionals. Thanks to the development of wireless sensors, apps can monitor physiological data (heartbeat, breathing, fetus hearth rate, glucose levels) and transmit them instantly to medical centers to get immediate support or medical contact.

Many apps providing data on fetus well-being (such as Baby Heart Monitors and Pregnancy Calculator) already exist, but without a direct connection or supervision with medical personnel, they are likely to become a source of anxiety rather than help (Tripp et al., 2014).

Smartphone technologies and apps, thanks to their always being in our pockets, may offer a new strategy to promote self-health practices more effectively than other existing material (Jihye and Iftekhar, 2016; Johnson, 2014). They are not simply an extension of traditional static forms of self-help, but a new way of using resources through a device in a variety of locations and even whilst multitasking.

Apps and social media are not simply sources of information; they also operate as performative devices in that they push women to act on and through their bodies via these devices (Johnson, 2014). They enable interactive and customized use more effective in promoting change in behavior than usual self-help tools (Hearn et al., 2014).

Last but not least, finding a pregnancy-related app on the Web is simple, low-cost and accessible to everyone. A quick Internet search with basic words (pregnancy, antenatal parent education, fetus, etc.) can be sufficient to find an app, and people can install these apps on their mobile devices without hassle and sometimes even for free.

In Table 2 we reported some examples of popular international pregnancy-related apps.

Apps and online resources may also play an important role in promoting psychological well-being of pregnant women. The availability of high-quality health information can decrease feelings of anxiety and stress born from the doubts and uncertainties that pregnancy naturally generates and increase a sense of control and self-efficacy in women. These new interactive and tailor-made tools are more likely to persuade women to change their lifestyles than are traditional tool kits. Training, monitoring and shaping functions can become a "good coach" in causing change.

*Table 2. Examples of mobile apps for pregnancy well-being*

| App/Developer | Main Features | Informing | Training | Monitoring | Shaping | Supporting | Linking |
|---|---|---|---|---|---|---|---|
| My Pregnancy Today – BabyCenter | • Free<br>• For IoS and Android<br>• Customizable<br>• English language | √ | √ | √ | √ | √ | |
| I'm Expecting – pregnancy app - MedHelp, Inc | • Free<br>• For IoS and Android<br>• Customizable<br>• English language | √ | | √ | √ | √ | |
| Dr. Miriam Stoppard Pregnancy - Dorling Kindersley | • Paid<br>• For IoS and Android<br>• Customizable<br>• English language<br>• Antenatal bonding functions | √ | √ | √ | √ | √ | |
| Healthy you, healthy baby - Ngala Organization | • Free<br>• For IoS (Android not available)<br>• Customizable<br>• English language<br>• Activities during pregnancy to the first 18 months of motherhood | √ | | √ | √ | √ | |
| Happy Pregnancy Ticker – Softcraft system and solutions private limited | • Free<br>• For IoS and Android<br>• Customizable<br>• English language | √ | √ | √ | √ | √ | √ |
| I'm Pregnant - Kolsoft | • Free<br>• For IoS and Android<br>• Customizable<br>• English language | √ | √ | | √ | | √ |

Apps are becoming a guide for pregnant women, and for this reason it is important to guarantee content quality and reliability to avoid increases in anxiety or misleading interpretation of data.

E-health and m-health still have great potential available to exploit, but healthcare professionals are fundamental in supporting this process. It would be good if care providers became an integral part of this system; they could protect women from e-health practice risks and promote e-health and mobile e-health both by filling the information gap and guiding women in online searches (Tripp et al., 2014; Bert et al., 2013; Romano, 2007).

## BenEssere Mamma, The Application

In recent years, many mobile apps for mental health have been developed and have demonstrated good potential for stress and anxiety management (Preziosa et al., 2009; Villani et al., 2012; Villani et al., 2013; Repetto et al., 2013). Typically they include several relaxation training approaches, but recently meditation has also been successfully included in self-help interventions supported by new technologies (Warnecke et al., 2011; Sharma et al., 2012; Cavanagh et al., 2013; Ahtinen et al., 2013; Chittaro and Vianello, 2014; Ly et al., 2014).

Nowadays, thanks to new mobile technologies like the Internet, social networks and mobile applications, it is possible to reach more and more mothers-to-be than through traditional methods. Pregnant women's ability to easily find information, give suggestions and tips and support each other in this delicate and magical life phase has helped reduce risks and dangers for them and for their unborn children.

Starting from these premises, the app BenEssere Mamma was developed to help pregnant women better manage anxiety and stress, especially in the last trimester of pregnancy, and better cope with childbirth.

BenEssere Mamma consists of a brief self-help protocol containing mindfulness meditation and guided imagery exercises delivered through a smartphone to reduce stress during pregnancy and to restore levels of energy and well-being. The creators of the app intend it to be a response to the desire of pregnant women to promote their wellness without investing too much time in courses that sometimes barely fit into working life (women are entitled to maternity leave starting two months prior to the expected date of delivery). The app aims to help women recognize, bring out and use their resources that are designed to promote awareness of their potential in addressing problems and difficulties related to pregnancy and childbirth. It is a personal empowerment app: a four-week self-help program that includes daily relaxation exercises to reduce anxiety and perceived stress level of pregnant women.

Reducing anxiety and negative mood can reduce the risk of postnatal depression. The application includes activities and materials that can be divided into the following areas:

- An *informative area*, to increase knowledge about stress, relaxation and its salutary effects:
    - The "Good to Know" section, containing explanations about stress, pregnancy and relaxation practices;
    - "Other practices," (see Figure 1) consisting of first-hand descriptions of the relaxation exercises and explanations about how they function;
- An *emotional awareness area*, called the "mood journal:" in this section it is possible to record notes on emotional state, thoughts and events to become aware of what influences mood and thus develop confidence in one's own ability to change negative emotional states and the correlated physiological activation. Expectant mothers are guided with positive emoticons (see Figure 1) to recognize and assess their mood day-by-day to improve awareness of their emotional state and

what affects it. This daily practice allows women to recognize when their negative moods subside and to identify possible events, feelings, thoughts and emotions that influence it. The objective is to develop a different way of thinking about their minds. Thanks to meditation exercises and daily mood mapping, pregnant women can realize the variability of their moods and consciously accept and recognize the link between mood, emotions and thoughts, sometimes unwanted. In this way it is possible to start breaking the usual and automatic routine that perpetuates difficulties and issues. Discovering what affects women's state of mind allows them to avoid behaviors and automatic thoughts that lead to a recurrence of the disorder; for example, focusing attention on the present moment rather than keeping minds on the past or the future. Awareness can help expectant mothers recognize early symptoms of post-partum or pregnancy depression and ask for support as soon as possible.

- An *experiential area*, called "your path:" a set of 20 daily exercises, each lasting about 10 minutes (5 days a week for 4 weeks), such as breath meditation, visualizations and listening to music/natural sounds. Several types of exercises are proposed to allow users to experiment with different practices and find the one they like best.
    - **Breathing Meditation:** These practices invite users to sit in a calm and peaceful location and focus their attention on breath and bodily movement (particularly of the chest and belly). When the mind wanders, the mother-to-be is invited to notice what distracted her and then return to observing her breathing. This practice consists of mindful breathing and thought distancing. In terms of mindful breathing, participants learned how to direct their attention to the sensations of breathing and to notice when their mind wandered away; in terms of thought distancing, participants had to try to perceive thoughts as ''events'' in their minds, simply observing the process of thought.
    - **Body Scan Exercises:** To strengthen the connection between the mind and the body, which is essential in facilitating childbirth. Body scan meditation is a form of Vipassana meditation that helps to expand mind/body awareness, release tension and quiet the mind. It is an effective meditation technique for strengthening concentration, focusing attention, relaxing the breath and making body-mind connection stronger.
    - **Imagery and Positive Visualizations:** Which can be considered a way the mind uses to communicate with the body (in some way this represents the biological connection between mind and body). It is really important for pregnant women to recover their body-mind connection so they will be able to cope with fear, pain and fatigue during childbirth. Different typologies of visualizations are proposed within the app:
        - **Safe Place Visualizations:** That invite a pregnant woman to imagine herself in a quiet, peaceful and secure place to rest and to release anxieties, worries and thoughts, allowing her to come out of this imagery with a sense of comfort and refreshment. For example, mothers-to-be were encouraged to imagine "a luminous sphere" and visualize the image's form, color and flow, and to focus attention on how they are feeling. The voice guide suggested desired psychological states and emotions (e.g., "You feel calm, You feel relaxed, Your body is calm and relaxed, also your baby is relaxed") to induce them. These images may mediate the communication between perception, emotion and physiological change and may induce a positive physiological process such as reducing the stress reaction and related stress symptoms (Schaub et al., 1995)

- **Baby in Womb Meditations:** Are exercises designed to create particular imagery during a state of direct connection with the baby to strengthen the relationship between mother and child. This connection can prepare mother and child for the childbirth, an event that marks the end of one past (pregnancy) and the beginning of a new one (motherhood).
- **Inner Smile Meditations:** Are designed to start a developed, healthy and loving relationship with themselves. These exercises create a strong mind-body connection and can relax both the body and and mind. The aim of constant practice is to improve the ability to accept oneself, exactly as one is, to promote self-esteem as well as love and acceptance for others.

- A *professional support link*, to take care of questions or doubts, is provided through the button "SOS" (the "contact me" section). Women can send an e-mail asking for information or psychological orientation to a psychologist, in addition to a range of information about stress, pregnancy and techniques for mental and physical relaxation.

Social support functions at the moment have not been implemented to avoid the risk of increased anxiety due to emotional contagion, which is common in mom-to-be communities. In the future, the app could be enhanced by including a virtual community that would be constantly monitored and supervised by health professionals (midwives, psychologists, doctors, etc.).

The app BenEssere Mamma strives to be a complement to existing courses in childbirth preparation, offering techniques to manage anxiety, stress and fear of childbirth and to allow future moms to better

*Figure 1. App home page, the other relaxing practices menu and mood diary emoticons*

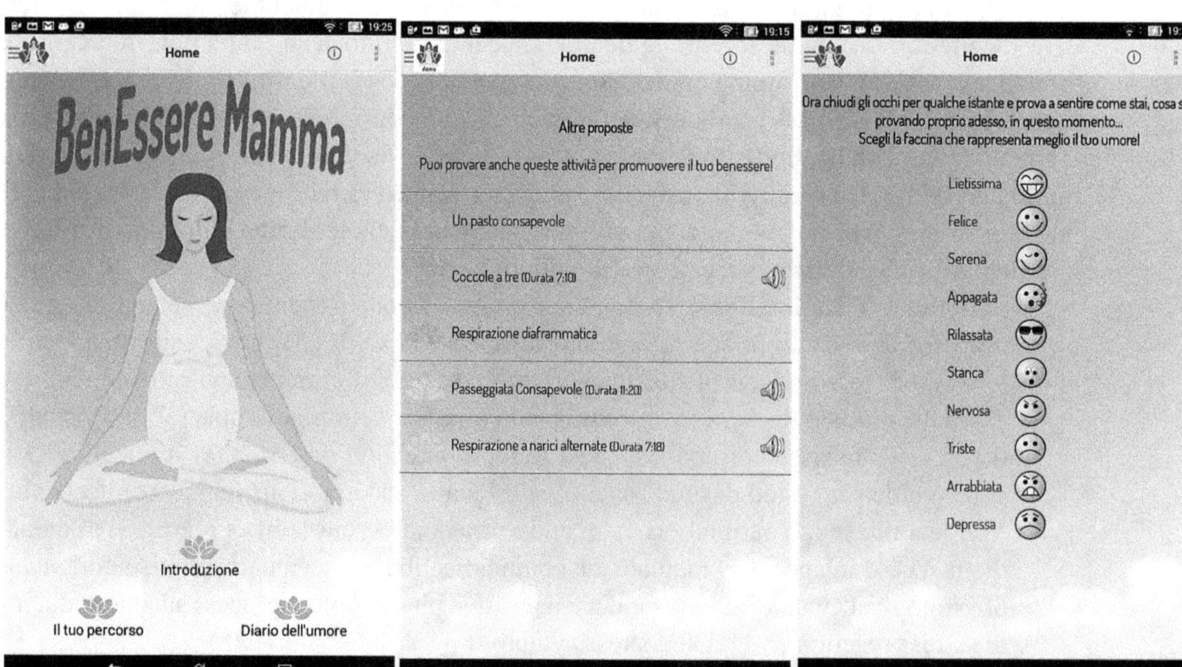

enjoy the experience of becoming mothers without forcing them to attend a course with fixed times and places.

Through practice, mothers-to-be can increase awareness of the present moment and of thoughts, feelings and body sensations. Mindfulness can help them, both during pregnancy and during labor, to deal with their feelings in a conscious way and to avoid reacting automatically on the basis of habits and rigid behavioral patterns.

Daily practice is critical to transform mindfulness meditation in a real habit, a way of being and living, and pregnant users will become able to relax more and more quickly and on demand.

Thanks to BenEssere Mamma, expectant mothers can practice meditation when and where they want, acquiring day-by-day familiarity with meditation and their constant changes, increasing confidence in their abilities and developing greater awareness of their own emotional states and confidence in their ability to generate positive emotional states.

BenEssere Mamma aims to help mothers-to-be develop critical skills useful in promoting the health of women and their children. Greater emotional awareness and confidence in personal abilities can help women accept their emotional state. It is fundamental to change the Western culture model that considers it unacceptable for pregnant women and new mothers to be sad, angry, unhappy, worried and distressed. Sadness, anxiety, and distress are often a part of the transition to motherhood, and women have to live these emotional experiences and ask for help if they need to be supported. Women who are more aware of their psychological status can accept their supposedly "inadequate" emotions and thus feel comfortable asking for professional help without waiting for months. Thanks to this app, emotions, both good and bad, can become familiar and acceptable as a part of this special time.

Additionally, emotional awareness and self-confidence can make depressive symptoms more recognizable and thus reduce depression risk. Postnatal depression is the most frequent complication occurring after pregnancy and affects about 10–15% of new mothers in Western countries; it can even evolve into puerperal psychosis, with an incidence of 0.2%, usually in the first weeks after childbirth but also after a few months.

Some studies have affirmed that symptoms of depression can be common and severe during pregnancy. Watson et al. declared that 23% of women with postnatal depression showed symptoms during pregnancy (Watson et al., 1984). Thus, it is important to understand, recognize and treat antenatal depression (Evans et al., 2001).

By increasing their mindfulness about their capabilities and self-esteem, women will be able to more quickly recognize the symptoms of depression and deal with them from the beginning, thereby avoiding negative consequences on the bond between mother and newborn. BenEssere Mamma can make women familiar with mood variability and help them to manage anxiety and negative emotions during pregnancy, reducing the risk of ante- and post-natal depression.

## FUTURE RESEARCH DIRECTIONS

Despite the growing recent literature about the emergency model of pregnancy care, wherein technologies are included and the scientific rationale of this approach seems to confirm the potentialities, to our knowledge very few studies have investigated the outcomes of many websites and pregnancy-related apps.

Given the paucity of contributions in this field, future research should use controlled studies to test the short-term and long-term outcomes of these services to well-being during pregnancy and to specific disease prevention, particularly for depression. Furthermore, research about possible inconveniences and negative effects of online and mobile services should be considered.

Thus, BenEssere Mamma at the moment represents a good proposal that has been tested to verify its effectiveness in promoting psychological well-being and positive affective state and in reducing anxiety, stress, negative mood and post-natal depression risk through controlled trials.

## CONCLUSION

Pregnancy is a complex phase in a woman's life characterized by physiological and psychological changes that can enhance anxiety or negative emotional states and favor risky behaviors (Lindgren, 2001).

Women's well-being during pregnancy is important for them as well as for the development of the child and the course of the pregnancy (Dayan et al., 2002; Hoffman & Hatch, 2000; Dunkel-Schetter, 1998; Austin et al., 2007; Grant et al., 2008).

By following the three levels of well-being identified by Keyes and Lopez (2002)—high emotional well-being, high psychological well-being, and high social well-being—this chapter proposes three critical aspects to take into consideration in order to improve quality of life and well-being during pregnancy. These aspects include the importance of positive affective states, the need to enhance the psychological skills of mothers in regulating their affective states through relaxation and meditation protocols, and the role of social support given by several persons (professionals as well as family, friends, co-workers and others).

Today, new technologies are becoming emergent tools to meet these needs. Thanks to their ubiquity, multimodality, interactivity, ease of use and sociality, new technologies allow pregnant women to communicate with each other and with health professionals, to share information, to constantly monitor their pregnancy status, to assume and maintain correct and healthy behaviors and to develop personal skills to better deal with impending childbirth and motherhood; they can even learn to relieve their stress in an interactive and fast way (Tripp et al., 2014; Peyton et al., 2014).

Many websites and pregnancy-related apps are already available in the market, and the popularity of these services amongst pregnant women indicates a shift towards patient empowerment within maternity care provision.

Although the Internet and mobile devices offer several advantages, up to now very few self-help interventions have been tested. Thus, it is not possible at the moment to come to a conclusion about the effectiveness of this approach.

At the end of the chapter, an Italian app (BenEssere Mamma) developed by the authors and intended to help pregnant women promote and take care of their well-being was described. Specifically, the app proposes an intervention based on the three levels of well-being. The goal of this app, which includes a four-week self-help intervention based on daily relaxation and meditation exercises, is to increase women's confidence in their abilities to generate positive emotional states and help them to develop new coping skills and a greater awareness of their own emotional states.

Making women better informed and more self-efficacious in managing their psychological state and their behavior represents an important goal. Prompted by positive technologies, mothers-to-be can become more engaged in care. This emerging model of pregnancy care will make the lives of pregnant women easier and more fulfilling and could also be critical in reducing possible healthcare and social costs.

## ACKNOWLEDGMENT

This work was partially supported by the Italian funded project "VRehab. Virtual Reality in the Assessment and TeleRehabilitation of Parkinson's Disease and Post-Stroke Disabilities" - RF-2009-1472190.

## REFERENCES

*500m people will be using healthcare mobile applications in 2015*. (2015). Research2guidance. Retrieved from http://research2guidance.com/500m-people-will-be-usinghealthcare-mobile-applications-in-2015/

Adolfsson, A., Linden, K., Sparud-Lundin, C., Larsson, P. G., & Berg, M. (2014). A web-based support for pregnant women and new mothers with type 1 diabetes mellitus in Sweden (MODIAB-Web): Study protocol for a randomized controlled trial. *Trials*, *15*(1), 513. doi:10.1186/1745-6215-15-513 PMID:25543854

Ahsan, A., & Raihan, A. (2013, December). Understanding m-health impact among Aponjon (MAMA Bangladesh) subscribers through a phone survey in Bangladesh. *Proceedings of the Sixth International Conference on Information and Communications Technologies and Development: Notes* (*Vol. 2,* pp. 1-4). ACM.

Ahtinen, A., Mattila, E., Välkkynen, P., Kaipainen, K., Vanhala, T., Ermes, M., & Lappalainen, R. (2013). Mobile mental wellness training for stress management: Feasibility and design implications based on a one-month field study. *JMIR mHealth and uHealth, 1*(2).

Akbarzade, M., Rafiee, B., Asadi, N., & Zare, N. (2015). The Effect of Maternal Relaxation Training on Reactivity of Non-Stress Test, Basal Fetal Heart Rate, and Number of Fetal Heart Accelerations: A Randomized Controlled Trial. *International journal of community based nursing and midwifery, 3*(1), 51.

Ammaniti, M. (1996). *Maternità e gravidanza: studio delle rappresentazioni materne*. Raffaello Cortina.

Austin, M. P., Tully, L., & Parker, G. (2007). Examining the relationship between antenatal anxiety and postnatal depression. *Journal of Affective Disorders*, *101*(1), 169–174. doi:10.1016/j.jad.2006.11.015 PMID:17196663

Barclay, L., Everitt, L., Rogan, F., Schmied, V., & Wyllie, A. (1997). Becoming a mother—an analysis of women's experience of early motherhood. *Journal of Advanced Nursing*, *25*(4), 719–728. doi:10.1046/j.1365-2648.1997.t01-1-1997025719.x PMID:9104667

Bartholomew, M. K., Schoppe-Sullivan, S. J., Glassman, M., Kamp Dush, C. M., & Sullivan, J. M. (2012). New parents' Facebook use at the transition to parenthood. *Family Relations*, *61*(3), 455–469. doi:10.1111/j.1741-3729.2012.00708.x PMID:23671354

Bastani, F., Hidarnia, A., Kazemnejad, A., Vafaei, M., & Kashanian, M. (2005). A randomized controlled trial of the effects of applied relaxation training on reducing anxiety and perceived stress in pregnant women. *Journal of Midwifery & Women's Health*, *50*(4), e36–e40. doi:10.1016/j.jmwh.2004.11.008 PMID:15973255

Bastani, F., Hidarnia, A., Montgomery, K. S., Aguilar-Vafaei, M. E., & Kazemnejad, A. (2006). Does relaxation education in anxious primigravid Iranian women influence adverse pregnancy outcomes?: A randomized controlled trial. *The Journal of Perinatal & Neonatal Nursing*, *20*(2), 138–146. doi:10.1097/00005237-200604000-00007 PMID:16714913

Beddoe, A. E., & Lee, K. A. (2008). Mind-Body Interventions during Pregnancy. *Journal of Obstetric, Gynecologic, and Neonatal Nursing*, *37*(2), 165–175. doi:10.1111/j.1552-6909.2008.00218.x PMID:18336440

Beebe, K. R., Lee, K. A., Carrieri-Kohlman, V., & Humphreys, J. (2007). The Effects of Childbirth Self-Efficacy and Anxiety during Pregnancy on Prehospitalization Labor. *Journal of Obstetric, Gynecologic, and Neonatal Nursing*, *36*(5), 410–418. doi:10.1111/j.1552-6909.2007.00170.x PMID:17880311

Bert, F., Gualano, M. R., Brusaferro, S., De Vito, E., de Waure, C., La Torre, G.,... & Carubia, L. (2013). Pregnancy e-health: a multicenter Italian cross-sectional study on Internet use and decision-making among pregnant women. *Journal of epidemiology and community health*, jech-2013.

Bribing, G. (1959). Some considerations of the psychological process in pregnancy. *The Psychoanalytic Study of the Child*, *14*, 113–119.

Buitelaar, J. K., Huizink, A. C., Mulder, E. J., de Medina, P. G. R., & Visser, G. H. (2003). Prenatal stress and cognitive development and temperament in infants. *Neurobiology of Aging*, *24*, S53–S60. doi:10.1016/S0197-4580(03)00050-2 PMID:12829109

Campbell, S. B., Morgan-Lopez, A. A., Cox, M. J., & McLoyd, V. C. (2009). A latent class analysis of maternal depressive symptoms over 12 years and offspring adjustment in adolescence. *Journal of Abnormal Psychology*, *118*(3), 479–493. doi:10.1037/a0015923 PMID:19685946

Cavanagh, K., Strauss, C., Cicconi, F., Griffiths, N., Wyper, A., & Jones, F. (2013). A randomised controlled trial of a brief online mindfulness-based intervention. *Behaviour Research and Therapy*, *51*(9), 573–578. doi:10.1016/j.brat.2013.06.003 PMID:23872699

Chittaro, L., & Vianello, A. (2014). Computer-supported mindfulness: Evaluation of a mobile thought distancing application on naive meditators. *International Journal of Human-Computer Studies*, *72*(3), 337–348. doi:10.1016/j.ijhcs.2013.11.001

Cogill, S. R., Caplan, H. L., Alexandra, H., Robson, K. M., & Kumar, R. (1986). Impact of maternal postnatal depression on cognitive development of young children. *BMJ*, *292*(6529), 1165–1167. doi:10.1136/bmj.292.6529.1165 PMID:3085767

Collins, N. L., Dunkel-Schetter, C., Lobel, M., & Scrimshaw, S. C. (1993). Social support in pregnancy: Psychosocial correlates of birth outcomes and postpartum depression. *Journal of Personality and Social Psychology*, *65*(6), 1243–1258. doi:10.1037/0022-3514.65.6.1243 PMID:8295121

Cooper, P. J., Tomlinson, M., Swartz, L., Landman, M., Molteno, C., Stein, A., & Murray, L. et al. (2009). Improving quality of mother-infant relationship and infant attachment in socioeconomically deprived community in South Africa: Randomised controlled trial. *BMJ (Clinical Research Ed.)*, *338*(Apr. 14), b974. doi:10.1136/bmj.b974 PMID:19366752

Costa, D. D., Rippen, N., Dritsa, M., & Ring, A. (2003). Self-reported leisure-time physical activity during pregnancy and relationship to psychological well-being. *Journal of Psychosomatic Obstetrics and Gynaecology*, *24*(2), 111–119. doi:10.3109/01674820309042808 PMID:12854395

Cuijpers, P., Donker, T., van Straten, A., Li, J., & Andersson, G. (2010). Is guided self-help as effective as face-to-face psychotherapy for depression and anxiety disorders? A systematic review and meta-analysis of comparative outcome studies. *Psychological Medicine*, *40*(12), 1943–1957. doi:10.1017/S0033291710000772 PMID:20406528

Cummings, E. M., & Davies, P. T. (1994). Maternal depression and child development. *Journal of Child Psychology and Psychiatry, and Allied Disciplines*, *35*(1), 73–112. doi:10.1111/j.1469-7610.1994.tb01133.x PMID:8163630

Cutrona, C. E. (1984). Social support and stress in the transition to parenthood. *Journal of Abnormal Psychology*, *93*(4), 378–390. doi:10.1037/0021-843X.93.4.378 PMID:6512084

Danaher, B. G., Milgrom, J., Seeley, J. R., Stuart, S., Schembri, C., Tyler, M. S., & Lewinsohn, P. et al. (2013). MomMoodBooster web-based intervention for postpartum depression: Feasibility trial results. *Journal of Medical Internet Research*, *15*(11), e242. doi:10.2196/jmir.2876 PMID:24191345

Davis, E. P., Glynn, L. M., Schetter, C. D., Hobel, C., Chicz-Demet, A., & Sandman, C. A. (2007). Prenatal exposure to maternal depression and cortisol influences infant temperament. *Journal of the American Academy of Child and Adolescent Psychiatry*, *46*(6), 737–746. doi:10.1097/chi.0b013e318047b775 PMID:17513986

Dayan, J., Creveuil, C., Herlicoviez, M., Herbel, C., Baranger, E., Savoye, C., & Thouin, A. (2002). Role of anxiety and depression in the onset of spontaneous preterm labor. *American Journal of Epidemiology*, *155*(4), 293–301. doi:10.1093/aje/155.4.293 PMID:11836191

Declercq, E. R., Sakala, C., Corry, M. P., & Applebaum, S. (2007). Listening to Mothers II: Report of the Second National US Survey of Women's Childbearing Experiences: Conducted January–February 2006 for Childbirth Connection by Harris Interactive® in partnership with Lamaze International*. *Journal of Perinatal Education*, *16*(4), 9–14. doi:10.1624/105812407X244769 PMID:18769512

Dover, S. (2012). Study: Number of smartphone users tops 1 billion. *CBSNews*. Retrieved from http://www.cbsnews.com/8301-205_162-57534583/study-numberof-smartphone-users-tops-1-billion

Duncan, L. G., & Bardacke, N. (2010). Mindfulness-based childbirth and parenting education: Promoting family mindfulness during the perinatal period. *Journal of Child and Family Studies*, *19*(2), 190–202. doi:10.1007/s10826-009-9313-7 PMID:20339571

Dunkel-Schetter, C. (1998). Maternal stress and preterm delivery. *Prenatal and Neonatal Medicine*, *3*, 39–42.

Dunkel Schetter, C. (2011). Psychological science on pregnancy: Stress processes, biopsychosocial models, and emerging research issues. *Annual Review of Psychology*, *62*(1), 531–558. doi:10.1146/annurev.psych.031809.130727 PMID:21126184

Dunkel-Schetter, C., Sagrestano, L. M., Feldman, P., & Killingsworth, C. (1996). Social support and pregnancy. In Handbook of social support and the family (pp. 375-412). Springer US. doi:10.1007/978-1-4899-1388-3_16

Dunn, C., Hanieh, E., Roberts, R., & Powrie, R. (2012). Mindful pregnancy and childbirth: Effects of a mindfulness-based intervention on women's psychological distress and well-being in the perinatal period. *Archives of Women's Mental Health, 15*(2), 139–143. doi:10.1007/s00737-012-0264-4 PMID:22382281

Field, T., Diego, M., & Hernandez-Reif, M. (2006). Prenatal depression effects on the fetus and newborn: A review. *Infant Behavior and Development, 29*(3), 445–455. doi:10.1016/j.infbeh.2006.03.003 PMID:17138297

Field, T., Diego, M. A., Hernandez-Reif, M., Schanberg, S., & Kuhn, C. (2004). Massage therapy effects on depressed pregnant women. *Journal of Psychosomatic Obstetrics and Gynaecology, 25*(2), 115–122. doi:10.1080/01674820412331282231 PMID:15715034

Field, T., Hemandez-Reif, M., Hart, S., Theakston, H., Schanberg, S., & Kuhn, C. (1999). Pregnant women benefit from massage therapy. *Journal of Psychosomatic Obstetrics and Gynaecology, 20*(1), 31–38. doi:10.3109/01674829909075574 PMID:10212885

Field, T., Hernandez-Reif, M., Diego, M., Schanberg, S., & Kuhn, C. (2006). Stability of mood states and biochemistry across pregnancy. *Infant Behavior and Development, 29*(2), 262–267. doi:10.1016/j.infbeh.2005.12.009 PMID:17138281

Fredrickson, B. L. (2001). The role of positive emotions in positive psychology: The broaden-and-build theory of positive emotions. *The American Psychologist, 56*(3), 218–226. doi:10.1037/0003-066X.56.3.218 PMID:11315248

Gao, L. L., Larsson, M., & Luo, S. Y. (2013). Internet use by Chinese women seeking pregnancy-related information. *Midwifery, 29*(7), 730–735. doi:10.1016/j.midw.2012.07.003 PMID:22958935

Gedde-Dahl, M., & Fors, E. A. (2012). Impact of self-administered relaxation and guided imagery techniques during final trimester and birth. *Complementary Therapies in Clinical Practice, 18*(1), 60–65. doi:10.1016/j.ctcp.2011.08.008 PMID:22196576

Grant, K. A., McMahon, C., & Austin, M. P. (2008). Maternal anxiety during the transition to parenthood: A prospective study. *Journal of Affective Disorders, 108*(1), 101–111. doi:10.1016/j.jad.2007.10.002 PMID:18001841

Green Paper on mobile-health (mHealth). (2014, June). Brussels, Belgium.

Haga, S. M., Drozd, F., Brendryen, H., & Slinning, K. (2013). Mamma mia: a feasibility study of a Web-based intervention to reduce the risk of postpartum depression and enhance subjective well-being. *JMIR research protocols, 2*(2).

Haug, T., Nordgreen, T., Öst, L. G., & Havik, O. E. (2012). Self-help treatment of anxiety disorders: A meta-analysis and meta-regression of effects and potential moderators. *Clinical Psychology Review, 32*(5), 425–445. doi:10.1016/j.cpr.2012.04.002 PMID:22681915

Hearn, L., Miller, M., & Lester, L. (2014). Reaching perinatal women online: The Healthy You, Healthy Baby website and app. *Journal of Obesity*, 2014. PMID:24872891

Hernández-Martínez, C., Val, V. A., Murphy, M., Busquets, P. C., & Sans, J. C. (2011). Relation between positive and negative maternal emotional states and obstetrical outcomes. *Women & Health*, *51*(2), 124–135. doi:10.1080/03630242.2010.550991 PMID:21476173

Hipwell, A. E., Goossens, F. A., Melhuish, E. C., & Kumar, R. (2000). Severe maternal psychopathology and infant–mother attachment. *Development and Psychopathology*, *12*(02), 157–175. doi:10.1017/S0954579400002030 PMID:10847622

Hoffman, S., & Hatch, M. C. (2000). Depressive symptomatology during pregnancy: Evidence for an association with decreased fetal growth in pregnancies of lower social class women. *Health Psychology*, *19*(6), 535–543. doi:10.1037/0278-6133.19.6.535 PMID:11129356

Israel, B. A., Farquhar, S. A., Schulz, A. J., James, S. A., & Parker, E. A. (2002). The relationship between social support, stress, and health among women on Detroit's East Side. *Health Education & Behavior*, *29*(3), 342–360. PMID:12038743

Jihye, H., & Iftekhar, S. N. Comparison on the Use of Smartphone Application between International and Korean Pregnant Women.

Johnson, S. A. (2014). "Maternal Devices", Social Media and the Self-Management of Pregnancy, Mothering and Child Health. *Societies*, *4*(2), 330–350. doi:10.3390/soc4020330

Jones, L. (2012). Pain management for women in labour: An overview of systematic reviews. *Journal of Evidence-Based Medicine*, *5*(2), 101–102. PMID:22419342

Kabat-Zinn, J. (1994). *Wherever you go, there you are: Mindfulness meditation in everyday life*. New York: Hyperion.

Keyes, C. L. M., & Lopez, S. J. (2002). Toward a science of mental health: positive direction in diagnosis and interventions. In C. R. Snyder & S. J. Lopez (Eds.), *Handbook of Positive Psychology*. New York: Oxford University Press.

Lagan, B. M., Sinclair, M., & George Kernohan, W. (2010). Internet Use in Pregnancy Informs Women's Decision Making: A Web-Based Survey. *Birth (Berkeley, Calif.)*, *37*(2), 106–115. doi:10.1111/j.1523-536X.2010.00390.x PMID:20557533

Lagan, B. M., Sinclair, M., & Kernohan, W. G. (2011). What Is the Impact of the Internet on Decision-Making in Pregnancy? A Global Study. *Birth (Berkeley, Calif.)*, *38*(4), 336–345. doi:10.1111/j.1523-536X.2011.00488.x PMID:22112334

Lancaster, C. A., Gold, K. J., Flynn, H. A., Yoo, H., Marcus, S. M., & Davis, M. M. (2010). Risk factors for depressive symptoms during pregnancy: A systematic review. *American Journal of Obstetrics and Gynecology*, *202*(1), 5–14. doi:10.1016/j.ajog.2009.09.007 PMID:20096252

Larsson, M. (2009). A descriptive study of the use of the Internet by women seeking pregnancy-related information. *Midwifery*, *25*(1), 14–20. doi:10.1016/j.midw.2007.01.010 PMID:17408822

Lima-Pereira, P., Bermúdez-Tamayo, C., & Jasienska, G. (2012). Use of the Internet as a source of health information amongst participants of antenatal classes. *Journal of Clinical Nursing*, *21*(3-4), 322–330. doi:10.1111/j.1365-2702.2011.03910.x PMID:22093043

Lindgren, K. (2001). Relationships among maternal–fetal attachment, prenatal depression, and health practices in pregnancy. *Research in Nursing & Health*, *24*(3), 203–217. doi:10.1002/nur.1023 PMID:11526619

Lowe, N. K. (2002). The nature of labor pain. *American Journal of Obstetrics and Gynecology*, *186*(5), S16–S24. doi:10.1016/S0002-9378(02)70179-8 PMID:12011870

Lund, S., Nielsen, B. B., Hemed, M., Boas, I. M., Said, A., Said, K., & Rasch, V. (2014). Mobile phones improve antenatal care attendance in Zanzibar: A cluster randomized controlled trial. *BMC Pregnancy and Childbirth*, *14*(1), 29. doi:10.1186/1471-2393-14-29 PMID:24438517

Luxton, D. D., McCann, R. A., Bush, N. E., Mishkind, M. C., & Reger, G. M. (2011). mHealth for mental health: Integrating smartphone technology in behavioral healthcare. *Professional Psychology, Research and Practice*, *42*(6), 505–512. doi:10.1037/a0024485

Ly, K. H., Trüschel, A., Jarl, L., Magnusson, S., Windahl, T., Johansson, R., & Andersson, G. et al. (2014). Behavioural activation versus mindfulness-based guided self-help treatment administered through a smartphone application: A randomised controlled trial. *BMJ Open*, *4*(1), e003440. doi:10.1136/bmjopen-2013-003440 PMID:24413342

Mathiesen, K. S., Tambs, K., & Dalgard, O. S. (1999). The influence of social class, strain and social support on symptoms of anxiety and depression in mothers of toddlers. *Social Psychiatry and Psychiatric Epidemiology*, *34*(2), 61–72. doi:10.1007/s001270050113 PMID:10189811

Melzer, K., Schutz, Y., Soehnchen, N., Othenin-Girard, V., de Tejada, B. M., Irion, O., & Kayser, B. et al. (2010). Effects of recommended levels of physical activity on pregnancy outcomes. *American Journal of Obstetrics and Gynecology*, *202*(3), 266–e1. doi:10.1016/j.ajog.2009.10.876 PMID:20022583

*mHealth App Developer Economics 2014: The State of the Art of mHealth App.* (2014). Research2guidance. Retrieved from http://research2guidance.com/r2g/mHealth-App-Developer-Economics-2014.pdf

mHealth: New Horizons for Health through Mobile Technologies: Based on the Findings of the Second Global Survey on eHealth (Global Observatory for eHealth Series, Volume 3) (2011). World Health Organization.

Miyata, K. (2002). Social support for Japanese mothers online and offline. *The internet in everyday life*, 520-548.

Monti, F., Fagandini, P., Agostini, F., Vettori, D., & La Sala, G. B. (2006). *La complessità della nascita: genitorialità e modalità di parto. La Sala GB, Iori V., Monti F., Fagandini P.(a cura di), La "normale" complessità del venire al mondo.* Milano: Guerini Studio.

Mulsow, M., Caldera, Y. M., Pursley, M., Reifman, A., & Huston, A. C. (2002). Multilevel factors influencing maternal stress during the first three years. *Journal of Marriage and the Family*, *64*(4), 944–956. doi:10.1111/j.1741-3737.2002.00944.x

Murray, L. (1992). The impact of postnatal depression on infant development. *Journal of Child Psychology and Psychiatry, and Allied Disciplines*, *33*(3), 543–561. doi:10.1111/j.1469-7610.1992.tb00890.x PMID:1577898

Murray, L., Fiori-Cowley, A., Hooper, R., & Cooper, P. (1996). The impact of postnatal depression and associated adversity on early mother-infant interactions and later infant outcome. *Child Development*, *67*(5), 2512–2526. doi:10.2307/1131637 PMID:9022253

Murray, L., Sinclair, D., Cooper, P., Ducournau, P., Turner, P., & Stein, A. (1999). The socioemotional development of 5-year-old children of postnatally depressed mothers. *Journal of Child Psychology and Psychiatry, and Allied Disciplines*, *40*(08), 1259–1271. doi:10.1111/1469-7610.00542 PMID:10604404

Narendran, S., Nagarathna, R., Narendran, V., Gunasheela, S., & Nagendra, H. R. R. (2005). Efficacy of yoga on pregnancy outcome. *Journal of Alternative and Complementary Medicine (New York, N.Y.)*, *11*(2), 237–244. doi:10.1089/acm.2005.11.237 PMID:15865489

Nasreen, H. E., Kabir, Z. N., Forsell, Y., & Edhborg, M. (2011). Prevalence and associated factors of depressive and anxiety symptoms during pregnancy: A population based study in rural Bangladesh. *BMC Women's Health*, *11*(1), 22. doi:10.1186/1472-6874-11-22 PMID:21635722

Newman, M. G., Szkodny, L. E., Llera, S. J., & Przeworski, A. (2011). A review of technology-assisted self-help and minimal contact therapies for anxiety and depression: Is human contact necessary for therapeutic efficacy? *Clinical Psychology Review*, *31*(1), 89–103. doi:10.1016/j.cpr.2010.09.008 PMID:21130939

Nickel, C., Lahmann, C., Muehlbacher, M., Pedrosa Gil, F., Kaplan, P., Buschmann, W., & Nickel, M. et al. (2006). Pregnant women with bronchial asthma benefit from progressive muscle relaxation: A randomized, prospective, controlled trial. *Psychotherapy and Psychosomatics*, *75*(4), 237–243. doi:10.1159/000092894 PMID:16785773

O'Connor, T. G., Heron, J., & Glover, V. (2002). Antenatal anxiety predicts child behavioral/emotional problems independently of postnatal depression. *Journal of the American Academy of Child and Adolescent Psychiatry*, *41*(12), 1470–1477. doi:10.1097/00004583-200212000-00019 PMID:12447034

O'Hara, M. W., & Swain, A. M. (1996). Rates and risk of postpartum depression-a meta-analysis. *International Review of Psychiatry (Abingdon, England)*, *8*(1), 37–54. doi:10.3109/09540269609037816

O'Higgins, A., Murphy, O. C., Egan, A., Mullaney, L., Sheehan, S., & Turner, M. J. (2013). The use of digital media by women using the maternity services in a developed country. *Irish Medical Journal*, *107*(10), 313–315. PMID:25556255

Oakley, A. (1992). Social support in pregnancy: Methodology and findings of a 1-year follow-up study. *Journal of Reproductive and Infant Psychology*, *10*(4), 219–231. doi:10.1080/02646839208403955

Oakley, A., Hickey, D., Rajan, L., & Rigby, A. S. (1996). Social support in pregnancy: Does it have long-term effects? *Journal of Reproductive and Infant Psychology*, *14*(1), 7–22. doi:10.1080/02646839608405855

Oakley, A., Rajan, L., & Grant, A. (1990). Social support and pregnancy outcome. *BJOG: An International Journal of Obstetrics & Gynaecology*, *97*(2), 155–162. doi:10.1111/j.1471-0528.1990.tb01741.x PMID:2317466

Parker, R. M., Dmitrieva, E., Frolov, S., & Gazmararian, J. A. (2012). Text4baby in the United States and Russia: an opportunity for understanding how mHealth affects maternal and child health. *Journal of health communication, 17*(sup1), 30-36.

Peyton, T. (2014, November). Pregnancy Ecologies As Teachable Moments For The Lifecourse: Changing The mHealth Design Paradigm. *Proceedings of the 18th International Conference on Supporting Group Work* (pp. 269-271). ACM. doi:10.1145/2660398.2660438

Peyton, T., Poole, E., Reddy, M., Kraschnewski, J., & Chuang, C. (2014, June). Every pregnancy is different: designing mHealth for the pregnancy ecology. *Proceedings of the 2014 conference on Designing interactive systems* (pp. 577-586). ACM. doi:10.1145/2598510.2598572

Pluess, M., Wurmser, H., Buske-Kirschbaum, A., Papousek, M., Pirke, K. M., Hellhammer, D., & Bolten, M. (2012). Positive life events predict salivary cortisol in pregnant women. *Psychoneuroendocrinology, 37*(8), 1336–1340. doi:10.1016/j.psyneuen.2012.01.006 PMID:22309824

Preece, J. (2001). Online communities: Usability, sociabilty, theory and methods. In *Frontiers of human-centered computing, online communities and virtual environments* (pp. 263–277). Springer London. doi:10.1007/978-1-4471-0259-5_18

Preziosa, A., Grassi, A., Gaggioli, A., & Riva, G. (2009). Therapeutic applications of the mobile phone. *British Journal of Guidance & Counselling, 37*(3), 313–325. doi:10.1080/03069880902957031

Repetto, C., Gaggioli, A., Pallavicini, F., Cipresso, P., Raspelli, S., & Riva, G. (2013). Virtual reality and mobile phones in the treatment of generalized anxiety disorders: A phase-2 clinical trial. *Personal and Ubiquitous Computing, 17*(2), 253–260. doi:10.1007/s00779-011-0467-0

Riva, G., Banos, R. M., Botella, C., Wiederhold, B. K., & Gaggioli, A. (2012). Positive technology: Using interactive technologies to promote positive functioning. *Cyberpsychology, Behavior, and Social Networking, 15*(2), 69–77. doi:10.1089/cyber.2011.0139 PMID:22149077

Romano, A. M. (2007). A changing landscape: Implications of pregnant women's Internet use for childbirth educators. *Journal of Perinatal Education, 16*(4), 18–24. doi:10.1624/105812407X244903 PMID:18769519

Roos, A., Faure, S., Lochner, C., Vythilingum, B., & Stein, D. J. (2013). Predictors of distress and anxiety during pregnancy. *The African Journal of Psychiatry, 16*(2), 118–122. PMID:23595531

Rotheram-Borus, M. J., Tomlinson, M., Gwegwe, M., Comulada, W. S., Kaufman, N., & Keim, M. (2012). Diabetes buddies peer support through a mobile phone buddy system. *The Diabetes Educator, 38*(3), 357–365. doi:10.1177/0145721712444617 PMID:22546740

Rotheram-Borus, M. J., Tomlinson, M., Swendeman, D., Lee, A., & Jones, E. (2012). Standardized functions for smartphone applications: Examples from maternal and child health. *International Journal of Telemedicine and Applications, 2012*, 21. doi:10.1155/2012/973237 PMID:23304136

Rubin, R. (1984). Maternal Identity and the Maternal Experience. *AJN The American Journal of Nursing, 84*(12), 1480. doi:10.1097/00000446-198412000-00030

Rush, J., Chalmers, I., & Enkin, M. (1991). Care of the new mother and baby. In I. Chalmers, M. Enkin, & M. Kierse (Eds.), *Effective Care in Pregnancy and Childbirth* (Vol. 2, pp. 1333–1346). Oxford: Oxford University Press.

Satyapriya, M., Nagendra, H. R., Nagarathna, R., & Padmalatha, V. (2009). Effect of integrated yoga on stress and heart rate variability in pregnant women. *International Journal of Gynaecology and Obstetrics: the Official Organ of the International Federation of Gynaecology and Obstetrics, 104*(3), 218–222. doi:10.1016/j.ijgo.2008.11.013 PMID:19110245

Schaub, B. G. (1995). Imagery in health care: Connecting with life energy. *Complementary Health Practice Review, 1*(2), 113–115.

Seligman, M. E. (2003). Fundamental assumptions. *The Psychologist, 16*(3), 126.

Seligman, M. E., & Csikszentmihalyi, M. (2000). Positive psychology: An introduction: Vol. 55. *No. 1* (p. 5). American Psychological Association.

Sethi, S., Campbell, A. J., & Ellis, L. A. (2010). The use of computerized self-help packages to treat adolescent depression and anxiety. *Journal of Technology in Human Services, 28*(3), 144–160. doi:10.1080/15228835.2010.508317

Sharf, B. F. (1997). Communicating breast cancer on-line: Support and empowerment on the Internet. *Women & Health, 26*(1), 65–84. doi:10.1300/J013v26n01_05 PMID:9311100

Sharma, V., Bauer, B., Prasad, K., Sood, A., & Schroeder, D. (2012). P02.197 Self help intervention to decrease stress and increase mindfulness: A pilot trial. *BMC Complementary and Alternative Medicine, 12*(Suppl. 1), 253. doi:10.1186/1472-6882-12-S1-P253 PMID:23237355

Smith, C. A., Levett, K. M., Collins, C. T., & Crowther, C. A. (2011). Relaxation techniques for pain management in labour. *The Cochrane Library*. PMID:22161453

Stern, D. N., Bruschweiler-Stern, N., & Freeland, A. (1998). *The birth of a mother*. London: Bloomsbury.

Stice, E., Ragan, J., & Randall, P. (2004). Prospective relations between social support and depression: Differential direction of effects for parent and peer support? *Journal of Abnormal Psychology, 113*(1), 155–159. doi:10.1037/0021-843X.113.1.155 PMID:14992668

Tamrat, T., & Kachnowski, S. (2012). Special delivery: An analysis of mHealth in maternal and newborn health programs and their outcomes around the world. *Maternal and Child Health Journal, 16*(5), 1092–1101. doi:10.1007/s10995-011-0836-3 PMID:21688111

Taylor, C. B., & Luce, K. H. (2003). Computer-and Internet-based psychotherapy interventions. *Current Directions in Psychological Science, 12*(1), 18–22. doi:10.1111/1467-8721.01214

Teixeira, J., Martin, D., Prendiville, O., & Glover, V. (2005). The effects of acute relaxation on indices of anxiety during pregnancy. *Journal of Psychosomatic Obstetrics and Gynaecology, 26*(4), 271–276. doi:10.1080/01674820500139922 PMID:16457423

Tietjen, A. M., & Bradley, C. F. (1985). Social support and maternal psychosocial adjustment during the transition to parenthood. *Revue canadienne des sciences du comportement [Canadian Journal of Behavioural Science], 17*(2), 109.

Tragea, C., Chrousos, G. P., Alexopoulos, E. C., & Darviri, C. (2014). A randomized controlled trial of the effects of a stress management programme during pregnancy. *Complementary Therapies in Medicine, 22*(2), 203–211. doi:10.1016/j.ctim.2014.01.006 PMID:24731890

Tripp, N., Hainey, K., Liu, A., Poulton, A., Peek, M., Kim, J., & Nanan, R. (2014). An emerging model of maternity care: Smartphone, midwife, doctor? *Women and Birth; Journal of the Australian College of Midwives, 27*(1), 64–67. doi:10.1016/j.wombi.2013.11.001 PMID:24295598

Tronick, E. Z., & Weinberg, K. (1999). *Le madri depresse ei loro bambini: l'insuccesso nella formazione degli stati di coscienza diadici. Murray, L., Cooper, P.(a cura di). Depressione del post-partum e sviluppo del bambino*. Roma: CIC Edizioni Internazionali.

Urech, C., Fink, N. S., Hoesli, I., Wilhelm, F. H., Bitzer, J., & Alder, J. (2010). Effects of relaxation on psychobiological wellbeing during pregnancy: A randomized controlled trial. *Psychoneuroendocrinology, 35*(9), 1348–1355. doi:10.1016/j.psyneuen.2010.03.008 PMID:20417038

Urizar, G. G. Jr, Milazzo, M., Le, H. N., Delucchi, K., Sotelo, R., & Muñoz, R. F. (2004). Impact of stress reduction instructions on stress and cortisol levels during pregnancy. *Biological Psychology, 67*(3), 275–282. doi:10.1016/j.biopsycho.2003.11.001 PMID:15294386

Vieten, C., & Astin, J. (2008). Effects of a mindfulness-based intervention during pregnancy on prenatal stress and mood: Results of a pilot study. *Archives of Women's Mental Health, 11*(1), 67–74. doi:10.1007/s00737-008-0214-3 PMID:18317710

Villani, D., Grassi, A., Cognetta, C., Toniolo, D., Cipresso, P., & Riva, G. (2013). Self-help stress management training through mobile phones: An experience with oncology nurses. *Psychological Services, 10*(3), 315–322. doi:10.1037/a0026459 PMID:23937091

Villani, D., & Riva, G. (2012). Does interactive media enhance the management of stress? Suggestions from a controlled study. *Cyberpsychology, Behavior, and Social Networking, 15*(1), 24–30. doi:10.1089/cyber.2011.0141 PMID:22032797

Vliet, H. V., & Andrews, G. (2009). Internet-based course for the management of stress for junior high schools. *The Australian and New Zealand Journal of Psychiatry, 43*(4), 305–309. doi:10.1080/00048670902721145 PMID:19296285

Voellmin, A., Entringer, S., Moog, N., Wadhwa, P. D., & Buss, C. (2013). Maternal positive affect over the course of pregnancy is associated with the length of gestation and reduced risk of preterm delivery. *Journal of Psychosomatic Research, 75*(4), 336–340. doi:10.1016/j.jpsychores.2013.06.031 PMID:24119939

Waring, M. E., Simas, T. A. M., Xiao, R. S., Lombardini, L. M., Allison, J. J., Rosal, M. C., & Pagoto, S. L. (2014). Pregnant women's interest in a website or mobile application for healthy gestational weight gain. *Sexual & Reproductive Healthcare, 5*(4), 182–184. doi:10.1016/j.srhc.2014.05.002 PMID:25433828

Warnecke, E., Quinn, S., Ogden, K., Towle, N., & Nelson, M. R. (2011). A randomised controlled trial of the effects of mindfulness practice on medical student stress levels. *Medical Education*, *45*(4), 381–388. doi:10.1111/j.1365-2923.2010.03877.x PMID:21401686

Watterson, J. L., Walsh, J., & Madeka, I. (2015). Using mHealth to Improve Usage of Antenatal Care, Postnatal Care, and Immunization: A Systematic Review of the Literature. *BioMed Research International, 2015*.

Wellman, B., & Frank, K. (2001). Network capital in a multilevel world: Getting support from personal communities. *Social capital: Theory and research* (pp. 233-273).

Williams, C., & Whitfield, G. (2001). Written and computer-based self-help treatments for depression. *British Medical Bulletin*, *57*(1), 133–144. doi:10.1093/bmb/57.1.133 PMID:11719913

Yali, A. M., & Lobel, M. (2002). Stress-resistance resources and coping in pregnancy. *Anxiety, Stress, and Coping*, *15*(3), 289–309. doi:10.1080/1061580021000020743

## KEY TERMS AND DEFINITIONS

**E-Health:** A general term for the use of information and communications technologies (ICT) in the healthcare promotion and medical fields.

**Empowerment:** Consists of a process of increasing personal resources and awareness of them to promote individual wellbeing and environment adaptation.

**Guided Imagery/Visualization:** A relaxation technique used to induce positive mental images, feelings and thoughts. Guided Imagery can be used by everyone: it is able to overcome barriers of education, class, race, gender and age. Because it involves all senses (not just sight) it is perceived as more pleasant and efficient. This practice is particularly powerful, as well as simpler than mindfulness meditation for most beginners.

**M-Health:** This term indicates the use of mobile and wireless technologies in health fields.

**Mindfulness:** A type of meditative technique that emphasizes an observant and nonreactive stance toward one's thoughts, emotions and body states. It involves purposeful attention to daily activities (e.g., mindfulness of eating).

**Mobile Application:** Software developed to be installed and run on mobile devices such as smartphones, PDAs or tablets. They can be both fun and useful, and they can be executed (run) on a mobile platform.

**Progressive Muscular Relaxation:** A relaxation technique of stress management developed by Edmund Jacobson in 1934, based on tensing and releasing tensions in the 16 different muscle groups. PMR (progressive muscular relaxation) programs include four sets of exercises: arms relaxation; face and shoulders relaxation; bust and legs relaxation. All exercises are based on two principles: contraction and relaxation, with the aim being to achieve a profound and aware state of calm.

**Smartphone:** An advanced mobile phone that includes mobile communication, a camera, a video camera, GPS system, a music player, Internet access, sensors and a range of multimedia capabilities in a single device. Several accessories are being developed to transform smartphones into "medical machines." They can become meters of blood glucose level, blood rate of oxygen, blood pressure and so on.

**Web-App:** This term is used to indicate any program stored on a remote server and delivered over the Internet through a browser interface. They are usable only with an Internet connection and use HTTP as communication protocol.

# Chapter 8
# Technology and Cognitive Empowerment for Healthy Elderly:
## The Link between Cognitive Skills Acquisition and Well-Being

**Silvia Serino**
*Istituto Auxologico Italiano, Italy*

**Elisa Pedroli**
*Istituto Auxologico Italiano, Italy*

## ABSTRACT

*The progressive growth of the ageing population represents opportunities as well as challenges. Consistently, the identification of effective cognitive empowerment programs in elderly population is now a worldwide health policy priority, specially for their preventive effect. In this chapter, within the paradigm of Positive Technology, the main focus will be on the use advanced technologies as effective tools for a new class of applications aimed at improving the traditional cognitive empowerment in elderly. Specifically, the attention will be devoted on how advanced technologies may be used to support elderly in reaching engaging and self-actualizing experiences. On the basis of the most recent evidence in literature, it will be discussed the possible advantages in using such advanced technologies for improving well-being in frail elderly: coupled with an increase in cognitive skills acquisition, the advantages may range increased self-efficacy and decreased subjective weakness, with a consequent improvement in both physical and cognitive performance.*

## INTRODUCTION

The ageing population (aged 65 and over) is projected to increase to 1.2 billion by 2025. According to the most recent demographic projections, there are 87.31 million elderly people in Europe (Lagiewka, 2012). The progressive growth of the ageing population represents opportunities as well as challenges. On one side, because of the substantial increase in life expectancy, the onset and prevalence of neuro-

DOI: 10.4018/978-1-4666-9986-1.ch008

degenerative disease will dramatically increase. To date, for example, Alzheimer's disease (AD) is the most common type of dementia, and it is estimated that the number of people affected will reach 81.1 million by 2040 (Ferri et al., 2006). On the other side, although ageing is usually related to physical and cognitive decline, many elderly individuals want to remain physically and cognitively healthy. Consistently, the identification of effective cognitive empowerment programs for healthy elderly populations is now a worldwide health policy priority.

The potential benefits of cognitive empowerment programs for individuals suffering from cognitive impairment and/or dementia have been increasingly recognized (Belleville et al., 2006; Bier et al., 2015; Buschert, Bokde, & Hampel, 2010; Jean, Bergeron, Thivierge, & Simard, 2010; Thivierge, Jean, & Simard, 2014). Moreover, the potentiality of cognitive empowerment programs is now accepted in healthy elderly populations as well (i.e., older individuals without current diagnosable cognitive impairment), especially for their preventive effect (see for example, Chapman et al., 2015; Kelly et al., 2014; Rebok et al., 2014; Willis et al., 2006).

An interesting recent study carried out by Hudson and colleagues (Hudson, Day, & Oliver, 2015) helps us understand why the definition of effective cognitive empowerment programs for healthy elderly populations may be particularly important. Indeed, Hudson and colleagues (Hudson et al., 2015) enrolled six older sedentary individuals in an exercise programme and interviewed them about their attitudes towards physical activity and their physical self-perceptions and identity. Participants' stories highlighted that while older adults may perceive exercise positively, their existing narratives of age-related decline may be resistant to change. The results of this study highlighted that it may be essential for all elderly people, cognitively impaired or not, to participate in cognitive empowerment programs since these kinds of activities may positively stimulate the elderly to change their attitudes towards age-related decline by increasing their self-efficacy. Indeed, what is crucial for a successful change is the increase in their sense of control. Participants at the beginning of the exercise programme described some existential challenges as well as their resolution of these. From this perspective, the possibility to participate in effective cognitive empowerment programs may become a resource both to delay cognitive impairment associated with ageing and to stimulate crucial cognitive skills fundamental to cope with the decline associated with an ageing body. The idea that cognitive empowerment programs can delay cognitive decline and improve sense of control in healthy older adults has dramatic consequences for its potential application. Cognitive intervention may help older individuals because they retain the cognitive capabilities to learn and apply sets of new strategies to improve their well-being. If designed properly, cognitive interventions may improve the cognitive functioning of elderly individuals and alleviate their anxiety resulting from their cognitive and physical difficulties related to both normal ageing and age-related disease.

The question is how to design and implement effective cognitive empowerment programs. To understand the role of cognitive empowerment programs for the elderly, the different types of traditional approaches will be presented alongside their specific characteristics in the following paragraph.

## COGNITIVE EMPOWERMENT FOR THE ELDERLY

Cognitive empowerment programs for elderly people can be generally included in the broader definition of "non-pharmacological interventions:" they directly or indirectly stimulate the cognitive functioning, as opposed to other interventions for elderly people that focus on emotion regulation (i.e., depressive symptoms) or physical frailty (i.e., fall prevention or weight loss) (Bahar-Fuchs, Clare, & Woods, 2013).

These interventions typically involve elders in different types of activities, ranging from specific cognitive training focused on a particular cognitive function to group-based intervention aimed at promoting the cognitive functioning in a variety of different social contexts that are relevant for daily life. The different types of cognitive empowerment programs may be complementary or not, and the choice of a particular training depends on the objectives and the cognitive profile of the individual.

To summarize and provide some useful guidelines, a recent Cochrane review (Bahar-Fuchs et al., 2013) classified the most used cognitive empowerment programs for the elderly into two main categories: "cognitive training" (or "retraining," or "brain training") and "cognitive rehabilitation." In the scientific literature, these definitions have often been used interchangeably, but in the aforementioned Cochrane review (Bahar-Fuchs et al., 2013), and in its previous version (Clare & Woods, 2003), it is possible to have an extensive description of these two related but distinct forms of cognitive empowerment programs.

The term "cognitive training" is used to describe the repeated practice of series of exercises in order to specifically stimulate targeted cognitive functions (e.g., attention, episodic memory, executive functions). Belleville (Belleville, 2008) defined cognitive training as "teaching theoretically motivated strategies and skills in order to optimize cognition functioning" (pg. 57). Cognitive training may be offered individually or in group sessions. During the training, the different exercises are specifically tailored according to individual performance and to the progress made. Another important assumption underlying these programs is that the cognitive abilities learnt during the training may be generalized to real-life situations. An interesting example was offered by Kaci Fairchild and Scogin (Kaci Fairchild & Scogin, 2010), who developed and tested a memory enhancement program for cognitively healthy elderly. In their study, 53 older adults were assigned to either a memory enhancement condition or a minimal social support condition. Results showed that participants who received the memory enhancement program had a significant improvement in their mnestic abilities, such as remembering names with faces, having fewer lapses in memory and not misplacing household objects, and feeling more confident about their memory.

On the other side, the term "cognitive rehabilitation," originally developed to indicate all programs used to help individuals with brain injuries achieve satisfactory social functioning within their daily context, is now used to refer to programs for people with cognitive impairments. Although the primary aim of cognitive rehabilitation is the development of new effective ways to restore/improve the cognitive functioning of individuals with cognitive impairment, this field has recognized the role of empowerment as a critical element of any treatment strategy. This implies a shift from a traditional medical perspective that focuses on illness, dependence and deficiency to a new integrated approach that focuses on supporting wellness, independence and competence. Indeed, the International Classification of Functioning Disability and Health (ICF) of the World Health Organization (WHO, 2003) defines disability as a "condition in which people are temporarily or definitively unable to perform an activity in the correct manner and/or at a level generally considered 'normal' for the human being." As underlined by Morganti and Riva (Morganti & Riva, 2004), this definition focuses not on deficits but on assets: a person is disabled when she/he is not able to fully exploit her/his relationship with everyday contexts. The emphasis in cognitive rehabilitation is not on a specific exercise, but rather on improving cognitive and social functioning: it is generally implemented in real-life settings with the crucial support of caregivers. Clare and colleagues (Clare et al., 2010) offered an interesting example of "cognitive rehabilitation" for patients suffering from AD. In their study, 69 individuals in the early stages of AD were enrolled in eight weekly individual sessions of cognitive rehabilitation consisting of personalized interventions to address individually relevant goals supported by components addressing practical aids and strategies, techniques for learning new information, practice in maintaining attention and concentration and techniques for stress management. This combined approach showed significant improvement in ratings of goal performance and satisfaction.

These two approaches to cognitive empowerment programmes are based on two different conceptual frameworks: a restorative approach and a compensatory approach (Ylvisaker, Hanks, & Johnson-Greene, 2002). In cognitive training implemented following a restorative approach ("use it or lose it," the well-known principle of brain plasticity), repeated exercises of increasing difficulty specifically targeting a cognitive function may accelerate synaptic growth and repair (Draganski et al., 2006; Hertzog, Kramer, Wilson, & Lindenberger, 2008). On the other hand, cognitive rehabilitation implemented following a compensatory approach exploits residual cognitive abilities of people with impaired cognitive domains.

It is important to acknowledge that under the "umbrella term" of "cognitive empowerment programme," both approaches can be used. But it is crucial to know that they have a different clinical rationale from which derives different peculiar techniques.

In Figure 1, the most peculiar features of the two most common approaches for developing an effective cognitive empowerment programme are summarized.

## The Role of Advanced Technologies for Cognitive Empowerment: A Recent Trend

The dramatic development in the Information and Communication Technology (ICT) sector has resulted in incredible change in the way we interact and live. One of the newest fields that benefits from the advances in technology is that of cognitive assessment and rehabilitation (Bohil, Alicea, & Biocca, 2011; Gaggioli & Riva, 2014; Rose, Brooks, & Rizzo, 2005). In this context, indeed, an increasing trend is the use of advanced technologies, from computer-based application to more sophisticated virtual-based

*Figure 1. The most peculiar features of the two most common approaches for cognitive empowerment programmes: cognitive training and cognitive rehabilitation*

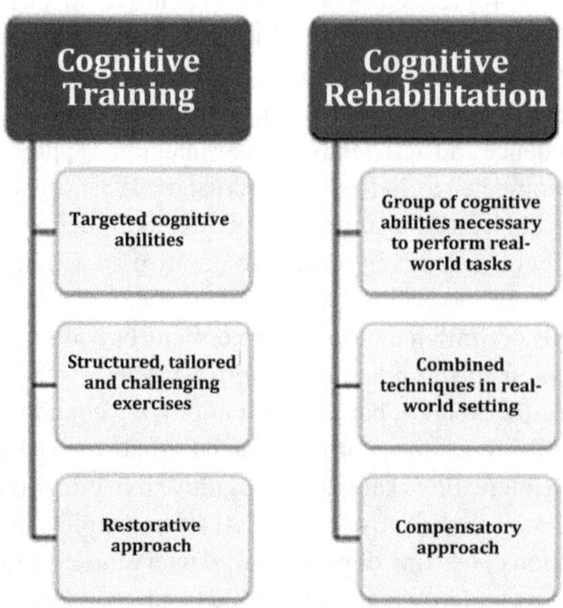

programmes, as functional tools for a new class of applications aimed to improve the traditional cognitive empowerment in the elderly (Barnes et al., 2009; Coyle, Traynor, & Solowij, 2014; García-Betances, Arredondo Waldmeyer, Fico, & Cabrera-Umpiérrez, 2015; García-Betances, Jiménez-Mixco, Arredondo, & Cabrera-Umpiérrez, 2015; Lampit, Hallock, & Valenzuela, 2014). What are the main advantages in using advanced technologies for supporting traditional cognitive empowerment? In general terms, the introduction of technology may offer a more flexible and personalized approach to traditional training programs.

First of all, computer-based cognitive empowerment programmes offer the chance to quantitatively measure behavior while maintaining strict control over stimulus delivery. Moreover, this kind of program allows cognitive exercises to be easily personalized to guarantee real-time performance feedback and an adjustment according to the user's ability level. Walinsky and colleagues (Wolinsky, Vander Weg, Howren, Jones, & Dotson, 2013) offered an interesting example of this great advantage by developing and testing a training programme for older adults focused on processing speed that could be easily delivered either in a clinical setting or at home using portable computers. In this programme, processing speed was improved by progressively reducing the time of exposure to stimuli for a correct identification. Interestingly, thanks to the use of technology, the training programme advanced automatically and in a controllable manner to a greater challenge when participants achieved a 75% success rate.

In the field of cognitive training and rehabilitation, Virtual Reality (VR) has been introduced to offer a completely new paradigm in which individuals (and, of course, patients) are no longer simply observers of stimuli appearing on a computer screen, but they are actively involved within ecologically valid virtual worlds (Riva, Mantovani, & Gaggioli, 2004). VR appears to be a suitable medium that offers several requirements for an effective cognitive empowerment program: repetitive practice, feedback about performance, multimodal stimulation and controlled and secure environments (Bohil et al., 2011; Riva et al., 2004; Schultheis & Rizzo, 2001). Peculiarly, it is possible to control and manipulate tailored exercises within meaningful, ecologically valid and engaging environments using virtual environments (Riva & Gaggioli, 2009).

It is interesting to report the words of McGee, who suggested that "older adults with impairments in memory and executive functioning could be presented with hierarchical rehabilitative challenges in a VE more efficiently and consistently than with traditional methods" (McGee et al., 2000). Indeed, one of the crucial features of the VR technology is the interactivity: immersive virtual environments incorporate a highly sensitive head and body tracking system. Interestingly, Optale and colleagues demonstrated how it is possible to exploit the interactivity of VR to stimulate the spatial functioning of older adults with cognitive impairment (Optale, Capodieci, Marin, Pastore, & Piron, 2007; Optale et al., 2001). They proposed and tested a cognitive rehabilitation memory training programme carried out on twelve patients suffering from mild cognitive impairments (Optale et al., 2007). This rehabilitation treatment consisted of three different listening experiences alternated with three different virtual experiences. The patients were invited to make an oral summary of their audio or VR experience to enhance their mnemonic abilities. During the immersive VR experience, patients were free to navigate in the environments. However, if the patients took a "wrong turn" and ended up at a dead-end, they were immediately transported back to that point along the path in the VR environment immediately before they took the "wrong turn."

After this brief overview of the potentiality of advanced technologies for integrating cognitive empowerment programmes for the elderly, the question is how to design and implement effective cognitive empowerment programmes exploiting the potentiality of new advanced technology.

New disciplines have been introduced, such as "gerontechnology", which refers to the "study of technology for ensuring good health, full social participation, and independent living throughout the entire life span" (Harrington & Harrington, 2000). However, continued technological advances, and progress in neuroscience and neurological research, require a new conceptual and practical framework. In this direction, a more comprehensive perspective is that of Positive Technology (Botella et al., 2012; Riva, Banos, Botella, Wiederhold, & Gaggioli, 2012; Riva & Gaggioli, 2015), which will be presented in the next section.

## AN INTRODUCTION TO POSITIVE TECHNOLOGY

To specifically design and deliver cognitive empowerment programmes, from the design of a tool to its introduction into the clinical practice after scientific validation, it is crucial to adopt a comprehensive framework that can provide scientifically validated guidelines for technological development that meets the needs of an ageing society.

Within this direction, Positive Technology is an emerging field that could be defined as the scientific and applied approach that exploits the potentiality of advanced technology for improving the quality of our personal experience (Botella et al., 2012; Riva et al., 2012; Riva & Gaggioli, 2015). As recently suggested by Riva and colleagues (Riva et al., 2012), the dramatic advancement in the ICT sector has challenged technology developers, designers and psychologists to reflect on how to develop positive technologies to promote well-being. More recently, it has also been suggested that positive technologies may play an important role in dealing with age-related decline by improving well-being of the elderly (Riva et al., 2014).

Why it is possible to reflect about "positive technologies" for elderly? What is well-being, and why is this concept useful for designing effective cognitive empowerment programmes for the elderly? The emerging discipline of Positive Psychology provides a critical framework to both define well-being and to understand how to use technology to develop cognitive empowerment programmes for the elderly. Positive Psychology can be broadly defined as the scientific study of well-being to understand human strength and virtues and to promote them to allow individuals, communities and societies to flourish (Delle Fave, Massimini, & Bassi, 2011; Ryan & Deci, 2001; Seligman & Csikszentmihalyi, 2000; Snyder, 2010). Within this perspective, it appears to be a really promising framework to develop advanced technologies for health. According to Seligman (Seligman, 2002), who is considered the father of Positive Psychology, the definition of a "good life" consists of three different aspects of life, which correspond to different constituents of well-being:

1. **The Pleasant Life:** Achieved through the presence of positive emotions;
2. **The Engaged Life:** Achieved through meaningful engagement in relevant activities that require the exploitation of individual strengths and virtues;
3. **The Meaningful Life:** Achieved through striving to connect to something greater than oneself.

Accordingly, it is possible to classify positive technologies according to their effects on these three aspects of well-being (see also Figure 2):

*Figure 2. Positive technology: how to use technology to promote well-being*

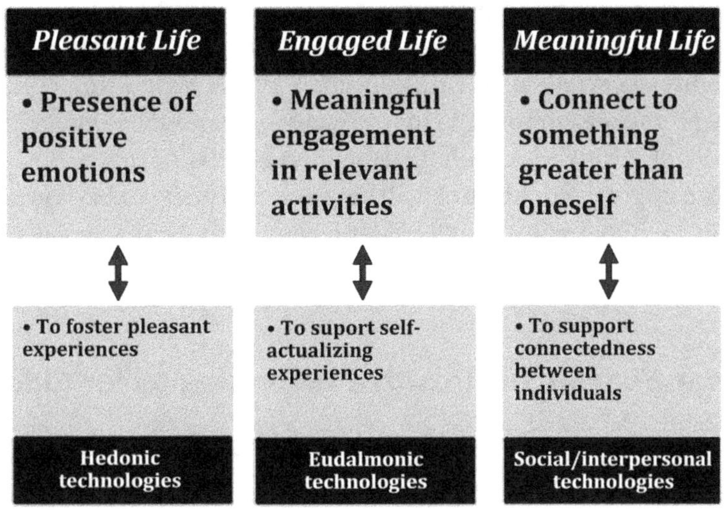


1. **Hedonic Positive Technologies:** Technologies used to foster positive emotions and pleasant experiences;
2. **Eudaimonic Positive Technologies:** Technologies used to support individuals in reaching engaging and self-actualizing experience;
3. **Social/Interpersonal Positive Technologies:** Technologies used to support and improve integration and connectedness between individuals and groups.

To further understand positive technologies and their role in improving well-being in the elderly, it is useful to introduce some relevant examples. A first crucial example of hedonic positive technology is the computer-based multi-media system recently developed and tested by Alm and colleagues (Alm et al., 2009). They started from the idea that interactive entertainment systems specifically designed for elderly individuals may engage them in activities that make life more enjoyable, thereby reducing depressive symptoms that may be associated with ageing and dementia. Their computer-based multimedia system was composed of three parts:

1. The entertainment system supplied engaging content in the form of interactive 3D games with simple, attractive and colorful interfaces;
2. The creative tool allowed a person to freely compose musical sounds independently of their musical skills;
3. The communication support system was designed to help the elderly communicate with their caregivers.

Within the Nostalgia Bits (NoBits) project, Gaggioli and colleagues gave us an example of social/interpersonal positive technology specially developed for the elderly. Indeed, the Nostalgia Bits (NoBits) project aimed at fostering social interaction between the elderly and children through collecting memories and increasing cross-sectional interactions and mentoring. They developed a web-based platform where tangible artifacts of an elderly person's life experience (e.g., photos, stories, personal documents) could be uploaded and thus become a meaningful resource to other generations and an "instrument" to connect elderly users with members of their own generation (Morganti, Riva, Bonfiglio, & Gaggioli, 2013). Findings collected from a user needs analysis conducted on 23 elderly and 310 children showed that both samples readily acceptedthe NoBits concept and that supporting collaborative reminiscing with social media is a promising approach to increase cross-generational interactions and mentoring.

Using the framework of Positive Technology (Botella et al., 2012; Riva et al., 2012; Riva & Gaggioli, 2015), in the following paragraph the attention will be specifically devoted to how advanced technologies that may be specifically used to support healthy elderly people in reaching engaging and self-actualizing experiences and how these experiences may be useful for improving traditional cognitive empowerment programmes.

## The Potentiality for Eudaimonic Positive Technologies for Elderly

Although ageing is typically associated with a decline in physical and cognitive health, this decline can be delayed with effective interventions. In the previous paragraph, it was suggested how positive technologies can be specifically used to support positive emotions and promote connectedness for the elderly (Riva et al., 2014). The two relevant examples presented help us to understand how technology may play an important role in structuring successful pleasant experiences for improving the quality of life for the elderly and improving the strength of their relationships. An improvement in the quality of personal experience, in terms of subjective well-being, can delay age-related decline (Diener & Chan, 2011).

The theory of flow (Csikszentmihalyi, 1991) provides a useful framework to define an "engaging and self-actualizing experience," as well as how they can be used to enable a positive change (Inghilleri, Riva, & Riva, 2015). Flow, or optimal experience, is a state of full engagement, deep concentration and action awareness, occurring during an activity perceived as highly self-rewarding, characterized by clear goals, unambiguous and immediate feedback and an altered sense of time. Specifically, flow is a positive state characterized by a perceived balance between high environmental opportunities for action (challenges) and adequate personal resources in facing them (skills).

Thanks to some key characteristics, Riva and colleagues suggested that advanced technologies, and specifically VR, could be possible sources of flow (Riva & Gaggioli, 2009). First of all, immersive and interactive technologies offer incredible opportunities for action (goals and rules): users are no longer just observers, but active participants within a wide range of increasingly challenging situations and tasks. Second, immersive and interactive technologies offer the chance for giving timing, appropriate and multimodal feedback to individuals based on their actions and behaviors. Within this perspective, Riva and colleagues introduced the strategy of "transformation of flow" (Riva & Gaggioli, 2009), suggesting the possibility to exploit the potentiality of using advanced technology for a new class of (positive) applications in mental health for the elderly. This strategy is based on the idea that, thanks to the continuous cognitive skills acquisition provided by an effective and interactive cognitive empowerment programme, an optimal experience (i.e., balance between skills and demands) is progressively reached and supported by the use of advanced technologies, and this state may be used to promote new and unexpected psychological resources.

Riva and colleagues (Riva et al., 2014) detailed the following steps for the development of eudaimonic positive technology applications for elderly that may integrate traditional cognitive programmes. The first suggested step is the development of an enriched environment containing functional real-world demands. An example was given by the Virtual Multiple Errands Test (VMET), a virtual version of the original

Multiple Errands Test (Shallice & Burgess, 1991) developed for an ecological evaluation of executive functions. The test comprised a virtual supermarket where participants were instructed to select and buy various products presented on shelves and to complete tasks that abided by certain rules (see Figure 3). A recent study showed that VMET was more sensitive in the early detection of executive deficits in a sample of elderly participants suffering from Parkinson's disease (Cipresso et al., 2014). One interesting example of the same approach was tested in a pilot study by Kizony and colleagues (Kizony, Korman, Sinoff, Klinger, & Josman, 2012). They used a modified version of the VMET (i.e., a shopping task) for the rehabilitation of the executive functions in a sample of seven participants with non-amnestic or multi-domain mild cognitive impairment. Although preliminary, results showed the potentiality of this kind of ecological task as a potentially effective tool for training the executive functioning in elderly people suffering from mild cognitive impairment.

The second step is the use of technology for developing interventions with tasks of increasing difficulty (challenges) that are matched to the cognitive level of the individual (skills). An example of a procedure showing increasing difficulty that is able to discriminate between the cognitive level of patients with mild cognitive impairment and patients with Alzheimer's disease has been recently proposed by Serino and colleagues (Serino, Morganti, Di Stefano, & Riva). Findings showed that patients with mild cognitive impairment performed significantly more poorly in the third trial of the first task, while patients with Alzheimer's disease performed significantly more poorly in the second task. A recent study by Kober and colleagues demonstrated the potentiality of VR in enhancing spatial abilities of neurological patients with focal brain lesions (Kober et al., 2013). They tested the efficacy of a verbally-guided passive navigation training in which participants were required to progressively learn the correct directions at each junction they had seen during the learning phase. Results showed that route-finding ability increased over the five VR sessions.

Finally, the third step is the cultivation of optimal experiences reached during the clinical session by linking the results obtained to the actual experience and skills during real life. The incredible develop-

*Figure 3. Screenshot of the virtual multiple errands test (VMET)*
*From Cipresso et al. (2014).*

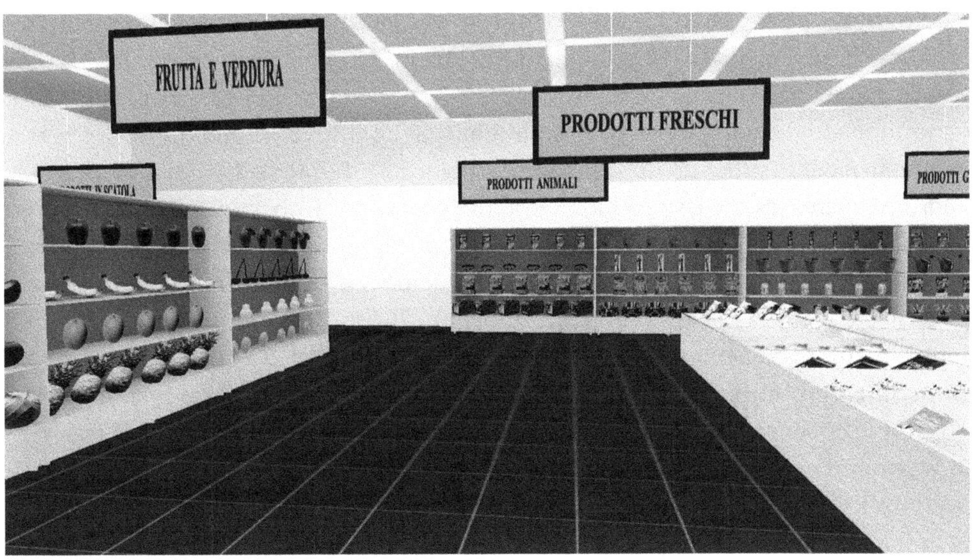

ment in mobile communications allows the diffusion of cognitive empowerment programmes via virtual environments implemented on mobile devices. This permits the extension of these immersive and interactive program at home to guarantee the continuity between virtual and real experience.

The expected benefit of this new class of eudaimonic positive technologies for the elderly is a functional reorganization of the brain produced by the broadening of the thought-action repertoire associated with an increase in self-efficacy.

## FRAIL ELDERLY: WHY USE POSITIVE TECHNOLOGIES FOR COGNITIVE EMPOWERMENT

In the last 30 years, research has tried to identify the most salient and earliest cognitive symptoms characterizing the cognitive decline associated with neurodegenerative diseases (Aarsland, Brønnick, & Fladby, 2011; Albert, 2011; Bastin & Salmon, 2014; Breitve et al., 2014; Hu et al., 2014; Petersen, 2011). Specifically, several studies from both genetic at-risk cohorts and clinically normal individuals suggest that the pathophysiology cascade of neurodegenerative diseases begins years before the diagnosis of dementia (Aarsland et al., 2011; Hu et al., 2014; Sperling et al., 2011).

In this direction, mild cognitive impairment may represent a useful clinical entity for detecting subtle signs of early cognitive decline (Petersen, 2004, 2011). Indeed, mild cognitive impairment refers to a cognitive decline that does not significantly impair cognitive functioning, i.e., it is used when an older person does not meet the criteria for dementia either because they lack two deficits in two different cognitive domains or because their cognitive deficits do not significantly affect their usual activities (Peterson, 2011). Evaluation for capturing the first sign of cognitive decline is usually done using standard clinical tests, such as the Mini-Mental State Examination (Folstein, Folstein, & McHugh, 1975) or the Montreal Cognitive Assessment Test (Nasreddine et al., 2005). This prompt neuropsychological evaluation is absolutely needed because older individuals with mild cognitive impairment were progressing more frequently to Alzheimer's disease compared to healthy age-matched controls (for a review, see Mitchell & Shiri-Feshki, 2009).

Associated with mild cognitive impairment is frailty, a condition defined as a multifaceted syndrome generally marked by the progressive decreased ability of an elderly individual to respond to stressors (Fried et al., 2001). As described by Fried (Fried et al., 2001), from a clinical perspective, frail older persons are characterized by height and muscle loss, physical exhaustion and weakness, slow gait and lower levels of activity and functionality. It is crucial to highlight that cognitive decline in frailty is not as evident as cognitive impairment in other neurodegenerative disorders, but recent crucial evidence has reported that this syndrome increases the risk of future cognitive decline (Robertson, Savva, & Kenny, 2013).

In this direction, a recent consensus panel proposed the identification of the so-called "cognitive frailty" as a heterogeneous clinical manifestation characterized by the simultaneous presence of both physical frailty and cognitive impairment (Kelaiditi et al., 2013). According to the recent clinical guidelines developed by the aforementioned consensus group (Kelaiditi et al., 2013), the key factors defining cognitive frailty are as follows: the presence of physical frailty and cognitive impairment and the concurrent exclusion of concurrent ad dementia. Consequently, identifying and treating frail people may be an effective way to prevent or delay dementia. More specifically, some recent evidence has established a link between frailty and cognitive domains such as executive function, attention and processing speed

(Boyle, Buchman, Wilson, Leurgans, & Bennett, 2010; Langlois et al., 2012; Macuco et al., 2012; Yassuda et al., 2012). However, today, a critical challenge has been to find new early innovative cognitive interventions to break the link between cognitive decline and frailty. To date, there are different traditional preventive approaches that may be considered for cognitively frail elderly people. These include promotion of physical activity, general cognitive stimulation, healthy dietary habits and good integrated lifestyles (i.e., smoking cessation, optimal daily sleep, promotion of positive emotions) (Desai, Grossberg, & Chibnall, 2010). Considering the suggested association between frailty and cognition, it is argued that positives technologies may play an important role in supporting the development of future cognitive empowerment programs for the elderly. On the basis of the most recent evidence in literature, in the following paragraph we will describe how eudaimonic positive technologies may integrate traditional cognitive training for frailty. Coupled with an increase in cognitive skills acquisition, the advantages may include improved mood, increased self-efficacy and decreased subjective weakness, with a consequent improvement in both physical and cognitive performance.

## The Role of Advanced Technologies for Cognitive Empowerment: A Recent Trend

The application of advanced positive eudaimonic technologies may yield to more ecologically valid protocols focused on the specific needs of different individuals and specifically intended to promote well-being in terms of engaging and self-actualizing experiences within challenging everyday life scenarios (Riva et al., 2014).

This is particularly relevant for frail older individuals, for whom prompt cognitive interventions may delay cognitive decline. Considering their concurrent physical early impairment (Fried et al., 2001), there is a need to develop cognitive empowerment programmes that reflect ecological situations in order to prompt the restoration of functional ability in their daily lives. Moreover, as explained before, recent studies have demonstrated that there is some cognitive weakness in frail individuals in some areas, namely executive functioning and attention processing (Boyle et al., 2010; Langlois et al., 2012; Macuco et al., 2012; Yassuda et al., 2012). On the basis of this evidence, Goal Management Training (Robertson, 1996) appears to be a promising cognitive empowerment programme for the stimulation of executive functioning in frail older individuals. Robertson (Robertson, 1996) developed the Goal Management Training (Robertson, 1996) as a theoretically-based intervention aimed at helping individuals be more and more effective at properly encoding intended goals by learning a mental checking system that enables them to maintain an active focus. Goal Management Training (GMT) is a structured cognitive training protocol based on Duncan's theory (Duncan, 1986, 1995; Duncan & Owen, 2000; Duncan et al., 2000) of disorganization of behavior following damage to the frontal lobes or to circuits that include frontal structures. In the "goal-neglect theory," Duncan argued that human behavior is goal-oriented since it is controlled by a list of goals or sub-goals. Individuals are able to formulate, store and check all these goals and sub-goals in order to effectively respond to environmental and/or internal demands. GMT can be generally defined as cognitive training for executive functions with two principal objectives: 1) improve awareness on behavior and its underlying goals; and 2) retain cognitive control when behavior becomes inconsistent with intended goals. The GMT trains individuals in five stages that characterise the most crucial elements for an effective rehabilitation of executive functions. In Stage 1, "STOP" participants are trained to ask themselves what they are doing at the moment and direct awareness towards relevant goals. In Stage 2, "DEFINE" participants are trained to define the main task and state the goals. In Stage 3, "LIST" participants are trained to list the steps necessary to achieve the main task. In Stage 4, "LEARN" participants are trained to encode and store goals and sub-goals. In Stage 5, "CHECK," the outcome of action is compared with the desired goal. Levine and colleagues (Levine et al., 2000) have demonstrated the clinical utility and efficacy of the GMT among patients with lesions in the frontal lobes.

GMT has been extensively developed, with different versions having been published ranging from a single session (Levine et al., 2000) to a 14-hour GMT training course for group rehabilitation in clinical settings (Levine et al., 2011). A very recent systematic review proposed by Krasny-Pacini and colleagues showed (Krasny-Pacini, Chevignard, & Evans, 2013) that comprehensive rehabilitation programs incorporating GMT, but also integrating other approaches, are effective in executive function rehabilitation following brain injury in adults.

However, as previously explained, the real challenge of cognitive training focusing on executive functions for frail older individuals is to improve the ability to participate in meaningful activities through transfer and generalization. For instance, if a cognitive rehabilitative intervention has been carried out at a rehabilitation center to improve executive abilities, it is important that the patient use these abilities in daily life activities such as preparation of a meal (generalization) at home (transfer). To address these needs, and to develop a programme that reflects ecological situations to prompt the restoration of functional ability in daily life, the use of advance virtual reality-based simulations has been proposed.

Following the guidelines of GMT, frail individuals with the use of VR may be composed of five stages: in Stages 1 and 2, frail people will be trained to direct awareness towards relevant goals and define the main task to achieve within virtual realistic environments. In Stage 3, people will be trained to list the steps necessary to achieve the main task, while in Stage 4 they will be trained to encode and store all the goals. In Stage 5, the outcome of action will be compared with the desired goal. To help frail people train their ability in formulating, storing and checking the goals necessary to perform a desired action, the VR-GMT protocol would be implemented in two virtual ecological environment real-life activities within ecological scenario (for example, purchasing an item or meal preparation). As suggested by Riva (Riva & Gaggioli, 2009; Riva et al., 2014), these enriched environments will contain functional real-world demands (for example, purchasing an item or meal preparation, including tasks of increasingly difficulty that will be progressively matched to the cognitive level of the individual). Then, as previously explained, it is crucial to cultivate the optimal experiences reached during the clinical session of GMT with VR by linking the results obtained to the actual experience and skills during real life. Within this perspective, the GMT with VR will be delivered on the following integrated devices: 1) a VR platform in the clinical setting that allows the chance to deliver secure and engaging cognitive exercises, and 2) a smartphone that allows the chance to deliver virtual-based cognitive exercises during daily life.

With this integrated technological platform, this kind of cognitive empowerment programme based on the principle of GMT may be a eudaimonic positive technology specifically designed for frail older people. Beyond specific improvements in executive functioning, the adoption of a eudaimonic positive technology exploiting the strategy of "transformation of flow" (Riva & Gaggioli, 2009) may range from increased self-efficacy (thanks to the continuous skills acquisition provided by the challenging virtual experiences) to decreased subjective weakness (thanks to the habituation to real-life scenarios provided by ecologically valid virtual environments), with a consequent improvement in both physical and cognitive performance.

## FUTURE RESEARCH DIRECTIONS

In the previous paragraphs, we argued that there is a "window of possibility" to develop a new class of applications that may enhance the traditional approaches used for cognitive empowerment in the elderly. In considering the future definition and testing of protocols using advanced technologies for improving well-being of the elderly, it is important to take into account the warnings of the above-mentioned recent Cochrane review about the efficacy of traditional cognitive programmes for patients suffering from mild AD and vascular dementia (Bahar-Fuchs et al., 2013). Conclusions about the efficacy of non-pharmacological interventions, especially about long-term effects, must still be viewed with caution due to the small number of randomized controlled trials. However, the findings available are promising and justify further studies in this direction.

Controlled studies testing the role of advanced positive technologies with a greater number of patients, appropriate control groups, a better definition of inclusion/exclusion criteria, standardized outcomes measures and follow-up measures are absolutely needed.

## CONCLUSION

Recently, the World Health Organization (WHO, 2001) developed a new framework of human functioning and disability to underline the interactive relationship between health conditions and psychological and environmental factors. Disability is defined as a term representing a condition in which individuals are temporarily or definitively unable to perform an "activity" in the correct manner and/or at a level generally considered "normal" for the human being. The emphasis given to the "activity" highlights the dynamic interactions between person and environment. By consequence, it also emphasises the key concept of "participation" as an important outcome of well-being. This definition is focused not on deficits but on assets: a person is disabled when she/he is not able to fully exploit her/his relationship with everyday contexts. Participation reduction refers to the social, familial, educational or other role disadvantages associated with a disability (e.g., failure in school or loss of a job because of a communication impairment). This comprehensive framework permits a deeper understanding of why the introduction of the concept of "empowerment" as a key factor in any cognitive/physical training strategy is needed when considering dynamic interactions between older people (with and without impairment) and his/her environment.

Within the theoretical paradigm of Positive Technology (Botella et al., 2012; Riva et al., 2012; Riva & Gaggioli, 2015), in this chapter it has been detailed how advanced technologies may enhance the traditional approaches used for cognitive empowerment in the elderly. After a brief presentation on how different positive technologies may be differently classified according to their effect in promoting different constituents of well-being, the focus will be specifically devoted to how advanced technologies (and particularly VR) may be used to support healthy elderly people in reaching engaging and self-actualizing experiences. The theory of flow (Csikszentmihalyi, 1991) provides an useful framework by which to define what constitutes an "engaging and self-actualizing experience," as well as how they can be used to enable a positive change to improve well-being (Inghilleri et al., 2015).

Thanks to the continuous cognitive skills acquisition provided by an effective and interactive cognitive empowerment programme, an optimal experience (i.e., balance between skills and demands) may be progressively reached and supported by the use of advanced technologies, and this state may be used to promote new and unexpected psychological resources (Riva & Gaggioli, 2009). This strategy, known as "transformation of flow," opens new interesting possibilities for developing innovative cognitive training able to exploit the potentiality of positive technologies to stimulate cognitive functioning in elderly people. An example is offered in the last section: a possible use of positive technologies for integrating a standard theoretically-based cognitive empowerment program for executive functioning in frail elderly has been presented.

In sum, as positive technologies may have an important role in the design, development and testing of cognitive empowerment programs for the elderly, future studies and controlled trials will be needed to deeply explore the potentiality of advanced technologies to meets the need of ageing society.

## ACKNOWLEDGMENT

This work was partially supported by the Italian funded project "VRehab. Virtual Reality in the Assessment and TeleRehabilitation of Parkinson's Disease and Post-Stroke Disabilities" - RF-2009-147219 and by the project "Design for All - SW integration and advance Human Machine Interfaces in design for Ambient Assisted Living" - CTN01_00128_297089

## REFERENCES

Aarsland, D., Brønnick, K., & Fladby, T. (2011). Mild cognitive impairment in Parkinson's disease. *Current Neurology and Neuroscience Reports*, *11*(4), 371–378. doi:10.1007/s11910-011-0203-1 PMID:21487730

Albert, M. S. (2011). Changes in cognition. *Neurobiology of Aging*, *32*, S58–S63. doi:10.1016/j.neurobiolaging.2011.09.010 PMID:22078174

Alm, N., Astell, A., Gowans, G., Dye, R., Ellis, M., Vaughan, P., & Riley, P. (2009). Engaging multimedia leisure for people with dementia. *Gerontechnology (Valkenswaard)*, *8*(4), 236–246. doi:10.4017/gt.2009.08.04.006.00

Bahar-Fuchs, A., Clare, L., & Woods, B. (2013). Cognitive training and cognitive rehabilitation for mild to moderate Alzheimer's disease and vascular dementia. *Cochrane Database of Systematic Reviews*, 6. PMID:23740535

Barnes, D. E., Yaffe, K., Belfor, N., Jagust, W. J., DeCarli, C., Reed, B. R., & Kramer, J. H. (2009). Computer-based cognitive training for mild cognitive impairment: Results from a pilot randomized, controlled trial. *Alzheimer Disease and Associated Disorders*, *23*(3), 205–210. doi:10.1097/WAD.0b013e31819c6137 PMID:19812460

Bastin, C., & Salmon, E. (2014). Early neuropsychological detection of Alzheimer's disease. *European Journal of Clinical Nutrition*, *68*(11), 1192–1199. doi:10.1038/ejcn.2014.176 PMID:25182019

Belleville, S. (2008). Cognitive training for persons with mild cognitive impairment. *International Psychogeriatrics*, *20*(01), 57–66. doi:10.1017/S104161020700631X PMID:17958927

Belleville, S., Gilbert, B., Fontaine, F., Gagnon, L., Ménard, É., & Gauthier, S. (2006). Improvement of episodic memory in persons with mild cognitive impairment and healthy older adults: Evidence from a cognitive intervention program. *Dementia and Geriatric Cognitive Disorders*, *22*(5-6), 486–499. doi:10.1159/000096316 PMID:17050952

Bier, N., Grenier, S., Brodeur, C., Gauthier, S., Gilbert, B., Hudon, C., & Belleville, S. et al. (2015). Measuring the impact of cognitive and psychosocial interventions in persons with mild cognitive impairment with a randomized single-blind controlled trial: Rationale and design of the MEMO+ study. *International Psychogeriatrics*, *27*(3), 511–525. doi:10.1017/S1041610214001902 PMID:25268968

Bohil, C. J., Alicea, B., & Biocca, F. A. (2011). Virtual reality in neuroscience research and therapy. *Nature Reviews. Neuroscience*, *12*(12), 752–762. PMID:22048061

Botella, C., Riva, G., Gaggioli, A., Wiederhold, B. K., Alcaniz, M., & Baños, R. M. (2012). The present and future of positive technologies. *Cyberpsychology, Behavior, and Social Networking*, *15*(2), 78–84. doi:10.1089/cyber.2011.0140 PMID:22149078

Boyle, P. A., Buchman, A. S., Wilson, R. S., Leurgans, S. E., & Bennett, D. A. (2010). Physical Frailty Is Associated with Incident Mild Cognitive Impairment in Comm Community-Based Older Persons. *Journal of the American Geriatrics Society*, *58*(2), 248–255. doi:10.1111/j.1532-5415.2009.02671.x PMID:20070417

Breitve, M. H., Chwiszczuk, L. J., Hynninen, M. J., Rongve, A., Brønnick, K., Janvin, C., & Aarsland, D. (2014). A systematic review of cognitive decline in dementia with Lewy bodies versus Alzheimer's. *Alzheimer's Research & Therapy*, *6*, 53. PMID:25478024

Buschert, V., Bokde, A. L. W., & Hampel, H. (2010). Cognitive intervention in Alzheimer disease. *Nature Reviews. Nephrology*, *6*(9), 508–517. PMID:20736983

Chapman, S. B., Aslan, S., Spence, J. S., Hart, J. J., Bartz, E. K., Didehbani, N., & DeFina, L. F. et al. (2015). Neural mechanisms of brain plasticity with complex cognitive training in healthy seniors. *Cerebral Cortex*, *25*(2), 396–405. doi:10.1093/cercor/bht234 PMID:23985135

Cipresso, P., Albani, G., Serino, S., Pedroli, E., Pallavicini, F., Mauro, A., & Riva, G. (2014). Virtual multiple errands test (VMET): A virtual reality-based tool to detect early executive functions deficit in Parkinson's disease. *Frontiers in Behavioral Neuroscience*. PMID:25538578

Clare, L., Linden, D. E. J., Woods, R. T., Whitaker, R., Evans, S. J., Parkinson, C. H., & Rugg, M. D. et al. (2010). Goal-oriented cognitive rehabilitation for people with early-stage Alzheimer disease: A single-blind randomized controlled trial of clinical efficacy. *The American Journal of Geriatric Psychiatry*, *18*(10), 928–939. doi:10.1097/JGP.0b013e3181d5792a PMID:20808145

Clare, L., & Woods, B. (2003). Cognitive rehabilitation and cognitive training for early-stage Alzheimer's disease and vascular dementia. *Cochrane Database of Systematic Reviews*, (4): CD003260. PMID:14583963

Coyle, H., Traynor, V., & Solowij, N. (2014). Computerized and virtual reality cognitive training for individuals at high risk of cognitive decline: Systematic review of the literature. *The American Journal of Geriatric Psychiatry*, *23*(4), 335–359. doi:10.1016/j.jagp.2014.04.009 PMID:24998488

Csikszentmihalyi, M. (1991). *Flow: The psychology of optimal experience* (Vol. 41). New York: Harper Perennial.

Delle Fave, A., Massimini, F., & Bassi, M. (2011). *Psychological selection and optimal experience across cultures: Social empowerment through personal growth* (Vol. 2). Springer. doi:10.1007/978-90-481-9876-4

Desai, A. K., Grossberg, G. T., & Chibnall, J. T. (2010). Healthy brain aging: A road map. *Clinics in Geriatric Medicine*, *26*(1), 1–16. doi:10.1016/j.cger.2009.12.002 PMID:20176289

Diener, E., & Chan, M. Y. (2011). Happy people live longer: Subjective well-being contributes to health and longevity. *Applied Psychology: Health and Well-Being*, *3*(1), 1–43. PMID:26286968

Draganski, B., Gaser, C., Kempermann, G., Kuhn, H. G., Winkler, J., Büchel, C., & May, A. (2006). Temporal and spatial dynamics of brain structure changes during extensive learning. *The Journal of Neuroscience*, *26*(23), 6314–6317. doi:10.1523/JNEUROSCI.4628-05.2006 PMID:16763039

Duncan, J. (1986). Disorganziation of behaviour after frontal lobe damage. *Cognitive Neuropsychology*, *3*(2), 271–290. doi:10.1080/02643298608253360

Duncan, J. (1995). Attention, intelligence and the frontal lobes. In M. S. Gazzaniga (Ed.), *The cognitive neurosciences* (pp. 721–733). Cambridge, MA: MIT Press.

Duncan, J., & Owen, A. M. (2000). Common regions of the human frontal lobe recruited by diverse cognitive demands. *Trends in Neurosciences*, *23*(10), 475–483. doi:10.1016/S0166-2236(00)01633-7 PMID:11006464

Duncan, J., Seitz, R. J., Kolodny, J., Bor, D., Herzog, H., Ahmed, A., & Emslie, H. et al. (2000). A neural basis for general intelligence. *Science*, *289*(5478), 457–460. doi:10.1126/science.289.5478.457 PMID:10903207

Ferri, C. P., Prince, M., Brayne, C., Brodaty, H., Fratiglioni, L., Ganguli, M., & Huang, Y. et al. (2006). Global prevalence of dementia: A Delphi consensus study. *Lancet*, *366*(9503), 2112–2117. doi:10.1016/S0140-6736(05)67889-0 PMID:16360788

Folstein, M. F., Folstein, S. E., & McHugh, P. R. (1975). "Mini-mental state": A practical method for grading the cognitive state of patients for the clinician. *Journal of Psychiatric Research*, *12*(3), 189–198. doi:10.1016/0022-3956(75)90026-6 PMID:1202204

Fried, L. P., Tangen, C. M., Walston, J., Newman, A. B., Hirsch, C., Gottdiener, J., & Burke, G. et al. (2001). Frailty in older adults evidence for a phenotype. *The Journals of Gerontology. Series A, Biological Sciences and Medical Sciences*, *56*(3), M146–M157. doi:10.1093/gerona/56.3.M146 PMID:11253156

Gaggioli, A., & Riva, G. (2014). Psychological treatments: Smart tools boost mental-health care. *Nature*, *512*(7512), 28–28. doi:10.1038/512028b PMID:25100471

García-Betances, R. I., Arredondo Waldmeyer, M. T., Fico, G., & Cabrera-Umpiérrez, M. F. (2015). A succinct overview of virtual reality technology use in Alzheimer's disease. *Name: Frontiers in Aging Neuroscience*, *7*, 80. PMID:26029101

García-Betances, R. I., Jiménez-Mixco, V., Arredondo, M. T., & Cabrera-Umpiérrez, M. F. (2015). Using Virtual Reality for Cognitive Training of the Elderly. *American Journal of Alzheimer's Disease and Other Dementias*, *30*(1), 49–54. doi:10.1177/1533317514545866 PMID:25107931

Harrington, T. L., & Harrington, M. K. (2000). *Gerontechnology: Why and How. Herman Bouma Foundation for Gerontechnology*. The Netherlands: Shaker Publishing B.V.

Hertzog, C., Kramer, A. F., Wilson, R. S., & Lindenberger, U. (2008). Enrichment effects on adult cognitive development can the functional capacity of older adults be preserved and enhanced? *Psychological Science in the Public Interest*, *9*(1), 1–65. PMID:26162004

Hu, M., Szewczyk-Królikowski, K., Tomlinson, P., Nithi, K., Rolinski, M., Murray, C., & Ben Shlomo, Y. (2014). Predictors of cognitive impairment in an early stage Parkinson's disease cohort. *Movement Disorders*, *29*(3), 351–359. doi:10.1002/mds.25748 PMID:24395708

Hudson, J., Day, M. C., & Oliver, E. J. (2015). A 'new life' story or 'delaying the inevitable'? Exploring older people's narratives during exercise uptake. *Psychology of Sport and Exercise*, *16*, 112–120. doi:10.1016/j.psychsport.2014.09.004

Inghilleri, P., Riva, G., & Riva, E. (2015). *Enabling Positive Change: Flow and Complexity in Daily Experience*. Warsaw: De Gruyter Open. doi:10.2478/9783110410242

Jean, L., Bergeron, M. È., Thivierge, S., & Simard, M. (2010). Cognitive intervention programs for individuals with mild cognitive impairment: Systematic review of the literature. *The American Journal of Geriatric Psychiatry*, *18*(4), 281–296. doi:10.1097/JGP.0b013e3181c37ce9 PMID:20220584

Kaci Fairchild, J., & Scogin, F. R. (2010). Training to Enhance Adult Memory (TEAM): An investigation of the effectiveness of a memory training program with older adults. *Aging & Mental Health*, *14*(3), 364–373. doi:10.1080/13607860903311733 PMID:20425656

Kelaiditi, E., Cesari, M., Canevelli, M., Van Kan, G. A., Ousset, P. J., Gillette-Guyonnet, S., & Provencher, V. et al. (2013). Cognitive frailty: Rational and definition from an (IANA/IAGG) international consensus group. *The Journal of Nutrition, Health & Aging*, *17*(9), 726–734. doi:10.1007/s12603-013-0367-2 PMID:24154642

Kelly, M. E., Loughrey, D., Lawlor, B. A., Robertson, I. H., Walsh, C., & Brennan, S. (2014). The impact of cognitive training and mental stimulation on cognitive and everyday functioning of healthy older adults: A systematic review and meta-analysis. *Ageing Research Reviews*, *15*, 28–43. doi:10.1016/j.arr.2014.02.004 PMID:24607830

Kizony, R., Korman, M., Sinoff, G., Klinger, E., & Josman, N. (2012, September 10-12). Using a virtual supermarket as a tool for training executive functions in people with mild cognitive impairment. *Paper presented at the 9th International Conference on Disability, Virtual Reality and Associated Technologies ICDVRAT*, Laval, France.

Kober, S. E., Wood, G., Hofer, D., Kreuzig, W., Kiefer, M., & Neuper, C. (2013). Virtual reality in neurologic rehabilitation of spatial disorientation. *Journal of Neuroengineering and Rehabilitation*, *10*(1), 17.

Krasny-Pacini, A., Chevignard, M., & Evans, J. (2013). Goal Management Training for rehabilitation of executive functions: A systematic review of effectiveness in patients with acquired brain injury. *Disability and Rehabilitation*. doi:10.3109/09638288.2013.777807 PMID:23597002

Lagiewka, K. (2012). European innovation partnership on active and healthy ageing: Triggers of setting the headline target of 2 additional healthy life years at birth at EU average by 2020. *Archives of Public Health*, *70*(1), 1–8. doi:10.1186/0778-7367-70-23 PMID:23088612

Lampit, A., Hallock, H., & Valenzuela, M. (2014). Computerized Cognitive Training in Cognitively Healthy Older Adults: A Systematic Review and Meta-Analysis. *PLoS Medicine*, *11*(11), e1001756. doi:10.1371/journal.pmed.1001756 PMID:25405755

Langlois, F., Vu, T. T. M., Kergoat, M. J., Chassé, K., Dupuis, G., & Bherer, L. (2012). The multiple dimensions of frailty: Physical capacity, cognition, and quality of life. *International Psychogeriatrics*, *24*(09), 1429–1436. doi:10.1017/S1041610212000634 PMID:22717010

Levine, B., Robertson, I. H., Clare, L., Carter, G., Hong, J., Wilson, B. A., & Stuss, D. T. et al. (2000). Rehabilitation of executive functioning: An experimental-clinical validation of goal management training. *Journal of the International Neuropsychological Society*, *6*(3), 299–312. doi:10.1017/S1355617700633052 PMID:10824502

Levine, B., Schweizer, T. A., O'Connor, C., Turner, G., Gillingham, S., Stuss, D. T., & Robertson, I. H. et al. (2011). Rehabilitation of executive functioning in patients with frontal lobe brain damage with goal management training. *Frontiers in Human Neuroscience*, *5*. doi:10.3389/fnhum.2011.00009 PMID:21369362

Macuco, C. R. M., Batistoni, S. S. T., Lopes, A., Cachioni, M., da Silva Falcão, D. V., Neri, A. L., & Yassuda, M. S. (2012). Mini-Mental State Examination performance in frail, pre-frail, and non-frail community dwelling older adults in Ermelino Matarazzo, São Paulo, Brazil. *International Psychogeriatrics*, *24*(11), 1725–1731. doi:10.1017/S1041610212000907 PMID:22652040

McGee, J. S., van der Zaag, C., Buckwalter, J. G., Thiebaux, M., Van Rooyen, A., Neumann, U., & Rizzo, A. A. et al. (2000). Issues for the assessment of visuospatial skills in older adults using Virtual Environment technology. *Cyberpsychology & Behavior*, *3*(3), 469–482. doi:10.1089/10949310050078931

Mitchell, A. J., & Shiri-Feshki, M. (2009). Rate of progression of mild cognitive impairment to dementia--meta-analysis of 41 robust inception cohort studies. *Acta Psychiatrica Scandinavica*, *119*(4), 252–265. doi:10.1111/j.1600-0447.2008.01326.x PMID:19236314

Morganti, F., & Riva, G. (2004). Ambient Intelligence in Rehabilitation. In G. Riva, F. Davide, F. Vatalaro, & M. Alcañiz (Eds.), *Ambient Intelligence: The evolution of technology, communication and cognition towards the future of the human-computer interaction* (pp. 283–295). Amsterdam: IOS Press.

Morganti, L., Riva, G., Bonfiglio, S., & Gaggioli, A. (2013). Building collective memories on the web: The Nostalgia Bits project. *International Journal of Web Based Communities*, *9*(1), 83–104. doi:10.1504/IJWBC.2013.051373

Optale, G., Capodieci, S., Marin, S., Pastore, M., & Piron, L. (2007). Multimedia memory- training nel declino cognitivo legato all'età, uno studio controllato e in follow-up. *Psicotech*, *2*, 33–45.

Optale, G., Capodieci, S., Pinelli, P., Zara, D., Gamberini, L., & Riva, G. (2001). Music-enhanced immersive virtual reality in the rehabilitation of memory-related cognitive processes and functional abilities: A case report. *Presence (Cambridge, Mass.)*, *10*(4), 450–462.

Petersen, R. C. (2004). Mild cognitive impairment as a diagnostic entity. *Journal of Internal Medicine*, *256*(3), 183–194. doi:10.1111/j.1365-2796.2004.01388.x PMID:15324362

Petersen, R. C. (2011). Mild cognitive impairment. *The New England Journal of Medicine*, *364*(23), 2227–2234. doi:10.1056/NEJMcp0910237 PMID:21651394

Rebok, G. W., Ball, K., Guey, L. T., Jones, R. N., Kim, H. Y., King, J. W., & Unverzagt, F. W. et al. (2014). Ten-year effects of the advanced cognitive training for independent and vital elderly cognitive training trial on cognition and everyday functioning in older adults. *Journal of the American Geriatrics Society*, *62*(1), 16–24. PMID:24417410

Riva, G., Banos, R. M., Botella, C., Wiederhold, B. K., & Gaggioli, A. (2012). Positive technology: Using interactive technologies to promote positive functioning. *Cyberpsychology, Behavior, and Social Networking*, *15*(2), 69–77. doi:10.1089/cyber.2011.0139 PMID:22149077

Riva, G., & Gaggioli, A. (2009). Rehabilitation as Empowerment: The Role of Advanced Technologies. In A. Gaggioli, E. A. Keshner, P. L. Weiss, & G. Riva (Eds.), *Technologies in Rehabilitation: Empowering Cognitive, Physical, Social and Communicative Skills through Virtual Reality, Robots, Wearable Systems and Brain-Computer Interfaces Advanced* (Vol. 145, pp. 3–22). Amsterdam: IOS Press.

Riva, G., & Gaggioli, A. (2015). Positive Change and Positive Technology. In P. Inghilleri, G.Riva, & R.E. (Eds.), Enabling Positive Change, Flow and Complexity in Daily Experience (pp. 39-49). Warsaw: De Gruyter Open. doi:10.2478/9783110410242.3

Riva, G., Gaggioli, A., Villani, D., Cipresso, P., Repetto, C., Serino, S., & Graffigna, G. et al. (2014). Positive Technology for Healthy Living and Active Ageing. *Studies in Health Technology and Informatics*, (203): 44–56. PMID:26630511

Riva, G., Mantovani, F., & Gaggioli, A. (2004). Presence and rehabilitation: Toward second-generation virtual reality applications in neuropsychology. *Journal of Neuroengineering and Rehabilitation*, *1*(9). PMID:15679950

Robertson, D. A., Savva, G. M., & Kenny, R. A. (2013). Frailty and cognitive impairment—a review of the evidence and causal mechanisms. *Ageing Research Reviews*, *12*(4), 840–851. doi:10.1016/j.arr.2013.06.004 PMID:23831959

Robertson, I. H. (1996). *Goal management training: A clinical manual*. Cambridge, UK: PsyConsult.

Rose, F. D., Brooks, B. M., & Rizzo, A. A. (2005). Virtual reality in brain damage rehabilitation [review]. *Cyberpsychology & Behavior*, *8*(3), 241–262. doi:10.1089/cpb.2005.8.241 PMID:15971974

Ryan, R. M., & Deci, E. L. (2001). On happiness and human potentials: A review of research on hedonic and eudaimonic well-being. *Annual Review of Psychology*, *52*(1), 141–166. doi:10.1146/annurev.psych.52.1.141 PMID:11148302

Schultheis, M. T., & Rizzo, A. A. (2001). The application of virtual reality technology in rehabilitation. *Rehabilitation Psychology*, *46*(3), 296–311. doi:10.1037/0090-5550.46.3.296

Seligman, M. E. P. (2002). *Authentic happiness: Using the new positive psychology to realize your potential for lasting fulfillment*. New York Free Press.

Seligman, M. E. P., & Csikszentmihalyi, M. (2000). *Positive psychology: An introduction* (Vol. 55). American Psychological Association.

Serino, S., Morganti, F., Di Stefano, F., & Riva, G. (2015). Detecting early egocentric and allocentric impairments deficits in Alzheimer's Disease: an experimental study with virtual reality. *Frontiers in Aging Neuroscience*, 7, 88.

Shallice, T., & Burgess, P. W. (1991). Deficits in strategy application following frontal lobe damage in man. *Brain*, *114*(2), 727–741. doi:10.1093/brain/114.2.727 PMID:2043945

Snyder, C. R. (2010). *Positive psychology: The scientific and practical explorations of human strengths*. Sage Publications.

Sperling, R. A., Aisen, P. S., Beckett, L. A., Bennett, D. A., Craft, S., Fagan, A. M., & Montine, T. J. et al. (2011). Toward defining the preclinical stages of Alzheimer's disease: Recommendations from the National Institute on Aging-Alzheimer's Association workgroups on diagnostic guidelines for Alzheimer's disease. *Alzheimer's & Dementia*, *7*(3), 280–292. doi:10.1016/j.jalz.2011.03.003 PMID:21514248

Thivierge, S., Jean, L., & Simard, M. (2014). A randomized cross-over controlled study on cognitive rehabilitation of instrumental activities of daily living in Alzheimer disease. *The American Journal of Geriatric Psychiatry*, *22*(11), 1188–1199. doi:10.1016/j.jagp.2013.03.008 PMID:23871120

WHO. (2003). *International Classification of Functioning*. Disability and Health.

Willis, S. L., Tennstedt, S. L., Marsiske, M., Ball, K., Elias, J., Koepke, K. M., & Stoddard, A. M. et al. (2006). Long-term effects of cognitive training on everyday functional outcomes in older adults. *Journal of the American Medical Association*, *296*(23), 2805–2814. doi:10.1001/jama.296.23.2805 PMID:17179457

Wolinsky, F. D., Vander Weg, M. W., Howren, M. B., Jones, M. P., & Dotson, M. M. (2013). A randomized controlled trial of cognitive training using a visual speed of processing intervention in middle aged and older adults. *PLoS ONE*, *8*(5), e61624. doi:10.1371/journal.pone.0061624 PMID:23650501

Yassuda, M. S., Lopes, A., Cachioni, M., Falcao, D. V. S., Batistoni, S. S. T., Guimaraes, V. V., & Neri, A. L. (2012). Frailty criteria and cognitive performance are related: Data from the FIBRA study in Ermelino Matarazzo, São Paulo, Brazil. *The Journal of Nutrition, Health & Aging*, *16*(1), 55–61. doi:10.1007/s12603-012-0003-6 PMID:22238002

Ylvisaker, M., Hanks, R., & Johnson-Greene, D. (2002). Perspectives on rehabilitation of individuals with cognitive impairment after brain injury: Rationale for reconsideration of theoretical paradigms. *The Journal of Head Trauma Rehabilitation*, *17*(3), 191–209. doi:10.1097/00001199-200206000-00002 PMID:12086574

## KEY TERMS AND DEFINITIONS

**Cognitive Rehabilitation:** Originally developed to indicate all programs used to help individuals with brain injury to achieve a satisfactory social functioning within their daily context, it is now used to refer to programs for people with cognitive impairments.

**Cognitive Training:** Repeated practice of series of exercises in order to specifically stimulate targeted cognitive functions.

**Empowerment:** (within a rehabilitation perspective) A key factor in any cognitive/physical training strategy is needed when considering dynamic interactions between older persons (with and without impairment) and his/her environment.

**Flow:** A state of full engagement, deep concentration and action awareness that occurs during an activity perceived as highly self-rewarding, characterized by clear goals, unambiguous and immediate feedback and an altered sense of time.

**Frailty:** A condition that can be defined as a multifaceted syndrome generally marked by a progressive decreased ability of an elderly individual to respond to stressors.

**Transformation of Flow:** A strategy based on an idea that an optimal experience (i.e., balance between skills and demands) is progressively reached and supported by the use of advanced technologies, and that this state may be used to promote new and unexpected psychological resources.

# Chapter 9
# Mindfulness as an Opportunity to Narrow the Grey Digital Divide

**Katherine Bercovitz**
*Harvard University, USA*

**Francesco Pagnini**
*Harvard University, USA*

## ABSTRACT

*With older adults living longer than ever before, more in this age demographic are seeking ways to stay engaged, happy, and healthy in the final decades of life following retirement. In this chapter, we discuss the many ways in which older adults can benefit from learning new technologies, including enjoying more functional independence, social connection, and cognitive engagement. We also discuss the barriers that prevent older adults from learning new technologies, including physical ailment and disability, skepticism over the benefits, and stereotype threat. Finally, we introduce the concept of Langerian mindfulness and how learning to be mindful as opposed to mindless can help older adults over these barriers.*

## INTRODUCTION

The U.S. Bureau of the Census (2011) reported that between the years 2000 and 2010, the rate of growth for the nation's 65-and-older sector surpassed the growth rate of the entire population. Similarly, in the European Union, the ratio of people above 65 years old to people between 15 and 64 years old is projected to increase from 25.4% to 53.5% between 2008 and 2060 (European Commission, 2009).

As a result, research has increasingly turned to improving well-being in later life, including investigations on how to preserve physical and cognitive functioning as well as psychological health (e.g., Cho, Martin, & Poon, 2014). This chapter will investigate some of the many ways technology can improve the lives of older adults and how a mindful approach can help this population overcome the barriers to technology usage.

DOI: 10.4018/978-1-4666-9986-1.ch009

# BACKGROUND

## Benefits to Using Technology

We are now in the digital age, a period of human history characterized by unprecedented advancements in information technology. The term "digital native" has been coined to describe those growing up inculcated in the digital world, while the term "digital immigrants" has been used to describe the rest of the population (Prensky, 2001). The introduction of these terms into everyday language reflects how technology usage has become part of our generational identities. Yet, the benefits to using this technology are not limited to digital natives, but instead can be enjoyed by everyone, including older adults (Peine, Rollwagen, & Neven, 2014). Enhancing quality of life of older adults is an important goal for positive psychologists. Technology can offer multiple avenues for the improvement of their well-being, providing that the barriers to usage are removed (Ranzijn, 2002).

In the next section, we will focus on three primary benefits in the older population, including functional independence, social connection, and cognitive engagement.

### Functional Independence

"Aging in place" (i.e. staying in one's own home into late adulthood) is a common goal for many people (e.g. American Association for Retired Persons, 2000; Shafer, 2000). However, this goal proves more difficult for those with a health condition or disability—both of which present problems for older adults. According to a 2006 report from the Centers for Disease Control and Prevention (CDC), 34% of American adults aged 65 or older have at least one health condition or disability. Thirty-seven percent of individuals aged 75 years or older reported three or more such conditions. These conditions may impede older adults from independently performing Activities of Daily Living (ADL), including bathing, using the toilet, and eating. Additionally, older adults living alone in their own homes are required to complete Instrumental Activities of Daily Living (IADL) including managing medication schedules and paying bills.

The benefits of "aging in place" are numerous. Financially, living at home is more cost-effective than full-time residential care (reviewed in Tang & Venables, 2000). In addition to its financial benefits, "aging in place" allows one to maintain independence and personal responsibility for daily activities. These factors have been experimentally determined to lead to health and longevity (Rodin & Langer, 1977).

Computer technology plays a large role in helping many older adults maintain functional independence in their own homes (Mynatt & Rogers, 2001). Specifically, technology supports older adults in completing everyday tasks and, when it becomes necessary, in aiding family members and caregivers in the home setting (Mynatt & Rogers, 2001). Technology can be used to provide memory aids (e.g. to provide reminders for following a medication schedule; Charness, Best, & Souders, 2012) and it can also be used to alert family members of falls (Rantz et al., 2013) or to allow children to check in on their elderly parents (Mynatt & Rogers, 2001).

One application of technology in the domain of functional independence is helping older adults avoid the two types of memory errors related to taking medications—scheduling errors and episodic errors (Hopkins, 2005). Scheduling errors occur when patients take a pill at the wrong time (e.g., 11 am instead of 9 am). Episodic errors occur when a patient forgets whether or not they have taken their medications, which can lead to accidental overdose. Costs due to medicine mismanagement in Americans 65 and older were estimated to reach around $887 million in 2005 (Field, Gilman, Subramanian, Fuller,

Bates, & Gurwitz, 2005). In response to these issues, special phone and tablet applications have been developed to help people track their medication schedule (e.g., MedCoach Medication Reminder™). Similarly, "smart" pill dispensers sound an alarm when it is time for patients to take the medication and do not stop until they are opened (e.g., the Swedish-designed Careousel™).

Another promising development to increased functional independence for older adults is telemedicine, a service in which health professionals help individuals monitor their health remotely (e.g., through the use of videoconference or telephone check-ups). The benefits of telemedicine include facilitating peer support, reducing the overall cost of health care, encouraging exercise habits, decreasing depression and chronic pain, and improving functional independence (discussed in Stronge, Rogers, & Fisk, 2007).

Even when older adults are functionally capable of staying in their own homes, family members do not always feel comfortable leaving them on their own. Mobile Personal Emergency Response Systems (MPERS) are designed with these worries in mind. This technology allows for individuals to check in on elderly family members to see if they need assistance. Providing family members with peace of mind is one key way in which technology can support the goal of "aging in place."

Older adults can utilize the advances of technology to help them reach the goal of living out their final years in their own homes and are relatively open to it (Mitzner et al., 2010), despite the common stereotype of the technophobic older adult. From alert systems that give peace of mind to concerned family members to developments in the domain of telemedicine, the goal of maintaining functional independence and "aging in place" seems more possible than ever before.

## Social Engagement

in addition to allowing older adults to maintain functional independence, technology can help older adults stay socially connected—online, in videoconferencing, and on the telephone. Social engagement in the senior years leads to many positive outcomes, including higher psychological well-being (Koropeckyj-Cox, 2002) and a longer life (House, Landis, & Umberson, 1988). Older adults who are more socially engaged are less prone to cognitive decline. Specifically, those who scored high on a social engagement index which included items like membership in groups and monthly contact with at least three friends or relatives showed decreased cognitive decline compared to those with lower scores (Cornoni-Huntley, Brock, Ostfeld, Taylor, & Wallace, 1986).

Technology has played an increasingly large role in helping older adults stay connected with other people. According to the Pew Internet and American Life Project from 2014, 27% of seniors (and 46% of online seniors) use a social network sites like Facebook (Smith, 2014). Using social media seems to encourage overall sociality. Of these individuals, 81% say that they have social interactions (online, over the telephone, or in-person) every day or nearly every day. This figure drops to 71% for those who are online without social network and 63% for those who are not online at all. In addition to connecting with younger generations that rely on these social networking sites for building and maintaining relationships, these sites allow elders to find and connect with those they haven't seen in many decades. Additionally, many sites are geared towards finding groups of people with similar interests to meet up and do interesting and engaging activities, even beginning romantic relationships (e.g. meetup.com and ourtime.com).

With society becoming more urbanized, younger people are increasingly moving out of their hometowns to join the urban workforce (*Millennials Continue Urbanization Of America, Leaving Small Towns*, 2014). Video chatting programs like Skype or Apple's FaceTime allow older people to see family members who now live far away. Technological advancements open opportunities for older adults to connect to strengthen their ties and expanding their network to other who enjoy the same types of activities.

### Cognitive Engagement

In the past, the primary mode of thought was that cognitive abilities steadily decline with age (e.g., processing speed; Salthouse, 1996) and that the aging brain is no longer plastic. These thoughts were reflected in the popular culture in statements like, "You can't teach an old dog new tricks." While neural plasticity is reduced as we age, this reduction is not as severe as initially supposed (see Greenwood, 2007 for a review).

There is much evidence for the "use it or lose it" hypothesis to cognitive aging. Specifically, this hypothesis states that in order to preserve cognitive faculties one must do stimulating and challenging mental activities as a form of brain exercise (Hertzog, Kramer, Wilson, & Lindenberger, 2009). This idea has reached broader audiences and spurred the success of a multi-million dollar industry offering brain-training games (e.g. www.Lumosity.com). While there is limited evidence for the transfer effects of these exercises (see Melby-Lervåg & Hulme, 2012 for a comprehensive meta-analysis), an intellectually stimulating lifestyle is linked to lower levels of cognitive decline. For example, in a longitudinal study (Wilson et al., 2003), older adults who reported the frequency of participation in seven intellectually stimulating activities (e.g. reading a magazine) showed reduced rates of cognitive decline over the interviews conducted every three years for an average of 5.3 years. There is also evidence that participation in stimulating mental activity is associated with reduced risk of developing incident dementia (e.g. Crowe, Andel, Pedersen, Johansson, & Gatz, 2003, Wang et al., 2013, Verghese et al., 2006).

Beyond the cognitively-engaging task of learning to use the machine, a personal computer provides a unique opportunity for older adults to stay cognitively active—from searching the web for new information to taking online courses and playing games. Online courses offer the opportunity to learn new knowledge, to access novel cultures and communities, and to satisfy an intellectual curiosity that doesn't cease upon retirement. It is also possible to learn new job skills. The number of available online courses and opportunities is increasing for everyone who has access to the internet, potentially including a vast number of retired older adults, who have more time to spend to satisfy their learning needs.

Video games are another technological product which may provide relevant benefits for people who play them, under certain circumstances (Granic, Lobel, & Engels, 2014). In particular, a research study (Anguera et al., 2013) showed that older adults who played a custom-designed video game (Neuroracer) improved sustained attention and multitasking abilities up to six months after the intervention. Moreover, active video games may provide light-intensity exercise, whether played while seated or standing, with physical benefits to older adults (Taylor et al., 2012), especially to those with more sedentary lifestyles. These video games can also help older adults improve balance (Lai et al., 2013), which is key to preventing falls.

Computer usage allows older adults to remain cognitively active, via gaming, internet surfing, and online learning. The very act of learning these skills provides excellent opportunity for cognitive engagement.

## Barriers to Usage

Having just outlined the many opportunities for older adults in the digital age, the question naturally follows: why are older people less likely than young people to use technology? Specifically, researchers have documented a "grey digital divide," in which older people are significantly less likely to adopt technology as compared to young adults (Millward, 2003). For example, Pew Research Center found that only 60% of older adults (aged 65+) have gone online (Smith, 2014), making them the age group least likely to have done so. While half of the general population owns a smartphone, only 18% of older adults own one. Breaking the figure down even further, in the second-quarter of 2014, 85% of Millennial (aged 18-24) own and 86% of young adults aged 25-34 own smartphone devices (Nielsen, 2014).

Among seniors who use the internet, 71% do so every day or almost every day. Younger, higher-income, more highly-educated seniors use the internet at rates approaching that of the general population. However, older adults who are less affluent and often facing health challenges or disabilities are not using digital tools and services. According to Pew Research Center, the barriers to the elderly using technology include physical challenges, skeptical attitudes towards the benefits of using technology, and difficulties learning to use these technologies (Smith, 2014). These barriers will be discussed in turn, together with our proposal for overcoming them. We suggest that a change in cognitive attitude may help older adults (and the rest of the population, when appropriate) to embrace the new experiences that technological advancements can offer. As reported elsewhere (Langer, 1989; 2000), most of the barriers rely on the use of previous categories and mindsets to navigate the present moment. Langer describes this reliance as "mindlessness" (Langer, 1989).

## SOLUTIONS AND RECOMMENDATIONS

### A Way to Overcome Barriers: Mindfulness

"Mindfulness" is a recurrent word and a trending topic in the contemporary psychological literature (Pagnini & Phillips, 2015). There are several approaches that have tried to define this concept, although we will refer to the definition of mindfulness provided by Ellen Langer, Harvard Professor of Psychology, who has studied it for more than 40 years (Langer, 1989). According to Langer, mindfulness is a multifaceted concept that can be summarized in the process of drawing novel distinctions (Langer & Moldoveanu, 2000). This process can deal with objects, people, feelings, thoughts or experiences. The act of noticing new things is the essence of mindfulness. It is described in opposition to "mindlessness," that is, the state of being entrapped in previous categories that were developed in the past. Mindlessness can be thought of as an "automatic pilot" that prevents us from fully engaging in the experience at hand, an experience that is by definition something novel. Being mindful allows us to be aware of this novelty (Langer, 1989). The epistemological background of Langerian mindfulness suggests a reality that is constantly changing and unpredictable. Using this logic, attempting to operate with previously-conceived mindsets and categories is mindless because things are always changing, even when those changes are subtle. In this view of reality, objects and experiences are not absolutes. Instead, they depend on the point of view that the person uses to look at them. These points of view can be changed. A mindful attitude allows people to understand that nothing "is" what it is, but it "could be" many things. For example, there are no "bad" or "good" events. Events are either positive or negative, depending on the eye of the beholder. The same event can be perceived positive or negative, or, both. Even if someone still feels the need to evaluate, a mindful suggestion could be that there is positivity inherent to negativity and vice versa.

A mindful approach is denoted by openness to experience, in particular in terms of a novelty-seeking attitude and with the ability of producing new contents and new views. Similarly, the construct of mindfulness is highly related to psychological flexibility, which refers to how a person is able to adapt to different situation and to shift his/her perspective (Kashdan & Rottenberg, 2010). Mindfulness is the essence of engagement, as engaged people are likely to notice more details about their specific relationship with the environment. Mindfulness refers to a psychological construct, although it is sometimes confused with the practice of meditation. This is a mindless mistake, as meditation is merely a way to improve mindfulness. It is neither the only path, nor the most accessible (Pagnini & Phillips, 2015). In fact, everybody experiences mindfulness and a mindful state of being is always available. It is enough, for example, to pay attention to novelty and to the present moment.

Several studies suggest a positive role of a mindful attitude toward stress, anxiety and depression, both in the general population and in clinical samples (Khoury, et al., 2013). Mindfulness is associated with higher quality of life and better psychological well-being (Keng et al., 2011). Moreover, mindfulness seems to be related to physical well-being and positive physiological functions. For example, people with Amyotrophic Lateral Sclerosis who are more mindful tend to have a slower course of the disease, in comparison to those who are less mindful (Pagnini, Phillips, Bosma, Reece, & Langer, 2015).

Especially relevant to this discussion, certain components of mindfulness seem to be associated with healthy aging. Openness to experience (Jackson, Hill, Payne, Roberts, & Stine-Morrow, 2012; Stephan, 2009), flexibility (Kangasniemi, Lappalainen, Kankaanpää, & Tammelin, 2014), and life engagement (Parisi, Stine-Morrow, Noh, & Morrow, 2009) are crucial elements for the well-being of all people, including older adults.

In the field of technology, a mindful attitude may promote the curiosity and the openness to the exploration of the unknown. Moreover, it improves the engagement, increasing the enjoyableness of the experience. Mindfulness can help to overcome technology barriers in several ways.

## Skeptical Attitudes

One of the barriers to the use of technology is skepticism. More than 35% of older adults that do not currently use the internet report a skeptical attitude about the benefits that it can bring to them (Smith, 2014). Additionally this same report found that thirty-five percent of non-internet users disagree that they are missing out on important information—an additional 18% of non-internet users strongly disagree.

As technological evolution has sped up over the past few decades, many older adults, in contrast with many young people, may have passively lived through the technical and social changes that society has experienced. One of the main difference between older adults and young people is that elderly were not exposed to high-tech opportunities when they were young. They often lack a sort of "technological imprinting", that is, the process of getting used to technology by using it spontaneously, as present-day children can do with tablets (Geist, 2012). By remaining disengaged from technological advancements, many elderly may have developed indifference (if not detachment) toward them (Chen & Chan, 2011). Many older adults are not aware that certain technologies may be very useful and that these can improve the quality of life of people (Coughlin, et al., 2007). To avoid the cognitive dissonance given by the rejection of the opportunity to use new technology and improve their own lives, some people may have developed a cognitive bias against the effectiveness of new equipment and techniques (Ahn, 2004). Biases are a great example of mindlessness: they are essentially the effect of relying on previous categories while considering a new situation. Past ideas that may have worked in previous contexts, when applied to the present situation, may therefore result in a bias. An example is the primacy effect, when the use of information considered early in the judgment process tends to be overweighed in the final judgment

(Hastie & Robyn, 2001). Memories (sometimes false or distorted memories) and similarities may play a similar role, distracting the person with present information and contextual peculiarities. Moreover, bias can be mindlessly maintained via confirmatory behavior. Consider the following mindless rational: If I believe that technology cannot have a positive role in my life, I'll stay away from it. In this way, I will not be exposed to potential benefits, but will have fewer opportunities to question my point of view. This is a self-confirmatory behavior, with a tautological content that ends in a self-fulfilling prophecy: eventually, technology does not lead to any good, because I haven't even given it the chance to prove otherwise.

All these points are related to a mindless attitude, when the person acts according to the sense our behavior made in the past, rather than the present and when he or she is stuck in a single, rigid perspective (Langer, 1989). Learning how to become mindful can help an individual overcome the mindless assumption that technology cannot provide any good or that it does not fit the person's needs. If the person begins to realize that the assumption may have been useful in the past for some reason, but that there is the possibility that it may not be true in the present, he or she can start questioning that irrational belief (Carson & Langer, 2006). When the mind is actively engaged in the present (i.e., noticing new things and being sensitive to the current context) it is easier to disassemble previous schemas and to fully join the opportunities that the experience allows in the present. These may include the enjoyment of what technological advancements may provide.

## Mindfulness and Physical Disability

According to the Pew Research Center report, two of every five report a "physical or health condition that makes reading difficult or challenging" or a "disability, handicap, or chronic disease that prevents them from fully participating in many common daily activities" (Smith, 2014). This group is less likely to go online, have broadband at home, and to own a digital device compared to seniors who do not face these challenges.

Mindfulness can be extremely useful in helping individuals with chronic illness and disability live a full life. Specifically, people can learn to be mindful of how the pain changes across contexts (Langer, 1989). While the word "chronic" indicates an incessant intrusion of symptoms, learning to notice that symptoms do not necessarily persist 100% of the time opens an individual to the possibility that certain contexts attenuate or worsen symptoms. Once an individual begins to notice such contexts, he/she can approach contexts that alleviate symptoms and avoid those which make it worse. Langer (1989) describes this concept as the Attention to Variability paradigm. For a practical example, consider an individual with chronic arthritic pain. The individual may learn to notice that he/she experiences more pain when typing for long periods of time or when relying more on one hand. The simple act of noticing the discomfort and the events that tend to precede it can help the sufferer adjust behavior for positive health outcomes. A mindful individual might find that typing at a slightly inclined angle reduces pain and thus buys a support pillow to place under the wrist. A mindful individual would continually re-evaluate the efficacy of the pillow and adjust when necessary. A mindful individual recognizes that products have many uses and is not caught up in a prototype of how one should use the product (i.e., premature cognitive commitments; Chanowitz & Langer, 1981). For example, a mindful individual is not committed to the idea that one must type with two hands. He or she will recognize cases in which typing with one hand is acceptable or even more appropriate than typing with two, sometimes. Similarly, a mindful individual would not be attached to the idea that typing an email should be done in a specific amount of time. Instead, they may realize that typing more slowly allows them to craft better emails and to think of better ideas in the process. It is then easy to see how someone without effective use of a hand (e.g., in the case of arthritis) can use a computer with the help of a mindful perspective.

Besides providing relief through micro-adjustments, capitalizing on the Attention to Variability strategy may allow an individual to feel more control over the situation and outcomes. There is much evidence that perceived control (i.e. feeling that you are in charge of the outcomes of a given situation helps those with chronic illness; e.g. Langer, 1989). For example, (Moser & Dracup, 1995) found that people recovering from a heart attack who felt that they had a high level of control over their situation were less anxious, depressed, and hostile. Indeed, adopting a mindful attitude holds much potential for those experiencing physical barriers to adopting technology.

## Mindfulness and Stereotypes

Researchers have shown that while people hold both positive and negative stereotypes towards the elderly, the negative are more prevalent in western society (e.g., Kite & Johnson, 1988; Levy & Langer, 1994). In the domain of cognitive aging, the dominant view in the field and society at large is that age-related cognitive decline is inevitable (e.g., Johnson, Hashtroudi, & Lindsay, 1993; Just & Carpenter, 1992; Salthouse, 1996). This decline is also associated with an assumption that it is difficult to "teach an old dog new tricks" and that older adults are technophobic. Indeed, the elderly tend to elicit disrespect because of this perceived lack of competence (Fiske, Cuddy, Glick, & Xu, 2002).

This perceived lack of competence extends into the domain of technology usage. This stereotype of technological incompetence is reflected in many domains of popular culture including commercials, cartoons, and programs including "Old People Using a Computer: The Game Show" featured on YouTube.com (https://www.youtube.com/watch?v=khhC5UkiNd4). These societal stereotypes of older people using technology were investigated in a research study asking participants to make judgments about a target person who was either a man or a woman, 25 or 75 years of age. Participants rated people 75 years of age as significantly less likely to succeed in a computer class (Ryan, Szechtman, & Bodkin, 1992). Older adults seem to internalize this stereotype, as many believe they are too old to learn the skills necessary to use a computer even before they have attempted to use one (Timmermann, 1998). In addition, Czaja and colleagues (2006) found that those who have lower self-efficacy and more anxiety toward the computer are less likely to use technology.

The negative content of these stereotypes has consequences not just for how older adults view themselves, but also for performance. For example, Levy (1996) found that subliminal exposure to "negative" age stereotypes (i.e., the words "decline", "dependent", "senile", "dying", "forgets") led to lower memory scores than those primed with positive age stereotypes (e.g., "guidance", "wise", "alert", "sage").

Research in stereotype threat sheds light on this issue. Older adults assigned to experimental conditions designed to maximize stereotype threat had significantly lower performance than older adults with less threat or young adult counterparts (Hess, Auman, Colcombe, & Rahhal, 2003). While some have focused on the inevitability of cognitive decline, others have focused on how age-related differences in cognition may have been exaggerated inadvertently through the framing of the task or the task, itself. For example, when the purpose of a task was framed in a memory-neutral way (learning facts) rather than emphasizing the memory component (to see how good one's memory is) age-related differences in the task were eliminated (Rahhal, Hasher, & Colcombe, 2001). Additionally, studies that have attempted to control for motivation show fewer age-related differences. For example, researchers found that older adults and younger adults remember the same amount of critical health information (e.g. severe allergens; Middlebrooks, McGillivray, Murayama, & Castel, 2015).

A mindful approach to learning technology is likely to attenuate stereotype threat. Specifically, a mindful person would learn to recognize and reject prescriptive messages about how they should be acting. Mindful individuals would be more apt to notice both the instances in which they struggle to use technology and the instances where they may excel at it. For example, one might notice that while they understand the mechanics about how to find information, they are slow to scan the page for specific information. A mindless individual may interpret slow processing speed as evidence confirming the bias that older adults are technologically incompetent. A mindful individual, however, would note that taking a few extra seconds or minutes to find relevant information may lead to new discoveries.

## FUTURE RESEARCH DIRECTIONS

The idea that mindfulness can help overcome the barriers that prevent many older adults from benefiting from technological advancements needs to be empirically tested. Despite direct clinical experience and the underlying scientific rationale seemingly confirming the hypothesis, to our knowledge no study has explored this opportunity. Given the paucity of contributions in this field, there are several options to investigate the relationship between mindfulness/mindlessness and technology usage in elderly. For example, future studies can begin from a cross-sectional analysis of the relationship among these elements. It is anticipated that older adults who use technology would be more mindful, flexible and open to new opportunities, also showing better cognitive functions. Considering the relationship that has been demonstrated between mindfulness and quality of life, it is expected that technological users may report, as a group, a better well-being than those who are reluctant to do so. Another kind of study that can provide useful insights is the longitudinal design. Following in time how the attitude toward technology may change in older adults, in the light of the construct of mindfulness, can help to understand how the barriers can be overcome. Finally, probably the most interesting and insightful research design that can contribute to this topic is the experimental one. The causal hypothesis that improving in mindfulness would improve the usage of technology can actually be tested almost only in that kind of study. Possible studies may randomly assign older adults who do not use technology in a mindfulness group or in an technological educational one. Improving in this kind of mindfulness does not require a long training, in contrast to other mainstream mindfulness-based interventions (e.g., Mindfulness-Based Stress Reduction, Mindfulness-Based Cognitive Therapy; Fjorback et al., 2011). A Langerian mindfulness training can easily be conducted in few sessions, or even condensed in one lecture (Carson & Langer, 2004; Phillips & Pagnini, 2014). This training includes simple exercises that allow the person to consider a reality that is in constant change, challenging previous cognitive schemas. For example, the simple process of noticing new aspects of a relationship, or paying attention to novel elements of a daily commute. In this model of mindfulness, noticing new things on purpose is the key to becoming present (Langer, 1989). The effects of that training could be compared to an educational training showing the consequences and the opportunities of technology.

## CONCLUSION

Innovation and technology have brought major changes in the society, creating new opportunities that were not even conceivable just a decade before. The high speed at which technology has grown allows it to diffuse more easily, eventually reaching more people than it did in the past. However, the innovation rate and the number of related changes may not be readily accepted by those who feel comfortable in their current views and not open to including new schemas. Remaining open to new opportunities that do not fit into our previous schema requires a certain amount of flexibility, openness and curiosity. In other words, it requires a mindful attitude.

## ACKNOWLEDGMENT

The study was supported by Università Cattolica del Sacro Cuore (D3.2).

## REFERENCES

AARP. (2000). *Fixing to stay: A national survey on housing and home modification issue---Executive summary*. Washington, D.C.: American Associtì for Retired Persons.

Ahn, M. (2004). *Older People's Attitudes toward Residential Technology: The Role of Technology in Aging in Place*. Virginia Polytechnic Institute and State University.

Anguera, J., Boccanfuso, J., Rintoul, J. L., Al-Hashimi, O., Faraji, F., Janowich, J., & Gazzaley, A. et al. (2013). Video game training enhances cognitive control in older adults. *Nature*, *501*(7465), 97–101. doi:10.1038/nature12486 PMID:24005416

Carson, S. L., & Langer, E. J. (2004). Mindful practice for clinicians and patients. In L. Haas (Ed.), *Handbook of primary care psychology* (pp. 173–186). New York, NY, USA: Oxford University Press.

Carson, S. L., & Langer, E. J. (2006). Mindfulness and self-acceptance. *Journal of Rational-Emotive & Cognitive-Behavior Therapy*, *24*(1), 29–43. doi:10.1007/s10942-006-0022-5

Centers for Disease Control and Prevention. (2006). *Health, United States, 2006, with chartbook on trends in the health of Americans*. Hyattsville, MD: U.S. Department of Health and Human Services, Centers for Disease Control and Prevention, National Center for Health Statistics.

Chanowitz, B., & Langer, E. J. (1981). Premature cognitive commitment. *Journal of Personality and Social Psychology*, *41*(6), 1051–1063. doi:10.1037/0022-3514.41.6.1051 PMID:6975812

Charness, N., Best, R., & Souders, D. (2012). Memory function and supportive technology. *Gerontechnology (Valkenswaard)*, *11*(1). doi:10.4017/gt.2012.11.01.006.00 PMID:24379752

Cho, J., Martin, P., & Poon, L. W. (2014). Successful Aging and Subjective Well-Being Among Oldest-Old Adults. *The Gerontologist*, *55*(1), 132–143. doi:10.1093/geront/gnu074 PMID:25112594

Cornoni-Huntley, J., Brock, D. B., Ostfeld, A. M., Taylor, J. O., & Wallace, R. B. (1986). *Established populations for epidemiologic studies of the elderly resource data book.* Washington, DC: U.S. Government Printing Office.

Coughlin, J. F., D'Ambrosio, L. A., Reimer, B., & Pratt, M. R. (2007, August). Older adult perceptions of smart home technologies: implications for research, policy & market innovations in healthcare. *Proceedings of the 29th Annual International Conference of the IEEE on Engineering in Medicine and Biology Society EMBS '07* (pp. 1810-1815). IEEE. doi:10.1109/IEMBS.2007.4352665

Crowe, M., Andel, R., Pedersen, N. L., Johansson, B., & Gatz, M. (2003). Does Participation in Leisure Activities Lead to Reduced Risk of Alzheimer's Disease? A Prospective Study of Swedish Twins. *The Journals of Gerontology. Series B, Psychological Sciences and Social Sciences*, *58*(5), 249–P255. doi:10.1093/geronb/58.5.P249 PMID:14507930

Czaja, S. J., Charness, N., Fisk, A. D., Hertzog, C., Nair, S. N., Rogers, W., & Sharit, J. (2006). Factors predicting the use of technology: Findings from the Center for Research and Education on Aging and Technology Enhancement (CREATE). *Psychology and Aging*, *21*(2), 333–352. doi:10.1037/0882-7974.21.2.333 PMID:16768579

European Commission. (2009). *2009 Ageing report: economic and budgetary projections for the EU-27 Member States (2008–2060).* Luxembourg: Office for Official Publications of the European Communities.

Field, T. S., Gilman, B. H., Subramanian, S., Fuller, J. C., Bates, D. W., & Gurwitz, J. H. (2005). The costs associated with adverse drug events among older adults in the ambulatory setting. *Medical Care*, *43*(12), 1171–1176. doi:10.1097/01.mlr.0000185690.10336.70 PMID:16299427

Fiske, S. T., Cuddy, A. J. C., Glick, P., & Xu, J. (2002). A model of (often mixed) stereotype content: Competence and warmth respectively follow from perceived status and competition. *Journal of Personality and Social Psychology*, *82*(6), 878–902. doi:10.1037/0022-3514.82.6.878 PMID:12051578

Fjorback, L. O., Arendt, M., Ørnbøl, E., Fink, P., & Walach, H. (2011). Mindfulness-Based Stress Reduction and Mindfulness-Based Cognitive Therapy–a systematic review of randomized controlled trials. *Acta Psychiatrica Scandinavica*, *124*(2), 102–119. doi:10.1111/j.1600-0447.2011.01704.x PMID:21534932

Granic, I., Lobel, A., & Engels, R. C. M. E. (2014). The benefits of playing video games. *The American Psychologist*, *69*(1), 66–78. doi:10.1037/a0034857 PMID:24295515

Greenwood, P. M. (2007). Functional plasticity in cognitive aging: Review and hypothesis. *Neuropsychology*, *21*(6), 657–673. doi:10.1037/0894-4105.21.6.657 PMID:17983277

Hertzog, C., Kramer, A. F., Wilson, R. S., & Lindenberger, U. (2009)... *Enrichment Effects on Adult Cognitive Development*, *9*(1), 1–65.

Hess, T. M., Auman, C., Colcombe, S. J., & Rahhal, T. (2003). The Impact of Stereotype Threat on Age Differences in Memory Performance. *The Journals of Gerontology. Series B, Psychological Sciences and Social Sciences*, *58*(1), 3–P11. doi:10.1093/geronb/58.1.P3 PMID:12496296

Hopkins, P. (2005). NT Clinical. *Nursing Times*, *101*(32). PMID:16119584

House, J. S., Landis, K. R., & Umberson, D. (1988). Social relationships and health. *Science*, *241*(4865), 540–545. doi:10.1126/science.3399889 PMID:3399889

Johnson, M. K., Hashtroudi, S., & Lindsay, D. S. (1993). Source monitoring. *Psychological Bulletin*, *114*(1), 3–28. doi:10.1037/0033-2909.114.1.3 PMID:8346328

Just, M., & Carpenter, P. (1992). A capacity theory of comprehension: Individual differences in working memory. *Psychological Review*, *99*(1), 122–149. doi:10.1037/0033-295X.99.1.122 PMID:1546114

Keng, S. L., Smoski, M. J., & Robins, C. J. (2011). Effects of mindfulness on psychological health: A review of empirical studies. *Clinical Psychology Review*, *31*(6), 1041–1056. doi:10.1016/j.cpr.2011.04.006 PMID:21802619

Kite, M. E., & Johnson, B. T. (1988). Attitudes Toward Older and Younger Adults : A Meta-Analysis. *Psychology and Aging*, *3*(3), 233–244. doi:10.1037/0882-7974.3.3.233 PMID:3268264

Koropeckyj-Cox, T. (2002). Beyond Parental Status. *Psychological Well-Being in Middle and Old Age*, *64*(November), 957–971.

Lai, C.-H., Peng, C.-W., Chen, Y.-L., Huang, C.-P., Hsiao, Y.-L., & Chen, S.-C. (2013). Effects of interactive video-game based system exercise on the balance of the elderly. *Gait & Posture*, *37*(4), 511–515. doi:10.1016/j.gaitpost.2012.09.003 PMID:23177921

Langer, E., & Moldoveanu, M. (2000). The construct of mindfulness. *The Journal of Social Issues*, *56*(1), 1–9. doi:10.1111/0022-4537.00148

Langer, E. J. (1989). *Mindfulness*: Addison-Wesley/Addison Wesley Longman.

Langer, E. J. (2000). Mindful learning. *Current Directions in Psychological Science*, *9*(6), 220–223. doi:10.1111/1467-8721.00099

Langer, E. J., & Rodin, J. (1976). Long-term Effects of a Control-relevant Intervention with the Institutionalized Aged. *Journal of Personality and Social Psychology*, *34*(2), 191–198. doi:10.1037/0022-3514.34.2.191 PMID:1011073

Levy, B. (1996). Improving memory in old age through implicit self-stereotyping. *Journal of Personality and Social Psychology*, *71*(6), 1092–1107. doi:10.1037/0022-3514.71.6.1092 PMID:8979380

Levy, B., & Langer, E. (1994). Aging free from negative stereotypes: Successful memory in China and among the American Deaf.

Melby-Lervåg, M., & Hulme, C. (2012). Is Working Memory Training Effective? A Meta-Analytic Review. *Developmental Psychology*, *49*(2), 270–291. doi:10.1037/a0028228 PMID:22612437

Middlebrooks, C. D., McGillivray, S., Murayama, K., & Castel, A. D. (2015). Memory for Allergies and Health Foods: How Younger and Older Adults Strategically Remember Critical Health Information. *The Journals of Gerontology. Series B, Psychological Sciences and Social Sciences*. doi:10.1093/geronb/gbv032 PMID:25975293

Millennials Continue Urbanization Of America, Leaving Small Towns. (2014). *National Public Radio.* Retrieved from http://www.npr.org/2014/10/21/357723069/millennials-continue-urbanization-of-america-leaving-small-towns

Milward, P. (2003). The 'grey digital divide': Perception, exclusion, and barriers of access to the Internet for older people. *First Monday*, *8*(7). doi:10.5210/fm.v8i7.1066

Mitzner, T. L., Boron, J. B., Fausset, C. B., Adams, A. E., Czaja, S. J., Dijkstra, K., & Sharit, J. et al. (2010). Older adults talk technology: Technology usage and attitudes. *Computers in Human Behavior*, *26*(6), 1710–1721. doi:10.1016/j.chb.2010.06.020 PMID:20967133

Mobile millennials: over 85% of generation Y owns smartphones. (2014). Nielsen. Retrieved from http://www.nielsen.com/us/en/insights/news/2014/mobile-millennials-over-85-percent-of-generation-y-owns-smartphones.html

Moser, D. K., & Dracup, K. (1995). Psychosocial recovery from a cardiac event : The influence of perceived control. *Heart and Lung: The Journal of Acute and Critical Care*, *24*(4), 273–280. doi:10.1016/S0147-9563(05)80070-6 PMID:7591794

Mynatt, E. D., & Rogers, W. (2001). Developing technology to support the functional independence of older adults. *Ageing International*, *27*(1), 24–41. doi:10.1007/s12126-001-1014-5

Pagnini, F., & Phillips, D. (2015). Being mindful about mindfulness. *The Lancet Psychiatry*, *2*(4), 288 - 289. doi:S2215-0366(15)00041-3

Pagnini, F., Phillips, D., Bosma, C., Reece, A., & Langer, E. (2015). Mindfulness, physical impairment and psychological well-being in people with amyotrophic lateral sclerosis. *Psychology & Health*, *30*(5), 503–517. doi:10.1080/08870446.2014.982652 PMID:25361013

Parisi, J. M., Stine-Morrow, E. A., Noh, S. R., & Morrow, D. G. (2009). Predispositional engagement, activity engagement, and cognition among older adults. *Neuropsychology, Development, and Cognition. Section B, Aging, Neuropsychology and Cognition*, *16*(4), 485–504. doi:10.1080/13825580902866653 PMID:19468932

Peine, A., Rollwagen, I., & Neven, L. (2014). The rise of the "innosumer"—Rethinking older technology users. *Technological Forecasting and Social Change*, *82*, 199–214. doi:10.1016/j.techfore.2013.06.013

Phillips, D., & Pagnini, F. (2014). A Mindful Approach to Chronic Illness. In A. Le, C. T. Ngnoumen, & E. Langer (Eds.), *The Wiley-Blackwell Handbook of Mindfulness* (pp. 852–863). London: Wiley-Blackwell. doi:10.1002/9781118294895.ch43

Prensky, M. (2001). Digital Natives, Digital Immigrants. *On the Horizon*, *9*(5), 1–6. doi:10.1108/10748120110424816

Rahhal, T., Hasher, L., & Colcombe, S. J. (2001). Instructional manipulations and age differences in memory: Now you see them, now you don't. *Psychology and Aging*, *16*(4), 697–706. doi:10.1037/0882-7974.16.4.697 PMID:11766922

Rantz, M. J., Skubic, M., Miller, S. J., Galambos, C., Alexander, G., Keller, J., & Popescu, M. (2013). Sensor technology to support Aging in Place. *Journal of the American Medical Directors Association, 14*(6), 386–391. doi:10.1016/j.jamda.2013.02.018 PMID:23562281

Ranzijn, R. (2002). The potential of older adults to enhance community quality of life: Links between positive psychology and productive aging. *Ageing International, 27*(2), 30–55. doi:10.1007/s12126-002-1001-5

Rodin, J., & Langer, E. J. (1977). Long-term Effects of a Control-relevant Intervention with the Institutionalized Aged. *J. Pers. Soc. Psycho.*, 35(12), 175–179.

Ryan, E. B., Szechtman, B., & Bodkin, J. (1992). Attitudes toward younger and older adults learning computers. *Journals of Gerontology: Psychological Science, 47*(2), 96–101. doi:10.1093/geronj/47.2.P96 PMID:1538074

Salthouse, T. (1996). The processing-speed theory of adult age differences in cognition. *Psychological Review, 103*(3), 403–428. doi:10.1037/0033-295X.103.3.403 PMID:8759042

Shafer, R. (2000). *Housing America's Seniors. Executive Summary*. Cambridge, MA: Joint Center for Housing Studies, Harvard University.

Smith, A. (2014). *Older Adults and Technology Use*. Retrieved from http://www.pewinternet.org/2014/04/03/older-adults-and-technology-use/

Stronge, A. J., Rogers, W. A., & Fisk, A. D. (2007). Human factors considerations in implementing telemedicine systems to accommodate older adults. *Journal of Telemedicine and Telecare, 13*(1), 1–3. doi:10.1258/135763307779701158 PMID:17288650

Tang, P., & Venables, T. (2000). "Smart" homes and telecare for independent living. *Journal of Telemedicine and Telecare, 6*(1), 8–14. doi:10.1258/1357633001933871 PMID:10824384

Taylor, L. M., Maddison, R., Pfaeffli, L. A., Rawstorn, J. C., Gant, N., & Kerse, N. M. (2012). Activity and energy expenditure in older people playing active video games. *Archives of Physical Medicine and Rehabilitation, 93*(12), 2281–2286. doi:10.1016/j.apmr.2012.03.034 PMID:22522217

Timmermann, S. (1998). The Role of Information Technology in Older Adult Learning. *New Directions for Adult and Continuing Education*, 1998(77), 61–72.

U.S. Bureau of the Census. (2010). Retrieved from http://www.census.gov/

Verghese, J., Levalley, A., Derby, C., Kuslansky, G., Katz, M., Hall, C., ... Lipton, R. B. (2006). Leisure activities and the risk of amnestic mild cognitive impairment in the elderly. Neurology, 66(6), 821–827.

Wang, H.-X., Jin, Y., Hendrie, H. C., Liang, C., Yang, L., Cheng, Y., & Gao, S. et al. (2013). Late life leisure activities and risk of cognitive decline. *The Journals of Gerontology. Series A, Biological Sciences and Medical Sciences, 68*(2), 205–213. doi:10.1093/gerona/gls153 PMID:22879456

Wilson, R. S., Bennett, D., Bienias, J. L., Mendes de Leon, C. F., Morris, M. C., & Evans, D. (2003). Cognitive activity and cognitive decline in a biracial community population. *Neurology, 61*(6), 812–816. doi:10.1212/01.WNL.0000083989.44027.05 PMID:14504326

## KEY TERMS AND DEFINITIONS

**Aging in Place:** Living in one's own home into late adulthood.

**Digital Native:** Someone who grew up immersed in a technological society and as a result are skilled in using technological products.

**Functional Independence:** The ability of a person to take care of him/herself without depending on the direct assistance of someone else.

**Grey Digital Divide:** The phenomenon in which older adults do not use technology to the same extent as younger population.

**Mindfulness:** The simple process of noticing new things.

**Mindlessness:** A mental state in which the person stuck in previous categories and schemas.

**Stereotype Threat:** The risk of confirming a negative stereotype of a group the person identifies with.

Section 4

# Positive Interventions:

## Games for Well-Being

# Chapter 10
# Hacking Well-Being:
## Can Serious Games Fit Positive Technology Framework?

**Luca Argenton**
*University of Milano-Bicocca, Italy*

**Andrea Zini**
*Università Cattolica del Sacro Cuore, Italy*

**Federica Pallavicini**
*University of Milano-Bicocca, Italy*

**Giacomo Garcea**
*Università Cattolica del Sacro Cuore, Italy*

**Gabriele Barone**
*Università Cattolica del Sacro Cuore, Italy*

**Andrea Zanacchi**
*Università Cattolica del Sacro Cuore, Italy*

**Fabrizia Mantovani**
*University of Milano-Bicocca, Italy*

## ABSTRACT

*Serious Games (SGs) have been able to shape new opportunities for human training and empowerment, imparting knowledge or skills in an engaging and motivating way to a new generation of learners. Further, they can be used to improve the quality of both individual and collective experience. In particular, SGs can nurture positive emotions promote engagement, as well as enhance social integration and connectedness. An in-depth analysis of each of these aspects will be presented in the chapter, with the support of concrete examples and case-analysis. Eventually, a game design practice will be discussed. Knowledge and awareness of hedonic, eudaimonic and social principles improve user-centered design models can be both fundamental to enhance learning effectiveness and retention and to improve players' well-being, contributing to the development of sustainable communities of practices.*

## INTRODUCTION

Serious Games (SGs) are digital games used for purposes other than mere entertainment (Susi et al., 2007). By fostering continuous learning experiences blended with entertaining affordances, SGs have been able to shape opportunities for human training and empowerment. They have in fact supported the creation of socio-technical environments (Fisher et al., 2005), where the interconnection between humans and technology encourages the emergence of innovative ways of thinking, creative practices, and both individual and collective development. SGs are able to match real and virtual experiences building contexts

DOI: 10.4018/978-1-4666-9986-1.ch010

that impart knowledge or skills in an engaging and motivating way (Zyda, 2005; Michael & Chen, 2006) to a new generation of learners grown up in a fully digitalized society. The use and effectiveness of SGs have been acknowledged in different areas, such as education, health, business and military both by the scientific literature and the concrete experience of players (Connolly et al., 2013; Wouters et al., 2013).

Further, SGs are able to address another important issue for the actual society: promoting health, wellness and happiness among individuals. As other technologies presented in the book, SGs have proven to be strongly related to maintaining and restoring good health (Brox et al., 2011; McCallum, 2012; Stapleton, 2004; Wattanasoontorn et al., 2013). For example, according to the taxonomy of Wattanasoontorn and colleagues (2013), SGs can support patients by monitoring health, detecting irregular symptoms, treating physical and mental issues and contributing to the rehabilitation process. Further, SGs can assist people to increase their well-being, physically, mentally and socially (Brooks et al., 2014).

That is why they can be considered as "Positive Technologies" (Argenton et al., 2014). This assumption opens a totally new perspective in the traditional digital gaming literature that has deeply investigated the negative impact of gaming, with respect to violence (Anderson et al., 2003; Gentile & Anderson, 2003; Wouters et al., 2013), addiction (Van Rooij et al., 2010; 2011) or social isolation (Colwell & Payne, 2000; Pezzeca, 2009).

Within this context, the aim of this chapter is to offer a theoretical framework about SGs as Positive Technologies, discussing how they can empower the quality of personal experience (Figure 1). In particular, we will discuss how SGs influence individual and interpersonal experiences by fostering positive emotions (hedonic level), promoting engagement (eudaimonic level), as well as enhancing social integration and connectedness (social level).

An in-depth analysis of each of these aspects will be presented in the chapter along with game design practices, with the support of concrete evidence and specific case-studies. Finally, an example of SG designed following the Positive Technologies principles will be presented: *Mind the* Game™.

*Figure 1. SGs as positive technologies*

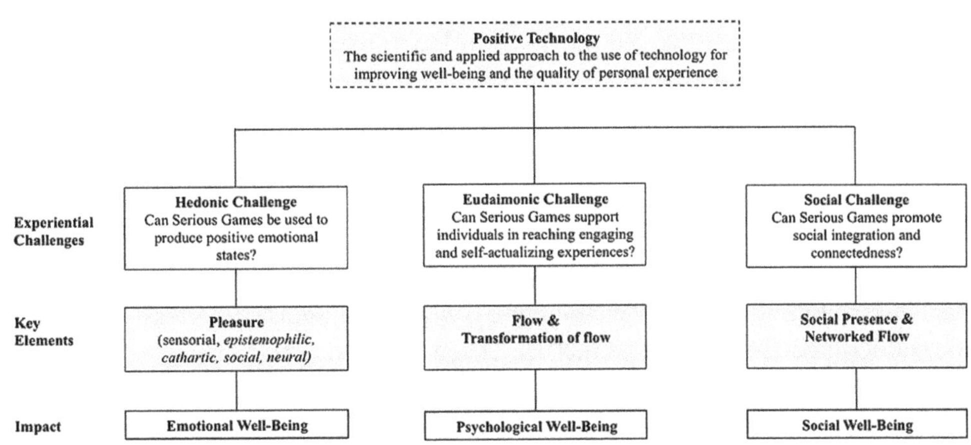

## CAN SERIOUS GAMES FIT THE POSITIVE TECHNOLOGY SCENARIO?

### The Hedonic Challenge

The hedonic side of Positive Technology analyses the ways technologies can be used to produce positive emotional states. Games can elicit several emotional states (Anolli et al., 2010). Many representations of players' affective states have been used in previous studies like anxiety, frustration, engagement, distress scales, and the valence-arousal space (Anderson & Ford, 1986; Freeman, 2004). However, SGs and games in general are strictly connected to positive emotions, and to a wide variety of pleasant situational responses that make gameplay the direct emotional opposite of depression (McGonigal, 2010). This is important, since one of the main principle and mechanism of game-based learning is learning through ''fun''. In the design of SGs, for this reason, great attention is given to entertainment mechanisms, The level of fun needed in SGs compared with purely videogame entertainment titles is still a subject of debate, as they are still debated methods for evaluating the level of enjoyment induced (Koster, 2014; Shaker et al., 2010; Mitgutsch, 2012).

At first, SGs can evoke a *sensorial pleasure* throughout graphics, usability, game aesthetic, visual and narrative stimuli. Secondly, SGs foster an *epistemophilic pleasure* by bridging curiosity with the desire of novelty within a protected environment where individuals can experience the complexity of their self, and developing mastery and control. In other words, they are able to recreate a "magic circle" (Huizinga, 1950) that enforces individual agency, self-confidence and self-esteem (Anolli et al., 2010), by sustaining a process of acknowledgement of personal ability to perform well, solve problems, and manage with difficulties. Hence, empowered by digital affordances, SGs can promote a dynamic equilibrium between excitement and security. Thirdly, SGs promote the *pleasure for victory* and, by supporting virtual interactions with real people, they nurture *social pleasure*, promoting collaborative and competitive dynamics, communication and sharing opportunities, even outside the context of the game (Anolli et al., 2010). Games have also been traditionally recognized as marked by a *cathartic pleasure* as they represent a relief valve for emotional tensions, anger and aggressiveness (Wouters et al., 2013). Finally, pleasure has a *neural* counterpart. An interesting example is that of dopamine, a neurotransmitter that affects the flow of information in the brain and that is often involved in pleasant experiences, as well as in different forms of addiction and learning. In a classic study made by Koepp and colleagues to monitor the effects of video games on brain activity, a significant increase of dopamine (found in a quantity comparable only to that determined by taking amphetamines) was measured (Koepp et al., 1998).

Moreover, knowledge and awareness of hedonic principles can be fundamental to enhance learning effectiveness and retention (Connolly et al., 2012). For example, recent studies have shown that students using SGs demonstrate deeper learning and spend roughly twice as much time, outside of class, on their homework (Coller & Scott, 2009).

From the perspective of game design, to make sure that the SG is able to provide fun to its players, is important to include entertainment game mechanisms, as role playing, collecting points, tile matching. Other mechanisms include also clear but challenging goals, rules, fantasy, progressive levels of difficulty, and feedback (Fullerton 2014; Baranowski, 2013; Deterding et al., 2011).

Good examples of SGs explicitly designed to foster positive emotion are *The Journey to Wild Divine*, *Eye Spy: the Matrix*, *Wham!*, and *Grow your Chi*!, developed in Dr. Baldwin's Lab at McGill University. In *The Journey to Wild Divine* the integration between usable biofeedback sensors and a computer software allows individuals to enhance their subjective wellbeing throughout a 3D graphic adventure. Here, wise mentors teach the skills to reduce stress, and increase physical and mental health.

*Eye Spy: the Matrix*, *Wham!,* and *Grow your Chi*! are indeed projects whose goal is to empower people with low self-esteem respectively by working on ignoring rejection information, throughout positive conditioning, or by focusing on positive social connections (Baccus et al., 2004; Dandeneau & Baldwin, 2004).

Another great example is *Mindlight,* developed by the GainPlay Studio in collaboration with the PlayNice Institute and Radboud University. The game realized for children aged 8-12, has been created on evidence-based principles of intervention with anxiety-disordered children and adults through the use of biofeedback. In the game, the main character, Little Arthur, has to deal with a scary and dark mansion where his grandmother has succumbed to shadows. In order to bring her back, Arthur has to use a Magical Hat, a neurofeedback headset the player wears when playing the game. Through the help of the Magical Hat, players learn to modulate their arousal by specific relaxation and mindfulness techniques that directly impact the game. Everything in the game (the environment, threats and puzzles) in fact responds to how the player is allocating his/her cognitive and emotional resources.

## The Eudaimonic Challenge

The eduaimonic challenge is related to the use of technology to engage people more actively in what they currently do. The theory of *flow* (Csikszentmihalyi, 1991) and *immersion*, extensively used to describe the main features of game experience (De Grove et al., 2010; Nacke & Lindley, 2009; Nacke & Lindley, 2008), are key elements to understand this challenge. According to Csikszentmihalyi,,individuals preferentially engage in opportunities for action associated with a positive, complex and rewarding state of consciousness, defined optimal experience or flow (Csikszentmihalyi, 1975; 1991).

Bergeron (2006) defined SGs as interactive computer applications, with or without a significant hardware component, that

1. Have challenging goals,
2. Are fun to play with and/or engaging,
3. Incorporate some concepts of scoring,
4. Impart to the player skills, knowledge, or attitude that can be applied in the real world.

Interestingly, all of these aspects can be easily overlapped to Csikszentmihalyi's theory of flow. Games are in fact "flow activities" (Csikszentmihalyi, 1991; 2000) as they are intrinsically able to provide enjoyable experiences (McGonigal, 2010), creating rules that require the learning of skills, defining goals, giving feedback, making control possible, and fostering a sense of curiosity and discovery.

In addition, the intrinsic potential of flow that characterizes SGs can be even empowered by (i) identifying an information-rich environment that contains functional real world demands; (ii) using the technology to enhance the level of presence of subjects in the environment, and (iii) allowing the cultivation, by linking this optimal experience to the actual experience of the subject (Ijsselsteijn & Riva, 2003). SGs should stimulate a mental focus on in-game dynamics, by providing a set of engaging, differentiated and worth-attending stimuli that limit the influence of external variables. Along with other aspects, concentration can result in hyperlearning processes that consist of the mental ability to totally focus on the task by using effective strategies aligned with personal traits (Csikszentmihalyi, 1991);

In order to develop a SG able to induce in players high level of immersion, it is important to look at game design elements, including for example (see also Fullerton, 2014; Baranowski, 2013; Sweetser & Wyeth, 2005):

- **Challenge:** As noted by Gee (Gee, 2003), who claims that the game experience should be "pleasantly frustrating", challenges have to match players' skills/level and to support their improvement throughout the game. During specific stages of the game, "Fish tanks" (stripped down versions of the real game, where gameplay mechanisms are simplified) and "Sand boxes" (versions of the game where there is less likelihood for things to go wrong) can support this dynamism;
- **Clear Goals:** Games should provide players with specific, measurable, achievable, responsible and time-bounded goals;
- **Storyline:** The targeted content needs to be intrinsically coupled with the fantasy context (or story) of the game in order to improve motivation, emotional attachment (Malone and Lepper 1987), and cognitive load (Sweller 1994). The storyline needs to be developed according to the specific skills to train in the target to player types audience (Bartle, 2003);
- **Feedback:** Players have to be supported by feedback on the progress they are making, on their action, and the ongoing situations represented in the virtual environment;
- **Control:** It is fundamental for players to experience a sense of control over what they are doing, as well as over the game interface, and input devices; players should feel a sense of control through endogenous feedback, in order to increase their motivation and engagement in the game (Paras, 2005).

On the one hand, numerous case studies have confirmed the usefulness of flow as SGs quality measure (Bellotti et al., 2013; Kiili et al., 2014; Kiili et al., in press). Moreover, results indicated that flow is an appropriate construct to assess the quality of game experience (Ermi & Mäyrä, 2005; Oksanen, 2014) and that its measurement can facilitate game evaluation and design practices (Bergeron, 2006; Kiili et al., 2014), especially for eudaimonic SGs.

On the other, there are SGs that have directly addressed the eudaimonic challenge. An example is *Reach Out Central* (ROC), developed by ReachOut.com. It is a Cognitive-Behaviour therapy game that encourages players to develop psychological well-being. Studied for young people aged 14-24, ROC is a single-player role play game with innovative 3D graphics and real-life scenarios and characters. Here, players can see how their decisions and reactions affect their moods, and apply skills they learn offline in their day-to-day lives. An evaluation conducted by Shandley and colleagues (Shandley, Austin, Klein, & Kyrios, 2010; Shandley, Klein, & Austin, 2008) found that ROC reduced psychological distress, alcohol use, and improved life satisfaction, resilience, and problem-solving abilities. Another great example is *SuperBetter,* developed by Jane McGonigal. *SuperBetter* helps people their life goals by working on personal resilience. The application of the aforementioned elements supports people being curious, optimistic and motivated and promotes high levels of user engagement.

## The Social Challenge

At the social level, the challenge for Positive Technology is concerned with the use of new media to support and improve the connectedness between individuals, groups, and organizations, and to create a mutual sense of awareness. Games should create opportunities for social interaction by supporting competition, collaboration, and sharing among players. Cantamesse and colleagues (Cantamesse, et al., 2011) examined the effect of playing the online game World of Warcraft (WoW), both on adolescents' social interaction and on the competence they developed on it. The in-game interactions, and in particular conversational exchanges, turn out to be a collaborative path of the joint definition of identities and social ties, with reflection on in-game processes and out-game relationships. At this level, SGs can also promote the development of a peak collaborative state experienced by the group as a whole and known as "networked flow" (Gaggioli, et al. 2013). Sawyer (2003, 2008), who referred to this state with the term of "group flow", identified several conditions that facilitate its occurrence: the presence of a common goal, close listening, complete concentration, control, blending egos, equal participation, familiarity, communication and the potential for failure. Group flow cannot be broken down into the work of individuals; rather, this phenomenon emerges from the interactions occurring within a group and is able to positively influence overall performance.

As noted by Gaggioli and colleagues (2013), networked flow occurs when high levels of presence and social presence are matched with a state of "liminality". In particular, three pre-conditions have to be satisfied:

- Group members share common goals and emotional experiences so that individual intentionality becomes a *we-intention* (Searle, 1983) able to inspire and guide the whole group;
- Group members experience a state liminality, a state of "being about" that breaks the homeostatic equilibrium previously defined;
- Group members identify in the ongoing activity the best affordances to overcome the situation of liminality.

Some studies have addressed the relationship between social presence and immersion in games finding controversial results (Cairns et al., 2013; Oksanen, 2014; Sweetser & Wyeth, 2005; Yoo & Alavi, 2001). On the one hand, there are those who claim that the presence of others, even mediated via online play, would require players to think about the other players and so draw their attention away from the thinking about the game, determining low level of immersion (Sweetser & Wyeth, 2005). Other studies have indeed highlighted the opposite. For example, Cairns et al. (2013) run three experiments that showed that players were more immersed when playing against another person than playing against a computer and that there was not significant different in the levels of immersion whether the other person was present in the room or not. Similarly, Oksanen (2014) found that the sociability of the environment strengthen the emergence of social presence and that it can also contribute to the formation of positive game experiences. Moreover, social presence has a specific role, particularly in collaborative games, to open communication, critical thinking, group cohesion, supportive interaction and negotiation (Kreijns et al., 2003, 2002). High levels of social presence are predictors of learning (Gunawardena, 1995) and they are correlated to high levels of enjoyment (Gajadhar et al., 2008), social interaction (Tu & McIsaac, 2002) and group cohesion (Yoo & Alavi, 2001).

These principles have been also used to support Participatory Design practices (Sanders, 2002), with users and other stakeholders playing a key role in all the stages relating to design, development and evaluation of a specific project (Corrigan et al., 2014). Participatory Design can improve communication, control of the project, innovation and creativity. Connoly and colleagues (Connolly et al., 2007) presented *SDSim Game*, a SG where a team has to manage and deliver a number of software development projects. In the game each player has a specific role, such as project manager, systems analyst, systems designer or team leader with specific tasks. During the game, the team is provided with background information and must produce an high-level product that addresses the clients' requirements and manage a limited amount of resources. To do so, players must move through game-levels, interact among them and 'talk' to the nonplayer characters (NPCs) in the game.

Good examples of specifically designed SGs can be found in the field of organizational management and education. For instance, *Everest V2* (2011), was developed by the Harvard Business School to promote leadership and team working, and *Woodment* (2010) was presented as an educational web-based collaborative multiplayer SG. Another example is *TeamUp* (2013) developed by The Barn in collaboration with the Delft University of Technology and Accenture (Mayer et al. 2013). SGs have shown to be effective also in supporting participative approaches. In these games, social presence and networked flow are fundamental (Brom et al., 2014).

Here below we will present a serious game that has been specifically designed to foster these states: *Mind the Game*™.

## MIND THE GAME™: A SERIOUS GAME TO PROMOTE NETWORKED FLOW

*Mind the* Game™ is a a multiplayer decision-making SG developed for a target of adult individuals to create a socio-technical environment (Fisher et al., 2005) where the interconnection between humans and technology encourages the emergence of collaboration and team working.

Embedding the potential of serious gaming, *Mind the Game*™ aims to expand the range of resources that groups can access in daily contexts, allowing a greater awareness of the skills possessed both individually and as a whole, and implementing an experiential learning process that supports shared optimal experiences. Hence, the game can be considered as a useful tool to promote collaboration and team working among individuals.

As a new medium aimed at facilitating change, the SG generates a virtual environment where groups can express their potential, dealing with a reality that constantly redefines the balance between challenges and skills. This was studied to create a virtuous circularity that promotes collective peak experiences and high levels of perceived effectiveness, both in an individual and collective sense.

### Technology

The interface, developed with Html5, is primarily textual, enriched multimodally by clips images, and animated graphics that make the game more interactive (Figure 2).

The game, studied for small groups of 5 people, provides the facilitator/the researcher with the ability to monitor the progress of the game. It is now embedded in a specific website that consists of a welcome page, a tutorial, and a questionnaire section to evaluate game experience.

### Sharing Goals and Emotional Experiences: Sport as a Narrative Tool

The narrative framework - especially in technological solutions based on a textual environment - is a core element for serious game design. Narratives have to be clear, straightforward, easy to understand and memorable to capture the interest of the player (Bateman, 2007; McQuiggan, et al., 2008). Therefore, the choice of plots and settings will be decisive to bring the group out of the comfort zone, nurturing

*Figure 2. The primarily textual interface of Mind the Game™ is enriched multimodally by clips, images, and animated graphics.*

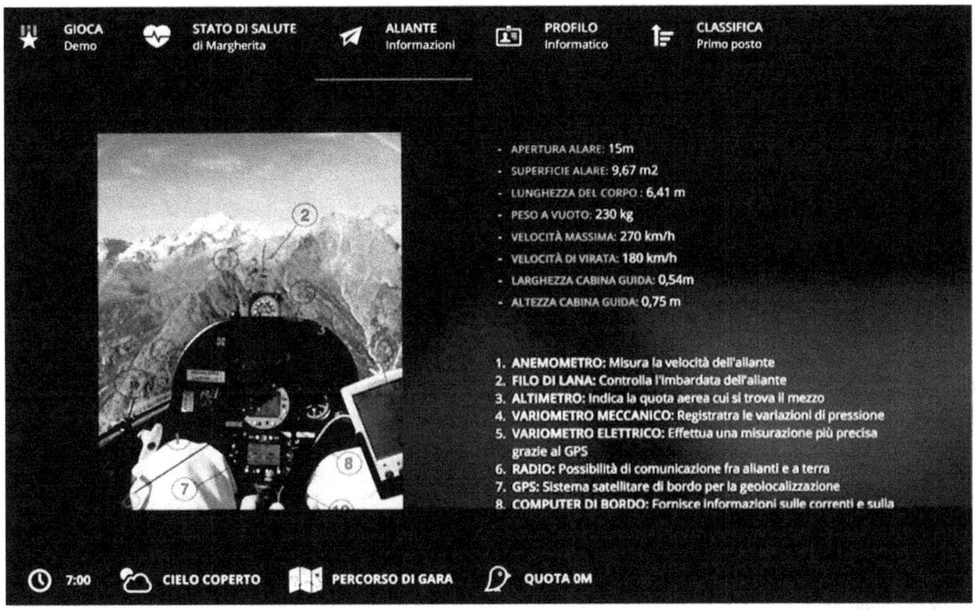
GIOCA
Demo
STATO DI SALUTE
di Margherita
ALIANTE
Informazioni
PROFILO
Informatico
CLASSIFICA
Primo posto
APERTURA ALARE: 15m
SUPERFICIE ALARE: 9,67 m2
LUNGHEZZA DEL CORPO : 6,41 m
PESO A VUOTO: 230 kg
VELOCITÀ MASSIMA: 270 km/h
VELOCITÀ DI VIRATA: 180 km/h
LARGHEZZA CABINA GUIDA: 0,54m
ALTEZZA CABINA GUIDA: 0,75 m
1. ANEMOMETRO: Misura la velocità dell'aliante
2. FILO DI LANA: Controlla l'imbardata dell'aliante
3. ALTIMETRO: Indica la quota aerea cui si trova il mezzo
4. VARIOMETRO MECCANICO: Registratra le variazioni di pressione
5. VARIOMETRO ELETTRICO: Effettua una misurazione più precisa grazie al GPS
6. RADIO: Possibilità di comunicazione fra alianti e a terra
7. GPS: Sistema satellitare di bordo per la geolocalizzazione
8. COMPUTER DI BORDO: Fornisce informazioni sulle correnti e sulla
7:00
CIELO COPERTO
PERCORSO DI GARA
QUOTA 0M

the onset of spontaneous behaviors, as well as promoting the emergence of we intentions (Searle, 1948), social presence and ingroup dynamics in multiplayer settings.

Moreover, the underlying potential of narratives can be amplified through the use of peculiar scenarios that have nothing to do with day by day experiences (Edery & Mollick, 2009). In this way, it is possible to modulate the impact of prior knowledge of player and to support common cognitive processes and knowledge sharing practices.

As a metaphor of life, sport is a powerful and effective training tool, capable of supporting learning and experiential transpositions. In particular, sport witnesses how beyond individual and team excellence there are challenges that do not end against the opponent, but in their relationship with the self.

According to the aforementioned considerations, we chose a little-known sport that could be used to promote networked flow: gliding. This is a discipline based on soaring flight, where, in the absence of the driving force of an engine, the pilot is required to take advantage of upward motions and movements of air masses (Brigliadori & Brigliadori, 2011). In fact, thanks to the overheating of the soil and the atmospheric layers close to it, the air creates connective vertical motions, called thermals, that support the flight. The development of the narrative plot structure on such a discipline can be particularly effective both because of an implicit and an explicit reason.

On the one hand, soaring flight embraces a deep archaic desire: the tension to the sky. Sky has represented a point of reference for a humanity that has begun to mature the dream of approaching it. Thus, before becoming the concrete possibility, outlined by the studies of Leonardo or by the efforts made by Wright and Montgolfier brothers, flight is synonym of purity and freedom, fantasy, hope, and imagination. It is the symbol of a challenge marked by a courageous and meaningful searching of the limit. On the other hand, as a sport, gliding implies competition and collaboration. The first concept is well reflected by the Grand Prix, a race in which pilots directly compete one another. The goal is to go throughout a task - a plot delimited by specific turning points that are placed so as to form a polygon – in the shortest time. Generally, the Grand Prix is structured among several days, implying different tasks from time to time.

The choice of an individual sport to promote group creativity and of team working may instead appear paradoxical. But it is not: individual excellence is the tip of the iceberg beneath which team effort and coordination always make the difference. The collaborative dimension of gliding is present because, despite the solo flight of the pilot, his/her staff can support each step of the race from the ground. In fact, parameters to be taken into consideration are extremely numerous and they require the intervention of professionals specifically trained. In particular, according to the model described by Brigliadori and Brigliadori (2011), five elements are fundamental:

- **Technical:** Managing an efficient flight and exploiting the energy available in the atmosphere in the best possible way, require specific skills: decision-making, problem-solving, control, and experience. Moreover, the maintenance of security and risk management are the foundation of successful flights.
- **Strategic:** The ability to take advantage of circumstances involves a process of decision-making able to take into account meteorological aspects, competitors, geography. The race is played on the ability to make the most from the opportunities that are revealed during the task.
- **Psychological:** Control of emotions, stress management, relaxation, high levels of concentration, resilience and self-efficacy are just some of the psychological components that may be decisive during a competition.
- **Athletic:** Pilots must take great care in athletic training, monitoring nutrition and fatigue management.
- **Meteorological:** Climate is a component whose analysis should be careful and meticulous in order to avoid unnecessary risks and make winning choices.
- **Organizational**: The athlete, together with the staff, is expected to prepare the race in every detail, monitoring equipment and logistics practices.

The sense of in-group belonging is first increased by the narrative framework, that immerses players in a collaborative environment. In this way, it is possible to encourage the emergence of a we-intention, whose genesis is the *conditio sine qua non* for the development and implementation of networked flow.

## Creating a Space of Liminality

With the support of a suggestive graphic environment and with an emotional clip, players are introduced to a letter written directly by "Sky Volaleggera", the main character of the game. After introducing herself, the pilot said to be in Australia where she will compete in the last gliding race of the season. Here she can realize her dream: winning for the first time the World Competition. By showing the characteristics of the race, the pilot explains that the task is going to be very technical and complicated, stressing that every detail can make an important difference.

Players begin to realize their role in the simulation: they will not be called to be an athlete or an opponent of the athlete, but a member of her team. Each player will in fact be assigned one of the following roles: team manager, strategist, technical expert, meteorologist or doctor.

The arrangement by which each character appears to the player is the same and tends to follow the systemic model proposed by Bowman (2010). It is marked by the definition of name, age, nationality, as well as the role played within the team and the tasks he/she has to preside. The player can then discover his/her background. This is realized on three levels, indicating aspects of the past, present and future. At the same time, the player can also view the individual goals of the character. Finally, there is a brief personality description. Further, during the game each player receives specific information according to his/her role that are not seen by his/her teammates.

It is then specified how, next to a shared goal (leading the athlete to win the World Competition), each character will be motivated by personal goals, different from those of the other participants. The team's score is indeed defined as a result of the following parameters:

- Score obtained in the race by the athlete. When completing a task, each group was given 1, 5 or 10 points according to the quality of the given answer. If players were not able to obtain more than 7 points in two subsequent challenges before task 4, the serious game stopped and subjects were not allowed to continue (failure). We coded as 1 a situation were the simulation was not completed and as 2 a situation were players could experience the complete game. Moreover, for those who completed the simulation, single scores were summed at the end of the game and coded as follow:
    - Total Score= 50: excellent performance.
    - 45 $\leq$ Total Score <49: good performance.
    - 41 $\leq$ Total Score <44: medium performance.
    - Total Score < 40: poor performance.
- Time Management as each task it time bounded. We consider the time (min) needed to complete each one of the five tasks and the game as a whole.

## Identifying a Common Activity to Overcome the Space of Liminality

When the intention is then transformed into action, the serious game becomes functional to stimulate a synergistic collaboration According to Steiner's model (1972), it is possible to distinguish:

- **Additive Tasks:** Referred to situations in which the final result is determined by the sum of individual contributions;
- **Compensatory Tasks:** Where the result is determined as an average of the contributions made by individual subjects;
- **Conjunctive Tasks:** Where the success of the group depends on the success of each member;
- **Disjunctive Tasks:** Where each member can promote a solution of their own, knowing that the success of the group depends on a single correct alternative;
- **Complementary Tasks:** That requires the sharing of knowledge, processes and methods so that the whole could exceed the sum of its single parts.

In line with this model, each task is designed according to a *complementary logic*, in an attempt to involve each player. Specifically, players are called upon to deal with distributed decision-making environments in which real success can not depend on free-riding efforts, but on the emergence of group phenomena, such as social facilitation, social labouring, and team thinking. Clearly, the effectiveness of the group will be marked by its specific characteristics, as well as on its communicative, emotional and hierarchical structure.

Collaboration and interdependency between participants are created by distributing different knowledge and resources to each player and triggering resource dependency among players (Oksanen, 2014; Price et al., 2003).

The tasks players have to solve are the following:

1. **Object Challenge:** Players needs to identify from a list of 15 objects the five most important tools that their pilot has to bring with her on-board.
2. **Medicine Challenge:** According to the information they receive, players have to select to best medicine for the athlete. The task is complicated by the fact that players have different and partly contradictory information.
3. **Map Challenge:** After a GPS breakdown, the pilot is not able to identify her position on the map. Players have to chronologically reorder the information they received and to solve subgroups puzzles to point on the map the right position of the glider.
4. **Strategy Challenge:** The final part of the race is approaching. Players have to decide whether going for a risky or a conservative strategy.
5. **Weather Challenge:** The team has just 10 minutes to understand the meteorological condition of the race and to support the athlete with the best option.

Each task is time bounded and players have to select an option before the time ends, otherwise the system automatically considers the task not completed. To successfully complete the simulation, at least four answers have to be given correctly.

## CONCLUSION

SGs are digital games used for purposes other than mere entertainment. By integrating different know-hows and experiences, SGs are able to contextualize user experience in stimulating and realistic environments (Bellotti et al., 2013) that foster practical learning experiences blended with ludic and engaging affordances.

In the present chapter we discussed the role of SGs as positive technologies. According to Positive Psychology theoretical framework and Positive Technology approach, we explored how these applications are able to promote hedonic well-being, eudaimonic well-being and social well-being.

Firstly, SGs can foster positive emotional states by enhancing the different forms of pleasure they are intrinsically made of. In particular, we discussed the importance of sensorial, epistemophilic, social, cathartic and neural pleasure.

Secondly, serious applications for computer game technologies can be associated with flow experiences and, thus, with eudaimonic well-being. Throughout high level of presence and flow, SGs can, in fact, promote optimal experiences marked by absorption, engagement, and enjoyment. Numerous studies have been realized to analyze the usefulness of flow as SGs quality measure (Bellotti et al., 2013; Kiili et al., 2014; Kiili et al., in press). Results indicated that flow is an appropriate construct to assess the quality of game experience (Ermi & Mäyrä, 2005; Oksanen, 2014) and that its measurement can facilitate game evaluation and design practices (Bergeron, 2006; Kiili et al., 2014), expecially for eudaimonic SGs.

Finally, SGs are able to increase connectedness and integration. To achieve such a complex goal they have to work on a mutual sense of awareness, as well as social presence and situations of liminality. In this way, groups can access high levels of social interaction and peak creative states, known as networked flow experiences, that are based on shared goals and emotions, collective intentions, and proactive behaviors. These experiences have a specific role, particularly in collaborative games, to open communication, critical thinking, group cohesion, supportive interaction and negotiation (Kreijns et al., 2003, 2002). High levels of social presence and networked flow are predictors of learning (Gunawardena, 1995) and they are correlated to high levels of enjoyment (Gajadhar et al., 2008), social interaction (Tu & McIsaac, 2002), and group cohesion (Yoo & Alavi, 2001). This result can be achieved by using storytelling and by presenting complimentary tasks.

On the one hand, knowledge and awareness of hedonic, eudaimonic and social principles can be both fundamental to enhance learning effectiveness and retention (Connolly et al., 2012). An effective balance of the three levels can support students not only to become active and engaged learners, but also to improve their well-being and contribute to the development of sustainable communities of practices.

On the other, the concrete application of Positive Technology principles may be fundamental to improve user-centered design models. One of the most important aspects to analyse when considering serious and computer games from a scientific point of view is game experience (Poels et al., 2007; Sweetser & Wyeth, 2005; Takatalo et al., 2008). Attempts to clearly define the construct are indeed scarce and the wide variety of games genres and the complex, subjective and dynamic nature of the idea of experience (Takatalo et al., 2008) makes it hard to find a common definition. However, many authors agree (Coller & Scott, 2009; De Kort et al., 2007; Ermi & Mäyrä, 2005) on the importance of elements like positive affects, flow and social presence that are central in the Positive Technology framework.

Despite the impressive growth of SGs applications, only a few of them have been tested and scientifically considered from an empirical point of view. This is a major challenge for future research and investigation. Positive Technology approach can address this issue not only by creating a concrete background for both theoretical and applied research, but also supporting game design processes.

## REFERENCES


Anderson, C. A., Berkowitz, L., Donnerstein, E., Huesmann, L. R., Johnson, J. D., Linz, D., & Neil, M. Malamuth, & Wartella, E. (2003). The influence of media violence on youth. *Psychological Science in the Public Interest*, *4*, 81–110. PMID:26151870

Anderson, C. A., & Ford, C. M. (1986). Affect of the Game Player: Short-Term Effects of Highly and Mildly Aggressive Video Games. *Personality and Social Psychology Bulletin*, *12*(4), 390–402. doi:10.1177/0146167286124002

Anolli, L., Mantovani, F., Confalonieri, L., Ascolese, A., & Peveri, L. (2010). Emotions in Serious Games: From Experience to Assessment. *International Journal of Emerging Technologies in Learning*, *5*, 7–16.

Argenton, L., Triberti, S., Serino, S., Muzio, M., & Riva, G. (2014). Serious Games as Positive Technologies for Individual and Group Flourishing. In A. L. Brooks, S. Brahnam, & L. C. Jain (Eds.), *Technologies of Inclusive Well-Being* (Vol. 536, pp. 221–244). Berlin: Springer International Publishing. doi:10.1007/978-3-642-45432-5_11

Armarego, J. (2002). Advanced software design: a case in problem-based learning. *Proceedings 15th Conference on Software Engineering Education and Training (CSEE&T 2002)* (pp. 57–65). doi:10.1109/CSEE.2002.995197

Baccus, J. R., Baldwin, M. W., & Packer, D. J. (2004). Increasing implicit self-esteem through classical conditioning. *Psychological Science*, *15*(7), 498–502. doi:10.1111/j.0956-7976.2004.00708.x PMID:15200636

Baker, A., Navarro, E. O., & Van Der Hoek, A. (2005). An experimental card game for teaching software engineering processes. *Journal of Systems and Software*, *75*(1-2), 3–16. doi:10.1016/j.jss.2004.02.033

Baranowski, T., Buday, R., Thompson, D., Lyons, E. J., Lu, A. S., & Baranowski, J. (2013). Developing games for health behavior change: Getting started. *GAMES FOR HEALTH: Research, Development, and Clinical Applications*, *2*(4), 183–190. doi:10.1089/g4h.2013.0048 PMID:24443708

Bartle, R. (2003). *Designing Virtual Worlds*. New Riders Games.

Bateman, C. M. (2007). *Game writing: narrative skills for video games*. Hingham, MA: Charles River Media.

Bellotti, F., Kapralos, B., Lee, K., Moreno-Ger, P., & Berta, R. (2013). Assessment in and of Serious Games: An Overview. *Advances in Human-Computer Interaction*, *4*, 1–11.

Bergeron, B. (2006). *Developing serious games*. Hingham, MA: Charles River Media.

Bowman, S. L. (2010). *The functions of role-playing games. How partecipants create community, solve problems and explore identity*. London, UK: McFarland & Copany Inc.

Brigliadori, L., & Brigliadori, R. (2011). *Competing in Gliders. Winning with your mind*. Pivetta Partners, Vedano al Lambro.

Brom, C., Buchtová, M., Šisler, V., Děchtěrenko, F., Palme, R., & Glenk, L. M. (2014). Flow, social interaction anxiety and salivary cortisol responses in serious games: A quasi-experimental study. *Computers & Education*, *79*, 69–100. doi:10.1016/j.compedu.2014.07.001

Brooks, A. L., Brahnam, S., & Jain, L. C. (2014). *Technologies of Inclusive Well-Being. Serious Games, Alternative Realities, and Play Therapy*. New York: Springer. doi:10.1007/978-3-642-45432-5

Brox, E., Fernandez-Luque, L., & Tøllefsen, T. (2011). Healthy Gaming – Video Game Design to promote Health. *Applied Clinical Informatics*, *2*(2), 128–142. doi:10.4338/ACI-2010-10-R-0060 PMID:23616865

Cairns, P., Cox, A. L., Day, M., Martin, H., & Perryman, T. (2013). Who but not where: The effect of social play on immersion in digital games. *International Journal of Human-Computer Studies*, *71*(11), 1069–1077. doi:10.1016/j.ijhcs.2013.08.015

Coller, B. D., & Scott, M. J. (2009). Effectiveness of using a video game to teach a course in mechanical engineering. *Computers & Education*, *53*(3), 900–912. doi:10.1016/j.compedu.2009.05.012

Colwell, J., & Payne, J. (2000). Negative correlates of computer game play in adolescents. *British Journal of Psychology*, *91*(3), 295–310. doi:10.1348/000712600161844 PMID:10958576

Connolly, T. M., Boyle, E. A., MacArthur, E., Hainey, T., & Boyle, J. M. (2012). A systematic literature review of empirical evidence on computer games and serious games. *Computers & Education*, *59*(2), 661–686. doi:10.1016/j.compedu.2012.03.004

Corrigan, S., Zon, G. D. R., Maij, A., McDonald, N., & Mårtensson, L. (2014). An approach to collaborative learning and the serious game development. *Cognition Technology and Work*, *17*(2), 269–278. doi:10.1007/s10111-014-0289-8

Csikszentmihalyi, M. (1975). *Beyond Boredom and Anxiety*. San Francisco: Jossey-Bass.

Csikszentmihalyi, M. (1991). *Flow: The psychology of optimal experience*. New York, NY: Harper Collins Publisher.

Csikszentmihalyi, M. (2000). Finding Flow. The Psychology of Engagement with Everyday Life. *Journal of Happiness Studies*, *1*(1), 121–123. doi:10.1023/A:1010032312178

Dandeneau, S. D., & Baldwin, M. W. (2004). The Inhibition of Socially Rejecting Information Among People with High Versus Low Self-Esteem: The Role of Attentional Bias and the Effects of Bias Reduction Training. *Journal of Social and Clinical Psychology*, *23*(4), 584–603. doi:10.1521/jscp.23.4.584.40306

De Grove, F., Van Looy, J., Courtois, C., & De Marez, L. (2010). I play, therefore I learn? Measuring the evolution of perceived learning and game experience in the design flow of a serious game. *Proceedings of meaningful play* (pp. 1–32). East Lansing: Michigan State University.

Deterding, S., Dixon, D., Khaled, R., & Nacke, L. (2011). From game design elements to gamefulness: defining gamification. *Proceedings of the 15th International Academic MindTrek Conference: Envisioning Future Media Environments* (pp. 9-15). ACM. doi:10.1145/2181037.2181040

Edery, D., & Mollick, E. (2009). *Changing the game: how video games are transforming the future of business*. Upper Saddle River, NJ: FT Press.

Ermi, L., & Mäyrä, F. (2005). Fundamental Components of the Gameplay Experience: Analysing Immersion. In S. De Castell & J. Jenson (Eds.), *Worlds in Play. International on Digital Games* (pp. 15–27). New York, NY: Peter Lang Publishing.

Fisher, G., Giaccardi, E., Eden, H., Sugimoto, M., & Ye, Y. (2005). Beyond binary choices: Integrating individual and social creativity. *International Journal of Human-Computer Studies*, *12*, 428–512.

Freeman, D. (2004). Creating emotion in games. *Computers in Entertainment*, *2*(3), 15. doi:10.1145/1027154.1027179

Fulleron, T. (2014). *Game Design Workshop: a Playcentric Approach to Creating Innovative Games*. Taylor & Francis Press.

Gaggioli, A., Riva, G., Milani, L., & Mazzoni, E. (2013). *Networked Flow: Towards an understanding of creative networks*. New York, NY: Springer. doi:10.1007/978-94-007-5552-9

Gajadhar, B., de Kort, Y. W., & IJsselsteijn, W. (2008). Shared Fun Is Doubled Fun: Player Enjoyment as a Function of Social Setting. In P. Markopoulos, B. de Ruyter, W. IJsselsteijn, & D. Rowland (Eds.), *Fun and Games SE - 11* (Vol. 5294, pp. 106–117). Berlin, Germany: Springer Berlin Heidelberg. doi:10.1007/978-3-540-88322-7_11

Gee, J. P. (2003). *What Video Games Have to Teach Us About Learning and Literacy* (2nd ed.). London, UK: Palgrave Macmillan.

Gentile, D. A., & Anderson, C. A. (2003). Violent video games: The newest media violence hazard. *Media Violence and Children*, 131–152.

Girard, C., Ecalle, J., & Magnan, A. (2013). Serious games as new educational tools: How effective are they? A meta-analysis of recent studies. *Journal of Computer Assisted Learning*, *29*(3), 207–219. doi:10.1111/j.1365-2729.2012.00489.x

Grasby, P. M., Koepp, M. J., Gunn, R. N., Lawrence, A. D., Cunningham, V. J., Dagher, A., & Bench, C. J. et al. (1998). Evidence for striatal dopamine release during a video game. *Nature*, *393*(6682), 266–268. doi:10.1038/30498 PMID:9607763

Gunawardena, C. N. (1995). Social Presence Theory and Implications for Interaction and Collaborative Learning in Computer Conferences. *International Journal of Educational Telecommunications*, *1*(2), 147–166.

Gunter, G. A., Kenny, R. F., & Vick, E. H. (2008). Taking educational games seriously: Using the RETAIN model to design endogenous fantasy into standalone educational games. *Educational Technology Research and Development*, *56*(5-6), 511–537. doi:10.1007/s11423-007-9073-2

Huizinga, J. (1950). *Homo Ludens: A study of the play - element in culture. A study of the element of play in culture*. London, UK: Routledge.

Ijsselsteijn, W., & Riva, G. (2003). Being There: The experience of presence in mediated environments. *Being There: Concepts. Effects and Measurement of User Presence in Synthetic Environments*, *10*, 14.

Kiili, K., Lainema, T., de Freitas, S., & Arnab, S. (2014). Flow framework for analyzing the quality of educational games. *Entertainment Computing*, *3*, 14–19.

Kiili, K., Perttula, A., Lindstedt, A., Arnab, S., & Suominen, M. (in press). Flow Experience as a Quality Measure in Evaluating Physically Activating Collaborative Serious Games. *International Journal of Serious Games*.

Koster, R. (2004). *Theory of fun for game design*. Paraglyph Press.

Kreijns, K., Kirschner, P. A., & Jochems, W. (2003). Identifying the pitfalls for social interaction in computer-supported collaborative learning environments: A review of the research. *Computers in Human Behavior*, *19*(3), 335–353. doi:10.1016/S0747-5632(02)00057-2

Kreijns, K., Kirschner, P. A., & Jochems, W. M. G. (2002). The sociability of computer-supported collaborative learning environments. *Journal of Educational Technology & Society*, *5*, 8–22.

Ligtenberg, A., de Vries, B., Vreenegoor, R., & Bulens, J. (2010). SimLandScape, a sketching tool for collaborative spatial planning. *URBAN DESIGN International*.

Malone, T. W., & Lepper, M. R. (1987). Making learning fun: A taxonomy of intrinsic motivations for Learning. In R. E. Snow & M. J. Farr (Eds.), *Aptitude, learning and instruction: Cognitive and affective process analyses* (pp. 223–253). Hillsdale: Erlbaum.

Mayer, I. S., van Dierendonck, D., van Ruijven, T., & Wenzler, I. (2013, October 23-25). Stealth Assessment of Teams in a Digital Game Environment. *Proceedings of the GALA 2013 Conference,* Paris (pp. 1–13). Springer. doi:10.1007/978-3-319-12157-4_18

McCallum, S. (2012). Gamification and serious games for personalized health. *Studies in Health Technology and Informatics*, *177*, 85–96. PMID:22942036

McGonigal, J. (2010). *Reality is broken*. New York, NY, USA: The Penguin Press.

McQuiggan, S. W., Rowe, J. P., Lee, S., & Lester, J. C. (2008). Story-Based Learning: The Impact of Narrative on Learning Experiences and Outcomes. *Intelligent Tutoring System, LNCS* (Vol. *5091*, 530–539). doi:10.1007/978-3-540-69132-7_56

Michael, D., & Chen, S. (2006). *Serious Games: Games That Educate, Train and Inform*. Boston: Thomson.

Mitgutsch, K., & Alvarado, N. (2012, May). Purposeful by design?: a serious game design assessment framework. *Proceedings of the International Conference on the foundations of digital games* (pp. 121-128). doi:10.1145/2282338.2282364

Myers, I. B. (1987). *Introduction to Type: A Description of the Theory and Applications of the Myers-Briggs Type Indicator*. Palo Alto: Consulting Psychologists Press.

Nacke, L., & Lindley, C. (2008). Boredom, Immersion, Flow - A pilot study investigating player experience. *Measurement*, *24*, 1–5.

Nacke, L., & Lindley, C. (2009). Affective ludology, flow, and immersion in a first-person shooter: Measurement of player experience. *The Journal of the Canadian Game Studies Association*, *3*(5), 37–42.

Oksanen, K. (2014). Subjective Experience and Sociability in a Collaborative Serious Game. *Simulation & Gaming*, *44*(6), 767–793. doi:10.1177/1046878113513079

Paras, B. (2005). Game, motivation, and effective learning: An integrated model for educational game design. In *Proceedings of DIGRA 2005 Conference Changing Views – Worlds in Play.*

Sanders, E. B. (2002). From User-Centered to Participatory Design Approaches. *Design and the social sciences: Making connections*, 1-8.

Sawyer, K. R. (2003). *Group creativity: Music, theatre, collaboration. New York, NY*. New York: Basic Books.

Sawyer, K. R. (2008). *Group genius: The creative power of collaboration*. New York, NY: Oxford University Press.

Searle, J. (1983). *Intentionality*. Cambridge: Cambridge University Press. doi:10.1017/CBO9781139173452

Shaker, N., Yannakakis, G., & Togelius, J. (2010). Towards Automatic Personalized Content Generation for Platform Games. *Proceedings of AIIDE 2010 - 6th. Digital Entertainment*.

Shandley, K., Austin, D., Klein, B., & Kyrios, M. (2010). An evaluation of "Reach Out Central": An online gaming program for supporting the mental health of young people. *Health Education Research*, *25*(4), 563–574. doi:10.1093/her/cyq002 PMID:20150530

Shandley, K., Klein, B., & Austin, D. (2008). The players' perspective of Reach Out Central: A therapeutic interactive online game. *E-Journal of Applied Psychology*, *4*(2), 51–55. doi:10.7790/ejap.v4i2.132

Slager, K., Ligtenberg, A., de Vries, B., & de Waard, R. S. (2007). Simlandscape: Serious Gaming in Participatory Spatial Planning. *Proceedings of the 10th AGILE International Conference on Geographic Information Science.*

Stapleton, A. J. (2004). Serious Games: Serious Opportunities. *Health Care*, *1*, 1–6.

Steiner, I. D. (1972). *Group process and productivity*. New York, NY: Academic Press.

Susi, T., Johanesson, M., & Backlund, P. (2007). *Serious Games - An Overview*. Skövde, Sweden: University of Skövde Press.

Sweetser, P., & Wyeth, P. (2005). GameFlow: A Model for Evaluating Player Enjoyment in Games. *Comput. Entertain.*, *3*(3), 1–24. doi:10.1145/1077246.1077253

Sweller, J. (1994). Cognitive load theory, learning difficulty and instructional design. *Learning and Instruction*, *4*(4), 295–312. doi:10.1016/0959-4752(94)90003-5

Takatalo, J., Nyman, G., & Laaksonen, L. (2008). Components of human experience in virtual environments. *Computers in Human Behavior*, *24*(1), 1–15. doi:10.1016/j.chb.2006.11.003

Tu, C.-H., & McIsaac, M. (2002). The Relationship of Social Presence and Interaction in Online Classes. *American Journal of Distance Education*, *16*(3), 131–150. doi:10.1207/S15389286AJDE1603_2

Van Rooij, A. J., Meerkerk, G.-J., Schoenmakers, T. M., Griffiths, M., & van de Mheen, D. (2010). Video game addiction and social responsibility. *Addiction Research and Theory*, *18*(5), 489–493. doi:10.3109/16066350903168579

Van Rooij, A. J., Schoenmakers, T. M., Vermulst, A. A., Van Den Eijnden, R. J. J. M., & Van De Mheen, D. (2011). Online video game addiction: Identification of addicted adolescent gamers. *Addiction (Abingdon, England)*, *106*(1), 205–212. doi:10.1111/j.1360-0443.2010.03104.x PMID:20840209

Wattanasoontorn, V., Boada, I., García, R., & Sbert, M. (2013). Serious games for health. *Entertainment Computing*, *4*(4), 231–247. doi:10.1016/j.entcom.2013.09.002

Wouters, P., van Nimwegen, C., van Oostendorp, H., & van der Spek, E. D. (2013). A meta-analysis of the cognitive and motivational effects of serious games. *Journal of Educational Psychology*, *105*(2), 249–265. doi:10.1037/a0031311

Yoo, Y., & Alavi, M. (2001). The Relationship of Social Presence and Interaction in Online Classes. *Management Information Systems Quarterly*, *25*(3), 371–390. doi:10.2307/3250922

Zyda, M. (2005). From Visual Simulation to Virtual Reality to Games. *Computer*, *38*(9), 25–32. doi:10.1109/MC.2005.297

# Chapter 11
# Video Games:
## Developing Resilience, Competence, and Mastery

**Jennifer G. Tichon**
*Griffith University, Australia*

**Dominicus Tornqvist**
*Griffith University, Australia*

## ABSTRACT

*Until recently, research on video games has been concerned largely with negative effects of play. Increasingly, however, a range of positive psychological effects of playing video games are being reported. Being able to identify positive impacts is an important step toward leveraging the huge appeal of game playing to aid psychological well-being. This chapter discusses a range of benefits associated with playing two genres of popular off-the-shelf video games as opposed to video games that have been constructed to specifically target education or teach health-related lessons. With the video game phenomenon set to have an ever-increasing impact across society on a global scale, knowledge of games that have the potential to meet positive psychological needs will be critical to leveraging positive outcomes from video game play.*

## INTRODUCTION

Video games often get a bad rap in both the research and the media for having a range of negative outcomes, including creating aggressive feelings, thoughts and behaviors in users. However, psychological research examining video games is presently undergoing a dramatic shift in focus. Until very recently, the preponderance of research in video games has been concern-focused, with studies aimed at identifying the potential negative effects of gaming. This has included the relationships between gaming and increased aggression, social isolation, and overuse, as well as association with poor performance at school (Gentile, Lynch, Linder, & Walsh, 2004; Fleming & Rickwood, 2001). Positive outcomes of computer games have generally been restricted to learning outcomes such as improved sensorimotor

DOI: 10.4018/978-1-4666-9986-1.ch011

skills (e.g. Green, Pouget, & Bavelier, 2010; Gozli, Bavelier, & Pratt, 2014). More recently, though, positive outcomes have been reported, such as improving healthy attitudes and behaviors (Greitmeyer, Osswald, & Brauer, 2010; Khalil, 2012).

A number of researchers have become intervention focused, hoping to harness the magnetic motivational appeal of video games to help relieve pain and stress, or customizing games for educational or health-related interventions (for a review, see Baranowski, Buday, Thompson, & Baranowski, 2008). These investigations often employ "serious games"—games that were designed explicitly to produce a specific benefit such as education. Increasingly, intervention-focused researchers are demonstrating that commercial games (designed just for fun rather than to promote wellbeing) can positively influence both psychological and physical wellbeing (Przybylski, Rigby, & Ryan, 2010). This chapter focuses on the ways in which two different genres of commercial games (role-playing games and sandbox games) can develop general-purpose skills of resilience and adaptation to master complex challenges in life.

## BACKGROUND

Although the goals of concern-focused and intervention-focused research are dissimilar, both share a descriptive research approach, in that the methods and theories they employ evaluate the extent to which video games exert positive, negative, or no influence on specified outcomes under a given set of circumstances. Less well understood and less widely studied are the mediating variables that underlie positive links. These include immersion/presence, interaction/movement, and motivation to play.

### Immersion/Presence

Immersion is an influential factor in both effective professional or "serious" games and games played for fun. It is has been shown to play a facilitative role in enhancing the effects of video games to positively affect players' self-esteem and affect (see, e.g., Granic, Lobel, & Engels, 2014; Przybylski, Rigby, & Ryan, 2010; Van Den Hoogen, IJsselsteijn, & De Kort, 2009). Immersion occurs when a player experiences a strong sense of presence in the game world. Immersion reflects an *illusion of nonmediation* between the player and the gaming context, so that the player feels directly embedded in the virtual environment and within the story that is happening there (Lombard & Ditton, 1997). The success or otherwise of a video game in immersing players shapes how the content of the game serves to influence player psychology. Prior research into video games has investigated presence through three subcomponents or subscales: *physical presence*, or feeling as if one is actually in the world; *emotional presence*, or feeling that game events have real emotional weight; and *narrative presence*, or having a personal investment in and engagement with the story (Ryan, Rigby, & Przybylski, 2006). Although these three components of immersion are thought to be highly collinear, they have different profiles within different games. Some games, for example, have little narrative but afford a strong physical sense of presence—such as a sport version of swordplay, like Wii fencing—while others, such as Wii's fantasy game *Legend of Zelda*, which embeds the swordplay within a full fantasy adventure—offer a much stronger narrative presence to the player.

Many game designers and players assume that a sense of immersion is based mainly on the fidelity of the graphics and sound provided by a virtual environment. However, prior research suggests that this is not the case (Tichon & Banks, 2006). Instead, the major predictor of presence is the degree to which a game is psychologically engaging. When players have their needs satisfied within the game, they are more phenomenologically embedded in the emotional, physical, and narrative elements of the game world (Przybylski et al., 2010; Ryan et al., 2006). Additionally, the work of Weinstein, Przybylski, and Ryan (2009) suggests that feeling physically present in a virtual context can intensify the carryover of the content of that context into real-world cognition and behavior.

## Interaction/Movement

The extent and degree to which a player must move to interact with a game has long been thought to have a direct influence on how immersed they become in the game world. Movement is important in terms of facilitating and increasing the amount of interaction between a player and game. The premise is that the more a player interacts, the more present in the game they will become. From a health perspective, increased movement is also of interest for overcoming the dangers of a sedentary lifestyle. From the perspective of game designers, movement is of key interest because it is believed to enhance how a player feels emotionally when they interact with the technology (Schell, 2008, Swink, 2009). However, despite some interesting experiments with using movement in interfaces to convey emotion (Sundström, Stahl, & Hook, 2005), there have been no sustained and systematic attempts to investigate movement-based interaction and its association with emotional changes throughout the game.

Game developers have led commercial distribution of movement-based interaction platforms. The tremendous success of Nintendo's Wii platform convinced game companies that movement was something players valued and wanted more of, and that it was a way to gain an even broader audience for gaming. Within gaming, the core definition of success for a game is that a person enjoys the game enough to keep playing it, rather than that it helps the person to achieve a specific training or task outcome. This puts a great deal of emphasis on how the experience feels—particularly the player's emotions.

Isbister (2011) has been investigating how movements evoke desired feelings for players. Despite the best attempts of developers, video games are not all created equal in this respect. For example, one dancing game might produce exhilaration and joy, while another might create tension and frustration, through the qualities of the movements players have to perform. Part of Isbister's work has been to develop methods to isolate and evaluate the impact of movement on how the player is feeling. These have had to account for the complex nature of games media, which use many components—animation, sound, and a reward system, among others—to contribute to their overall effect.

Isbister has found that vigorous higher degrees of movement lead to reports of higher arousal, and that players reported a greater sense of social connectedness when playing in the movement condition. In conjunction with the NYU Games for Learning Institute, which focuses on discovering and validating design patterns for building effective learning games, Isbister is investigating how the feel of movement mechanics can contribute to learning outcomes. Recent outcomes have demonstrated that striking "high-power" poses for just two minutes leads to changes in people's biochemistry (higher testosterone levels, lower cortisone levels) as well as greater risk tolerance when completing a sample task directly after play (Carney, Cuddy, & Yap, 2010). In essence, this research supports the popular view that one should pose as confident in order to feel confident. Studies have shown that being in a mildly positive mood enhances creativity (Isen, Daubman, & Nowicki, 1987); in a similar vein, Isbister's (2011) exploratory results suggest that the feel of movement can be used to produce a range of performance- and attitude-enhancing effects on task-based system interaction.

Looking at the effects of movement on both positive emotion and learning outcomes, it would seem that video games which use movement to interact with the game—and specifically a higher level and degree of movement—should result in better outcomes in terms of players' levels of self-esteem, self-mastery, and psychological resilience.

## The Need to Play

As mentioned, one of the most significant concerns about video game play is the selection of games available that contain highly violent content. However, research suggests that violent game content is not, on average, a significant motivator of play or source of enjoyment. In fact, although violent game content appeals more to players who are dispositionally high in aggression, violence was a weak and unreliable motivator of play or source of enjoyment even for them (Przybylski, Ryan, & Rigby, 2009; Przybylski et al., 2010). For most players, violent content was unrelated to game appeal. Significantly, within-person, between-games analyses have shown that play experiences that support the psychological need for autonomy and competence produce more enjoyable and more immersive play that enhances player self-esteem and affect (Przybylski et al., 2010).

According to Przybylski and colleagues' (2010) motivational model, based on self-determination theory (Ryan & Deci, 2000), "video games have the potential to enhance intrinsic motivation and short-term well-being insofar as they provide players with experiences that satisfy universal psychological needs" (Przybylski et al., 2010: 157). This perspective emphasizes motivational processes inherent in the structure of gaming contexts—that is, games are generally more or less appealing, and have a greater or lesser influence on player wellbeing, as a function of the extent to which the in-game experiences fulfil fundamental psychological needs. Research suggests that the broad appeal of games lies in the psychological need satisfaction that can be provided by play; that these motivational processes are robust predictors over and above differences in player demographics; and that they apply across game genres and content.

Psychological research also suggests that the fun element in video games may also be enjoyed most because it addresses psychological needs. Evidence suggests that video games meet many such needs. Mellou (1994) provides an overview of the progression of play research. Initially, it was dismissed as burning off excess energy when all other needs were satisfied. It was also seen as a form of imitation—of teaching children how to "do" adult activities. However, the range of benefits and motivations for play in adults has gradually been accumulating. It appears that there is no single purpose of play—no one psychological need that it has evolved to satisfy. Play encompasses many diverse, complex behaviors found in people at all stages of development, and those behaviors satisfy many different psychological needs.

Nacke, Bateman and Mandryk (2011) suggest that video game play satisfies a collection of needs to varying degrees, where some players might focus more heavily on different needs than others. For example, in this model, the Seeker enjoys wonder, curiosity, and discovery, while the Survivor enjoys the terror of danger. Play could also serve the psychological need of maintaining optimal sensory stimulation and cognitive arousal (Grodal, 2000). There are many other psychological needs that could be satisfied by play: catharsis, self-expression, or the contentment of productivity and progression. This chapter focuses on three primary areas of psychological need: competence, mastery and resilience.

Two genres of video game design that support positive psychological outcomes will be discussed. First, game designs will be explored that support the development of psychological resilience and improved self-esteem—specifically, video games in which a player's character must overcome adversity and in which the player's progress in the game is matched to gradually increased levels of challenge. These are generally referred to as role-playing games (RPG), with progressive difficulty levels. The second type of game genre discussed is referred to as Sandbox games. These games are designed purely for "fun," through exploratory play; no specific way exists to "win" the game. With no well-defined, ultimate goal, players find their own fun. Both role-play and exploratory play in video games have largely been overlooked in research, despite them having the potential to provide insight into the possible positive psychological outcomes of video game play.

## ROLE-PLAYING GAMES WITH PROGRESSIVE DIFFICULTY LEVELS

Role-playing games (RPG) are interactive worlds where players assume the role of a fictional character and determine their actions based on the mindset of their character. Players typically follow a set story-line, which involves successfully completing missions and achieving set goals:

*As the player completes quests and overcomes conflicts, his/her character advances in levels and becomes stronger. Typically as the player advances in levels, game challenges increase ... as a player becomes more proficient with the game and his/her character becomes tougher, the amount of experience or other metric needed to advance a level should be more than the amount needed on the previous level. (Bostan & Ogut, 2009: 2)*

RPG video games that involve overcoming many obstacles to get to the next level, and learning to "power up" by hitting or jumping on something that will provide the strength to keep going, share values similar to those of real life, where individuals need to learn to cope with a variety of stresses, keep on going, and learn along the way how to "bounce back up." All these skills are aspects of resilience.

Researchers and society alike are concerned with how people bounce back or recover from stress and adapt to stressful circumstances (Smith et al., 2008). Psychological resilience can ameliorate the effects of stress and promote recovery. The development of resilience also plays a key role in promoting health and preventing disease. While resilience research has focused primarily on the personal characteristics associated with effective coping, a few recent studies have investigated the effectiveness of targeted resilience training (Burton, Pakenham, & Brown, 2010) and its effects on both psychological and physical health. Games in which characters must overcome adversity through picking themselves up and trying again should exert an influence on the players' real-life behavior via changes in the individual's automatic self-concept. A resilient individual will be one for whom 'bouncing back' has become an automatic trait.

### Can Psychological Resilience Be Trained?

Over the past decade, resilience increasingly has become a focus of research in the behavioral and medical sciences. Resilience has been defined in a variety of ways, including as the ability to bounce back or recover from stress, to adapt to stressful circumstances, to not become ill despite significant adversity, and to function above the norm in spite of stress or adversity (Smith et al., 2008). In addition, there has been some debate as to whether the measures that have been developed to assess "resilience" have not focused on resilience itself, but rather on the factors and resources that make being resilient possible (Ahern, Kiehl, Sole, & Buyers, 2006). In 2008, Smith and colleagues developed a resilience scale for assessing the original and most basic meaning of the word resilience—to bounce or spring back—making the argument that the ability to bounce back or recover from stress is important to assess and study in its own right.

In current military training, resilience appears as a set of cognitive skills that anyone can develop, given the correct training. Founded in cognitive behavioral therapy, "resilience centres innovativeness, enterprise, responsibility and flexibility" (O'Malley 2010: 488). This shift from viewing resilience as being made up of elements of human attributes to reconfiguring it as a set of skills that can be learned is embodied in the programs of resilience training adopted by the US, Canadian, and Australian defense forces (O'Malley, 2010). Outside the military, most studies of resilience have focused on young people or individuals experiencing specific adverse circumstances, and have explored the personal characteristics associated with effective coping (Burton et al., 2009). The lack of investigation into whether resilience can be trained or enhanced in civilians, and how this might best be achieved, is surprising. In the area of preventative health, the potential of psychosocial resilience training to promote wellbeing has recently been investigated (Burton et al., 2009). Outdoor education philosophers have argued for some time that controlled exposure to challenge can also be used to train psychological resilience (Neill & Dias, 2012). Much adventure philosophy emphasizes the need for humans to encounter the boundaries of their physical and psychological possibilities in order to enhance their capacity to deal with everyday life.

The complexity of defining the construct of resilience has been recognized widely, and creates problems for developing an operational definition of resilience. Ryff and Keyes (1995) conceptualize resilience as a psychological quality that allows a person to cope with, and to respond effectively to, life stressors. This conceptualization focuses on resilience at the level of the individual, and does not include the availability of resources from family and community—which, although important, can alternatively be conceptualized as the resources that support resiliency. In a recent methodological review of 17 resilience measurement scales (Windle, Bennett, & Noyes, 2001), the Brief Resilience Scale was one of only three measures to receive the highest ratings across all quality criteria. This scale specifically avoids items that measure the resources that might facilitate a resilient outcome; instead, the scale was developed with a specific focus on bouncing back from stress.

## Performing under Stress: Computer-Based Training for Professionals

Computer-based training via both high-end simulators and PC-based game applications (referred to as serious games) has been used as a tool for training professionals for high-stress operations across the military, aviation, railway, and mining industries for many years (Tichon & Wallis, 2010). It has always been a goal of simulation training to expose trainees gradually to increasing levels of stress until they are able to tolerate a significantly higher stressful state before they start to withdraw effort. Simulation training works on the premise that a professional's confidence in their ability to cope under pressure can be strengthened through training, where they have been given the opportunity to experience mastery while in a highly aroused state—for example, they have been able to work through fear and successfully translate it into high goal performance (Driskell & Johnston, 1998). This is very similar to the inherent nature of video games designed to gradually increase challenges in line with a player's progress in the game. This gradual training effect is critical to gaming success: if players are under-challenged, they will become bored, but if they are over-challenged, they may become frustrated. Either effect will result in a loss of interest in the game (Przybylski et al., 2010).

Within professional training applications, content that deliberately influences emotion is an area that is receiving increasing attention. In simulator training for first responders to terrorist attacks, it was ascertained that higher levels of perceived emotional intensity were linked to more effective learning (Tichon, Hall, & Higlers, 2003; Hall et al., 2004). This indicates that emotion is a key variable in understanding the success of computer-based training to overcome stress. Additionally, research in psychology indicates that emotions play an essential role in the development of cognitive skills (Norman, 2004). Negative emotional states such as stress can have a negative effect on decision-making and problem-solving through causing undue anxiety or fear, overestimation of risks and avoidant choices (Peters, Lipkus, & Diefenbach, 2006).

Computer-based stress training provides lessons in how to draw on an optimal blend of reason and emotion. Trainees learn how to ignore their fear when fear isn't useful, and how to make quick, complicated decisions in the most fraught of situations (Lehrer, 2009). These training applications provide the opportunity to put these skills to the test by practicing the achievement of goals while under stress. A further aim of the proposed research is to investigate whether video games that support the development of increased competence via paced progress in a game where a player's character may be facing life-and-death challenges could be achieving similar psychological resilience training outcomes for game players.

Research into the impact of video games has revealed that exposure leads to automatic associations with the self—that is, players associate themselves with the same traits as their characters in the game. This occurs because game playing increases the automatic accessibility of traits associated with the self during the game, in the player's memory (Uhlmann & Swanson, 2004). Additionally, video games are designed to increase challenges gradually, in line with a player's progress in the game. This gradual exposure effect is critical to gamer motivation to stay in the game, and therefore to gaming success. It is also the same approach used in professional domains, where computer-based resilience training is designed to gradually expose trainees to increasing levels of stress (Driskell & Johnson, 1998). The goal is to provide the opportunity for trainees, through repetition, to gain confidence in their ability to maintain optimum performance under pressure. Are video games gradually training players to feel confident under pressure and through trait association? Equally, are players transferring these positive psychological effects to their real-world lives?

The pacing of challenges in games is designed so players can continually experience enhanced competence as they progress in the game, with challenges increasing in pace with player ability. In *Halo 3*, the internet is used to match players against one another on the basis of their history of in-game performance. The music game *Guitar Hero* uses an in-game audience of non-playing characters to provide continuous feedback, as these characters cheer and scream if the player performs well. These aspects of game play also appear to provide reinforcing aspects of personal strengths that correspond to a resilient personality—namely a sense of mastery and self-esteem.

Game players may learn resilience through unintended training and trait association outcomes of playing some video games. In a recent exploratory study of the Playstation blog Blog.us.playstation.com, it was found that, while the resilience topic was not specifically sought through the forum, over one-third of participants voluntarily discussed how experiences and lessons learned via game play had helped them to feel more resilient in real-life situations. Game players reported that popular off-the-shelf video games had gradually taught them, through challenges, to be confident in their abilities. Significantly, some players also reported transferring these positive psychological effects to their real-world lives (Tichon & Mavin, in press). Role-playing games where a player's character must overcome adversity do appear to exert an influence on their self-identity in the real world.

## SANDBOX GAMES AND EXPLORATORY PLAY

Games have been used in a variety of educational contexts (for reviews, see Clark, Tanner-Smith & Killingsworth, 2015; McClarty et al., 2012). While there are many forms of play in games, exploratory play is a behavior motivated by curiosity and the drive for competence and mastery (Jennings, Harmon, Morgan, Gaiter, & Yarrow, 1979; Keller, Schneider, & Henderson, 1994; Lorenz, 1981; Tornqvist, 2014). The capacity for spontaneous exploratory play to help development of one's understanding of a system has been observed in constructivist learning paradigms (e.g. Baytak, Land, & Smith, 2011; Mitra & Dangwal, 2010) and has received experimental support (e.g. see Cook, Goodman, & Schulz, 2011; Gopnik & Schulz, 2007).

In sandbox video games, it is asserted that the fun of playing them is derived entirely from the process of learning how to interact with and master the game system. Koster (2005) defines fun itself as the process of mastery. He argues that the development and eventual perfection of the strategy is the process that yields fun for players. Thus the primary appeal of a game lies not in being successful at pursuing one's goals, but rather in the process of *becoming* successful at the patterns the game demands. Koster (2005) points out that children are initially fascinated by tic-tac-toe. However, once they figure out the optimal strategy, every game ends in a draw and the game ceases to hold any interest for them. This observation would suggest that the process of learning is central to the fun of at least some games. The sandbox genre of video games also fosters an attitude of experimentation, metacognition, and creative problem solving via the low-risk environment of sandbox play. In particular, many design features of sandbox games relate to teaching how to adapt to complex systems.

Psychological research suggests that the "fun" element in these games may also be enjoyed because they address the key psychological needs of competency and mastery. Additionally, the quest to satisfy curiosity that underlies exploratory play also makes it a valuable learning mechanism. Curiosity is a powerful motivator that is "highly transient but, at the same time, quite intense" (Loewenstein, 1994: 86). It compels the player to make the item of interest the focus of their attention to absorb perceptual information (van Schijndel, Franse, & Raijmakers, 2010). Rubin (2001) considers exploratory behavior to be characterized by focusing perceptual attention upon a subject of interest to satisfy curiosity. Ruff and Saltarelli (1993) primarily distinguish exploratory and non-exploratory play by whether or not the player is focused intensely on the toy. However, learning about a system from passive observation alone, without interaction, ranges from difficult to impossible (Gopnik & Schulz, 2007; Gopnik & Wellman, 2012). Furthermore, play demands action—one cannot play without participating or interacting, as that would just be viewing, listening, or resting (Juul, 2005). This is where the motivation of mastery becomes integral to the sandbox video game genre. Exploratory play consists of impulsive interventions that test hypotheses and whittle away possible causal structures until only one remains. This play teaches the player about causality, and therefore about how to exert control. Thus curiosity and mastery combine to form an extremely useful behavior that is crucial to both educational and "fun" games.

Despite being systematic, exploratory play is also non-routine. It is a spontaneous behavior unconcerned with conforming to an ultimate goal or productive purpose for each impulsive intervention (Jennings et al., 1979; Schulz, Standing & Bonawitz, 2008). Although the interventions are informative, to the player they just seem like a string of unrelated fun things to try. All these characteristics of exploratory play match well with sandbox game play. The desire to satisfy curiosity and develop mastery of the system is a central motivation of play in sandboxes (Breslin, 2009; Stewart, 2014). It is also often described in terms of conducting impulsive interventions just to observe the results (Breslin, 2009; Calhoun, 2010).

The interventions during play in sandboxes are systematic and non-routine because the player goes to great lengths to find new ways to do things and new things to do (Calhoun, 2010). The interventions are not bound to any common, overarching goal, which is possibly the most defining and interesting characteristic of this form of play: Players seem to select an immediate goal and act upon it with no regard for the next goal but, once completed, a new goal is generated and the process starts over again. Thus the exploratory play found in sandbox games entails a combination of characteristics that produces just the right environment for unrestricted experimentation.

Sandbox games emphasize player agency and creativity, giving players open choice not only of what to do, but also how to accomplish it. This is a promising design philosophy in light of research indicating that when people are told what to do, it discourages exploration or experimentation (Bonawitz et al., 2011; Burns & Vollmeyer, 2002; Horner & Whiten, 2005). Players seem more eager to test hypotheses when they are given non-specific goals, or when they are presented with a hypothesis to test (Burns & Vollmeyer, 2002). Bonawitz and colleagues (2011) suggest that, since the efficiency of direct instruction comes at the cost of exploration, perhaps instruction should be reserved for contexts where the teacher has full knowledge of what the learner needs to know. In contexts where the teacher doesn't have sufficient knowledge or enough time to impart full knowledge, such as when dealing with a complex system that exhibits unpredictable, emergent behaviors, it may be better to provide no instructions so as to maximize the tendency to explore. This is the domain in which games for learning (particularly sandbox games) show most promise: teaching players how to adapt to novel complexity.

The difficulty students have in grasping complex processes in science could be due to an over-reliance on linear, narrative-like models of cause and effect. Learning through games, such as sandboxes, provide an opportunity to develop an individual's systems thinking skills (Morris, Croker, Zimmerman, Gill, & Romig, 2013). Due to the interactive nature of games, they may offer unique benefits for learning about complex systems and adapting to unscripted, emergent situations. Schell (2008) claims that it is necessary to be surprised in order to have fun. According to Breslin (2009), the question, "What happens if I do this?" is part of play, and "any sufficiently complex game can be considered a sandbox if one of the aims of the players is to explore the implications of the game's rules" (Breslin, 2009: 4). Sandbox games are particularly relevant to developing an emergent schema, since a core characteristic of the genre is emergent game play (Glean, 2005; Kickmeier-Rust & Albert, 2009; Stewart, 2014; Sweetser, 2008). Emergent game play is defined as a simple set of underlying rules that result in complex overall behavior (Sweetser, 2008). The aim is to have the game produce situations and events that surprise even the game designer. Varying the conditions and context like this can improve adaptability and the transfer of procedural knowledge to novel situations (Clark, 2009).

Games of emergence are in direct contrast to games of progression. In content-focused games of progression, the player sequentially plays through levels constructed by the game designer. In system-focused games of emergence, the encounters simply arise out of the rules of the game, and solutions to problems can be found by leveraging knowledge of the game rules to turn the situation to the player's favor. Data intensity runs the risk of players developing narrowly useful rote procedures for dealing with familiar problems. They might become very good at dealing with one set of challenges that they have played through many times, but they may not be good at much else. For example, in a racing game where the player has to do multiple laps of the same circuit, they might learn that to get around the sharp corner they should start to turn when they pass the red sign. This is a very narrow heuristic with no other applications. Compare this with a racing game that doesn't involve laps, but procedurally generates new road as needed. This would force the player to develop their general (improvisational) driving skills if they wanted to master the game. Thus maximally process-intensive games are more or less "walkthrough-proof." They don't allow players to rely on scenario-specific formulae to master the game. These games render direct instructions useless, in favor of strategies and skills.

Process-intensive games require that players create their own solutions to emergent problems, and sandbox games positively encourage this. Creative problem solving is enhanced by creating a low-stress, positive-affect environment (Baas, De Dreu, & Nijstad, 2008). Providing a playful environment that includes the freedom to fail is something at which sandboxes excel. It has also been found that gamers are generally more creative than non-gamers (Jackson et al., 2012), and Gallagher and Prestwich (2013) found that frequent gamers had better cognitive skills for cognitive adaptability than infrequent gamers. Players need to be open and adaptable when faced with surprising results in order to thrive in sandbox games. Squire, Barnett, Grant, and Higginbotham (2004) were able to get students to confront their misconceptions about electromagnetism by giving them direct interactive experience with a game on the subject.

A central skill in scientific thinking is metacognition—self-monitoring and self-regulating to identify and correct errors in one's thinking (Schneider, 2008). This ability to stop and figure out where things went wrong is valuable in a variety of domains, but importantly it is a necessary skill to succeed in most games. Gamers persist for longer with difficult problems (Ventura, Shute, & Zhao, 2013), and Ravaja and colleagues (2005) even found that positive affect resulted from failure events in games, which is consistent with the theory that play relies on the joy of the unexpected and the opportunity to improve. Hsu, Tsai and Wang (2012) were able to integrate self-explanation prompts into an educational game, and Kim, Park, and Baek (2008) found that games could be used to practice meta-cognitive skills. Barton and colleagues (2015) found a purpose-built game to be more effective than traditional instruction in helping students recognise and mitigate cognitive biases. Blumberg, Rosenthal, and Randall (2008) found that players who frequently articulated their thought processes also performed better, suggesting that self-monitoring has a natural benefit in gaming contexts. Gozli, Bavelier, and Pratt (2014) concluded that the benefits of game play are not in better sensorimotor control, but rather in accelerated sensorimotor learning—when they play, people aren't learning how to do all tasks better; they are learning how to learn. When faced with complex systems and emergent situations, a player cannot rely on rote procedures tailored to achieve a given goal with a given set of initial conditions; instead, the player is forced to develop strategies to quickly adapt to unforeseen circumstances, and to improvise a solution with whatever tools are to hand. Thus players may develop a set of *meta*strategies—strategies not for a particular system, but for quickly adapting to and developing new solutions for novel situations that they encounter. It is such game experiences that result in an increased sense of mastery and competence. In producing surprising and interesting situations, sandbox games are constantly developing players' metastrategies – an invaluable life skill when it comes to developing generalized competence.

## FUTURE RESEARCH DIRECTIONS

The cultural penetration of video games will only continue to increase. Therefore, an important agenda becomes that of employing new theoretical models and research designs to empirically explore these domains. New knowledge is needed to meaningfully inform more effective decisions from leaders in health and education arenas who are well placed to garner positive benefits from the widespread success of video games. Identifying the strengths of games will help those who are vulnerable to aggressive or addictive behaviors, and advance the basic science of what is going on when humans play.

Games in which characters must overcome adversity through picking themselves up and trying again should exert an influence on their real-life behavior via changes in the individual's automatic self-concept. The mediating variables that influence the ability of games to have this psychological impact are therefore most likely to be the same as those found in professional computer-based resilience training applications. They are immersion/presence and interaction/movement. Future research on the impact of video games should include these variables as moderating factors. It would seem that higher levels of emotional, physical, and narrative presence should correspond to higher scores on the self-esteem, self-mastery, and resilience scales.

Despite recent research indicating that games designed for "fun"—such as sandbox games—are linked to providing individuals with experiences that are meaningful and appreciated (Oliver et al., 2015), exploratory play in video games has been overlooked in many studies where it may have provided insight into the possible positive psychological outcomes of video game play. Sandbox games, which provide emergent play opportunities, appear to foster experimentation, metacognition, and creative problem solving. However, empirical examinations of the details are still under construction. Future research could compare the potential of games with traditional methods for increasing an individual's problem-solving and creative-thinking skills. Bogost's (2007) theory of procedural rhetoric is plausible: players pick up on the mechanics of games and what those mechanics are meant to represent in the real world, then go on to apply their mental model of the game to the real-world phenomena depicted. But this theory needs to be tested empirically. Chi, Roscoe, Slotta, Roy, and Chase (2011) demonstrated the effectiveness of direct instruction in helping students to develop an emergent schema and reduce misconceptions about complex processes in science. The next step is to compare such instructional methods to games with and without design features such as process intensity and sandbox game play to see whether they can help develop competence with novel complexity.

Similarly, while prior research has found that certain conditions improve people's ability to discard old models and adapt to a change in the system with which they are playing, it would be an important area of future research to extend these studies to establish whether the shift in people to be more adaptable and willing to change their mental models is lasting and transferrable. There is a gap in the literature concerning whether/how games can be used to create lasting improvements in curiosity, information foraging, and cognitive flexibility. There is great potential here, given the promise of games to increase people's creative problem solving, to explore further the use of games to actually train people to be more creative or have better general-purpose creative problem-solving skills.

## CONCLUSION

The effects of video games represent a contentious topic in society and in the media, with many legitimate concerns about the negative effects of game playing. Research has shown that video games are played extensively—for example, over 10 million players a week forgo other interests to invest more than 225 million hours in playing *World of Warcraft* (Przybylski et al., 2010). With more than 90% of individuals aged from 2 through 17 playing video games and sales of video games steadily increasing, their psychological effects are of great importance to both society and individual consumers. Recent shifts in video game research suggest some video games can have significant positive psychological effects, and there are as yet many untapped potential positive outcomes of video game play.

As discussed in this chapter, indications are that video games have a range of positive psychological effects. Research on games and player motivation derived from the psychological sciences has lagged behind the fast pace of developments in game design and the exponential expansion of game genres from which to choose. With the cultural penetration of video games constantly increasing, new approaches are needed to empirically explore and expand our understanding of both the positives and the negatives of immersion in these domains. More research on positive gaming is also required to support and inform decision-making around video gaming. If some video games can have more positive effects than others, then consumers and community leaders responsible for health and education policy decisions need this information. Currently, we are told what we should avoid about games, but not what games to choose for healthy outcomes.

The knowledge base in this field is severely restricted, and the potential benefits of video games remain largely unknown. Clearly, increasing knowledge in the area of potential positive aspects of popular video games is an important step toward supporting efforts to leverage the appeal of game playing to aid psychological wellbeing. Knowledge of popular off-the-shelf video games is primarily focused on problems of addiction and aggression. Yet examinations of video games for psychological health benefits are increasingly coming to the notice of health and education experts worldwide—although, in general, "games for health" have been designed specifically for a particular learning purpose. The study of computer games in wide community use in terms of positive psychological benefits still lags behind research targeting games specifically designed for educational and training purposes. This chapter has explored the positive psychological outcomes of play in the areas of resilience, competency, and autonomy. These outcomes have potential application across a number of areas of education and preventative health.

With the video game phenomenon set to have ever-increasing impact across society, more research to identify those games that can meet important psychological needs will be significant in its contribution to current efforts being undertaken to harness the widespread appeal of video games to leverage positive outcomes in society.

## REFERENCES


Ahern, N. R., Kiehl, E. M., Sole, M. L., & Byers, J. (2006). A review of instruments measuring resilience. *Issues in Comprehensive Pediatric Nursing*, *29*(2), 103–125. doi:10.1080/01460860600677643 PMID:16772239

Baas, M., De Dreu, C. K., & Nijstad, B. A. (2008). A meta-analysis of 25 years of mood-creativity research: Hedonic tone, activation, or regulatory focus? *Psychological Bulletin*, *134*(6), 779–806. doi:10.1037/a0012815 PMID:18954157

Baranowski, T., Buday, R., Thompson, D., & Baranowski, J. (2008). Playing for real: Video games and stories for health-related behavior change. *American Journal of Preventive Medicine*, *34*(1), 74–82. doi:10.1016/j.amepre.2007.09.027 PMID:18083454

Barton, M., Symborski, C., Quinn, M. M., Morewedge, C. K., Kassam, K. S., & Korris, J. H. (2015, May). The use of theory in designing a serious game for the reduction of cognitive biases. *Proceedings of the 2015 DiGRA International Conference DiGRA '15*, Digital Games Research Association.

Bateman, C. (2014). Empirical game aesthetics. In M. C. Angelides & H. Agius (Eds.), *Handbook of computer game studies* (pp. 411–442). Hoboken, NJ: John Wiley & Sons.

Baytak, A., Land, S. M. & Smith, B. K. (2011). Children as educational computer game designers: An exploratory study. *Turkish Online Journal of Educational Technology, 10*(4), 84–92.

Blumberg, F. C., Rosenthal, S. F., & Randall, J. D. (2008). Impasse-driven learning in the context of video games. *Computers in Human Behavior*, *24*(4), 1530–1541. doi:10.1016/j.chb.2007.05.010

Bogost, I. (2007). *Persuasive games: The expressive power of videogames*. Cambridge, MA: MIT Press.

Bonawitz, E., Shafto, P., Gweon, H., Goodman, N. D., Spelke, E., & Schulz, L. (2011). The double-edged sword of pedagogy: Instruction limits spontaneous exploration and discovery. *Cognition*, *120*(3), 322–330. doi:10.1016/j.cognition.2010.10.001 PMID:21216395

Bostan, B., & Öğüt, S. (2009). In pursuit of optimal gaming experience: Challenges and difficulty levels. *Paper presented at the Entertainment=Emotion Conference*, Spain. Retrieved from https://scholar.google.com/citations?view_op=view_citation&hl=en&user=JDYxzV0AAAAJ&citation_for_view=JDYxzV0AAAAJ:W7OEmFMy1HYC

Breslin, S. (2009). The history and theory of sandbox game play. *Gamasutra*. Retrieved from http://www.gamasutra.com/view/feature/4081/the_history_and_theory_of_sandbox_.php

Burns, B. D., & Vollmeyer, R. (2002). Goal specificity effects on hypothesis testing in problem solving. *Quarterly Journal of Experimental Psychology*, *55A*(1), 241–261. doi:10.1080/02724980143000262 PMID:11873850

Burton, N. W., Pakenham, K. I., & Brown, W. J. (2009). Evaluating the effectiveness of psychosocial resilience training for heart health, and the added value of promoting physical activity: A cluster randomized trial of the READY program. *BMC Public Health*, *9*(1), 247–255. doi:10.1186/1471-2458-9-427 PMID:19930615

Calhoun, A. (2010). A sociopathic comedy of errors, player cruelty in open world games and developer savviness. *Gamasutra*. Retrieved from http://www.gamasutra.com.blogs/AndrewCalhoun/20101018/88273/A_Sociopathic_Comedy_of_Errors_Player_Cruelty_in_ Open_World_Games_and_Developer_Savviness

Carney, D. R., Cuddy, A. J. C., & Yap, A. J. (2010). Power posing: Brief nonverbal displays affect neuroendocrine levels and risk tolerance. *Psychological Science*, *21*(10), 1363–1368. doi:10.1177/0956797610383437 PMID:20855902

Chi, M. T. H., Roscoe, R. D., Slotta, J. D., Roy, M., & Chase, C. C. (2011). Misconceived causal explanations for emergent processes. *Cognitive Science*, *36*(1), 1–61. doi:10.1111/j.1551-6709.2011.01207.x PMID:22050726

Clark, D., Tanner-Smith, E., & Killingsworth, S. (2014). *Digital games, design and learning: A systematic review and meta-analysis (executive summary)*. Menlo Park, CA: SRI International.

Cook, C., Goodman, N. D., & Schulz, L. E. (2011). Where science starts: Spontaneous experiments in preschoolers' exploratory play. *Cognition*, *120*(3), 341–349. doi:10.1016/j.cognition.2011.03.003 PMID:21561605

Driskell, J. E., & Johnston, J. H. (1998). Stress exposure training. In J. A. Cannon-Bowers & E. Salas (Eds.), *Making decisions under stress: Implications for individual and team training* (pp. 191–217). Washington, DC: American Psychiatric Association. doi:10.1037/10278-007

Fleming, M. J., & Rickwood, D. J. (2001). Effects of violent versus non-violent video games on children's arousal, aggressive mood, and positive mood. *Journal of Applied Social Psychology*, *31*(10), 2047–2071. doi:10.1111/j.1559-1816.2001.tb00163.x

Gallagher, P. S., & Prestwich, S. H. (2013). Can game design be leveraged to enhance cognitive adaptability? Electronic Journal of e-Learning, (Special Edition on Games Based Learning).

Gentile, D. A., Lynch, P. J., Linder, J. R., & Walsh, D. A. (2004). The effects of violent video game habits on adolescent hostility, aggressive behaviors, and school performance. *Journal of Adolescence*, *27*(1), 5–22. doi:10.1016/j.adolescence.2003.10.002 PMID:15013257

Glean, N. (2005). Growing complex games. *Paper presented at DiGRA conference Changing Views: Words in Play*, Vancouver.

Gopnik, A., & Schulz, L. E. (2007). *Causal learning: Psychology, philosophy and computation*. Oxford: Oxford University Press. doi:10.1093/acprof:oso/9780195176803.001.0001

Gopnik, A., & Wellman, H. M. (2012). Reconstructing constructivism: Causal models, Bayesian learning mechanisms, and the theory. *Psychological Bulletin*, *138*(6), 1085–1108. doi:10.1037/a0028044 PMID:22582739

Gozli, D. G., Bavelier, D., & Pratt, J. (2014). The effect of action video game playing on sensorimotor learning: Evidence from a movement tracking task. *Human Movement Science*, *38C*, 152–162. doi:10.1016/j.humov.2014.09.004 PMID:25318081

Granic, I., Lobel, A., & Engels, R. C. (2014). The benefits of playing video games. *The American Psychologist*, *69*(1), 66–78. doi:10.1037/a0034857 PMID:24295515

Green, C. S., Pouget, A., & Bavelier, D. (2010). Improved probabilistic inference as a general learning mechanism with action video games. *Current Biology*, *20*(17), 1573–1579. doi:10.1016/j.cub.2010.07.040 PMID:20833324

Greitemeyer, T., Osswald, S., & Brauer, M. (2010). Playing prosocial video games increases empathy and decreases schadenfreude. *Emotion (Washington, D.C.)*, *10*(6), 796–802. doi:10.1037/a0020194 PMID:21171755

Grodal, T. (2000). Video games and the pleasures of control. In D. Zillman & P. Vorderer (Eds.), *Media entertainment: The psychology of its appeal* (pp. 197–213). Mahwah, NJ: Lawrence Erlbaum.

Hall, R. H., Wilfred, L. M., Higlers, M. G., Leu, M. C., Walker, C. P., & Hortenstine, J. M. (2004). Virtual terrorist attack on the computer science building: Design and evaluation of a research methodology. *Presence-Connect, 4*(4). Retrieved from http://lite.mst.edu/documents/vr_affect_presence_connect_2004.pdf

Horner, V., & Whiten, A. (2005). Causal knowledge and imitation/emulation switching in chimpanzees (Pan troglodytes) and children (Homo sapiens). *Animal Cognition*, *8*(3), 164–181. doi:10.1007/s10071-004-0239-6 PMID:15549502

Hsu, C. Y., Tsai, C. C., & Wang, H. Y. (2012). Facilitating third graders' acquisition of scientific concepts through digital game-based learning: The effects of self-explanation principles. *The Asia-Pacific Education Researcher*, *21*(1), 71–82.

Isbister, K. (2011). Emotion and motion: Games as inspiration for shaping the future of interface. *Interaction*, *18*(September–October), 24–27. doi:10.1145/2008176.2008184

Isen, A. M., Daubman, K. A., & Nowicki, G. P. (1987). Positive affect facilitates creative problem-solving. *Journal of Personality and Social Psychology*, *52*(6), 1122–1131. doi:10.1037/0022-3514.52.6.1122 PMID:3598858

Jackson, L. A., Witt, E. A., Games, A. I., Fitzgerald, H. E., von Eye, A., & Zhao, Y. (2012). Information technology use and creativity: Findings from the Children and Technology Project. *Computers in Human Behavior*, *28*(2), 370–376. doi:10.1016/j.chb.2011.10.006

Jennings, K. D., Harmon, R. J., Morgan, G. A., Gaiter, J. L., & Yarrow, L. J. (1979). Exploratory play as an index of mastery motivation: Relationships to persistence, cognitive functioning, and environmental measures. *Developmental Psychology*, *15*(4), 386–394. doi:10.1037/0012-1649.15.4.386

Juul, J. (2005). *Half-real: Video games between real rules and fictional worlds*. Cambridge, MA: MIT Press.

Keller, H., Schneider, K., & Henderson, B. B. (Eds.). (1994). *Curiosity and exploration*. Berlin: Springer-Verlag. doi:10.1007/978-3-642-77132-3

Khalil, G. E. (2012). When losing means winning: The impact of conflict in a digital game in young adults' intentions to get protected from cancer. *Games for Health Journal*, *1*(4), 279–286. doi:10.1089/g4h.2012.0017 PMID:26191631

Kickmeier-Rust, M. D., & Albert, D. (2009). Emergence in digital educational games: A world of incidents in a universe of rules. *Proceedings of the 3rd European Conference on Game Based Learning* (p. 220). Academic Conferences Limited.

Kim, B., Park, H., & Baek, Y. (2009). Not just fun, but serious strategies: Using meta-cognitive strategies in game-based learning. *Computers & Education*, *52*(4), 800–810. doi:10.1016/j.compedu.2008.12.004

Koster, R. (2005). *A theory of fun for game design*. Scottsdale, AZ: Paraglyph Press.

Lehrer, J. (2009.) "Deliberate calm" guided US airways crew. *The Los Angeles Times*. Retrieved from http://www.latimes.com/la-oe-lehrer17-2009jan17-story.html

Loewenstein, G. (1994). The psychology of curiosity: A review and reinterpretation. *Psychological Bulletin, 116*(1), 75–98. doi:10.1037/0033-2909.116.1.75

Lombard, M., & Ditton, T. (1997). At the heart of it all: The concept of presence. *Journal of Computer-Mediated Communication, 3*(2). Retrieved from http://onlinelibrary.wiley.com/doi/10.1111/j.1083-6101.1997.tb00072.x/full

Lorenz, K. (1981). Exploratory behavior or curiosity. In K. Lorenz & R. W. Kickert (Eds.), *The foundations of ethology* (pp. 325–335). New York: Springer-Verlag. doi:10.1007/978-3-7091-3671-3_18

McClarty, K. L., Orr, A., Frey, P. M., Dolan, R. P., Vassileva, V., & McVay, A. (2012). *A literature review of gaming in education.* Upper Saddle River, NJ: Pearson.

Mellou, E. (1994). Play theories: A contemporary review. *Early Child Development and Care, 102*(1), 91–100. doi:10.1080/0300443941020107

Mitra, S., & Dangwal, R. (2010). Limits to self-organising systems of learning—the Kalikuppam experiment. *British Journal of Educational Technology, 41*(5), 672–688. doi:10.1111/j.1467-8535.2010.01077.x

Morris, B. J., Corker, S., Zimmerman, C., Gill, D., & Romig, C. (2013). Gaming science: The 'gamification' of scientific thinking. *Frontiers in Psychology, 4*, 607. doi:10.3389/fpsyg.2013.00607 PMID:24058354

Nacke, L. E., Bateman, C., & Mandryk, R. L. (2011). BrainHex: Preliminary results from a neurobiological gamer typology survey. *Proceedings of the 10th International Conference on Entertainment Computing* (pp. 288–293). Berlin: Springer. doi:10.1007/978-3-642-24500-8_31

Neill, J. T., & Dias, K. L. (2012). Adventure education and resilience: The double-edged sword. *Journal of Adventure Education and Outdoor Learning, 2*(1), 35–42.

Norman, D. A. (2004). *Emotional design: Why we love or hate everyday things.* New York: Basic Books.

O'Malley, P. (2010). Resilient subjects: Uncertainty, warfare and liberalism. *Economy and Society, 39*(4), 488–509. doi:10.1080/03085147.2010.510681

Oliver, M. B., Bowman, N. D., Woolley, J. K., Rogers, R., Sherrick, B. I., & Chung, M.-Y. (2015). Video games as meaningful entertainment experiences. *Psychology of Popular Media Culture.* Retrieved15May2015. doi:10.1037/ppm0000066

Peters, E., Lipkus, I., & Diefenbach, M. A. (2006). The functions of affect in health communications and in the construction of health preferences. *Journal of Communication, 56*(Suppl. 1), s140–s150. doi:10.1111/j.1460-2466.2006.00287.x

Przybylski, A. K., Rigby, C. S., & Ryan, R. M. (2010). A motivational model of video game engagement. *Review of General Psychology, 14*(2), 154–166. doi:10.1037/a0019440

Przybylski, A. K., Ryan, R. M., & Rigby, C. S. (2009). The motivating role of violence in video games. *Personality and Social Psychology Bulletin, 35*(2), 243–259. doi:10.1177/0146167208327216 PMID:19141627

Ravaja, N., Saari, T., Laarni, J., Kallinen, K., Salminen, M., Holopainen, J., & Jarvinen, A. (2005). The psychophysiology of video gaming: Phasic emotional responses to game events. Retrieved from http://www.digra.org/wp-content/uploads/digital-library/06278.36196.pdf

Rubin, K. H. (2001). *The play observation scale (POS)*. Ontario, Canada: University of Waterloo.

Ruff, H. A., & Saltarelli, L. M. (1993). Exploratory play with objects: Basic cognitive processes and individual differences. *New Directions for Child and Adolescent Development*, *59*(59), 5–16. doi:10.1002/cd.23219935903 PMID:8483525

Ryan, R. M., & Deci, E. L. (2000). Self-determination theory and the facilitation of intrinsic motivation, social development and well-being. *The American Psychologist*, *55*(1), 68–78. doi:10.1037/0003-066X.55.1.68 PMID:11392867

Ryan, R. M., Rigby, C. S., & Przybylski, A. K. (2006). The motivational pull of video games: A self-determination theory approach. *Motivation and Emotion*, *30*(4), 347–364. doi:10.1007/s11031-006-9051-8

Ryff, C. D., & Keyes, C. L. M. (1995). The structure of psychological well-being revisited. *Journal of Personality and Social Psychology*, *69*(4), 719–727. doi:10.1037/0022-3514.69.4.719 PMID:7473027

Schell, J. (2008). *The Art of Game Design: A Book of Lenses*. Amsterdam: Elsevier/Morgan Kaufmann.

Schneider, W. (2008). The development of metacognitive knowledge in children and adolescents: Major trends and implications for education. *Mind, Brain, and Education*, *2*(3), 114–121. doi:10.1111/j.1751-228X.2008.00041.x

Schulz, L. E., Standing, H. R., & Bonawitz, E. B. (2008). Word, thought, and deed: The role of object categories in children's inductive inferences and exploratory play. *Developmental Psychology*, *44*(5), 1266–1276. doi:10.1037/0012-1649.44.5.1266 PMID:18793061

Smith, B. W., Dalen, J., Wiggins, K., Tooley, E., Christopher, P., & Bernard, J. (2008). The brief resilience scale: Assessing the ability to bounce back. *International Journal of Behavioral Medicine*, *15*(3), 194–200. doi:10.1080/10705500802222972 PMID:18696313

Squire, K., Barnett, M., Grant, J. M., & Higginbotham, T. (2004). Electromagnetism supercharged! Learning physics with digital simulation games. *Proceedings of the 6th International Conference on Learning Sciences* (pp. 513–520). Mahwah, NJ: Lawrence Erlbaum.

Stewart, B. (2014). *Dynamics vs. mechanics: A pre-analysis of watch dogs*. Retrieved from [REMOVED HYPERLINK FIELD]http://www.gamasutra.com/blogs/BartStewart/20140423/216090/Dynamics_vs_Mechanics_A_PreAnalysis_of_Watch_Dogs.Php

Sundstrom, P., Stahl, A., & Hook, K. (2005). eMoto-affectively involving both body and mind. Proceedings of CHI 05 extended abstracts. ACM: New York.

Sweetser, P. (2008). *Emergence in games*. Boston, MA: Charles River Media.

Swink, S. (2009). *Game feel: A game designer's guide to virtual sensation*. Amsterdam: Morgan Kaufmann/Elsevier.

Tichon, J., & Banks, J. (2006). Virtual reality exposure therapy: 150-degree screen to desktop PC. *Cyberpsychology & Behavior, 9*(4), 480–487. doi:10.1089/cpb.2006.9.480 PMID:16901251

Tichon, J., Hall, R., & Higlers, M. G. (2003). Education and training in virtual environments for disaster management. *Proceedings of the World Conference on Educational Multimedia, Hypermedia & Telecommunications* (pp. 1191–1194). Honolulu.

Tichon, J., & Mavin, T. (in press). Powering up and bouncing back: Videogames teach resilience. *Games for Health Journal.*

Tichon, J., & Wallis, G. (2010). Stress training and simulator complexity: Why sometimes more is less. *Behaviour & Information Technology, 29*(5), 459–466. doi:10.1080/01449290903420184

Tornqvist, D. (2014). Exploratory play in simulation sandbox games: A review of what we know about why players act crazy. *International Journal of Game-Based Learning, 4*(2), 78–95. doi:10.4018/ijgbl.2014040105

Uhlmann, E., & Swanson, J. (2004). Exposure to violent video games increases automatic aggressiveness. *Journal of Adolescence, 27*(1), 41–52. doi:10.1016/j.adolescence.2003.10.004 PMID:15013259

Van Den Hoogen, W. M., IJsselsteijn, W. A., & De Kort, Y. A. (2009). Effects of sensory immersion on behavioural indicators of player experience: Movement synchrony and controller pressure. In *Breaking new ground: innovation in games, play, practice and theory. Proceedings of the 2009 Digital Games Research Association Conference* (pp. 1–6). London: Brunel University.

van Schijndel, T. J. P., Franse, R. K., & Raijmakers, M. E. J. (2010). The exploratory behavior scale: Assessing young visitors' hands-on behavior in science museums. *Science Education, 94*(5), 794–809. doi:10.1002/sce.20394

Ventura, M., Shute, V., & Zhao, W. (2013). The relationship between video game use and a performance-based measure of persistence. *Computers & Education, 60*(1), 52–58. doi:10.1016/j.compedu.2012.07.003

Weinstein, N., Przybylski, A. K., & Ryan, R. M. (2009). Can nature make us more caring? Effects of immersion in nature on intrinsic aspirations and generosity. *Personality and Social Psychology Bulletin, 35*(10), 1315–1329. doi:10.1177/0146167209341649 PMID:19657048

Windle, G., Bennett, K. M., & Noyes, J. (2011). A methodological review of resilience measurement scales. *Health and Quality of Life Outcomes, 9*(8). Retrieved from http://www.hqlo.com/content/9/1/8 PMID:21294858

## KEY TERMS AND DEFINITIONS

**Competence:** A motivational drive to become maximally effective at exerting intentional control over a system.

**Curiosity:** A transient but intense motivation to collect specific information.

**Emergence:** A phenomenon where a simple set of rules gives rise to complex overall behaviour.

**Exploratory Play:** A series of impulsive but systematic, non-repeating interventions, driven by curiosity and the need for competence, that generate information about a novel system's causal structure.

**Mastery:** Possessing a comprehensive knowledge or skill in a particular subject or activity.

**Metacognition:** Self-monitoring and self-regulating to identify and correct errors in one's thinking.

**Motivation:** Factors that initiate and sustain the desire and energy to remain interested and committed to a goal-orientated behavior.

**Process Intensity:** In the context of game design, the proportion of the game's content that is the result of algorithms, relative to the proportion that is handcrafted by artists and level designers. The opposite of data intensity.

**Psychological Resilience:** The ability to bounce back or recover from stress.

**Sandbox Game:** A genre that provides players with broad or no goals, and sufficient complexity to enable them to approach problems in a variety of different ways. A genre where the primary mode of play is not concerned with pursuing specific goals, but rather with exploring the systems of the game.

# Chapter 12
# This Drives Me Nuts!
## How Gaming Technologies Can Elicit Positive Experiences by Means of Negative Emotions

**Stefano Triberti**
*Università Cattolica del Sacro Cuore di Milano, Italy*

## ABSTRACT

*Video games are an interesting example of technologies/media able to generate complex emotions. Indeed, part of the emotions commonly arising in the experience of video gamers are quite negative. On the one hand, video gamers may feel frustration and anger due to the difficulty of the gameplay. On the other hand, they may experience sadness, anxiety and fear due to the immersion into emotionally rich narratives. Yet, video gamers seem to appreciate gaming technologies generating negative emotions, and the research on media frequently highlights a counterintuitive positive relation between negative affect and enjoinment/well-being outcomes. Starting from these premises, the present chapter is aimed to review the negative emotions typical of video games, in order to understand in what ways they can concur in generating an overall positive experience. Then, the chapter discusses implications for research on video games as positive technologies, namely technologies able to promote well-being in their users.*

## INTRODUCTION

You are a flower. Well, sort of. You have small feet to move and big cartoon-like eyes. Your main goal, after an adventurous journey, is to rescue a princess from prison. In order to do this, you jump from one platform to another, avoiding obstacles and beating enemies by means of jumps on their heads. This is the actual first-part of the storyline (and gameplay) of *Eversion*, a video game developed and produced by Zaratustra Productions in 2008. Judging the video game by this brief description, it appears as a quite typical example of a Super Mario-style 2-D platform game. But if you proceed through the game, something weird happens. While the flower-like protagonist remains unvaried, the environment around him gradually changes. During the first levels of the game, it is funny, colorful, cheerful, and accompanied by cute music. As the game progresses, the environments gradually become darker, creepy if not disturbing; the music becomes cacophonous and unsettling; as the difficulty increases, the enemies become

DOI: 10.4018/978-1-4666-9986-1.ch012

horrendous in their appearance and clearly express evil intentions towards the protagonist. Moreover, the very end of the game, when the protagonist succeeds in saving the princess, is notably cruel and unexpected, implying that nothing, even the princess herself, is what it seems to be.

Among others, *Eversion* is an interesting example of a video game with peculiar features. Although it is not a horror game in an absolute sense, it generates a bad feeling because a game genre typically characterized by nice and inoffensive properties is suddenly filled with horrific, tragic, and cynical contents. A not really positive ending is provided to the player, who has to be satisfied with a bitter smile at most. In the end, it is possible to say that *Eversion* elicits negative emotions and an unpleasant experience in its users.

Despite this, the game generated quite positive reactions. At the moment the present chapter is been writing, *Eversion* has 669 user reviews on the *Steam* video game platform and 627 of them (93.7%) are labeled as "positive/recommended." How is this possible? How can a video game generate a positive experience and a consequential positive evaluation, if it has been created with the purpose of generating a disturbing sensation? Actually, this question relies on a very classic problem for the human sciences applied to the study of media: understanding the "pleasures" associated with tragedy, horror, and catastrophic elements in media content has been a topic of interest from Aristotle to our times. Probably, this problem can be even more complex for what is regarded as an interactive medium such as the video game. Indeed, first of all, a video game entails the possibility of failure, and as such it possibly represents a continuous occasion for the player to confront his own inadequacy; secondly, the horrific and tragic elements may be even stronger in their emotional effects than traditional media. Indeed, the interactive narration of the video game can be not only more immersive than the ones of other media but it also involves the possibility for the user to feel *first-person responsibility* for what happens.

Yet, video gamers still evaluate horrific and tragic video games as positive experiences, so that they commonly tend to be considered as good products worth trying and recommending to friends. This implies that a video game may be a positive technology, that is, a technology/means able to guarantee positive experiences to its users. Surprisingly, in some cases this happens independently of the actual emotional content of the video game, which can be substantially negative.

Starting from these premises, the purpose of this chapter is to analyze video games as positive technologies, taking into account the inherent complexity of their abilities in promoting hedonic experiences among their users. Precisely, as this introduction already touched on, video games are able to elicit emotions, both positive and negative. Actually, as will be explained in the following sections, negative emotions are a fundamental component of video game playing, which deserve to be properly analyzed. Indeed, negative emotions are: (a) a potential component of any game instance which is characterized by difficulty, challenge and the possibility of continuous failure for the player; and (b) a fundamental feature of some precise video games and video game genres. However, the present chapter will argue that negative emotions are not an obstacle to the use of video games to promote well-being. On the contrary, they potentially constitute an innovative resource, which should be properly mastered instead of opposed, in order to discover the true potentialities of video games as positive media.

## POSITIVE TECHNOLOGY

Technology is often referred to as negative in terms of user experience. Numerous philosophers and social scientists have studied technology as a risk for social life, because use of technology can contribute to alienating/substituting natural communication and relationship building (Mcluhan, 1994; Sproull & Kiesler, 1986). Additionally, technological instruments may be seen as able to extend our abilities to the point that it becomes dangerously easy to overcome ethical principles and values (Ellul, 1967; Heidegger, 1977; Postman, 1993).

On the other hand, Positive Technology (Riva, Baños, Botella, Wiederhold, & Gaggioli, 2012) is a theoretical paradigm useful for orienting research, technology analysis/evaluation, and design based on new media's distinctive properties for promoting human well-being. Indeed, it is possible to conceptualize technologies as a fundamental resource to promote health and well-being. According to this new paradigm, the quality of experience should become the main guiding principle for the design and the implementation of new technologies. Elaborating on the main concepts of Positive Psychology (Seligman & Csikszentmihalyi, 2000; Seligman, 2002), the authors identified three domains for the positive technological applications:

- **Hedonic Technologies:** Promoting pleasant emotions in the users;
- **Eudaimonic Technologies:** Supporting the users in the achieving of engaging and self-actualizing experiences; and
- **Social/Interpersonal Technologies:** Enhancing the integration between individuals, groups and societies.

The first domain is the one of interest here. Hedonic technologies are related to the generation and support of positive emotions in the technology users. According to the Broaden-and-Build Theory (Fredrickson, Danner, & Snowdon, 2003) positive emotions (such as joy, interest, commitment, gratitude, etc.) broaden an individual's momentary mindset, making possible the generation of personal resources. In a broader sense, positive emotions are related to longer and healthier living (Fredrickson, 2000). Research in the field of Hedonic Technologies has demonstrated that interactive simulation technologies are particularly suitable for fostering positive emotional states. For example, virtual reality obtained remarkable results in fostering and manipulating joy and relaxation (Baños et al., 2012; Grassi, Gaggioli, & Riva, 2009; Riva et al., 2007). According to Serino and colleagues (2013) the main features of virtual reality able to induce positive moods are interactivity and manipulability, in that they contribute to improving users' motivation and allow the technology design to be tailored to the user's exact intentions and needs.

In this sense, video games and serious games (a term that identifies video games designed for educational purposes) proved to be useful technological tools for inducing positive emotional states (Anolli, Mantovani, Confalonieri, Ascolese, & Peveri, 2010; Argenton, Triberti, Serino, Muzio, & Riva, 2014). According to Frome (2007), this is possible thanks to four factors: narrative (roleplaying and feeling the emotions of fictional characters), gameplay (frustration-satisfaction cycle related to losing and winning), simulation (experiencing new and engaging activities simulated by the game), and aesthetics (considering the game design as a piece of art). In general, interaction and interface features of new technologies can be designed with the goal of generating pleasurable experiences, according to a "Hedonomics" approach (Hancock, Pepe, & Murphy, 2005; Hsee, Hastie, & Chen, 2008).

However, a deeper look at gaming technologies shows that this field is more complex than it seems. The next section will include a brief overview of the research on video games related to the emotions experienced by the game players.

## VIDEO GAMES AND EMOTIONS

The literature on emotions experienced while playing video games can be regarded as composed of two main scenarios. The first is concerned with the effects of violent video games. Indeed, the widespread research on this important topic has touched on the study of emotions too. Since the studies by Albert Bandura and colleagues (Bandura, Ross, & Ross, 1963; Bandura, 1978; Touhey & Bandura, 1975), who demonstrated that people may systematically imitate violent behavior after having seen it as demonstrated by another person (a model), a plethora of studies began to analyze the effects of violent media on the behavior of the spectators. According to some authors (Anderson & Dill, 2000; Anderson, 2004), video games are more dangerous than other media in promoting behavioral imitation, basically because of their identification and interactive features. According to them, the emotional domain (along with the cognitive and the behavioral ones) is crucial in the context of violent video games' effects. Specifically, the authors suggest that a violent video game may generate negative emotions in the player (anger), which may persist even after the in-game experience, influencing the player's behavior in everyday life.

In this context, research on violent video games has entailed the consideration of players' emotions, usually based on psychophysiological measurements. However, the results of different researchers appear often uncertain or even contradictory. The first studies, using tonic physiological measures, showed that violent video games promoted physiological arousal related to negative emotions (anger and anxiety) (Anderson & Bushman, 2001; Ballard & Wiest, 1996).

Other studies entailed phasic physiological measures, with the goal of analyzing emotional responses to specific events happening inside the game instances. Some researchers (Baldaro et al., 2004) found differences between psychophysiological activations in response to violent/non-violent video games, with the first ones appearing related to increasing in systolic blood pressure and measures associated with state anxiety. However, some studies with similar methods and experimental design found no significant differences for what was regarded as players' arousal (Ivory & Kalyanaraman, 2007), while others highlighted that physiological and self-reported emotional responses may vary strongly among players depending on their own expertise with video game playing (Ivarsson, Anderson, Åkerstedt, & Lindblad, 2013): For example, gamers high-exposed to violent games reported positive feelings after playing in the context of the experiment, while low-exposed gamers reported sadness.

Ravaja and colleagues (Ravaja, Turpeinen, Saari, Puttonen, & Keltikangas-Järvinen, 2008) analyzed facial EMG activity and skin conductance in response to precise emotionally-salient events during video game experience (e.g., killing an opponent). The authors found unexpected activations, with the players showing negative emotions in response to the opponent killing, and positive emotions in response to the wounding/dying of their own character. These results have been confirmed by more recent research (Kivikangas & Ravaja, 2013). The authors argue that similar results may be interpreted as empathetic responses; however, they also speculate on the inherent difficulty in distinguishing between the emotions provoked by the video game and the ones related to the real environment/situation the players are in. Also Weber and colleagues (Weber, Behr, Tamborini, Ritterfeld, & Mathiak, 2009) highlighted considerable variation in emotional responses to in-game events, and emphasized the importance of gaming styles and gamers' personal interpretations of the game content in any attempts to understand the effects on behavior.

Similarly, contradictory and paradoxical results appear quite common in the other main scenario of the field too, which is the study of the experience of video games in order to understand their engagement/enjoinment properties. Some authors discussed the importance of deepening the affective/

emotional outcomes of video game playing, in addition to the more obvious cognitive and technical/motor ones, in that they support learning and behavioral change (Connolly, E.A. Boyle, MacArthur, Hainey, & Boyle, 2012; Garris, Ahlers, & Driskell, 2002). Numerous studies report a causal relation between playing preferred video games and experiencing improvements in mood and positive emotions (Russoniello, O'Brien, & Parks, 2009; Richard M. Ryan, Rigby, & Przybylski, 2006); indeed, pleasure and fun often come out as one of the main reasons to play video games (Chou & Tsai, 2007; Connolly et al., 2012; Yee, 2006). Furthermore, recent research involving fMRI (Cole, Yoo, & Knutson, 2012), which analyzed the brain activity during the onset, the offset, and the interactive gameplay of a serious video game, revealed activation of the reward-related mesolimbic neural circuits. However, according to McGonigal (2011), video games are able to promote not only the most simple pleasant experiences, but also the most complex and varied positive emotions. An example is the feeling of *fiero*, an Italian word the author uses to indicate the intense pride one may experience after having overcame a huge obstacle or difficulty. Numerous authors tried to understand what aspects of video game playing present opportunities for the experience of complex positive emotions. According to Granic and colleagues (Granic, Lobel, & Engels, 2014), video games constitute a resource to learn and to exercise individuals' abilities of emotion regulation. Indeed, video games often move players to try strategies and approaches different from those already established in their own habits, in order to overcome the constantly-varying game challenges. This would help players to enact reappraisals (re-evaluations) of the situation from the point of view of their own emotional response too, teaching them the benefits of dealing with anxiety, frustration, and stress in adaptive ways. Similarly, other authors (Przybylski, Weinstein, Murayama, Lynch, & Ryan, 2012) emphasize video game peculiarities in terms of self-exploration thanks to the use of avatars. They found that positive emotions related to game experience were mediated by the perceived convergence between in-game-self and ideal-self, that is, how much the players felt that the avatars were similar to their own desired renditions of the Self. This effect was stronger for those players who experienced a discrepancy between their real and ideal selves. In other words, the players were more motivated to play games that provided them with the opportunity to embody their ideal characteristics.

Schneider and colleagues (Schneider, Lang, Shin, & Bradley, 2004) demonstrated that adding a storyline to a first-person shooter video game generated a significant increase in the sense of presence, identification with characters, and physiological arousal; despite this, self-reported arousal was not affected. In other studies (Klimmt, Rizzo, Vorderer, Koch, & Fischer, 2009), the video game eliciting negative emotions associated with suspense obtained the highest level of enjoinment. Also immersion has been found as possibly related to negative emotions (Jennett et al., 2008); recent reviews state that future research should consider the role of negative emotions in engaging players in games in more detail (Boyle, Connolly, Hainey, & Boyle, 2012). However, it is interesting to note that, while the research from some years ago used video games as stimuli to promote positive engagement, more recent research (Lobel, Granic, & Engels Rutger, 2014) has begun to use video games as stressful stimuli, in order to investigate negative emotions and coping.

In the field of emotion studies, appraisal theories try to understand what aspects of the cognitive evaluation of the emotional stimuli may influence the final experience of the emotion. One of these aspects is "goal conduciveness," namely the evaluation of whether a stimulus or event helps or hinders one to obtain a desired goal. According to Scherer's conception (Aue, Flykt, & Scherer, 2007; Aue & Scherer, 2008), goal conduciveness should be considered as a construct different and independent from pleasantness, that is, an emotion may be more or less intense (also in its measurable psychophysiological correlates) because the event that generated it is particularly important for the subject's personal goal.

This has not a clear relation with the event being inherently pleasant or not. The research on this topic involving video games (van Reekum et al., 2004) seems to confirm this theory: goal conduciveness of in-game events has been shown to predict gamers' physiological responses, while in game events' pleasantness/unpleasantness obtained no significant results. Commenting on these results in their review, Boyle and colleagues (Boyle et al., 2012) argue that physiological correlates often do not confirm our intuitions that people "simply" prefer pleasant to unpleasant events.

In the end, the literature briefly reviewed here shows that the research topic of video games and emotions is still filled with contradictions and inconsistencies. On the one hand, traditional research on violent video games hypothesized that this kind of video games elicited negative emotions, but also positive emotions have been observed during violent games playing; on the other hand, the research on engagement and enjoinment has often found that those players who actually enjoyed the games, then also report negative emotions.

In general, a number of authors (Boyle, Connolly, & Hainey, 2011; Jansz, 2005; Triberti, Villani, & Riva, 2015) agree in considering video games as laboratory-like environments, used by players to experiment with different roles, social behavior and, of course, emotions. Starting from this perspective, this chapter presents an analysis of the phenomenon of negative emotions in the context of video game playing, in order to understand

1. How and why they are promoted by video games, and
2. What are their effects in terms of the gamer's overall experience.

## VIDEO GAMES AND *NEGATIVE* EMOTIONS

Considering the studies cited in the previous section, it appears that negative emotions are a common experience in the context of video game playing. But what exactly are these negative emotions? In general, they could be divided into two main categories:

- **Negative Emotions Related to Gameplay:** (Usually anger and frustration); they are typically due to the game's difficulty and to the gamer's transient sense of inability/inadequacy in managing the video game challenge.
- **Negative Emotions Related to Narration/Storyline:** (Usually sadness, anxiety and fear); they are typically associated with the tragic or horrific contents that some video game narratives feature.

In the next sections, the two groups of emotions will be described separately, focusing on how and why they are established in the players' experience. Then, for every set of emotions an explanation is given of how it is possible that positive experiences tend to result from the "more simple" negative emotions, that is, how technology giving negative emotions can become a hedonic positive technology.

### Gameplay Negative Emotions

Some studies about motivations for playing video games (Przybylski, Rigby, & Ryan, 2010; Przybylski, Ryan, & Rigby, 2009), based on self-determination theory (Ryan & Deci, 2000), emphasized that video games constitute a resource for the players to satisfy their fundamental needs for well-being, such as autonomy, competence, and relatedness. Such a claim implies that video games are not only a form of media that is fun and interesting to watch and play, but possibly an occasion for encountering complex experiences that challenge a person's abilities. In order to achieve this goal, games have to be stimulating, difficult, and physically and/or intellectually demanding. They have to make the player *fail* sometimes, and move the player to try again and again.

Juul (2013) argues that video games can be properly considered the "art of failure." Indeed, other media such as novels and movies can represent failure, but it is always the failure of someone else; Juul says that failure depicted in fiction helps us to feel smart and successful. We can identify with heroes and protagonists who succeed; moreover, we are completely free to convince ourselves that we would be able to avoid the failure of a protagonist, if we would be in his shoes. In the context of video games, this is impossible. They are precisely designed to make us fail, and especially to provide us clear feedback about our exclusive responsibility for the failure.

Something that is not clearly explained by the idea of video game engagement as based on self-determination theory is, given that humans have a natural need for activities able to make them feel strong and competent, why do video game players engage in activities designed to make them feel incompetent and systematically fail? Juul explains this phenomenon as the paradox of failure, which he considers inherent in video games and essential for their production:

1. We generally avoid failure.
2. We experience failure when playing games.
3. We seek out games, although we will experience something that we normally avoid.

The paradox is essential in the sense that failure is not a secondary effect of video games that we have to patiently tolerate, such as a necessary evil; it is something we actively look for. Video gamers often return to games that make them fail a lot, while they are more likely to abandon games that

1. Do not make them fail enough, or
2. Do not provide clear feedback about the failure being related to (some of) their lack of ability and/or precise errors in the action.

Indeed, the absence (or a low rate) of failure coincides with a corresponding lowering of the enjoinment to be experienced when the game is completed (Lorentz, 2014).

In this sense, failure is related to precise negative emotions. James Paul Gee (2005) maintains that video games lower the experience of failure, in that they always allow the player to start again the failed action or at least the game level. He sees this characteristic of video games as a positive aspect from an educational point of view, in that it teaches the value of risk-taking and a positive attitude towards trying again to reach a desired goal. However, failure is never a positive experience from the subjective point of view of the loser.

As previously noted, failure, and especially repeated failure, is associated with increasing negative emotions. Frustration and anger typically are established in the experience of the player who is failing, and they potentially increase if the failure is repeated in the context of the same challenge. Moreover, failure has a detrimental effect on our self-efficacy, that is, one's cognitions about his or her own capacity to enact behaviors for a given objective (Bandura, 1977, 1982).

How can these negative emotions lead to positive experiences? This happens thanks to the "promise" of video games. According to Juul (2013), this is what games do: They promise us that we can overtake and resolve a sense of personal inadequacy... an inadequacy that they have produced in us in the first place.

The possibility of failure, and the consequential sense of inadequacy, constitute the necessary intermediate step through the success, and the consequential sense of having overcome one's own limits. Moreover, it is only through the experience of *direct interaction* that one can feel the emotions related to the experience of failure (frustration and anger) and, consequently, a pleasant emotional relief when the emotion-eliciting stimulus has been re-appraised thanks to a final success.

From the point of view of Human Computer Interaction, failure in video games is in all respects considered as a *breakdown* (Gilleade & Dix, 2004). This word identifies a moment in which a given technology/interface ceases to be "invisible" or "transparent" (Flores, Graves, Hartfield, & Winograd, 1988; Pallavicini et al., 2013; Winograd & Flores, 1986) A breakdown occurs when the stream of interaction is interrupted by some type of malfunction in the system, and the user has to recruit conscious cognitive processes to find the cause of the perceived error. Breakdowns have been considered in the field of Human Computer Interaction as a resource to measure difficulty of use (Bødker, 1996; Spagnolli, Gamberini, & Gasparini, 2002), but other studies suggest that they can be also a resource for the design of complex systems such as video games (Gaver, Beaver, & Benford, 2003; Gilleade & Dix, 2004). Indeed, breakdowns imply that the user stops his own action and reflects on different strategies/approaches of interaction in order to achieve greater empowerment, enjoinment, and even learning.

The element of failure may help to explain some of the problems for another well-known account of video games as positive experiences, namely the one based on *flow*. Flow, the psychological state of total absorption inside an ongoing activity, is typically related to an overall positive affect (Riva et al., 2012; Ullén et al., 2012). The concept introduced by Csikszentmihalyi (Csikszentmihalyi, 2002; 1988; Nakamura & Csikszentmihalyi, 2002) is quite prevalent in video game research (Argenton et al., 2014; Cowley, Charles, Black, & Hickey, 2008; Jin, 2012; Kaye & Bryce, 2012). As an example, Keller and Bless (2008) used a computer game to provide an experimental demonstration of the challenge-skill balance hypothesis of the flow concept. Indeed, players in the condition with the video game adapting to their own skills were the ones experiencing an optimal experience. Moreover, recent neuropsychological research on video game playing showed that the components of flow can be associated with specific neural activations that have been observed in the players (Klasen, Weber, Kircher, K.A. Mathiak, & Mathiak, 2012). Some authors have even proposed tables highlighting the characteristics of flow, and

*Table 1. Comparison between psychological flow characteristics and video games characteristics*

| Flow Element | Game Element |
|---|---|
| A challenging task | The complete game experience |
| Ability to concentrate on the task | Immersion; fantasy worlds that draw the gamer in |
| Task has clear goals | Survival, collection of points, solving the puzzle, etc. |
| Feeling of full control | Familiarity/skill with controller, genre conventions, game-play mechanics |
| Immediate feedbacks to action | Rewards and penalties |
| Altered sense of time | "Years" played out in hours, battles conducted in minutes; temporally-independent environments |

the corresponding elements typically present in video games. Table 1 shows a simplified version of such proposals, based on Jones (1998) and Cowley and colleagues (2008):

Actually, when failure "comes into play," these conceptions seem somewhat partial or even simplistic. On the one hand, video games appear as a perfect candidate for understanding flow, in that they surely feature peculiar elements that, as pointed out by these approaches, can be easily associated with the characteristics of flow. However, the experience of video games is not so simple in reality. It is possible to consider critically the comparisons of Table 1. Indeed, video gamers do not spend their time inside pleasant and fluent streams of interaction. On the contrary, depending on the characteristics of the game they are playing, they may encounter situations in which their experience of interaction is brutally interrupted (breakdowns), and failure emerges as a signal of their own inability/inadequacy. Failure is something more than "penalties," in that it literally stops the game, rather than indicating the proper action to complete it. Moreover, failure occurs often when the goals of a single action are not clear (the player is not able to proceed in the game, and he continues to fail, because he doesn't understand what course of action must be enacted. (e.g., "Where do I have to go? What do I have to do in order to kill this monster? How can I solve this puzzle?"). Finally, familiarity with controller and game mechanics is not always something that can be taken for granted, but rather something the player has to learn by means of trial and error.

Does this mean that video games are not really able to promote flow? This is a serious possibility. Or maybe, the theory of flow itself needs to be enhanced with more complex reflections. Recent accounts of the phenomenon (Løvoll & Vittersø, 2014; Vittersø, 2004) reject the hypothesis of skills/challenges balance, showing that situations in which challenges are in balance with skills can produce feelings of boredom or disinterest. On the contrary, the authors suggest that situations in which high challenges are either higher or lower than skills are more associated with the experience of flow. This seems to explain more adequately the case of video games; typically, challenges *vary* over time while playing a video game, and this is probably the video game feature providing surprise, interest, and real room for improvement, all of these possibly relating to an optimal experience.

## Narrative Negative Emotions

The case of negative emotions related to narrative is quite different. As noted in the previous paragraph, gameplay-related negative emotions arise from the fact that experiencing failure and difficulty entails a sense of inability/inadequacy for the player, possibly lowering his or her self-efficacy. These emotions are related to the video game as an interactive medium that challenges a person's skills.

In addition to that, it is important to remember that video games often have content in them, that is, they are more or less complex pieces of narration. They feature characters, situations, and events; they can be more or less "cinematic," depending on the amount of scenes that happen independently of gamers' commands, showing avatars and/or non-playable characters involved in dramatic action.

At least three negative emotions are typically related to the structure and to the content of narrative.

*Sadness* is the emotion experienced in the face of unpleasant events, typically involving the sensation of irrevocable loss (Lazarus, 1994). According to appraisal theories, sadness emerges when the cognitive evaluation of an event highlights low pleasantness, low goal conduciveness, and low coping potential (Frijda, 1993). *Anxiety* is an emotion activated by the expectation of an impending encounter that involves a threat to oneself or others. In the context of a media production, anxiety has been recognized as engaging the player's attention and, despite the negative hedonic valence of the experience, motivating the player to remain and/or to return in front of the screen in order to watch how a problematic situation is resolved by the narrative. This is the concept of *suspense* (Hartmann, 2011; Klimmt et al., 2009), which is the reason for the use of strategic interruptions of story segments to constitute a common expedient for promoting engagement in modern dramas—the narrative feature known as the *cliffhanger* (Baranowski & Buday, 2008). Anxiety that is directed to a specific event, increases in intensity and is characterized by an episodic activation is commonly regarded as *fear* (Repetto & Riva, 2011). Indeed, while enjoying media, people are more likely to be scared while already in a state of anxiety (Vachiratamporn, Legaspi, Moriyama, Fukui, & Numao, 2015).

For the sake of simplification, here these three emotions—sadness, anxiety, and fear—are considered as prototypical of specific types of video gaming. While almost absent in the context of casual gaming (Juul, 2009), they are quite frequent for those "hardcore" gamers who prefer to engage themselves in games characterized by dramatic and complex narrative contents.

Sad and tragic contents appear to be more and more widespread in the context of commercial video games. According to Juul (2013), video games constitute the occasion to make the media viewers experience a totally-new type of tragedy. Indeed, thanks to their interactive features, video games make it possible for one not only to identify with tragic actions but also to feel responsible for possible wrong choices and disastrous consequences of action.

Then, how is it that media-conveyed sadness can promote a positive experience in the viewer? This problem is very ancient, involving the contribution of many authors throughout classic and modern philosophy. David Hume described what he called the paradox of tragedy: "It seems as unaccountable pleasure which the spectators of a well-written tragedy receive from sorrow, terror, anxiety, and other passions that are in themselves disagreeable and uneasy" (*Of Tragedy*). Indeed, many studies involving different types of media, from movies to music to video games, highlighted a counterintuitive positive relation between an increased experienced sadness and an increase in enjoyment (Ahn, Jin, & Ritterfeld, 2012; de Wied, Zillman, & Ordman, 1994; Hanich, Wagner, Shah, Jacobsen, & Menninghaus, 2014; Vuoskoski & Thompson, 2012).

The first type of positive emotion that can emerge from a negative narrative are emotions related to the medium as a piece of art. For example, as Plantinga (2009) observes, one may be scared by the dinosaurs of *Jurassic Park*, but still be amused by the technology used to design and animate them: these are labeled *artifact emotions*. Similar to this concept is the philosophical proposal that maintains that catastrophic events have some features in common with the experience of beauty (such as novelty, magnitude, identification of a scheme, etc.), so that assisting to violent or destructive actions may generate an experience of aesthetic contemplation (Allen & Greenberger, 1978). However, the concept of artifact emotions seems insufficient to explain the complexity of a positive experience related to a medium, since they are clearly indirect emotions, independent by the content of the drama.

The more classic account of how negative emotions may transform into positive emotions is the concept of *catharsis*. Aristotle is somewhat vague about this concept in the *Poetics*, but it seems clear that he assumes expressing an emotion (for example, crying out loud because of identification in a tragedy) allows the spectator to let go of or release the emotion itself, to let it profusely come out of the body, therefore leaving space for another, positive emotional activation. It has been observed that the concept of catharsis is based on a "hydraulic" idea of emotions (Scheff, 1979), as if there were something like a container of emotional experience that could be filled, purged, and filled again with different material. Modern psychology challenged the concept of catharsis, since expression of emotion does not lead to the lowering of the emotion itself. On the contrary, for example, expressing anger tends to make one more rather than less angry (Bushman, 2002).

Other emotions that may be experienced while enjoying a narrative have the distinctive characteristic of being consistent with the emotions expressed by the fictional characters. For example, a suspenseful situation in a movie may at some point engage the viewer to feel and share the objectives and the feelings of the protagonist whose own life is in danger. While the protagonist is clearly experiencing fear, suddenly the viewer may feel something very close to fear also. The fundamental difference between the protagonist and the viewer is that the viewer's life is not in danger, and this aspect is a fundamental part of the cognitive appraisal of the situation and therefore a distinctive characteristic of the emotional experience. This is the reason why these emotions are labeled *sympathetic* (Feagin, 1983), and not *empathic* (Plantinga, 2009). They are surrogates of the emotional experience detected in the fictional characters. Here it is possible to state an interesting point about video games. Again Plantinga (2009), whose interest is in movies, observes that some emotions are not prone to be featured in sympathetic experiences. For example, the sense of guilt and shame are possible, he says, only if the spectator should also be the director or the screenwriter of the movie. Otherwise these emotions, that are typical of one evaluating his or her own actions, cannot be properly experienced by spectators; that is, one can share the fear or the sadness of a character, but will always be external to the experience of guilt and/or shame, because of lacking responsibility for the character's actions and the events in the narration.

However, the case regarding video games is very different. Actually, there is research about video gamers feeling a sense of guilt for immoral actions they have just performed in video game playing (Hartmann, Toz, & Brandon, 2010; Hartmann & Vorderer, 2010; Hartmann, 2011). Maybe, this allows media psychology to speculate about a greater range of possible sympathetic experiences in the case of the video game as a medium.

In the context of efforts in the literature to explain the paradox of tragedy, the concept of *meta-emotions* has been introduced (Mayer & Gaschke, 1988; Oliver, 1993). A meta-emotion is basically an emotion felt in response to the feeling of another emotion (Bartsch, Vorderer, Mangold, & Viehoff, 2008; Koven, 2011; Mitmansgruber, Beck, Höfer, & Schüßler, 2009). The concept of meta-emotions highlights the capacity to feel specific second-level emotional responses, along with cognitive appraisals, that deserve to be analyzed and treated differently from the first-level emotions that promote them. The concept of meta-emotions has been considered already in the field of video games study (Madeira, Arriaga, Adrião, Lopes, & Esteves, 2015); indeed, also enjoinment can be considered a meta-emotion. However, as the authors say, experimental research on meta-emotions in video games is still missing throughout the literature. For now, research on traditional media (or on media considered from a general viewpoint) can be used to understand what meta-emotions are and how they work.

Feagin (1983) noted that people normally do not feel pleasure due to their sympathetic responses to tragedies in real life. The point with fiction is that because the suffering is fictional, no one really suffers. So, viewers are allowed to examine their own feelings without regard for other people. According to Feagin, when viewers examine their own emotions in the context of tragedy (showing that they care for the welfare of other people and deplore the immoral forces that make them suffer), they are reminded of their common humanity, thus reducing the sense of aloneness. More recently, Hofer and Wirth (2012) confronted sad films with positive/negative endings, showing that in the case of negative endings meta-appraisal processes (Schramm & Wirth, 2010) mediated the relationship between sadness and enjoyment. In their research, the most important component of meta-appraisal was norm compatibility, that is, the sadness experienced by the participants was evaluated by them as a proper response from the point of view of social and cultural values. Apparently, this played an important role in the transformation of sadness (first level, sympathetic emotion) in enjoinment (second level, meta-emotion).

Another field of research highlights that sad narratives often feature characters embodying profound moral virtues such as courage, sacrifice, abnegation, and wisdom. Kohlberg (1971) believed that morality was the main function of tragedies. Thanks to their moral virtue contents, sad narratives promote a direct emotional response that can be conceived as the opposite of social disgust, and is typically triggered by the witnessing of acts of human beauty and virtue (Haidt, 2000, 2003; Plantinga, 2009). *Elevation* is a precise emotion characterized not only by specific sets of stimuli able to generate it but also by a unique physical response, namely the "lump in throat" (Oliver, Hartmann, & Woolley, 2012), as the autonomic nervous system reaction is often called.

Morality is an increasingly recurring feature of video games (Weaver & Lewis, 2012). Usually, it constitutes a gameplay affordance in that players are allowed to decide to interpret good or evil characters (Triberti et al., 2015). Sometimes, video games depicting sad but morally salient stories are able to provide elevation in the players. For example *Shadow of the Colossus* (Team ICO, Sony Computer Entertainment, 2005) communicates both the determination and the sense of guilt of the young warrior who, in order to save his lover's life, is obligated to hunt and kill giant and powerful yet innocent creatures. Likewise, *Red Dead Redemption* (Rockstar San Diego, Rockstar Games, 2010) is well known for its tragic and touching finale featuring the heroic self-sacrifice of the protagonist. Indeed, elevation contents have been recognized along all types of media, included video games (Oliver et al., 2012).

Another important account of how emotionally-negative contents in media may generate positive outcomes is related to the so-called *post-viewing social gratifications*. In a famous experiment, Zillman and colleagues (Zillmann, Weaver, Mundorf, & Aust, 1986) sent pairs of participants to see a violent horror movie. One member of every pair was a collaborator of the experimenters, and he/she was instructed to behave in a precise way while viewing the movie; showing either courage, indifference, or fear. After the movie, the experimenters interviewed the participants and discovered that the males considered more attractive the female companions who acted afraid and in need of protection, while the female participants considered more attractive the courageous male companions. Although this experiment was not centered on emotions, it shows how appreciation of negative content in media can be related to positive outcomes that are independent of the content itself: Especially, young people may use violent/horror/disturbing media to reinforce their belonging to a social role, such as a rite of passage (Twitchell, 1995; Westerfelhaus & Alan Brookey, 2004).

It is interesting to note how similar practices are present in video games. More and more video game players engage in the shooting of the so-called reaction videos to be shared on online video platforms and social networks, in order to show to others their reactions while playing horror/violent video games (Triberti & Argenton, 2015).

## IMPLICATIONS FOR VIDEO GAMES AS POSITIVE TECHNOLOGIES

As an introduction, video games were first presented as positive technologies, that is, technologies that can be used to promote positive experiences in people. Next in focus are hedonic technologies, the field of positive technologies related to the promotion of positive emotions. The thesis of the present chapter is that hedonic technologies allow some kinds of positive emotional experiences to be generated by the preliminary experience of simpler negative emotions. From the point of view of mere interaction with digital media (gameplay emotions) or exploration of their emotional content and meaning (narrative emotions) video games constitute an interesting example of how hedonic technologies may evolve towards something more complex and rich than simple tools able to elicit basic emotional states.

Considering the review above, gameplay negative emotions typical of video games have been shown to be positive in the sense that they are related to the "promise" of video games: They allow the player to overcome the failure and the related sense of inadequacy they produce in the first place.

Positive technology interventions using video games to support self-efficacy and empowerment of abilities in people should not propose interactive technologies that are too easy to interact with. Doing so would probably preserve in the user the experience of negative emotions, but at the same time they would not really leave room for improvement. On the contrary, video games are an interactive virtual reality-based technology that feature challenge as a fundamental characteristic. Moreover, the challenge that a video game presents to the player should probably not be designed as an identical, specular counterpart of some measurement of the player's ability. According to recent research on the flow concept (Løvoll & Vittersø, 2014; Vittersø, 2004), unbalance and variance among high challenges may be more likely to generate an optimal experience. This aspect clearly has interesting implications for the creation of both hedonic and eudaimonic positive technologies, in that breakdowns, difficulty, and ambiguity can be considered a novel resource for design (Gaver et al., 2003).

With regard to narrative negative emotions, positive technology interventions can be directed to replacing the experience of a person with a digital experience (Riva et al., 2012). Virtual reality-based interventions, for example, can replace a negative real-experience of a person with a positive digital one. This entails, for instance, health-care technologies used to promote stress relief and relaxation (Serino et al., 2013; Villani, Preziosa, & Riva, 2006; Villani & Riva, 2012) and also technologies for patient centered healthcare, which do not address a specific pathology but are concerned with patients' well-being (Triberti & Liberati, 2014). Experimental research has shown that adding a storyline to virtual reality empowers its effectiveness in promoting sense of presence, that is the sensation of *being there* (Gorini, Capideville, De Leo, Mantovani, & Riva, 2011; Schultze, 2010), and consequently its effectiveness as a medium conveying a complex experience (Juan et al., 2006; Rigby & Ryan, 2011; Triberti, Repetto, & Riva, 2014).

Narrative negative emotions contribute to making a narration effective. Indeed, narrations feature events and characters, but also conflicts, obstacles, and difficulties—sometimes also tragedies—, which will probably generate negative reactions both in the characters and the viewers/players. Otherwise, a narration would be ineffective in conveying interesting content that may have positive effects on people. Indeed, narration is able not only to convey emotions and meanings but also is strictly related to behavioral change (Baranowski & Buday, 2008; Lu, Baranowski, Thompson, & Buday, 2012); that is, it has a strong persuasive power.

According to Lu and colleagues (Lu et al., 2012), narrative contents may influence people thanks to three features:

- First, immersion in the narrative promotes suspension of disbelief, that is, in order to enjoy a story people are more likely to modify their cognitive evaluation of a situation, in terms of the information's adherence to truth and plausibility; this has proven to reduce the generation of counterarguments and to enhance motivation.

- Second, the narrative experience can become a personal experience. A well-crafted narrative may generate the impression of having a first-person experience of the narrative content (in some cases, this results even in delusive memories).
- Third, narrative may generate strong affection for the characters and, as a consequence of an alone effect, a positive attitude towards the ideas/values expressed by them.

Moreover, the peculiar emotion labeled *elevation*, related to the media portrayals depicting moral virtues, is quite recurring in the context of media that generate negative emotions. Elevation is not only an inner experience, but it facilitates the rise of motivations to *embody* the moral virtues, this way modifying behavior, such as becoming a better person and helping others (Oliver et al., 2012). Pursuing virtue has a precise effect on well-being (Huta & Ryan, 2010), in that it relates to one finding meaning in life, improvements in elevating experiences such as awe and inspiration, and general well-being outcomes that tend to last longer than the ones typical of pure hedonism.

In the context of positive technology interventions, the use of complex narratives featuring complex characters, able to generate elevation and other possible emotions influencing motivations and future behavior of the users, should be taken into consideration as an innovative resource.

## FUTURE RESEARCH DIRECTIONS

The ability of video games to generate emotions in their players, and possibly positive emotions, proves that they can be considered positive technologies. However, as this contribution points out, these positive experiences may emerge against a background of complex emotional states, sometimes entailing initial responses that are substantially negative. To date, almost all of the research showing that media content is able to promote positive experiences based on negative emotions (namely the paradox of tragedy) has been carried out on traditional media, ranging from literature and music to cinema and television. Future research should focus on the new media of video games, in order to experimentally verify whether meta-emotions actually emerge or not in this peculiar type of interactive content delivery. This could be done using experimental designs entailing multiple research methods (psychophysiological measures, ad-hoc questionnaires, qualitative interviews) able to capture the complexity of affective states that cannot be reduced to the immediate responses to single in-game stimuli. Moreover, meta-emotions and other high level emotional states such as awe and elevation can be the result of re-appraisals performed at a later time or considering the media as an organic product. Therefore, another guideline for future research would be to study video games as completed by the players as a whole, not limiting analysis to the responses to single instances or scenes. Finally, the research on video games could benefit of being theoretically grounded on the more complex conception of media related emotions emerging from the literature on more traditional media, especially in order to correctly interpret the recurring, contradictory results on the hedonic outcomes of video game playing.

## CONCLUSION

Video games are becoming an increasingly important part of global entertainment and media. The increasing number of people using video games, in different contexts and on multiple platforms, contribute to making them a fundamental topic of research. Moreover, as the present contribution (partially) shows, video games are able to convey emotions in multiple and complex ways; precisely, such as the highest examples coming from other media, they are able to generate positive experiences, desirable outcomes, and even pleasant affect, starting from the generation of simple emotions which may be essentially negative. In the end, it seems inadequate to explain video games' hedonic features based on simple, monodimensional theories of emotions and engagement; for example, the concept of enjoinment itself should probably not be considered as necessarily grounded on positive emotions. On the contrary, enjoying a videogame, similar to enjoying a movie or a book, means passing through multifaceted and dynamic emotional experiences. Future research should identify the emotional possibility of video game playing (for example, considering features related to gameplay mechanics, and features related to immersion into narratives), also in order to identify the exact potentialities of video games to promote behavior modification and positive experiences.

## REFERENCES

Ahn, D., Jin, S. A. A., & Ritterfeld, U. (2012). Sad movies don't always make me cry the cognitive and affective processes underpinning enjoyment of tragedy. *Journal of Media Psychology*, *24*(1), 9–18. doi:10.1027/1864-1105/a000058

Allen, V. L., & Greenberger, D. B. (1978). An Aesthetic Theory of Vandalism. *Crime and Delinquency*, *24*(3), 309–321. doi:10.1177/001112877802400305

Anderson, C. (2004). An update on the effects of playing violent video games. *Journal of Adolescence*, *27*(1), 113–122. doi:10.1016/j.adolescence.2003.10.009 PMID:15013264

Anderson, C., & Bushman, B. J. (2001). Effects of violent video games on aggressive behavior, aggressive cognition, aggressive affect, physiological arousal, and prosocial behavior: a meta-analytic review of the scientific literature. *Psychological Science: A Journal of the American Psychological Society*, 12, 353–359. doi:10.1111/1467-9280.00366

Anderson, C. A., & Dill, K. E. (2000). Video games and aggressive thoughts, feelings, and behavior in the laboratory and in life. *Journal of Personality and Social Psychology*, *78*(4), 772–790. doi:10.1037/0022-3514.78.4.772 PMID:10794380

Anolli, L., Mantovani, F., Confalonieri, L., Ascolese, A., & Peveri, L. (2010). Emotions in Serious Games: From Experience to Assessment. *International Journal of Emerging Technologies in Learning*, *5*(SI3), 7–16. doi:10.3991/ijet.v5s3.1496

Argenton, L., Triberti, S., Serino, S., Muzio, M., & Riva, G. (2014). Serious games as positive technologies for individual and group flourishing. In A. L. Brooks, S. Brahnam, & L. C. Jain (Eds.), *Technologies and Inclusive Well-Being* (Vol. 536, pp. 6–12). Berlin, Heidelberg: Springer; doi:10.1007/978-3-642-45432-5_11

Aue, T., Flykt, A., & Scherer, K. R. (2007). First evidence for differential and sequential efferent effects of stimulus relevance and goal conduciveness appraisal. *Biological Psychology*, *74*(3), 347–357. doi:10.1016/j.biopsycho.2006.09.001 PMID:17052833

Aue, T., & Scherer, K. R. (2008). Appraisal-driven somatovisceral response patterning: Effects of intrinsic pleasantness and goal conduciveness. *Biological Psychology*, *79*(2), 158–164. doi:10.1016/j.biopsycho.2008.04.004 PMID:18495321

Baldaro, B., Tuozzi, G., Codispoti, M., Montebarocci, O., Barbagli, F., Trombini, E., & Rossi, N. (2004). Aggressive and non-violent videogames: Short-term psychological and cardiovascular effects on habitual players. *Stress and Health*, *20*(4), 203–208. doi:10.1002/smi.1015

Ballard, M., & Wiest, R. (1996). Mortal Kombat (tm): The Effects of Violent Videogame Play on Males' Hostility and Cardiovascular Responding. *Journal of Applied Social Psychology*, *26*(8), 717–730. doi:10.1111/j.1559-1816.1996.tb02740.x

Bandura, A. (1977). Self-efficacy: Toward a unifying theory of behavioral change. *Psychological Review*, *84*(2), 191–215. doi:10.1037/0033-295X.84.2.191 PMID:847061

Bandura, A. (1978). Social learning theory of aggression. *Journal of Communication*, *28*(3), 12–29. doi:10.1111/j.1460-2466.1978.tb01621.x PMID:690254

Bandura, A. (1982). Self-efficacy mechanism in human agency. *The American Psychologist*, *37*(2), 122–147. doi:10.1037/0003-066X.37.2.122

Bandura, A., Ross, D., & Ross, S. A. (1963). Imitation of film-mediated aggressive models. *Journal of Abnormal and Social Psychology*, *66*(1), 3–11. doi:10.1037/h0048687 PMID:13966304

Baños, R. M., Etchemendy, E., Castilla, D., García-Palacios, A., Quero, S., & Botella, C. (2012). Positive mood induction procedures for virtual environments designed for elderly people. *Interacting with Computers*, *24*(3), 131–138. doi:10.1016/j.intcom.2012.04.002

Baranowski, T., Buday, R., Thompson, D. I., & Baranowski, J. (2008). Playing for real: Video games and stories for health-related behavior change. *American Journal of Preventive Medicine*, *34*(1), 74–82. doi:10.1016/j.amepre.2007.09.027 PMID:18083454

Bartsch, A., Vorderer, P., Mangold, R., & Viehoff, R. (2008). Appraisal of Emotions in Media Use: Toward a Process Model of Meta-Emotion and Emotion Regulation. *Media Psychology*, *11*(1), 7–27. doi:10.1080/15213260701813447

Bødker, S. (1996). Applying activity theory to video analysis: how to make sense of video data in human-computer inter- action. In B. Nardi (Ed.), *Context and consciousness. Activity theory and human computer interaction* (pp. 147–174). Cambridge, USA: Mit Press.

Boyle, E., Connolly, T. M., & Hainey, T. (2011). The role of psychology in understanding the impact of computer games. *Entertainment Computing*, *2*(2), 69–74. doi:10.1016/j.entcom.2010.12.002

Boyle, E. A., Connolly, T. M., Hainey, T., & Boyle, J. M. (2012). Engagement in digital entertainment games: A systematic review. *Computers in Human Behavior*, *28*(3), 771–780. doi:10.1016/j.chb.2011.11.020

Bushman, B. J. (2002). Does Venting Anger Feed or Extinguish the Flame? Catharsis, Rumination, Distraction, Anger, and Aggressive Responding. *Personality and Social Psychology Bulletin*, *28*(6), 724–731. doi:10.1177/0146167202289002

Chou, C., & Tsai, M.-J. (2007). Gender differences in Taiwan high school students' computer game playing. *Computers in Human Behavior*, *23*(1), 812–824. doi:10.1016/j.chb.2004.11.011

Cole, S., Yoo, D., & Knutson, B. (2012). Interactivity and reward-related neural activation during a serious videogame. *PLoS ONE*, *7*(3), e33909. doi:10.1371/journal.pone.0033909 PMID:22442733

Connolly, T. M., Boyle, E. A., MacArthur, E., Hainey, T., & Boyle, J. M. (2012). A systematic literature review of empirical evidence on computer games and serious games. *Computers & Education*, *59*(2), 661–686. doi:10.1016/j.compedu.2012.03.004

Cowley, B., Charles, D., Black, M., & Hickey, R. (2008). Toward an understanding of flow in video games. *Computers in Entertainment*, *6*(2), 1. doi:10.1145/1371216.1371223

Csikszentmihalyi, M. (1988). The flow experience and its significance for human psychology. In M. Csikszentmihalyi & I. S. Csikszentmihalyi (Eds.), *Optimal experience: Psychological studies of flow in consciousness*. Cambridge: Cambridge University press. doi:10.1017/CBO9780511621956.002

Csikszentmihalyi, M. (2002). *Flow: The Classic Work on How to Achieve Happiness*. London: Rider.

De Wied, M., Zillman, D., & Ordman, V. (1994). The role of empathic distress in the enjoyment of cinematic tragedy. *Poetics*, *23*(1-2), 91–106. doi:10.1016/0304-422X(94)00010-4

Ellul, J. (1967). *The technological society*. New York: A.A. Knopf.

Feagin, S. L. (1983). The pleasures of tragedy. *American Philosophical Quarterly*, *20*(1), 95–104.

Flores, F., Graves, M., Hartfield, B., & Winograd, T. (1988). Computer systems and the design of organizational interaction. *ACM Transactions on Information Systems*, *6*(2), 153–172. doi:10.1145/45941.45943

Fredrickson, B. L. (2000). Cultivating positive emotions to optimize health and well-being. *Prevention & Treatment*, *3*(1). doi:10.1037/1522-3736.3.1.31a

Fredrickson, B. L., Danner, D., & Snowdon, D. (2003). The Value of Positive Emotions. *American Scientist*, *91*(4), 330–335. doi:10.1511/2003.4.330

Frijda, N. H. (1993). *Appraisal and beyond: Special issue of Cognition and Emotion*. Hillsdale, NJ: Erlbaum.

Frome, J. (2007). Eight Ways Videogames Generate Emotion. *Paper presented at DIGRA,* Tokyo, Japan (pp. 831–835).

Garris, R., Ahlers, R., & Driskell, J. E. (2002). Games, motivation, and learning: A research and practice model. *Simulation & Gaming*, *33*(4), 441–467. doi:10.1177/1046878102238607

Gaver, W., Beaver, J., & Benford, S. (2003). Ambiguity as a resource for design. *Paper presented at CHI - Designing Design,* Fort Lauderdale, USA (pp. 233–240). doi:10.1145/642611.642653

Gee, J. P. (2005). Good Video Games and Good Learning. *Phi Kappa Phi Forum, 85*, 33–37. doi:10.1177/1555412008317309

Gilleade, K. M., & Dix, A. (2004). Using frustration in the design of adaptive videogames. *Proceedings of the 2004 ACM SIGCHI International Conference on Advances in Computer Entertainment Technology - ACE '04* (pp. 228–232). doi:10.1145/1067343.1067372

Gorini, A., Capideville, C. S., De Leo, G., Mantovani, F., & Riva, G. (2011). The role of immersion and narrative in mediated presence: The virtual hospital experience. *Cyberpsychology, Behavior, and Social Networking*, *14*(3), 99–105. doi:10.1089/cyber.2010.0100 PMID:20649451

Granic, I., Lobel, A., & Engels, R. C. M. E. (2014). The benefits of playing video games. *The American Psychologist*, *69*(1), 66–78. doi:10.1037/a0034857 PMID:24295515

Grassi, A., Gaggioli, A., & Riva, G. (2009). The green valley: The use of mobile narratives for reducing stress in commuters. *Cyberpsychology & Behavior*, *12*(2), 155–161. doi:10.1089/cpb.2008.0156 PMID:19275475

Haidt, J. (2000). The Positive emotion of elevation. *Prevention & Treatment*, *3*(1). doi:10.1037/1522-3736.3.1.33c

Haidt, J. (2003). Elevation and the Positive Psychology of Morality. In C. L. M. Keyes & J. Haidt (Eds.), *Flourishing: Positive psychology and the life well-lived*. Washington, DC, USA: American Psychological Association. doi:10.1037/10594-012

Hancock, P., Pepe, A., & Murphy, L. (2005). Hedonomics: The power of positive and pleasurable emotions. *Ergonomics in Design*, *13*(1), 8–14. doi:10.1177/106480460501300104

Hanich, J., Wagner, V., Shah, M., Jacobsen, T., & Menninghaus, W. (2014). Why we like to watch sad films. The pleasure of being moved in aesthetic experiences. *Psychology of Aesthetics, Creativity, and the Arts*, *8*(2), 130–143. doi:10.1037/a0035690

Hartmann, T. (2011). Not so moral responses to media entertainment? *Media Psychology*, *23*(1), 24–28. doi:10.1027/1864-1105/a000028

Hartmann, T., Toz, E., & Brandon, M. (2010). Just a Game? Unjustified Virtual Violence Produces Guilt in Empathetic Players. *Media Psychology*, *13*(4), 339–363. doi:10.1080/15213269.2010.524912

Hartmann, T., & Vorderer, P. (2010). It's Okay to Shoot a Character: Moral Disengagement in Violent Video Games. *Journal of Communication*, *60*(1), 94–119. doi:10.1111/j.1460-2466.2009.01459.x

Heidegger, M. (1977). *The Question Concerning Technology and Other Essays*. New York, USA: Garland Pub.

Hofer, M., & Wirth, W. (2012). It's Right to Be Sad. *Journal of Media Psychology: Theories, Methods, and Applications*, *24*(2), 43–54. doi:10.1027/1864-1105/a000061

Hsee, C. K., Hastie, R., & Chen, J. (2008). Hedonomics: Bridging Decision Research With Happiness Research. *Perspectives on Psychological Science*, *3*(3), 224–243. doi:10.1111/j.1745-6924.2008.00076.x PMID:26158937

Huta, V., & Ryan, R. M. (2010). Pursuing Pleasure or Virtue: The Differential and Overlapping Well-Being Benefits of Hedonic and Eudaimonic Motives. *Journal of Happiness Studies*, *11*(6), 735–762. doi:10.1007/s10902-009-9171-4

Ivarsson, M., Anderson, M., Åkerstedt, T., & Lindblad, F. (2013). The effect of violent and nonviolent video games on heart rate variability, sleep, and emotions in adolescents with different violent gaming habits. *Psychosomatic Medicine*, *75*(4), 390–396. doi:10.1097/PSY.0b013e3182906a4c PMID:23645706

Ivory, J. D., & Kalyanaraman, S. (2007). The effects of technological advancement and violent content in video games on players' feelings of presence, involvement, physiological arousal, and aggression. *Journal of Communication*, *57*(3), 532–555. doi:10.1111/j.1460-2466.2007.00356.x

Jansz, J. (2005). The emotional appeal of violent video games for adolescent males. *Communication Theory*, *15*(3), 219–241. doi:10.1111/j.1468-2885.2005.tb00334.x

Jennett, C., Cox, A. L., Cairns, P., Dhoparee, S., Epps, A., Tijs, T., & Walton, A. (2008). Measuring and defining the experience of immersion in games. *International Journal of Human-Computer Studies*, *66*(9), 641–661. doi:10.1016/j.ijhcs.2008.04.004

Jin, S.-A. A. (2012). "Toward Integrative Models of Flow": Effects of Performance, Skill, Challenge, Playfulness, and Presence on Flow in Video Games. *Journal of Broadcasting & Electronic Media*, *56*(2), 169–186. doi:10.1080/08838151.2012.678516

Jones, M. G. (1998). Creating Electronic Learning Environments : Games, Flow, and the User Interface. *Proceedings of Selected Research and Development Presentations at the National Convention of the Association for Educational Communications and Technology (AECT)* (pp. 205–214).

Juan, M. C., Baños, R., Botella, C., Pérez, D., Alcaníiz, M., & Monserrat, C. (2006). An Augmented Reality System for the Treatment of Acrophobia: The Sense of Presence Using Immersive Photography. *Presence (Cambridge, Mass.)*, *15*(4), 393–402. doi:10.1162/pres.15.4.393

Juul, J. (2009). *A Casual Revolution: Reinventing Video Games and Their Players*. Cambridge: MIT Press.

Juul, J. (2013). *The art of failure. An essay on the pain of playing videogames*. Cambridge: MIT Press.

Kaye, L. K., & Bryce, J. (2012). Putting the fun factor into gaming: The influence of social contexts on experiences of playing videogames. *International Journal of Internet Science*.

Keller, J., & Bless, H. (2008). Flow and regulatory compatibility: An experimental approach to the flow model of intrinsic motivation. *Personality and Social Psychology Bulletin*, *34*(2), 196–209. doi:10.1177/0146167207310026 PMID:18212330

Kivikangas, J. M., & Ravaja, N. (2013). Emotional responses to victory and defeat as a function of opponent. *IEEE Transactions on Affective Computing*, *4*(2), 173–182. doi:10.1109/T-AFFC.2013.12

Klasen, M., Weber, R., Kircher, T., Mathiak, K., & Mathiak, K. (2012). Neural contributions to flow experience during video game playing. *Social Cognitive and Affective Neuroscience*, *7*(4), 485–495. doi:10.1093/scan/nsr021 PMID:21596764

Klimmt, C., Rizzo, A., Vorderer, P., Koch, J., & Fischer, T. (2009). Experimental evidence for suspense as determinant of video game enjoyment. *Cyberpsychology & Behavior, 12*(1), 29–31. doi:10.1089/cpb.2008.0060 PMID:19025464

Kline, F. M. (1981). Catharsis in Healing, Ritual and Drama. *The Journal of Clinical Psychiatry*. doi:10.2307/2068827

Kohlberg, L. (1971). Moral psychology and the study of tragedy. In S. Weintraub & P. Young (Eds.), *Directions in Literary criticisms*. University Park, USA: Pennsylvania State University Press.

Koven, N. S. (2011). Specificity of meta-emotion effects on moral decision-making. *Emotion (Washington, D.C.), 11*(5), 1255–1261. doi:10.1037/a0025616 PMID:21942703

Lazarus, R. (1994). *Emotion and adaptation*. New York, USA: Oxford University Press.

Lobel, A., Granic, I., & Engels Rutger, C. M. E. (2014). Stressful Gaming, Interoceptive Awareness, and Emotion Regulation Tendencies: A Novel Approach. *Cyberpsychology, Behavior, and Social Networking, 17*(4), 222–227. doi:10.1089/cyber.2013.0296

Lorentz, P. (2014). Why Failing in Games is a Positive Aspect of Play: A Review of Jesper Juul's The Art of Failure. *Journal of Game Criticism, 1*(2).

Løvoll, H. S., & Vittersø, J. (2014). Can Balance be Boring? A Critique of the "Challenges Should Match Skills" Hypotheses in Flow Theory. *Social Indicators Research, 115*(1), 117–136. doi:10.1007/s11205-012-0211-9

Lu, A. S., Baranowski, T., Thompson, D., & Buday, R. (2012). Story Immersion of Videogames for Youth Health Promotion: A Review of Literature. *Games for Health Journal, 1*(3), 199–204. doi:10.1089/g4h.2011.0012 PMID:24416639

Madeira, F., Arriaga, P., Adrião, J., Lopes, R., & Esteves, F. (2015). Emotional Gaming. In Y. Baek (Ed.), *Psychology of Gaming*. New York, USA: Nova Science Publishers.

Mayer, J. D., & Gaschke, Y. N. (1988). The experience and meta-experience of mood. *Journal of Personality and Social Psychology, 55*(1), 102–111. doi:10.1037/0022-3514.55.1.102 PMID:3418484

McGonigal, J. (2011). *Reality is broken*. New York, USA: Penguin.

Mcluhan, M. (1964). The Medium is the Message. *Understanding Media, 14*, 7–23.

Mitmansgruber, H., Beck, T. N., Höfer, S., & Schüßler, G. (2009). When you don't like what you feel: Experiential avoidance, mindfulness and meta-emotion in emotion regulation. *Personality and Individual Differences, 46*(4), 448–453. doi:10.1016/j.paid.2008.11.013

Nakamura, J., & Csikszentmihalyi, M. (2002). The concept of flow. In C. R. Snyder & S. J. Lopez (Eds.), *The handbook of positive psychology*. Oxford: Oxford University Press.

Oliver, M. B. (1993). Exploring the Paradox of the Enjoyment of Sad Films. *Communication, 19*(3), 315–342. doi:10.1111/j.1468-2958.1993.tb00304.x

Oliver, M. B., Hartmann, T., & Woolley, J. K. (2012). Elevation in Response to Entertainment Portrayals of Moral Virtue. *Human Communication Research*, *38*(3), 360–378. doi:10.1111/j.1468-2958.2012.01427.x

Pallavicini, F., Cipresso, P., Raspelli, S., Grassi, A., Serino, S., Vigna, C., & Riva, G. et al. (2013). Is virtual reality always an effective stressor for exposure treatments? Some insights from a controlled trial. *BMC Psychiatry*, *13*(1), 52. doi:10.1186/1471-244X-13-52 PMID:23398927

Plantinga, C. (2009). *Moving viewers: American Film and the Spectator's Experience*. Oakland, USA: University of California Press.

Postman, N. (1993). *Technopoly: The Surrender of Culture to Technology*. New York, USA: Vintage.

Przybylski, A. K., Rigby, C. S., & Ryan, R. M. (2010). A motivational model of video game engagement. *Review of General Psychology*, *14*(2), 154–166. doi:10.1037/a0019440

Przybylski, A. K., Ryan, R. M., & Rigby, C. S. (2009). The motivating role of violence in video games. *Personality and Social Psychology Bulletin*, *35*(2), 243–259. doi:10.1177/0146167208327216 PMID:19141627

Przybylski, K., Weinstein, N., Murayama, K., Lynch, M. F., & Ryan, R. M. (2012). The Ideal Self at Play: The Appeal of Video Games That Let You Be All You Can Be. *Psychological Science*, *23*(1), 69–76. doi:10.1177/0956797611418676 PMID:22173739

Ravaja, N., Turpeinen, M., Saari, T., Puttonen, S., & Keltikangas-Järvinen, L. (2008). The psychophysiology of James Bond: Phasic emotional responses to violent video game events. *Emotion (Washington, D.C.)*, *8*(1), 114–120. doi:10.1037/1528-3542.8.1.114 PMID:18266521

Repetto, C., & Riva, G. (2011). From virtual reality to interreality in the treatment of anxiety disorders. *Neuropsychiatry*, *1*(1), 31–43. doi:10.2217/npy.11.5

Rigby, S., & Ryan, R. (2011). *Glued to games: how video games draw us in and hold us spellbound*. New York, USA: ABC-CLIO.

Riva, G., Baños, R. M., Botella, C., Wiederhold, B. K., & Gaggioli, A. (2012). Positive technology: Using interactive technologies to promote positive functioning. *Cyberpsychology, Behavior, and Social Networking*, *15*(2), 69–77. doi:10.1089/cyber.2011.0139 PMID:22149077

Riva, G., Mantovani, F., Capideville, C. S., Preziosa, A., Morganti, F., Villani, D., & Alcañiz, M. et al. (2007). Affective interactions using virtual reality: The link between presence and emotions. *Cyberpsychology & Behavior*, *10*(1), 45–56. doi:10.1089/cpb.2006.9993 PMID:17305448

Russoniello, C. V., O'brien, K., & Parks, J. M. (2009). EEG, HRV and Psychological Correlates while Playing Bejeweled II: A Randomized Controlled Study. *Annual Review of Cybertherapy and Telemedicine*, *7*(1), 189–192. doi:10.3233/978-1-60750-017-9-189 PMID:19592761

Ryan, R. M., & Deci, E. L. (2000). Self-determination theory and the facilitation of intrinsic motivation, social development, and well-being. *The American Psychologist*, *55*(1), 68–78. doi:10.1037/0003-066X.55.1.68 PMID:11392867

Ryan, R. M., Rigby, C. S., & Przybylski, A. (2006). The motivational pull of video games: A self-determination theory approach. *Motivation and Emotion*, *30*(4), 347–363. doi:10.1007/s11031-006-9051-8

Schneider, E., Lang, A., Shin, M., & Bradley, S. D. (2004). Death with a Story: How Story Impacts Emotional, Motivational, and Physiological Responses to First-Person Shooter Video Games. *Human Communication Research*, *30*(3), 361–375.

Schramm, H., & Wirth, W. (2010). Exploring the paradox of sad-film enjoyment: The role of multiple appraisals and meta-appraisals. *Poetics*, *38*(3), 319–335. doi:10.1016/j.poetic.2010.03.002

Schultze, U. (2010). Embodiment and presence in virtual worlds: A review. *Journal of Information Technology*, *25*(4), 434–449. doi:10.1057/jit.2010.25

Seligman, M. E., & Csikszentmihalyi, M. (2000). Positive psychology. An introduction. *The American Psychologist*, *55*(1), 5–14. doi:10.1037/0003-066X.55.1.5 PMID:11392865

Seligman, M. E. P. (2002). Positive psychology, positive prevention, and positive therapy. In C. R. Snyder & S. J. Lopez (Eds.), *The handbook of positive psychology*. Oxford, United Kingdom: Oxford University Press.

Serino, S., Cipresso, P., Gaggioli, A., & Riva, G. (2013). The Potential of Pervasive Sensors and Computing for Positive Technology: The Interreality Paradigm. In S. Mukhopadhyay & O. Postolache (Eds.), *Pervasive and Mobile Sensing and Computing for Healthcare. Smart Sensors, Measurement and Instrumentation* (Vol. 2, pp. 207–232). New York, USA: Springer. doi:10.1007/978-3-642-32538-0_10

Serino, S., Triberti, S., Villani, D., Cipresso, P., Gaggioli, A., & Riva, G. (2013). Toward a validation of cyber-interventions for stress disorders based on stress inoculation training: A systematic review. *Virtual Reality (Waltham Cross)*, *18*(1), 73–87. doi:10.1007/s10055-013-0237-6

Spagnolli, A., Gamberini, L., & Gasparini, D. (2002). Situated Breakdown Analysis for the Evaluation of a Virtual Environment. *PsychNology Journal*, *1*(1), 5–17. PMID:12322671

Sproull, L., & Kiesler, S. (1986). Reducing Social Context Cues: Electronic Mail in Organizational Communication. *Management Science*, *32*(11), 1492–1512. doi:10.1287/mnsc.32.11.1492

Touhey, J. C., & Bandura, A. (1975). Aggression: A Social Learning Analysis. *Contemporary Sociology*, *4*(2), 169. doi:10.2307/2062223

Triberti, S., & Argenton, L. (2015). Eros, Thanatos e Pixel: lo scandalo nei videogiochi e i suoi effetti psicologici. In L. Papale & F. Alinovi (Eds.), *Virtual Erotico*. Milan, Italy: Unicopli.

Triberti, S., & Liberati, E. G. (2014). Patient Centered Virtual Reality: An Opportunity to Improve the Quality of Patient's Experience. In P. Cipresso & S. Serino (Eds.), *Virtual Reality: Technologies, Medical Applications and Challenges*. New York, USA: Nova Science.

Triberti, S., Repetto, C., & Riva, G. (2014). Psychological factors influencing the effectiveness of virtual reality-based analgesia: A systematic review. *Cyberpsychology, Behavior, and Social Networking*, *17*(6), 335–345. doi:10.1089/cyber.2014.0054 PMID:24892195

Triberti, S., Villani, D., & Riva, G. (2015). Moral positioning in video games and its relation with dispositional traits: The emergence of a social dimension. *Computers in Human Behavior*, *50*, 1–8. doi:10.1016/j.chb.2015.03.069

Twitchell, J. (1995). *Dreadful Pleasures: An Anatomy of Modern Horror*. Oxford, United Kingdom: Oxford University Press.

Ullén, F., de Manzano, Ö., Almeida, R., Magnusson, P. K. E., Pedersen, N. L., Nakamura, J., & Madison, G. et al. (2012). Proneness for psychological flow in everyday life: Associations with personality and intelligence. *Personality and Individual Differences*, *52*(2), 167–172. doi:10.1016/j.paid.2011.10.003

Vachiratamporn, V., Legaspi, R., Moriyama, K., Fukui, K., & Numao, M. (2015). An analysis of player affect transitions in survival horror games. *Journal on Multimodal User Interfaces*, *9*(1), 43–54. doi:10.1007/s12193-014-0153-4

Van Reekum, C. M., Marije, C., Johnstone, T., Banse, R., Etter, A., Wehrle, T., & Scherer, K. R. (2004). Psychophysiological responses to appraisal dimensions in a computer game. *Cognition and Emotion*, *18*(5), 663–688. doi:10.1080/02699930341000167

Villani, D., Preziosa, A., & Riva, G. (2006). Coping with stress using virtual reality: A new perspective. *Annual Review of Cybertherapy and Telemedicine*, *4*, 25–32.

Villani, D., & Riva, G. (2012). Does Interactive Media Enhance the Management of Stress? Suggestions from a Controlled Study. *Cyberpsychology, Behavior, and Social Networking*, *15*(1), 24–30. doi:10.1089/cyber.2011.0141 PMID:22032797

Vittersø, J. (2004). Subjective well-being versus self-actualization: Using the flow-simplex to promote a conceptual clarification of subjective quality of life. *Social Indicators Research*, *65*(3), 299–331. doi:10.1023/B:SOCI.0000003910.26194.ef

Vuoskoski, J. K., & Thompson, W. F. (2012). Who Enjoys Listening to Sad Music and Why? *Music Perception: An Interdisciplinary Journal*, *29*(3), 311–317. doi:10.1525/mp.2012.29.3.311

Weaver, A. J., & Lewis, N. (2012). Mirrored Morality: An Exploration of Moral Choice in Video Games. *Cyberpsychology, Behavior, and Social Networking*. doi:10.1089/cyber.2012.0235 PMID:23017118

Weber, R., Behr, K.-M., Tamborini, R., Ritterfeld, U., & Mathiak, K. (2009). What Do We Really Know About First-Person-Shooter Games? An Event-Related, High-Resolution Content Analysis. *Journal of Computer-Mediated Communication*, *14*(4), 1016–1037. doi:10.1111/j.1083-6101.2009.01479.x

Westerfelhaus, R., & Alan Brookey, R. (2004). At the unlikely confluence of conservative religion and popular culture: Fight club as heteronormative ritual. *Text and Performance Quarterly*, *24*(3-4), 302–326. doi:10.1080/1046293042000312788

Winograd, T., & Flores, F. (1986). *Understanding Computers and Cognition: A New Foundation for Design*. Wilmington, USA: Intellect Books.

Yee, N. (2006). Motivations for play in online games. *Cyberpsychology & Behavior*, *9*(6), 772–775. doi:10.1089/cpb.2006.9.772 PMID:17201605

Zillmann, D., Weaver, J. B., Mundorf, N., & Aust, C. F. (1986). Effects of an opposite-gender companion's affect to horror on distress, delight, and attraction. *Journal of Personality and Social Psychology*, *51*(3), 586–594. doi:10.1037/0022-3514.51.3.586

## KEY TERMS AND DEFINITIONS

**Artifact Emotions:** Emotions elicited by the contemplation of an artifact/medium as a piece of art, independently by its content.

**Breakdown:** An experience of malfunction during a human-technology interaction. It features the technology suddenly becoming no more "transparent", and the user recruiting conscious cognitive processes to repair the failed action.

**Catharsis:** The idea according to which expressing a negative emotion allows one to "let it go", this way leaving space in him/herself for a subsequent positive emotion (the term comes from Aristotle).

**Elevation:** A specific emotion felt in response to the depiction of heroism and human virtues, characterized by the specific physical activation "lump in throat".

**Flow:** The feeling of total absorption into an ongoing activity, also called optimal experience.

**Meta-Emotion:** An emotion felt in response to the feeling of another emotion.

**Positive Technology:** A theoretical paradigm guiding research, intervention and technology design, focused on the use of new technologies for providing well-being.

**Sympathetic Experience:** Feeling an emotion quite similar to the one showed by another (in this context, a character in a media-conveyed narration).

**Video Game:** An interactive technology/medium designed for entertainment purposes. It is usually based on non-immersive virtual reality. It usually features game rules and mechanics and/or a narrative content.

# Chapter 13
# Serious Games and Gamified Tools for Psychological Intervention:
## A Review

**Unai Diaz-Orueta**
*Nesplora Technology & Behavior, Spain*

## ABSTRACT

*Mobile technologies and technological advances in behavioral assessment have found their way in common healthcare practices. However, there are still few studies about videogame-based interventions to support concrete psychological treatments. While the market for self-help mobile apps is continuously increasing, in most cases, they are a mere digitalization of texts contained in self-help books and do not take advantage of the interactive and playful potential of devices on which they are offered. Nevertheless, a number of health games have been developed for children and adults for a variety of therapeutic purposes. The current chapter provides an overview of the state-of-the-art serious games currently available as psychological interventions across popular delivery formats (virtual reality environments, online and PC videogames). Where available, evidence about their efficacy is reported. These serious games have the potential to complement traditional psychological interventions and improve psychological wellbeing for people of all ages.*

## INTRODUCTION

Humans play games in all cultures with different goals: to learn new skills, to feel a sense of achievement, to interact with friends and family, etc. (Krebs, 2013). In this sense, digital games are just a new expression of this old method of social interaction and a subset of digital games is the serious games genre, which can make the player experience different levels of *presence* and *immersion* (two concepts we will revisit in this chapter) within the game environment.

In recent years, serious games, or videogames for purposes other than mere entertainment, have received increased attention and dissemination, mainly due to their proved impact in the areas of military training (Yildrim, 2010), education, and stroke and physical rehabilitation. In 2010, synergies between

DOI: 10.4018/978-1-4666-9986-1.ch013

videogame industry and other sectors such as education, defense, medicine, health, work security, activism, culture, or inclusion generated a profit of 1.5 million Euros (IDATE, 2010), with an expected annual increase of 47% until 2015.

In a recent literature review, Rahmani and Boren (2012) analyzed electronic databases published between January 2000 and April 2012 searching for Randomized Control Trials (RCTs) examining the potential of videogames on health outcomes. Their analysis found that most of the studies showed promising results using videogames in healthcare, with potential uses for pain management, diagnostics, education, physical rehabilitation, cognitive loss prevention, and so forth.

'Serious Games,' or 'Game-Based Learning,' are terms used interchangeably for digital play experiences developed for the broader purpose of training and behavior change (Connolly, Boyle, MacArthur et al., 2012). In society today, we find serious games in just about any setting—from corporate, healthcare, and government to non-governmental organizations, non-profits, and education. Moreover, games, once regarded as mere stimuli or something to be blamed for increasing aggressive behaviors (Nap & Díaz-Orueta, 2014), are now known to be persuasive and motivating digital tools capable of positively affecting training, learning, and skill acquisition. For example, Shin, Heard, Suo, and Chow (2012) studied the brains of people playing the game *Counter-Strike* (CS) (Valve Software, Bellevue, WA) using an EEG alpha asymmetry index and found that overall results were consistent with the hypothesis that predominantly positive emotional reactions were elicited from playing the CS game and concurred with positive subjective ratings of happiness. Even the *TETRIS* puzzle game can be used as a non-invasive cognitive resource for crisis intervention after traumatic events; more specifically, it produced a significant reduction in flashback frequency over one week, and these results were in agreement with a clinical measure of Post-Traumatic Stress Disorder (PTSD) symptomatology (Holmes, James, Coode-Bate & Deeprose, 2009). In summary, serious games are defined as games with a purpose beyond mere entertainment that are designed specifically for the goal of training and behavior change in different domains (either education, healthcare or others as stated above). Among those, we may find specific games targeting behavioral change in the context of a psychological intervention or treatment (such as treatment for mood disorders such as depression or anxiety, anger management, identification and prevention of bullying behaviors, etc.)

Regarding psychological interventions, there are many features in game structure and mechanics that can be used successfully when planning a therapeutic treatment. Most existing game worlds easily can be adapted by changing the scenery, complexity, avatar, controls, etc., with a patient or therapist using these variables to easily personalize the game and make it compatible with the clients' abilities and needs. As Nap and Díaz-Orueta (2014) stated referring to rehabilitation gaming (but the same could be applied to psychological treatment), not only can the patient or therapist adapt the game, but also the game itself can automatically adapt to the clients' progress. Therefore, the whole virtual environment, including the characters, scenery, and even the storyline, can be adapted to the player's specific needs and abilities.

This chapter will focus on the existing serious games for psychological intervention, an area that has not received as much attention as physical or stroke rehabilitation by serious game developers. This is possibly because physiological or medical signs of progress and efficacy are easier to be measured than psychological changes (a problem that will be constant in any type of psychological intervention when compared to other types of health, medical, or rehabilitative interventions). The current review provides updated information on the existing games in different formats such as virtual reality environments, or online games with a special emphasis on serious games for the PC platform, as they include the most heterogeneous features and have the most game-like enjoyable graphic environments (i.e., they look like entertainment videogames, not like mere treatment applications or programs). Where possible, evidence will be discussed on their efficacy and ongoing development, all of which aim to provide support for traditional psychological interventions and a significant improvement in quality of life and psychological healthcare for people of all ages.

## BACKGROUND: THE RELEVANCE OF GAMIFICATION AND SERIOUS GAMES FOR PSYCHOLOGICAL INTERVENTION

The current section provides an overview on what is known about how game-based interventions and game features may be relevant for psychological and/or psychotherapeutic intervention. An increasing body of research suggests that moderate game play can contribute to positive emotions and emotional stability and that positive mental wellbeing has been associated with game play as a means of relaxation and stress reduction (Jone, Scholes, Johnson, Katsikitis, & Carras, 2014). It has also been found that casual videogame play may address psychological and somatic symptoms associated with depression (Russionello, Fish, & O'Brien, 2013). At the end of the last century, Gardner (1991) claimed that using videogames in psychotherapy sessions provided common ground between himself and his younger clients as well as excellent behavioral observation opportunities to gain relevant information about the children's repertoire of: (1) problem-solving strategies, (2) ability to perceive and recall subtle cues, (3) foresee consequences of behaviors and act on them, (4) eye-hand coordination, (5) release of aggression and control, and (6) ability to deal with frustration. Wilkinson et al. (2008) discussed studies that showed that digital games (more specifically, a NASA patent on ADHD intervention via biofeedback that modulated 'off-the-shelf' digital games and Sony PlayStation games such as skateboarding or adventure games) can also help to reduce Attention Deficit Hyperactivity Disorder (ADHD) symptoms as much as conventional interventions. Furthermore, the participants stated that the game intervention was far more enjoyable than existing methods.

In combination with the technology's ability to create accurate spatial, situation or mechanical simulations, digital games can be transformed into highly engaging and sophisticated training tools (Alexiou, Schippers, & Oshri, 2012). Game-based learning and interventions seem to be at least as effective as conventional instructional media (Honka, Kaipainen, Hietala, & Saranummi, 2011). However, relatively few studies on the usage of games for psychological intervention have been conducted, and the evidence in the area is still scarce. Goh, Ang, and Tan (2008) discussed how mental health professionals can explore and take advantage of the diffusion of computer games to help the treatment of mental illness and highlighted the need for considering the potential users' characteristics, such as gender, culture, socioeconomic status as well as needs and expectations. A more recent review on the serious games to support psychotherapeutic treatments reported improvements in terms of elevated self-esteem, higher self-efficacy, increased knowledge, awareness of the illness, adherence to treatment and problem solving skills, and enhanced outcome on cognitive and behavioral aspects of aggression (Santamaría, Soto, Fernández-Aranda, Krug, Forcano, Gunnard et al., 2011).

According to Baranowski, Buday, Thompson et al. (2013), game-based learning and interventions have been defined by means of the identification of their principles (intrinsic motivation, learning through "fun," contextualized learning, self-reliance, and experiential learning) and mechanics (rules, clear and challenging goals, fantasy, progressive levels of difficulty, interactivity, player control, uncertainty, feedback, and social components). Although it is not that clear which are the most relevant ingredients necessary to implement and maintain behavior change in their target population, especially among children, emphasis has been put on basic psychological needs (autonomy, competence, relatedness), characters, and a personally relevant storyline to enhance attention and depth of information processing (Ryan, Rigby, & Przybylski, 2006). According to Buckley & Anderson (2006), games are useful motivational tools when the player has control over the game, he can play at his own ability level and speed, and when the game provide immediate feedback and rewards (as they increase the frequency of the rewarded behavior in the game, and generate more positive attitudes towards the content of the game). Parker, Jimmieson and Amiot (2009) found that people with a high desire of control are more satisfied with their performance and show better execution and maintenance in their tasks than others with less desire of control. In modern video games, reward systems also provide social meaning within and outside of games (Reeves & Read, 2009; Salen & Zimmerman, 2004).

Moreover, there is discussion about major issues to be taken into account when deciding which channel and technology to use for serious game development. Baranowski et al. (2013) stated that this decision depends on (1) how many targeted participants you want to reach in an easy and inexpensive way, (2) which platform allows the programming flexibility or features you need to develop for the game, (3) where the target participant will play (i.e. on the bus, in a classroom, at home, etc.) and (4) when they will play (i.e. school or work time, leisure time, etc.). In addition, the game should be created using technology that will have the broadest reach to the targeted participants in the future, not in the immediate past, as the latter may lead to invest effort in developing in a platform or device that may become obsolete when the game is finally available to the target participants.

In the following sections, virtual reality environments and serious videogames that can mainly be reached and used on a desktop computer or laptop environment are presented. The different examples provided were selected based on the availability of the description about their features and goals. For all of them, when available, evidence about their efficacy for the purposes for which they were developed will be presented. This availability may lead to some SG to be presented with more detail and consistence, while others would require a closer approach.

## SERIOUS GAMES FOR PSYCHOLOGICAL INTERVENTION

### Psychological Intervention in the Format of Virtual Environments

The current section presents the primary virtual reality based games that have been developed for psychological treatment, mainly towards conditions such as Post-Traumatic Stress Disorder (PTSD), phobias, treatment-related pain and anxiety, or other mental health problems. The main justification for the inclusion of VR in a chapter of serious games is that it fulfills two requirements:

1. Some structured VR environments may add value to traditional psychological intervention by providing users with safe environments for training and skills acquisition (e.g. learning of coping skills to deal with phobias, fear, anxiety, etc.) and reproducing realistic environments for treatment that should otherwise be faced by the patient in probably less safer and effective, but 'traditional' ways (for example, in Desensitization Therapy, the patient tries to 'imagine' the feared stimuli – snakes, roaches, spiders, etc.– but many times the patient is not good imagining feared stimuli and there is no guarantee that he is actually imagining them properly; also, in the Flooding technique,

the patient has to deal face-to-face with the feared stimuli – e.g. real snakes or spiders in the same room, which may lead to over sensitization if therapy is not carried out properly (Leitenberg, 1990).

2. They may be presented in the format of games with the same core ingredients described by McGonigal, (2011) (i.e. goal, rules, feedback system, and voluntary participation), thus motivating and engaging the patient for treatment.

What makes Virtual Reality environments so suitable to be used as tools for psychological intervention? According to Riva, Botella, Baños et al. (2015), the sense of *presence* provided by VR technologies can be a critical advantage, as it may provide the person a place where he/she can be placed in and live the experience. According to Mantovani and Castelnuovo (2003), the learning potential of virtual reality training relies on the possibility for learners to make a number of significant first-person experiences and to fail in a safe and protected environment, within an experience that should seem real and engaging to participants, as if they were present right there in the virtual environment, both from the emotional and cognitive point of view. These authors collect different definitions about the sense of presence pointing to a multi-dimensional construct, "a subjective feeling depending on many environmental, contextual and personal characteristics and factors" and with "at least eight different ways to consider "presence" (spatial presence, sensory presence, social realism, engagement, social presence, co-presence, social actor within the medium, medium as social actor)" (Mantovani & Castelnuovo, 2003, p. 171).

Used appropriately, it is possible to target a specific cognitive system without any significant change in the therapeutic approach. For instance, VR may help the therapist confront a phobic patient with the feared stimuli, or on the contrary may be used to isolate the patient from the external world and help him/her in practicing the right actions. In this sense, hi-tech and immersive VR can be an effective new kind of learning tool, since trainees in virtual environments can have multi-sensory experience including visual, auditory and to some extend haptic and tactile cues (Mantovani & Castelnuovo, 2003). In sum, the possibility of structuring a large amount of realistic controlled stimuli and, simultaneously, of monitoring the possible responses generated by the user of the technology offers a considerable increase in the likelihood of therapeutic effectiveness, as compared to traditional procedures, according to Riva et al. (2015).

Together with presence, another ingredient of VR is what is known as *immersion*. According to Baranowski, Buday, Thompson and Baranowski (2008), immersion takes place when the game or the VR environment captures a player's full attention, as if the player were actually part of the VR or game environment. Finally, in order to talk about VR environments as potential serious games, we need to keep in mind the four key traits that define all games according to McGonigal (2011): goal, rules, feedback system, and voluntary participation. The *goal* is the specific outcome that players will work to achieve, focusing their attention and continually orienting their participation throughout the game, thus providing players with a sense of purpose. *Rules* place limitations on how players can achieve the goal, pushing players to explore previously uncharted possibility spaces, unleashing creativity, and fostering strategic thinking. *Feedback* is what McGonigal defines as real-time feedback, ''a promise to the players that the goal is definitely achievable, and it provides motivation to keep playing'' (2011, p. 21). *Voluntary participation* requires that everyone who is playing the game knowingly and willingly accepts the goal, the rules, and the feedback, and the freedom to enter or leave a game at will ensures that intentionally stressful and challenging work is experienced as safe and pleasurable activity. Finally, for a game to be engaging in any format, including VR environment, it is mandatory to check whether it allows "flow"—the state of optimal experience (Csikszentmihalyi, 1975; Csikszentmihalyi & Csikszentmihalyi, 1988), a basic concept which has been successfully adopted in videogame design when trying to match the player's skills and the game's difficulty level (if the game is too easy, the player will be bored; if the game is too difficult, the player will be frustrated). In a flow state, the players are fully engaged with the task at hand, actions are performed automatically, and an optimal balance between skills and challenge is reached. In terms of the application of VR to therapy, exposure therapy, a traditional methodology of the cognitive behavioral therapy approach, has been combined lately with Virtual Reality, leading to VRET (Virtual Reality Exposure Therapy), which has been used for specific phobias, such as acrophobia, claustrophobia, fear of flying, fear of driving, arachnophobia, as well as anxiety disorders such as social phobia, panic disorders with agoraphobia and PTSD (Gamberini, Barresi, Majer, & Scarpetta, 2008; Scozzari & Gamberini, 2011; Riva et al., 2015). According to Riva (2005), the rationale behind its use is that in VR the patient is intentionally confronted with the feared stimuli while allowing the anxiety to attenuate. Thus, because avoiding a dreaded situation reinforces all phobias, each exposure to it actually lessens the anxiety through the processes of habituation and extinction. The success of virtual reality games on PTSD led Rizzo, Pair, Graap, et al. (2006) to successfully use the Full Spectrum Warrior graphic assets as a Virtual Environment for the treatment of Iraq War military service personnel diagnosed with PTSD. VRET has also been used by active duty service members who served in Iraq and Afghanistan, and results show that, of those who completed post-treatment assessment, 75% had experienced at least a 50% reduction in PTSD symptoms. They no longer met DSM-IV criteria for PTSD at post treatment; average PTSD scores decreased by 50.4%, depression scores by 46.6%, and anxiety scores by 36%; and, these improvements were maintained at follow up (McLay, Graap, Spira, et al., 2012).

One of the most interesting pioneer studies on using VR for PTSD is the one by Difede and Hoffman (2002). These authors showed the effectiveness of VR exposure therapy for PTSD in a case study with a patient who suffered from World Trade Center (WTC) PTSD, which was triggered by an intense experience or repeated exposure to the WTC attack in New York (September 11, 2001). In this report, the authors reported significant reduction of PTSD symptoms (90%) by exposing the patient to explosions, sound effects, virtual people jumping from the burning buildings, towers collapsing, and dust clouds. As the patient in the study had failed to improve after traditional imaginal exposure therapy, results were attributed partly to the increased realism of the VR images as compared to the mental images the patient could generate by imagination. Wiederhold and Wiederhold (2003) summarized advantages of VRET compared to *in vivo* exposures as follows: no loss of patient confidentiality, no safety issues, more flexibility (possibility to practice repeatedly with one aspect of exposure), it is realistic enough –but it is not actually "real" –to have patients willing to try treatment (as there is no real exposure to feared items); and, less time involved (i.e., cost-effective). In a very recent review, Riva et al. (2015) examine the role of VRET in a diverse series of phobias (achrophobia, claustrophobia, small animal phobia, flying phobia, driving phobia, public speaking disorder, panic disorder and agoraphobia), as well as in eating and pain disorders, The main conclusion for most of the studies revised by them is the need of more controlled studies with larger samples and comparable treatment conditions with regard to number of sessions and length of sessions in order to draw firmer conclusions.

With regards to pain treatment, the use of VR games is based on a distraction of the thought processes in the brain, including pain experiences. According to Gold, Kant, Kim, & Rizzo (2005), people can experience combinations of visual, auditory, and tactile stimuli that help to ''immerse'' the individual into the computer generated reality and create a sense of presence within the environment. In this way, the more immersed, the more that person feels like a part of the virtual world. Hoffman, Patterson, Soltani et al. (2009) stated that psychological factors such as attention can influence how much acute pain the patients report, and it is expected that, with VR, the patient becomes so distracted while interacting with objects in immersive virtual worlds that he or she has less attention available to process pain.

Based on distracting processes, Diaz-Orueta, Alvarado, Gutiérrez, et al. (2012) presented the usability study of a newly developed and commercialized virtual environment for pain and anxiety distraction—*Isla Calma*) (in English, *Peaceful Island*) (see Figure 1). *Isla Calma* is an introspection of an island where the player must explore and give life to some scenarios that need interaction with the user. In this way, participants get immersed in a situation demanding their attention, thus minimizing situations of pain and anxiety. In a recent study with patients at dental clinics (Diaz-Orueta, Climent, & Banterla, 2014), it was found that 82% of the experimental group (who received dental intervention together with "Isla Calma") compared to a control group (people undergoing a classical dental treatment) reported a significant reduction of anxiety and fear linked to dental intervention, which is subcategorized in fear of the consultation, fear of the instruments, and fear of the procedures. On the contrary, in the control group, levels of anxiety and fear were maintained. Interestingly, with regards to the time spent in the intervention, patients using IC perceived the intervention shorter than it really was, while patients not using IC perceived the dental intervention as longer than it really was. *Isla Calma* is an efficient intervention for acute pain distraction, although some limitations still need to be addressed. The applicability of the intervention for chronic pain conditions such as fibromyalgia and chronic asthenia was less successful. In a joint project developed by Nesplora and the Fibromyalgia Association of Zaragoza in Spain, the sample of women who participated was more concerned with perfect performance rather than letting themselves go and enjoying the island. The focus on control shown by these patients was that none of them were able to relax and distract from pain. In conclusion, further research is needed to address which specific elements of Isla Calma are efficient and which clinical interventions beyond the dental setting can be extrapolated.

Also, it is interesting to focus in the VR applications for other mental health problems, such as psychotic disorders. As described by Landgraf, Krebs, Olié et al. (2010), psychotic symptoms in schizophrenia

*Figure 1. Screenshot of Isla Calma*
*© Nesplora, Technology and Behavior.*

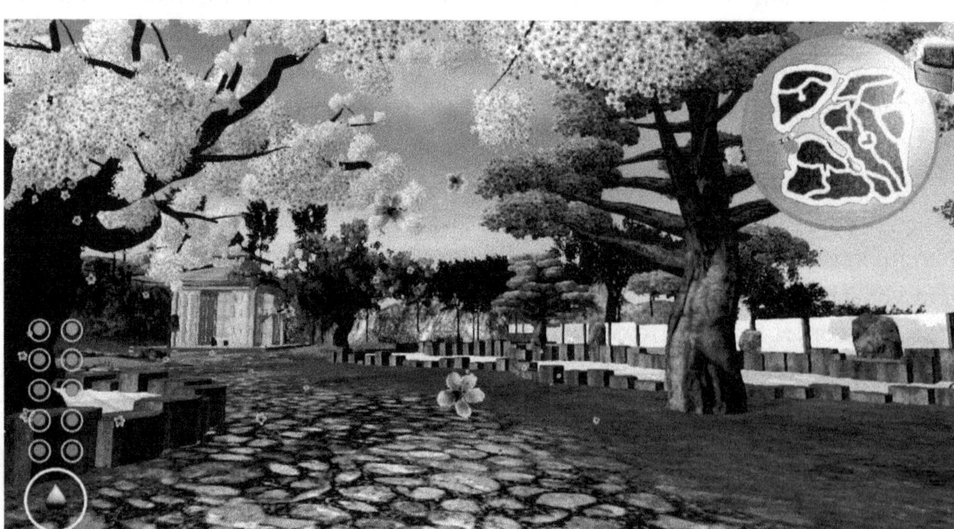

patients encompass the difficulty to distinguish between the respective points of view of self and others and they proved, by means of a virtual reality environment, that schizophrenia patients' adoption of an egocentric perspective is preserved, while adopting an allocentric point of view and switching between egocentric and landmark-centered perspectives were impaired. This use of VR helped Landgraf et al. (2010) understand that perturbations in non-egocentric referencing and transferring efficiently between different referential systems might contribute to altered personal and social world comprehension in schizophrenia.

One study that has properly described the use of VR in the understanding of schizophrenia and psychotic disorders is the one by Freeman (2008). This authors states that VR allows one of the key variables in understanding psychosis (i.e. social environments) to be controlled, providing exciting applications to research and treatment. More specifically, he sets out seven applications of virtual social environments to schizophrenia:

1. Symptom assessment,
2. Identification of symptom markers,
3. Establishment of predictive factors,
4. Tests of putative causal factors,
5. Investigation of the differential prediction of symptoms,
6. Determination of toxic elements in the environment, and
7. Development of treatment.

For the purpose of this chapter, we will focus on the latter. According to Freeman, the use of VR encompasses with emerging cognitive-behavioral interventions for psychosis, by means of three applications:

- Learning to cope with symptoms as they occur: a variety of coping strategies could be tried out for learning how to remain engaged in a social situation even when symptoms occur.
- Demonstrate how emotional state affects hallucinations by having the individual enter VR after a mood manipulation (up or down).
- Exposure to persecutory fears (the same way as in anxiety disorders): VR experiments are likely to feel safer and easier to the patient than tests of fears in real life and could precede them.

Virtual environments developed for social phobia, claustrophobia, and agoraphobia are likely to be applicable to psychosis, but all these types of studies are yet to be carried out. Moreover, validating scenarios developed for psychosis against the real life equivalents would be an issue of added value.

## Psychological Intervention in the Format of PC, Laptop, or Online Videogames

Most of the games described in the following section are based on the cognitive behavioral therapy (CBT) paradigm—the theoretical model underlying the most effective treatment for mood disorders, including depression, anxiety—and work with self-esteem and self-efficacy. The most remarkable advantages of serious games using the CBT paradigm are discussed and, where available, evidence on their efficacy is presented. Details on each game will be presented according to the available information about their description and efficacy.

## Game Based CBT for Children and Adolescents: Treating Anxiety, Depression, and Fears in Youngsters

According to Brezinka (2008), one of the most innovative uses of computer games is for child psychotherapy. By including therapeutic concepts within video games, children can be offered attractive electronic homework assignments that enable them to rehearse and repeat basic psychoeducational concepts they have learned during therapy sessions.

*Treasure Hunt* was the first serious game for children based on principles of cognitive behavior modification (Brezinka, 2008). It is an interactive adventure game with six levels, each of which corresponds to a certain step in cognitive-behavioral treatment. The game takes place on an old ship inhabited by Captain Jones, Felix, the ship's cat, and Polly, the ship's parrot. Captain Jones has found an old treasure map in the hull of his ship. To solve its mystery, he needs the help of a child. Tasks take place in different parts of the ship—on the deck, in the galley, in Captain Jones' dining room, and in the shipmates' bunks. Each task corresponds to a certain step in cognitive behavioral treatment, implying a linear structure for the game. For each completed task, the child receives a sea star reward. The old treasure map has a dark spot in the shape of a sea star at six important places. The child and Captain Jones will only be able to read what is written there when they place the missing sea star on the map. After having solved all the tasks, the last mission consists of a recapitulation of the previous exercises. Once the child has solved this last problem, he/she will find out where the treasure is buried. One of the most interesting parts of the game consists of hunting unhelpful (automatic) thoughts by means of an ego-shooter. The child has to catch a flying fish to be able to read the unhelpful thought written on it and replace it by a helpful one. Before joining Captain Jones on the final search for the treasure, the child receives a sailor's certificate that summarizes what he/she has learned through the game. The certificate is signed by Captain Jones and the therapist. Consequently, this game is not a self-help game but a complementary therapeutic game to be used with the guidance of a psychotherapist.

Another noteworthy project to treat anxiety by means of gaming was *Relax to Win* from the MindGames team at Media Lab in Europe (Sharry, McDermott, & Condron, 2003). *Relax to Win* is a two-player competitive game that uses biofeedback to control a dragon in a race. The more a player relaxes, as measured by the galvanic skin response (GSR), the faster the dragon moves, i.e., the player wins by learning to relax. According to the authors, the game has proved to be engaging to children and motivates them to become curious on how they relax and to learn new relaxation skills. Future research and development in relaxation gaming should add additional measurements besides GSR. A combination of measurements is preferred because some people have little variation in their GSR between relaxation and stress, while others always have a high conductive skin response, irrespective of their emotional status. Furthermore, an increase in the measured level of conductance cannot explain the type of emotion that is triggered, and therefore future research could combine ECG measurements, heart rate variability, facial expressions, et cetera, as a more valid indicator of relaxation.

A recent study by Khanna & Kendall (2012) examined the feasibility, acceptability and effects of *Camp Cope-a-Lot*, a computer-assisted cognitive behavioral therapy for anxiety. Forty-nine children with anxiety disorder were randomly assigned to one of three groups (CCAL, individual CBT or computer-assisted education, support and attention). Independent diagnostic interviews and self-report measures were completed at pre and post treatment and 3-month follow-up. Results showed that children playing *Camp Cope-A-Lot* (70%) and those undergoing Individual CBT (81%) showed significantly better gains than the others (19%) in the remission of their principal anxiety diagnosis—a series of gains that were maintained at follow-up, with no significant differences between ICBT and CCAL. Findings support the feasibility, acceptability, and beneficial effects of *Camp Cope-A-Lot* for anxious young individuals.

Knoe, Lentini, Cummings et al. (2011) studied the efficacy of an active feedback game called *The Journey of Wild Divine* with 24 children diagnosed with Attention Deficit Hyperactivity Disorder (ADHD), who were taught to manipulate their heart rate using breathing techniques taught during the game, showing that they demonstrated significant reductions in behavioral symptoms such as anxiety and stress. The study by Knoe et al. (2011) is, as the author's state, the first to test the effects of biofeedback-assisted relaxation training with a video game format for anxious children and young adults. The 8-session protocol that was implemented with combined relaxation training and practice with a psycho-educational intervention about relaxation and stress. According to the authors, further longitudinal studies with larger samples are needed to replicate these findings and to examine whether these changes last over time.

Depression is a common disorder among adolescents, and it has been demonstrated that it can be treated as effectively with individual therapy or with specialized computerized therapy. One of the games for the treatment of depression and anxiety in children is David Gnatenborough's *Island* (O'Dwyer-O'Brien, Coyle, Coyle, & O'Reilly, 2011), which is a CBT based therapy game for children between 9 and 13 years of age who experience anxiety and depression. *Island* is designed to be played in the therapy sessions together with the therapists. An alternative is the *SPARX* game developed by Merry, Stasiak, Shepherd et al. (2012). This group tried to evaluate whether a new computerized cognitive behavioral therapy intervention called *SPARX* (Smart, Positive, Active, Realistic, X-factor thoughts) could reduce depressive symptoms in adolescents seeking therapeutic help for their depression as much as traditional CBT treatment. With a multi-center study design including 24 primary healthcare sites in New Zealand, they recruited 187 adolescents between ages 12 and 19 (94 allocated to *SPARX*, with seven modules delivered for 2-7 weeks, and 93 to the usual treatment, with traditional, face-to-face counseling delivered by trained counselors and clinical psychologists).

As described by Merry et al. (2012), *SPARX* (see Figure 2) is an interactive fantasy game designed to deliver cognitive behavioral therapy for the treatment of clinically significant depression. It utilizes both first person instruction and a three dimensional interactive game where the young person chooses an avatar and undertakes a series of challenges to restore the balance in a fantasy world dominated by GNATs (Gloomy Negative Automatic Thoughts). The game consists of seven modules (levels), which are completed sequentially. At the beginning and end of each module, the user interacts in first person with a "guide," who puts the game into context, provides education, gauges mood, and sets and monitors real-life challenges (equivalent to homework). Young people who are not improving are prompted to seek help from their referring clinicians. *SPARX* is supplemented by a paper notebook with summaries of each module and spaces to add comments about the challenges completed.

In another study, one hundred and seventy adolescents (85 in each group) completed the treatment and were assessed immediately after the intervention, and almost all ($n$=168, 2 less in the *SPARX* group) were assessed at the three month follow-up point (Merry, Stasiak, Shepherd et al., 2012). Results indicated that remission rates were significantly higher using *SPARX* (more specifically, 44% of the participants who completed at least 4 "homework" modules showed a complete remission compared with the 26% of total remissions in the treatment as usual group), and all secondary measures (depression rating scales, and various mood and feelings questionnaires including Kazdin hopelessness scale and Spence children's anxiety scale, among others) supported similar results for both types of interventions.

*Figure 2. Screenshot of SPARX*

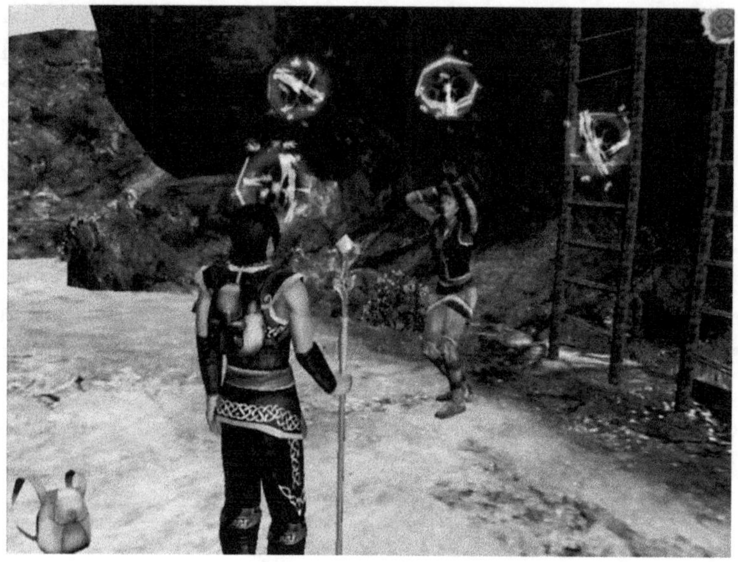

Szczesna, Grudzinski, Grudzinski et al. (2011) presented a prototype of the game *Mission - Master Your Fear* (see Figure 3), a psychoeducational game for preschool children where they can learn how to manage different kinds of fears (fear of weather occurrences, public performance, doctors), ways to overcome those fears, and ways to strengthen the feeling of security and courage. This game has cognitive, behavioral and developmental elements and is based on principles of behavior modification. This game provides guidance with exercises where players can practice how to manage children with different kinds of fears: fear of darkness, weather occurrences, public performance, et cetera. The game takes place in a zoo. With the help of animals, a player can learn how to deal with strong emotions and to learn ways to overcome fear (in the form of game, "magically").

*Figure 3. Mission: Master your Fear*

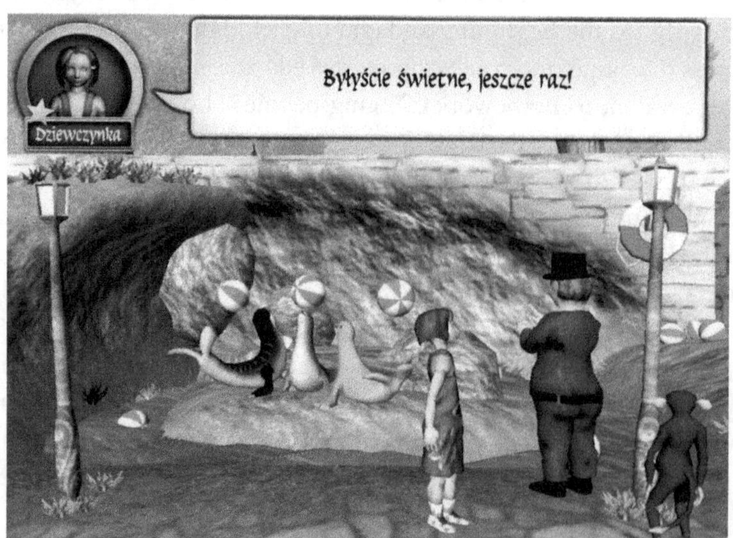

The scenario of the game consists of five main episodes each with specific therapeutic goals. In each episode the player has to find a way to help animals overcome theirs fears and strong emotions. Episode one is an introduction to the game. To better identify with the game character, a player can pick a boy or a girl character. The player gets to know the main characters of the game, the director of the zoo (who is the guide of the game and gives advice and support to a player) and the monkey (who is an assistant of the director and also helps throughout the game). The player, the director and the monkey are going to help animals overcome their fears. The player is packing a briefcase with equipment, which can be used to overcome different fears. In every episode, the player has to help an animal overcome fear so the children learn: (a) what is fear and what is its meaning, (b) in what situations we can feel fear, (c) what we can be afraid of, and (d) how to identify symptoms of fear. In scenes with animals, the player is learning different "magical" ways to overcome fear—e.g., by turning attention by singing, reciting a rhyme, by drawing fear and next decorating it, by drawing fear and next burying it, or by eating something good. Throughout the game, the player can go to the journal mode where he/she can write his/her impressions and their ideas for managing fears. Because this game is directed to children who cannot yet write in the journal, the game allows for "writing" via pictographs. This journal can provide the base for further conversations with the parents or a specialist. The game also creates a detailed log with a record about the player's activity during the game. This also may be a valuable element in the session with a specialist.

## Game-Based CBT for Adults

One biofeedback based-game was presented by Fernández-Aranda, Jiménez-Murcia, Santamaria et al. (2012), who developed and evaluated a serious video game designed to remediate attitudinal, behavioral, and emotional processes of patients with impulse-related disorders. The video game was created and developed within the European research project *PlayMancer*. It aims to prove the potential capacity to change underlying attitudinal, behavioral, and emotional processes of patients with impulse-related disorders. As described by Fernández-Aranda et al. (2012), new interaction modes such as emotion recognition from speech and face and physiological reactions were provided, while specific impulsive reactions were elicited. The video game uses biofeedback to help patients learn relaxation skills, acquire better self-control strategies, and develop new emotional regulation strategies. Recently, it has been used successfully been to improve emotional regulation, increase heart rate variability, and reduce respiratory rate and impulsivity measure in a series of cases with eating disorders (e.g. bulimia nervosa) (Fagundo, Santamaría, Forcano, et al., 2013).

With a different purpose of regulating and gaining emotional control, the *RAGE-Control* game (Kahn, Ducharme, Rotenberg, & Gonzalez-Heydrich, 2013) takes the user's emotional arousal as an input. Based on the classic arcade game *Space Invaders*, if the emotional arousal is above a certain threshold, the ship starts to fire "blanks"—that is, it can no longer fire at the aliens and it starts to move randomly as if it is out of control. The ship remains in this state until the player regains emotional control (measured through heart rate, which is an excellent proxy for emotional arousal in seated players). At the beginning, the player chooses a heart rate threshold for playing the game with the help of a therapist. Once they do it, they have to keep a balance between succeeding in the game and applying relaxation skills to keep themselves under a threshold. Results between an experimental and a control group showed that patients in the *RAGE-control* treatment intervention decreased significantly in their frequency of feeling angry, and additionally, they improved control over their heart rate during game play, inferring that, while playing, the players showed increased ability to keep emotionally low.

## Attention Deficit Hyperactivity Disorder (ADHD): Specific Game-Based Applications for Children

According to Diaz-Orueta, Iriarte, Climent, and Banterla (2012), attention deficit/hyperactivity disorder (ADHD) is a chronic mental health disorder with distinct behavioral manifestations in childhood, adolescence, and adulthood. It may be characterized by attentional lability, impulsive behavioral style, sterile hyperactivity, and fragility of the mechanisms of adaptation to the environment, all of those without any other psychopathological problems that justify the presence of these symptoms. As Diaz-Orueta, Garcia-Lopez, Crespo-Eguilaz et al. (2014) stated, neuropsychological evaluation has increasingly become part of the protocol in an efficient approach to the understanding and appropriate diagnosis of this pathology. In relation to this, Nesplora (www.nesplora.com) has developed a neuropsychological test with the appearance of a game that prevents children from avoiding the need to undergo neuropsychological evaluation to evaluate their attention and motor activity. The test is called AULA, and it consists of an evaluation test that employs Virtual Reality to facilitate diagnosis of Attention Deficit Disorder with and without Hyperactivity. The AULA system analyses the behavior of a child in the context of a virtual classroom. The tool is perceived initially as a game, in which the child performs a task while typical distractors of a classroom are presented to him or her (see Figure 4). The AULA test evaluates factors determining the existence of ADHD, such as sustained attention, impulsivity, divided visual and auditory attention, excessive motor activity, and a tendency to distraction (by means of a movement sensor). After the test, the system provides an evaluation report that helps the clinician perform a more accurate and reliable diagnosis.

In the area of specific intervention for ADHD, two games are noteworthy in the specific target of symptoms of this disorder. The first one, *Plan-It Commander* (www.planitcommander.com), resulted from the cooperation of the pharmaceutical firm Janssen Pharmaceutical/Healthy Solutions (part of Johnson & Johnson), the Yulius Academie, a mental health care institute, the Flemish Society for Parents

*Figure 4. AULA VR test*
*© Nesplora, Technology and Behavior.*

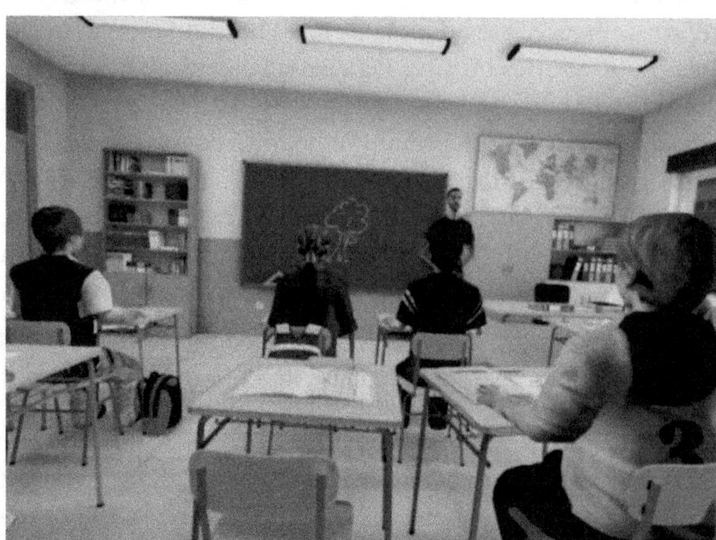

of Children with ADHD, and the Ranj serious game company from the Netherlands. The game takes the form of an adventure game and centers on a situation involving considerable problems, a solution to which must be sought. Within the overall narrative, the player practices dealing with problematic aspects of ADHD in subgames. Furthermore, he/she will learn to enlist the right help from his/her team at the right time. There is also ample room for interaction within an internal community. Children can watch and rate each other's actions, can help one another and give advice. The time that the children can spend on the game has been limited to a well-considered maximum number of minutes a day. With some of the studies currently in progress, the initial user survey yielded positive responses. A playable version of ten missions has been available since September 2012, and, in June 2013, the Dutch version of the game became commercially available. After that, a clinical follow-up study is planned to measure the progress of a new group of over 200 children playing the full version of the game, which will concentrate on the impact of the game on the children's day-to-day lives.

The latest developments in the ADHD management area is the game *Braingame Brian* (Prins, Brink, Dovis et al., 2013), a computerized training game for three Executive Functions (EF): visuospatial Working Memory (WM), inhibition, and cognitive flexibility, embedded in an extensive, game-like world. One may choose to train one, two, or all three EFs. *Braingame Brian*, named after the main character Brian (see Figure 5), consists of 25 training sessions of about 40–50 minutes each. Every training session contains two blocks of three training tasks in a fixed order. The first training task is always a WM training task; the second and third task, an inhibition training task and a cognitive flexibility task, are presented in changing order. During each session, the three training tasks are performed twice, which results in a total training time of about 30 minutes per session. Over a period of 5 weeks, the child trains and plays the total of 25 sessions. Each day of training, the child plays one session of approximately 40–50 minutes (30 minutes of training and 10–20 minutes of walking around in the world). After each block of training tasks, the difficulty level of the training task is automatically adjusted to the child's level of performance.

The game world has seven different worlds—the area around the house of Brian's parents, the village, the uninhabited island, the backlands, the beach, the swamp, and the subterranean laboratory. All

*Figure 5. Screenshot of BrainGame Brian*

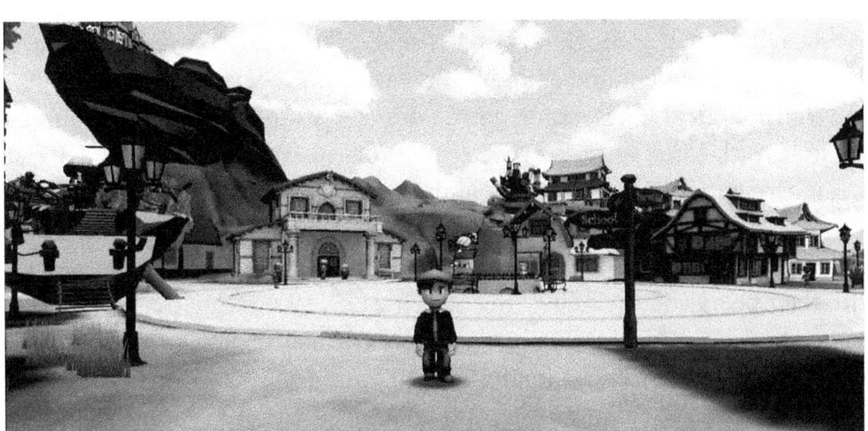

characters living in these worlds have a problem. Brian helps them to solve these problems by doing the training tasks, and by doing so, he invents all kinds of handy machines.

Walking around in the world and seeing the inventions are the child's reinforcement for initiating and completing the training tasks. To enhance the child's motivation, each completed block of training tasks results in an enhanced game world and extra powers for Brian. Before, after, and in between training tasks, the child can walk around in the world.

From the first to the last session, the game world becomes more and more elaborate, and every completed block of training results in extra powers for Brian. With these extra powers, Brian can create inventions to help people in the village solve their problems, which makes them happier.

Thus, completing training sessions not only results in a more elaborate game world and more powers for Brian but also in happier people in the village. An additional external reinforcement system—receiving points for completing sessions—is used to even further raise the child's motivations to do the training.

With regards to its efficacy, Prins et al. (2013) performed a pilot study, and results showed that the children in the EF training condition significantly improved on parent-rated EFs (BRIEF total score = 27) and ADHD behaviors (Inattention and Hyperactive-impulsivity subscales of the Disruptive Behavior Problems Scale = 28), both in the total sample and in the subsample treated with methylphenidate. Effects were maintained at follow-up. It should be noted that the design of this first evaluation study did not control for expectation and nonspecific treatment effects, and future research should further examine the efficacy of *Braingame Brian* with placebo-controlled designs. Finally, according to its authors, at this point *Braingame Brian* is not to be considered a stand-alone treatment module, but one that should be added, combined, or integrated with existing, empirically supported treatments for ADHD such as parent and teacher training programs, and/or medication, to fully have its therapeutic impact.

## Serious Games Providing Improvements in Self-Esteem and Self-Efficacy

According to Santrock (2010), 'self-esteem' refers to the global assessment of the self, performed by any person, while 'self-efficacy' (the judgment or beliefs a person has about his/her own abilities) is parceled for each activity (e.g. self-efficacy in math, self-efficacy when establishing a relationship, self-efficacy with computers, etc.) (Bandura, 1997; Delgado-Egido & Contreras-Felipe, 2009). Keeping this distinction in mind, with regards to self-esteem and self-efficacy in children, a serious game specifically designed for diabetes control was successful in reducing emergency visits by a 77% after diabetic children had the game at home for 6 months, compared to a control group of youngsters who played an entertainment no-health-related videogame (Lieberman, 2001). Similar results were found for games related to asthma self-management and smoking prevention. Lieberman (2001) states that even if not directly targeting psychological goals, some games directed to manage diabetes and asthma may have an impact on children, as children suffering these conditions also suffer from low self-esteem. By means of these games, Lieberman (2001) stated that children may be more aware about their own abilities to control the symptomatology and prevent crises, thus increasing both their self-efficacy with regards to their competence to control their condition and their overall self-esteem by keeping them more active and engaged with their peers and their daily life activities.

Another noteworthy project for children is *Monité* (www.monite.org), a trans-media project intended to prevent behaviors related to bullying situations (see Figure 6). It has 5 main axes (a 3D videogame, a manual for parents and teachers, videos, a tale, and a Webpage to share game experiences and reinforce learning). The 3D videogame is targeted for children aged between 6 and 10 years, and its objective is to prevent bullying related behaviors. This is not done explicitly but in a funny and highly playable way. The main character, Monité, is the involuntary guardian of the spiral galaxy named Cocrópolix composed of different planets, some habitable and some not. The distance between planets changes during the year, and the creation of this singular galaxy was due to the enormous explosion of a star. All seems to indicate that the violence of the explosion made some elements fall over those planets, but some affirm that the existence of life depends on the will of a villain, the doctor Solid Malicious Drax, known as SMD. The game starts with Monité riding his bike on his home planet, the Raining Planet, not expecting what the near future may bring. Suddenly, his friend Radium tells him that SMD is terrifying the population of the planet, throwing many clones of himself and peculiar objects over the planet. While Radium is telling this, suddenly, a spaceship appears. It is SMD, who kidnaps Radium and takes him away. The first thing that Monité will have to do is to find and liberate his friend from the evil Solid Malicious Drax. Monité is expected to overcome different challenges that will take him through four different planets (Raining Planet, Clown Planet, Indifferent Planet, and Electro Planet). These challenges will allow the child, but also parents and teachers, to work in different psychoeducational contents about bullying from different perspectives. The tool is expected to be played with the educational support from parents and teachers for a better processing of learning, with the ultimate goal to acquire better adaptation responses from all the potential agents implied in a bullying situation—the aggressor, the victim and the passive witnesses. An increase in self-efficacy for social situations (stimulating the adoption of coping strategies with relation to empathy, assertiveness, and peer support) and overall self-esteem (by improving social relationships with peers and their view about how they function in daily life both inside and outside the school environment) is expected, though not yet confirmed. The first part of the game and its corresponding complementary materials have been commercially available in Spain since March 2015.

As an example for the intervention in self-efficacy and self-esteem in adults Procci, Bowers, Wong and Andrews (2013) developed and evaluated a serious game to teach deploying military personnel about available mental health resources and coping skills, as well as to determine whether the inclusion of mini-games improved learning outcomes. The Web-based serious game played by the experimental group was called *Walk in My Shoes*, which takes 2 to 3 hours to be played in its entirety. The game includes seven mini-games, some of them designed to rely heavily on information learned in *Walk in My*

*Figure 6. Image from the game Monité for bullying prevention*

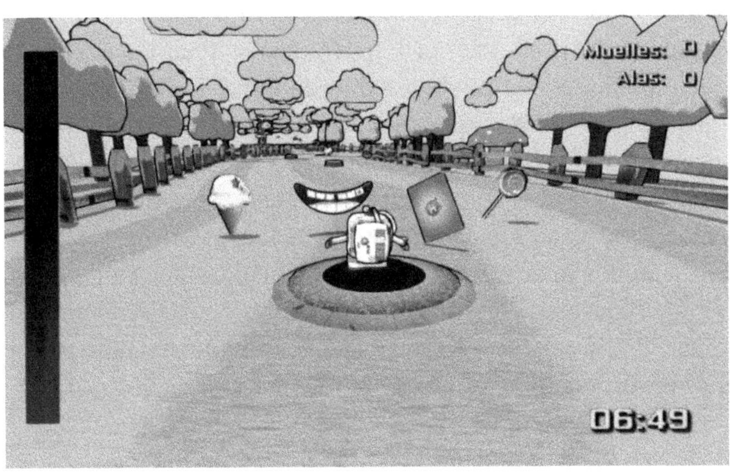

*Shoes*, and some designed as sequels to scaffold the instructional material. For example, "Devil's Advocate" is a mini-game for practicing the cognitive restructuring method. Players take control of Judith, a supernatural being whose job it is to help repair the broken thoughts of soldiers. It is a stealth-based game, so players must place Judith behind the unsuspecting soldier without being seen. From there, the player can enter the brain of the soldier and must identify the specific type of negative automatic thought that he or she is experiencing. Identification is only the first step, so in the mini game's sequel, "Devil's Advocate 2," the player must not only sneak up on the soldier, but also analyse the automatic thought and replace it with a functional thought. Results of this study showed that participants who played mini-games as part of a serious game featuring relevant information demonstrated an improvement in declarative knowledge about mental health resources whereas those who received irrelevant information did not. This suggests that the gains are not simply a consequence of simply playing a game, but of playing a game that delivers appropriate information and provides opportunities for practice. Exposure to *Walk in My Shoes* resulted in both increased knowledge regarding coping skills and an increase in the participants' reported level of deployment self-efficacy. Again, the results support the hypothesis that the game-based training program is effective, and participants who experienced the game reported increased self-efficacy for the trained material.

## Serious Games for Intervention in Dementia

While most of the serious games presented so far have addressed psychological interventions for children and younger adults, the development of serious games for healthy older adults who enjoy a normal cognitive aging or who are undergoing a neurodegenerative process in the brain is scarce, but relatively recent and it is increasing. In many cases, as stated by McCallum and Boletsis (2013), there are no dementia specific serious games, but a reorientation of games previously designed for entertainment which are now used to target cognitive function in older people with dementia. Whether the effect of those games is long lasting or transferable to players' daily life must be determined in future studies.

One of the most recent and clear contributions in terms of psychological intervention in people with dementia is *What Remains?* (Cadamuro & Visch, 2013), a game developed in the context of a wider project that investigates how to change human behavior by designing game elements. In *What Remains?*, the challenge is to persuade patients suffering from Alzheimer's disease (AD) to tell stories of the lives that could be used to facilitate the care home intake procedure and to personalize caregiving, in what can be called a game-based reminiscence therapy intervention. In this sense, the game provides the player with three interactive phases in which they can generate story elements, connect them to generate a story, and capture them into a diary that can be used by caregivers. The pictorial categories in the game include family, jobs, hobbies, pets, favorite food, religion, things they did not like to do, things they do like, holidays, and memories. Moreover, pictures of objects mentioned by the patient or those that may provoke restlessness to them may also be collected. Pictures inserted into objects may be placed on a virtual table in front of the patient and serve as a motivational game for storytelling. The patient connects these pictorial elements, and this interaction motivates them to tell the stories that connect the pictures. *What Remains?* allows a high level of control to players but the stories and outcomes are unpredictable, a fact that triggers older adults' relatives and caretakers in understanding AD patients thoughts and autobiographical stories of the patients.

## FUTURE RESEARCH DIRECTIONS

In the case of virtual reality environments, pilot studies with small to moderate incidental samples are the norm (like for *VRET* or *Isla Calma*), but no evidence has been found of any randomized controlled trial to prove the treatment effect of any of these developments.When it comes to the area of serious games, most of them have been validated and efficacy have been shown with small to moderate incidental samples. The only exception is *SPARX*, with a well established randomized controlled trial. Some of them are current trials in progress (*Plan-it commander*, *Braingame Brian*) and others like *Monité* are in the final stages but still in need to be tested.

The interest in the future of serious games for health interventions is increasing. At the European Union, under the scope of the Horizon 2020 funding program, cooperation project calls are including topics related to gamification and more explicitly to serious game interventions in some of the program calls.

It is clear that more randomized controlled trials (RCTs) are needed to demonstrate the efficacy of game-based interventions. The achievement of evidence-based serious games interventions is, in many cases, more a goal than a reality, as there is a clear need to evaluate several games that are designed as psychological interventions and compare their efficacy with traditional interventions and control interventions (either psycho-educational or placebo interventions) in order to be able to start to speak about evidence-based game interventions. These remarks are in line with a recent review by Horne-Moyer, Moyer, Messer, and Messer (2014), which report that methodological concerns including the lack of randomized controlled trials (RCT) for many electronic games designed for therapy is the main gap that needs to be filled.

The main challenges of these evaluations are

1. To convince psychotherapy professionals who are still reluctant about the advantages of implementing serious games and game-based therapeutic interventions with their patients,
2. Develop experimental designs with meaningful sample sizes, and
3. Report on the achievements and limitations that are needed to overcome by the integration of game-based interventions within real psychotherapeutic contexts.

In addition, one of the greatest challenges is the need of identifying which concrete game elements are more suitable and likely to produce a therapeutic achievement. In other words, to determine which game elements are efficient and valid for obtaining psychotherapeutic response. Beyond a pre-post experimental design that states that a particular game is useful or not, what would be really interesting to understand is which specific ingredients or features of a particular game can be extrapolated as rules of efficacy to other game-based interventions to be designed in the future. This means not only to include game interventions as companion tools for the therapeutic setting (i.e. as an external aid for patient's 'homework' between sessions) but to study games to further analyze how they can be integrated within the professional-patient therapeutic relationship during treatment sessions. In addition, as it was not possible to extract any clear conclusion from the reviewed literature, there is a clear need to specify what game formats may be the most appropriate for each diagnosis. For example, is it the same to treat depression with a mobile app or with an immersive virtual reality environment? What are the potentials for each specific format in each specific disorder? Answers to these questions remain uncertain.

Another potential gap in the existing literature is to know which specific socio-demographic factors affect game play and, hence, could affect the effectiveness of a particular game-based intervention.

Yee (2006) found that male players are more interested in achievement, while female players are more interested in the social aspects of a game. However, Begy and Consalvo (2011) have recently reported that female players are exceptionally attracted by achievement-related content in the Facebook game *Faunasphere*, which conflicts with Yee's finding. In addition, concerning age, Diaz-Orueta, Facal, Nap, and Ranga (2011) found that the main interests shared among senior participants in serious games were to highlight the social aspect of the gaming experience, to experience challenge in games, to combine cognitive and physical activity, and to acquire specific abilities or skills. Two components were commonly agreed on in the participating countries—challenge (as a basic foundation for the game development, with participants asking for challenging, fun-to-play games with increasing difficulty) and socialization (i.e., participants clearly noting that they wanted to play with others and not necessarily against others). However, even with available evidence, further research is needed to address how other socio-demographic factors such as culture and socioeconomic status impact gamification in this context, including varying levels of access to technology, adoption, and adherence to treatment programs.

According to the present overview, there is still another gap that needs to be covered by the industry. There is a considerable difference between the amount of resources that can be invested in a videogame for entertainment and in a serious game, in terms of playability, marketing capacities, and effective business plans that could make serious games attractive for the general public. Gamification in healthcare will be possible as long as games developers and health and social care providers would be able to communicate properly the advantages and cost-effectiveness of implementing gamification and serious gaming in the healthcare sector. The costs of treatments for many neurodegenerative, brain-related diseases, are covered by public administrations. Given this situation, although intuition and early results suggest that gamifying certain types of intervention via virtual reality environments, telemedicine, and games for health could significantly reduce costs, this is still an issue to be solved—not only in the scientific community but also among healthcare professionals, general public, and public administration. We are talking about stakeholders that need to address the gamification of healthcare and games for health as a strategic industrial sector that could, in the end, imply significant savings in healthcare and social care costs. In other words, only time will tell whether gamification of healthcare can reach the status of priority for policymakers and public administrations and governments, especially when they have to decide the budget priorities in a context of global economic crisis.

## CONCLUSION

The current chapter provided an overview of serious games as a means of obtaining health, educational, training and therapeutic outcomes. After a brief introduction to the state-of-the-art research about the benefits of games in terms of health outcomes, a review of the main target formats (virtual reality environments and PC games) for the development of serious games for health have been presented. Many game developments need to move forward and promote the implementation of further studies with larger samples, as mere feasibility and acceptability studies with small incidental samples may not be enough to guarantee an expansion of these games as a health solution that may be prescribed by healthcare professionals. Efforts are needed to plan and carefully design randomized controlled trials that allow to identify if games are efficient as aids for psychological treatment, and more in-depth research will be needed to clarify which specific aspects of these games are the ones that work (is it the design, the graphics, the narrative or the story they tell, or is it something else?) so rules or lessons can be established about what is needed for a serious game to be effective in the area of psychological intervention and generalize and extend the knowledge among serious game developers. In this chapter, most of the software examples described cannot be considered evidence-based games, as many are still under current analysis and undergoing trials, and some are still under development. However, they helped us to provide an insight into the past, the present and the future of gamification and serious games for psychological intervention.

There is still a lot of progress to be made in the development of rigorous empirical research that may provide more evidence for some of the serious games for psychological intervention still under development. A common declaration found across many psychological research articles is that "future longitudinal studies with larger samples and randomized controlled trials will be needed." As this is a main symptom for psychological research, it can be generalized for serious games that aim to be a reference for psychological research and intervention. Luckily, the increasing social awareness of the potentialities of serious games for many healthcare interventions will eventually make it possible that the number of longitudinal and randomized controlled trials increase in the near future.

As other areas of healthcare, particularly in medicine for areas like stroke and cancer treatment, find success in the progressive integration of gaming and gamification in daily care practice, psychology may also obtain benefits. Skepticism is reasonably established on the lack of solid evidence that exists so far, but it is expected that ongoing trials will provide higher amounts of evidence on the utility of these type of game-based applications for psychological intervention. Time will tell if this is just a wave or a fashion, or if, as it seems, serious games for health interventions, including psychological intervention, are here to stay.

## REFERENCES

Alexiou, A., Schippers, M., & Oshri, I. (2012). Positive Psychology and Digital Games: The Role of Emotions and Psychological Flow in Serious Games Development. Psychology (Savannah, Ga.), 3(12A), 1243–1247.

Bandura, A. (1997). Self-Efficacy: The Exercise of Control. New York: Freeman.

Baranowski, T., Buday, R., Thompson, D. I., & Baranowski, J. (2008). Playing for Real: Video Games and Stories for Health-Related Behavior Change. American Journal of Preventive Medicine, 34(1), 74–82.

Baranowski, T., Buday, R., Thompson, D., Lyons, E.J., Lu, A.S., & Baranowski, J. (2013). Developing Games for Health Behavior Change: Getting Started. Games for Health Journal, 2(4), 183–190. doi:10.1089/g4h.2013.0048 PubMed doi:10.1089/g4h.2013.0048 PMID:24443708

Baranowski, T., Lieberman, D., Buday, R., Peng, W., Zimmerli, L., Wiederhold, B., & Kato, P. M. (2013). Videogame Mechanics in Games for Health. Games for Health Journal, 2(4), 194–204. doi:10.1089/g4h.2013.0617 PubMed doi:10.1089/g4h.2013.0617 PMID:26192223

Begy, J., & Consalvo, M. (2011). Achievements, Motivations and Rewards in Faunasphere. Game Studies, 11(1). Retrieved from http://gamestudies.org/1101/articles/begy_consalvo

Brezinka, V. (2008). Treasure Hunt – a serious game to support psychotherapeutic treatment of children. In S. K. Andersen, M.C.A. Klein, S. Schulz, J. Aarts, & M.C. Mazzoleni (Eds.), eHealth Beyond the Horizon – Get IT There (pp. 71–76). Amsterdam: IOS Press.

Buckley, K. E., & Anderson, C. A. (2006). A theoretical model of the effects and consequences of playing videogames. In P. Vorderer & J. Bryant (Eds.), Playing video games –motives, responses and consequences (pp. 363–378). Mahwah, NJ: LEA.

Cole, S. W., Yoo, D. J., & Knutson, B. (2012). Interactivity and Reward-Related Neural Activation during a Serious Videogame. PLoS ONE, 7(3), e33909. doi:10.1371/journal.pone.0033909 PubMed doi:10.1371/journal.pone.0033909 PMID:22442733

Connolly, T. M., Boyle, E. A., MacArthur, E., Hainey, T., & Boyle, J. M. (2012). A systematic literature review of empirical evidence on computer games and serious games. Computers & Education, 59(2), 661–686. doi:10.1016/j.compedu.2012.03.004 doi:10.1016/j.compedu.2012.03.004

Csikszentmihalyi, M. (1975). Beyond boredom and anxiety. San Francisco, CA: Jossey-Bass.

Csikszentmihalyi, I., & Csikszentmihalyi, M. (1988). Optimal experience: Psychological studies of flow in consciousness. New York, NY: Cambridge University Press. doi:10.1017/CBO9780511621956 doi:10.1017/CBO9780511621956

Delgado-Egido, B., & Contreras-Felipe, A. (2009). Desarrollo social y emocional. En B. Delgado Egido (Ed.). (2011). Psicología del desarrollo: desde la infancia a la vejez [Social and emotional development]. (Vol. 2, pp. 35-66). Spain: McGraw-Hill.

Diaz-Orueta, U., Alvarado, A., Gutiérrez, D., Climent, G., & Banterla, F. (2012). "Isla Calma", a Novel Virtual Reality Environment for Pain and Anxiety Distraction: Report on Usability, Acceptability, and Subjective Experience. Games for Health Journal, 1(5), 353–361. doi:10.1089/g4h.2012.0037 PubMed doi:10.1089/g4h.2012.0037 PMID:26192002

Diaz-Orueta, U., Banterla, F., & Climent, G. (2014). (in press). Isla Calma: Distracción del miedo al dolor y la ansiedad mediante realidad virtual [Isla Calma: pain and anxiety distraction by means of virtual reality]. Revista de Ansiedad y Estrés, 20(2-3), 127–141.

Diaz-Orueta, U., Facal, D., Nap, H. H., & Ranga, M. M. (2012). What is the key for older people to show interest in playing digital learning games? Initial qualitative findings from the LEAGE project on a multicultural European sample. Games for Health Journal, 1(2), 115–123. doi:10.1089/g4h.2011.0024 PubMed doi:10.1089/g4h.2011.0024 PMID:26193185

Diaz-Orueta, U., Garcia-Lopez, C., Crespo-Eguilaz, N., Sánchez-Carpintero, R., Climent, G., & Narbona, J. (2014). AULA virtual reality test as an attention measure: Convergent validity with Conners' Continuous Performance Test. Child Neuropsychology, 20(3), 328–342. doi:10.1080/09297049.2013.792332 PubMed doi:10.1080/09297049.2013.792332 PMID:23638628

Diaz-Orueta, U., Iriarte, Y., Climent, G., & Banterla, F. (2012). AULA: An ecological virtual reality test with distractors for evaluating attention in children and adolescents. Journal of Virtual Reality, 5(2), 1–20.

Difede, J., & Hoffman, H. (2002). Virtual reality exposure therapy for World Trade Center Post Traumatic Stress Disorder. Cyberpsychology & Behavior, 5(6), 529–535. doi:10.1089/109493102321018169 PubMed doi:10.1089/109493102321018169 PMID:12556115

Fagundo, A.B., Santamaría, J.J., Forcano, K., Giner-Bartolomé, C., Jiménez-Murcia, S., Sánchez, I. et al. (2013). Video game therapy for emotional regulation and impulsivity control in a series of treated cases with bulimia nervosa. European Eating Disorders Review: the journal of the Eating Disorders Association, 21(6), 493-499.

Fernández-Aranda, F., Jiménez-Murcia, S., Santamaría, J. J., Gunnard, K., Soto, A., Kalapanidas, E.,... Penelo, E. (2012). Video games as a complementary therapy tool in mental disorders: PlayMancer, a European multicentre study. Journal of Mental Health (Abingdon, England), 21(4), 364–374. doi:10.3109/09638237.2012.664302 PubMed doi:10.3109/09638237.2012.664302 PMID:22548300

Freeman, D. (2007). Studying and treating schizophrenia using virtual reality: A new paradigm. Schizophrenia Bulletin, 34(4), 605–610. doi:10.1093/schbul/sbn020 PubMed doi:10.1093/schbul/sbn020 PMID:18375568

Gamberini, L., Barresi, G., Majer, A., & Scarpetta, F. (2008). A game a day keeps the doctor away: A short review of computer games in mental healthcare. Journal of Cyber Therapy and Rehabilitation, 1(2), 127–145.

Gardner, J. E. (1991). Can the Mario Bros. help? Nintendo games as an adjunct in psychotherapy with children. Psychotherapy (Chicago, Ill.), 28(4), 667–670. doi:10.1037/0033-3204.28.4.667 doi:10.1037/0033-3204.28.4.667

Goh, D. H., Ang, R. P., & Tan, H. C. (2008). Strategies for designing effective psychotherapeutic gaming interventions for children and adolescents. Computers in Human Behavior, 24(5), 2217–2235. doi:10.1016/j.chb.2007.10.007 doi:10.1016/j.chb.2007.10.007

Holmes, E. A., James, E. L., Coode-Bate, T., & Deeprose, C. (2009). Can Playing the Computer Game ''Tetris'' Reduce the Build-Up of Flashbacks for Trauma? A Proposal from Cognitive Science. PLoS ONE, 4(1), e4153. doi:10.1371/journal.pone.0004153 PubMed doi:10.1371/journal.pone.0004153 PMID:19127289

Honka, A., Kaipainen, K., Hietala, H., & Saranummi, N. (2011). Rethinking Health: ICT-Enabled Services to Empower People to Manage Their Health. IEEE Reviews in Biomedical Engineering, 4, 119–139. doi:10.1109/RBME.2011.2174217 PubMed doi:10.1109/RBME.2011.2174217 PMID:22273795

Horne-Moyer, H. L., Moyer, B. H., Messer, D. C., & Messer, E. S. (2014). The Use of Electronic Games in Therapy: A Review with Clinical Implications. Current Psychiatry Reports, 16(12), 520. doi:10.1007/s11920-014-0520-6 PubMed doi:10.1007/s11920-014-0520-6 PMID:25312026

IDATE. (2010): Serious games. A 10 billion euro market in 2015. Idate News, 518. Montpellier, France.

Jones, C. M., Scholes, L., Johnson, D., Katsikitis, M., & Carras, M. C. (2014). Gaming well: Links between videogames and flourishing mental health. Frontiers in Psychology, 5, 1–8. doi:10.3389/fpsyg.2014.00260 PubMed doi:10.3389/fpsyg.2014.00260 PMID:24744743

Kahn, J., Ducharme, P., Rotenberg, A., & Gonzalez-Heydrich, J. (2013). "RAGE-Control": A Game to Build Emotional Strength. Games for Health Journal, 2(1), 53–57. doi:10.1089/g4h.2013.0007 PubMed doi:10.1089/g4h.2013.0007 PMID:26196556

Khanna, M. S., & Kendall, P. C. (2010). Computer-Assisted Cognitive Behavioral Therapy for Child Anxiety: Results of a Randomized Clinical Trial. Journal of Consulting and Clinical Psychology, 78(5), 737–745. doi:10.1037/a0019739 PubMed doi:10.1037/a0019739 PMID:20873909

Knox, M., Lentini, J., Cummings, T. S., McGrady, A., Whearty, K., & Sancrant, L. (2011). Game-based biofeedback for paediatric anxiety and depression. Mental Health in Family Medicine, 8, 195–203. PubMed PMID:22942901

Krebs, J. (2013). Moral dilemmas in serious games. Proceedings of the 2013 International Conference on Advanced ICT (pp. 232-236).

Landgraf, S., Krebs, M. O., Olié, J. P., Committeri, G., van der Meer, E., Berhtoz, A., & Amado, I. (2010). Real world referencing and schizophrenia: Are we experiencing the same reality? Neuropsychologia, 48(10), 2922–2930. doi:10.1016/j.neuropsychologia.2010.05.034 PubMed doi:10.1016/j.neuropsychologia.2010.05.034 PMID:20540956

Leitenberg, H. (1990). Handbook of Social and Evaluation Anxiety. New York: Springer Science. doi:10.1007/978-1-4899-2504-6 doi:10.1007/978-1-4899-2504-6

Mantovani, F., & Castelnuovo, G. (2003). Sense of presence in virtual training: enhancing skills acquisition and transfer of knowledge through learning experience in virtual environments. In G. Riva, F. Davide, & W. A. IJsselsteijn (Eds.), Being There: Concepts, effects and measurement of user presence in synthetic environments (pp. 167–181). Amsterdam: Ios Press.

McCallum, S., & Boletsis, C. (2013). Dementia Games: A Literature Review of Dementia-Related Serious Games. Serious Games Development and Applications, LNCS (Vol. 8101, pp. 15–27). doi:10.1007/978-3-642-40790-1_2 doi:10.1007/978-3-642-40790-1_2

McLay, R. N., Graap, K., Spira, J., Perlman, K., Johnston, S., Rothbaum, B. O.,... Rizzo, A. (2012). Development and Testing of Virtual Reality Exposure Therapy for Post-Traumatic Stress Disorder in Active Duty Service Members Who Served in Iraq and Afghanistan. Military Medicine, 177(6), 635–642. doi:10.7205/MILMED-D-11-00221 PubMed doi:10.7205/MILMED-D-11-00221 PMID:22730837

Merry, S. N., Stasiak, K., Shepherd, M., Frampton, C., Fleming, T., & Lucassen, M. F. (2012). The effectiveness of SPARX, a computerised self-help intervention for adolescents seeking help for depression: Randomised controlled non-inferiority trial. British Medical Journal, 344(apr18 3), e2598. doi:10.1136/bmj.e2598 PubMed doi:10.1136/bmj.e2598 PMID:22517917

Nap, H. H., & Diaz-Orueta, U. (2014). Rehabilitation Gaming. In J. Bishop (Ed.), Gamification for Human Factors Integration: Social (pp. 122–147). Hershey, PA, USA: Education, and Psychological Issues. doi:10.4018/978-1-4666-5071-8.ch008 doi:10.4018/978-1-4666-5071-8.ch008

O'Dwyer-O'Brien, A., Coyle, S., Coyle, D., & O' Reilly, G. (2011, July). Gnatenborough's Island: A C-CBT adaption for young people with internalising disorders. Paper presented at the British Association for Behavioural and Cognitive Psychotherapies 39th Annual Conference, UK.

Parker, S., Jimmieson, N., & Amiot, C. (2009). The Stress buffering effects of control on task satisfaction and perceived goal attainment: An experimental study of the moderating influence of desirability of control. Applied Psychology, 58(4), 622–652. doi:10.1111/j.1464-0597.2008.00367.x doi:10.1111/j.1464-0597.2008.00367.x

Prins, P. J., Brink, E. T., Dovis, S., Ponsioen, A., Geurts, H. M., de Vries, M., & van der Oord, S. (2013). "Braingame Brian": Toward an Executive Function Training Program with Game Elements for Children with ADHD and Cognitive Control Problems. Games for Health Journal, 2(1), 44–49. doi:10.1089/g4h.2013.0004 PubMed doi:10.1089/g4h.2013.0004 PMID:26196554

Procci, K., Bowers, C., Wong, C., & Andrews, A. (2013). Minigames for Mental Health: Improving Warfighters' Coping Skills and Awareness of Mental Health Resources. Games for Health Journal, 2(4), 240–246. doi:10.1089/g4h.2013.0014 PubMed doi:10.1089/g4h.2013.0014 PMID:26192227

Rahmani, E., & Boren, S. A. (2012). Videogames and Health Improvement: A Literature Review of Randomized Controlled Trials. Research, Development, and Clinical Applications, 1(5), 331–341. PubMed PMID:26191999

Reeves, B., & Read, J. L. (2009). Total engagement: Using games to change the way people work and businesses compete. Boston: Harvard Business School.

Riva, G., Botella, C., Baños, R., Mantovani, F., García-Palacios, A., Quero, S.,... Gaggioli, A. (2015). Presence-inducing media for mental health applications. In M. Lombard, F. Biocca, J. Freeman, W. Ijsselsteijn, & R. Schaevitz (Eds.), Inmersed in Media: Telepresence Theory, Measurement & Technology (pp. 283–332). New York: Springer. doi:10.1007/978-3-319-10190-3_12 doi:10.1007/978-3-319-10190-3_12

Rizzo, A., Pair, J., Graap, K., Manson, B., McNerney, P. J., Wiederhold, B.,.... (2006). A Virtual Reality Exposure Therapy Application for Iraq War Military Personnel with Post Traumatic Stress Disorder: From Training to Toy to Treatment. In M. Roy (Ed.), NATO Advanced Research Workshop on Novel Approaches to the Diagnosis and Treatment of Posttraumatic Stress Disorder (pp. 235-250). Washington DC: IOS Press.

Russoniello, C. V., Fish, M., & O'Brien, K. (2013). The Efficacy of Casual Videogame Play in Reducing Clinical Depression: A Randomized Controlled Study. Games for Health Journal, 2(6), 341–346. doi:10.1089/g4h.2013.0010 PubMed doi:10.1089/g4h.2013.0010 PMID:26197075

Ryan, R., Rigby, S., & Przybylski, A. (2006). The motivational pull of video games: A self-determination theory approach. Motivation and Emotion, 30(4), 347–363. doi:10.1007/s11031-006-9051-8 doi:10.1007/s11031-006-9051-8

Salen, K., & Zimmerman, E. (2004). Rules of Play: Game Design Fundamentals. Cambridge: MIT Press.

Santamaría, J. J., Soto, A., Fernández-Aranda, F., Krug, I., Forcano, L., Gunnard, K.,.... (2011). Serious games as additional psychological support: A review of the literature. Journal of Cyber Therapy and Rehabilitation, 4(4), 469–476.

Santrock, J. (2010). Psicología del desarrollo en la infancia, 7ª Ed [Developmental Psychology in Childhood, 7th Edition –Book In Spanish. Colombia: Mc-Graw Hill Interamericana.

Scozzari, S., & Gamberini, L. (2011). Virtual Reality as a Tool for Cognitive Behavioral Therapy: A Review. In S. Brahnam & L. C. Jain (Eds.), Advanced Computational Intelligence Paradigms in Healthcare 6. Virtual Reality in Psychotherapy, Rehabilitation, and Assessment, SCI (Vol. 337, pp. 63–108). Berlin: Springer-Verlag.

Sharry, J., McDermott, M., & Condron, J. (2003). Relax To Win: Treating children with anxiety problems with a biofeedback video game. Eisteach, 2, 22–26.

Shin, M., Heard, R., Suo, C., & Chow, C. M. (2012). Positive Emotions Associated with ''Counter-Strike'' Game Playing. Games for Health Journal, 1(5), 342–347. doi:10.1089/g4h.2012.0010 PubMed doi:10.1089/g4h.2012.0010 PMID:26192000

Szczesna, A., Grudzinski, J., Grudzinski, T., Mikuszewski, R., & Debowski, A. (2011, November 16-18). The Psychology Serious Game Prototype for Preschool Children. Paper presented at the IEEE 1st International Conference on Serious Games and Applications for Health (SeGAH), Braga, Portugal.

Wiederhold, B. K., & Wiederhold, M. D. (2003). A New Approach: Using Virtual Reality Psychotherapy in Panic Disorder with Agoraphobia. Psychiatric Times. Retrieved from http://www.psychiatrictimes.com/articles/new-approach-using-virtual-reality-psychotherapy-panic-disorder-agoraphobia

Wilkinson, N., Ang, R. P., & Goh, D. H. (2008). Online video game therapy for mental health concerns: A review. The International Journal of Social Psychiatry, 54(4), 370–382. doi:10.1177/0020764008091659 PubMed doi:10.1177/0020764008091659 PMID:18720897

Yee, N. (2006). The labor of fun: How video games blur the boundaries of work and play. Games and Culture, 1(1), 68–71. doi:10.1177/1555412005281819 doi:10.1177/1555412005281819

Yildirim, S. (2010, June). Serious Game Design for Military Training. Paper presented at the Games Design and Research Conference, Volda University College, Volda, Norway.

## KEY TERMS AND DEFINITIONS

**Cognitive-Behavioral Therapy:** Psychological intervention therapy aimed to focus on changing negative thoughts, usually exaggerations or distortions of reality done by a person, in order to improve the emotional and behavioral outcome. Changing negative thoughts emotion and behavior improve. It is the psychological intervention on anxiety and depression with more empirical evidence on its efficacy.

**Flow:** A state of balance in the game experience, in which the player feels that his/her skills are completely in agreement with the game's difficulty level. Lower difficulty would lead to boredom (as the game would be too easy) and higher difficulty would lead to frustration (as the game would be too difficult according to the player's skills).

**Game-Based Learning:** Any learning process which uses games as a resource or mean to reach the learning results.

**Self-Efficacy:** Personal expectations about the ability to succeed in specific situations.

**Serious Games:** Games that are developed for the purpose of training, learning, and skill acquisition.

**Virtual Reality:** An interactive simulated environment that can induce physical presence and can be accessed by means of a head mounted display and data gloves.

# Section 5

# Positive Interventions:
## Cognition and Stress

# Chapter 14
# Positive Technology for Helping People Cope with Stress

**Daniela Villani**
*Università Cattolica del Sacro Cuore, Italy*

**Pietro Cipresso**
*Università Cattolica del Sacro Cuore, Italy & I.R.C.C.S. Istituto Auxologico Italiano, Italy*

**Andrea Gaggioli**
*Università Cattolica del Sacro Cuore, Italy & I.R.C.C.S. Istituto Auxologico Italiano, Italy*

**Giuseppe Riva**
*Università Cattolica del Sacro Cuore, Italy & I.R.C.C.S. Istituto Auxologico Italiano, Italy*

## ABSTRACT

*The emerging convergence of new technologies and health care is offering a new approach to support effective interventions. This chapter aims to describe how Positive Technology can help people cope with stress in several contexts. On the one hand, the potential capacity of sensor technologies to offer individuals the technology with which to monitor certain biological signals known to be associated with stress might serve to promote engagement with a mediated experience for stress management. On the other hand, the chapter focuses on the hedonic and eudaimonic experiences supported by technology in terms of inducing positive affective states and supporting personal growth by teaching strategies to reduce stress and enhance well-being. To further connect mediated experiences with real ones, the Interreality approach (IR) allows for the combination of assessment and intervention as inseparable parts of the general process of coping with stress.*

## INTRODUCTION

Stress is currently a growing problem that affects many people and significantly worsens their quality of life (Cohen, Janicki-Deverts, & Miller, 2007). Stress has various definitions that all converge upon the notion of "strain" or "the nonspecific response of the body to any demand placed upon it" (Selye, 1956).

According to Cohen et al. (Cohen et al., 2007), psychological stress occurs when people perceive that environmental demands tax or exceed their adaptive capacity. Thus, stressful experiences are con-

DOI: 10.4018/978-1-4666-9986-1.ch014

ceptualized as person-environment transactions whose result is dependent on the impact of the external stimulus at three levels:

1. **Primary Appraisal:** i.e., A person's judgment about the significance of a stimulus as stressful, positive, controllable, challenging or irrelevant;
2. **Secondary Appraisal:** Which address what one can do about the situation;
3. **Problem Management Phase:** Which is aimed at regulation of the external stimulus.

According to these levels, it's evident that there is no ''best'' stress response: an optimal adaptation to environmental demands requires the ability to flexibly use coping strategies depending on the particular context and the specific stressors. In order to effectively manage stress, it is crucial to help people change the way they see the events and to learn to use coping skills.

While the mind and body's responses to stress can be helpful and adaptive in the short-term (McEwen, 1998), repeated or long-term activation of the stress response can damage the body over time (McEwen & Stellar, 1993; Seeman, Singer, Rowe, Horwitz, & McEwen, 1997), and the effects of chronic stress are common and costly (Kalia, 2002). Indeed, chronic stress is associated with lowered immune functioning, impaired memory, chronic headaches, cardiac disease and premature aging of genes, among others (Hammen, 2005; Kiecolt-Glaser, McGuire, Robles, & Glaser, 2002; Leserman et al., 2002; McEwen, 2006; Rozanski, Blumenthal, & Kaplan, 1999). Psychological stress has been linked empirically with dysregulation of facets of the human immune system. A recent review that focused on the effects of stress on inflammation in clinical populations has demonstrated that stress exposure can increase the likelihood of developing disease, as well as exacerbate pre-existing conditions (Morey, Boggero, Scott, & Segerstrom, 2015). For example, in persons with a particular genetic disposition, as well as high level of trait anxiety, repeated and early exposure to stress may result in a decreased threshold for developing anxiety (Jackson, Knight, & Rafferty, 2010; Lupien, McEwen, Gunnar, & Heim, 2009). Stressful events influence the pathogenesis of physical diseases by causing continuous negative affective states (potentially leading to feelings of anxiety and depression), which in turn may induce changes in the emotional circuitry of the brain that can contribute to stress-related psychopathology (Davidson, Jackson, & Kalin, 2000).

The range of considerable problems related to stress highlights the importance of successfully managing stress.

Is it possible to live and live well under stress? To answer this question Antonovsky proposed the salutogenesis model (Antonovsky, 1987, 1996), which deals with the issue of stress from a whole different perspective. According to Antonovsky, daily life is constantly subject to the micro- and macro-stressors that prevent a person from achieving a state of homeostasis. However, the vast majority of people are able to maintain a balanced relationship with the environment. In some cases, even under the most challenging circumstances, people succeed in developing, growing and achieving increasingly intense levels of well-being.

Pathogenesis and salutogenesis are seen as complementary approaches. On the one hand, pathogenesis focuses on discovering the causes and precursors of disease and identifying disease risk factors. On the other hand, salutogenesis represents a model or framework focused on discovering the causes and origins of health and wellness (Latin *salus* = "health;" Greek *genesis* = "origins") (Antonovsky, 1979) and looks prospectively at how to create, enhance and improve physical, mental and social well-being. This paradigm focuses on locating and developing personal and social resources and adaptive tendencies, which result in effective coping behaviour and growth. Strümpfer (Strümpfer, 1995) suggested that there are six significant salutogenic strengths: the sense of coherence, hardiness, learned resourcefulness, potency, internal locus of control and self-efficacy. The salutogenic paradigm and its constructs developed from various personality theories emphasising personality growth, wellness and optimal psychological functioning (Antonovsky, 1987; Strümpfer, 1995).The work started by Antonovsky has been further developed within Positive Psychology, an emerging field that is defined as the scientific study of ordinary, positive and subjective human strengths, virtues, experiences and functioning (Seligman & Csikszentmihalyi, 2000; Sheldon & King, 2001).The progressive convergence between the objectives of Positive Psychology and the impressive advances of Information and Communication Technologies (ICTs) has led toward a new paradigm that has been named Positive Technology. This is a scientific and applied approach to the use of advanced technology for improving the quality of our personal experience (Botella et al., 2012; Riva, Banos, Botella, Wiederhold, & Gaggioli, 2012).Within this framework, this chapter aims to describe how interactive technologies can be effectively used in the assessment of stress and to support interventions for stress management. Proposals about how to combine assessment and interventions and integrate technology in these processes (Pallavicini, Gaggioli, et al., 2013; Riva, 2009a; Riva, Banos, et al., 2012) will be described at the end of the chapter.

## PSYCHOLOGICAL ASSESSMENT OF STRESS SUPPORTED BY NEW TECHNOLOGIES

Typically, two main approaches are used to assess psychological stress in naturalistic conditions: the first is based on self-reporting of participants' subjective experiences and perception of stressful events; the second approach is based on sensing physiological signals associated with the stress response.

The first approach includes self-report questionnaires, such as the psychological stress measure (PSM) (Di Nuovo, Rispoli, & Genta, 2000; Lemyre & Tessier, 1988) or the perceived stress scale (PSS) (Cohen, 1986), the experience sampling method and the day reconstruction method.

The experience sampling method (ESM), also known as ecological momentary assessment (EMA), is a naturalistic observation technique that allows the capturing of participants' thoughts, feelings and behaviours at multiple times across a range of situations as they occur in the natural environment (Csikszentmihalyi & Larson, 1987). In a typical ESM study, participants are asked to fill out a form when prompted by an acoustic signal. Thanks to repeated sampling, a number of surveys are collected from each participant throughout the day, thus providing an ecologically valid and highly detailed description of the subjective quality of experience. ESM has been applied to study a wide range of behaviours and experiences, including daily stress (Serino et al., 2012). However, this procedure has high costs and places a significant burden on the participant (Scollon et al. 2003), thus limiting its practical applicability as a stress monitoring technique.

A less expensive and time-consuming approach for assessing experience and affect in everyday life is the day reconstruction method (DRM), developed by Kahneman and colleagues (Kahneman, Krueger, Schkade, Schwarz, & Stone, 2004). It involves the retrospective recall of the study period as a continuous sequence of episodes, which are rated on a series of affect scales. DRM reports have been validated against experience sampling data, showing that this technique allows the identification of changes in affect over the course of the day with almost the same accuracy as ESM (Kahneman et al., 2004; A. A. Stone et al., 2006). However, since DRM respondents are asked to reconstruct the previous day by completing a structured self-administered questionnaire, this method is potentially susceptible to recall biases. Furthermore, it has been suggested that using retrospective measures as proxies for actual experience may result in weaker or inconsistent results, particularly when tested in connection to biologic pathways (Conner & Barrett, 2012).

The second strategy to assess stress in everyday situations is based on the analysis of physiological correlates of this experience. Psychological stressors are linked with the activation of two main neuro-physiological pathways that are involved in the maintenance of homeostasis: the hypothalamic-pituitary-adrenocortical (HPA) axis and the sympathetic-adrenal medullary system (SAM). One of the most investigated biomarker in the first system is salivary cortisol, which, together with catecholamines, is one of the end products of HPA activation (Kirschbaum & Hellhammer, 1989; G. E. Miller, Chen, & Zhou, 2007). However, due to significant between- and within-individual variation in the diurnal secretion of cortisol, the measurement of the magnitude of cortisol response is a difficult procedure that requires the application of advanced statistical approaches such as multilevel models (Hruschka, Kohrt, & Worthman, 2005; Ice, Katz-Stein, Himes, & Kane, 2004). With respect to the SAM system, heart rate variability (HRV), defined as the variation over time of the period between consecutive heartbeats, is increasingly regarded as a potentially convenient and non-invasive marker of autonomic activation associated with psychological stressors (Orsila et al., 2008). The normal variability in heart rate (HR) is controlled by the balancing activation of the (acceleratory) sympathetic and of the (deceleratory) parasympathetic branches of the autonomic nervous system. However, in stressful events or contexts, there is a trend towards increased sympathetic control and reduced vagal tone, which is associated with decreased HRV (Berntson & Cacioppo, 2004).

Higher HRV has been also associated with the availability of context- and goal-based control of emotions (Thayer, Ahs, Fredrikson, Sollers, & Wager, 2012). Based on this preliminary evidence, several authors have been experimenting with wearable heart monitors for the identification of stress levels from HRV, in both healthy and clinical populations. For example, Kim and colleagues (Kim, Seo, Cho, & Cho, 2008) used HRV patterns to discriminate between subjects reporting high and low levels of stress during the day, with an overall accuracy of 66.1%. In a similar study, Melillo et al. (Melillo, Bracale, & Pecchia, 2011) compared within-subject variations of short-term HRV measures using short-term ECG recordings in students undergoing university examination. By applying Linear Discriminant Analysis on nonlinear features of HRV for automatic stress detection, these authors were able to obtain a total classification accuracy of 90%. Kimhy and colleagues (Kimhy et al., 2009) investigated the relationship between stress and cardiac autonomic regulation in a sample of psychotic patients, using experience sampling in combination with cardiac monitoring. They found that momentary increases in stress were significantly associated with an increase in sympathovagal balance and parasympathetic withdrawal. In addition to studies that have examined the association between HRV and stress during waking hours, other recent research has proposed the use of HRV patterns during sleep as a supplement to the analysis of subjective assessments and voice messages collected during the workday (Muaremi, Arnrich, & Tröster, 2013). Results, though preliminary, have been encouraging.

As previously discussed, a fundamental issue in the measurement of stress in everyday life is that this response is idiosyncratic because it depends on an individual's perception of challenges and the skills that he/she can use to face those challenges. As a consequence, any approach aimed at inferring stress levels from "honest" physiological signals should take care not to overlook the role played by the subjective appraisal of the situation. Furthermore, since HRV values are characterized by high interindividual variability, it is important that the system be tailored to individual characteristics (Cinaz, Arnrich, La Marca, & Tröster, 2013; Morris et al., 2010).

One possible approach to developing adaptative systems for stress recognition has been suggested by Morris and Guilak (Morris et al., 2010). The strategy proposed by these authors involves identifying a subject's baseline and stress threshold in the lab by elicitation of sympathetic and parasympathetic responses, and then using this information to differentiate between stress and nonstress in daily life. A first attempt to implement this approach was performed by Cinaz and colleagues (Cinaz et al., 2013). These authors measured participants' sympathetic and parasympathetic responses during three different levels of mental workload (low, medium and high) in a controlled laboratory setting. Then they investigated whether the data collected in this calibration session were appropriate to discriminate between the corresponding workload levels that occurred during office work. To this end, individual HRV responses of each workload level were used to train the models and test the trained models on the data collected while the subjects performed normal office work, using a mobile ECG logger. Afterward, a multiple regression analysis was applied to model the relationship between relevant HRV features and the subjective ratings of perceived workload; resulting predictions were correct for six out of the seven subjects.

A possible integration between the above presented approaches is PsychLog (Gaggioli et al., 2013), a mobile experience sampling platform designed for research in mental health, which allows simultaneous collection of psychological, physiological (ECG) and motion activity data. PsychLog proposed the Italian adaptation of the ESM questionnaire applied by Jacobs and colleagues (Jacobs et al., 2007) for studying the immediate effects of stressors on mood. Specifically, psychological data are collected from surveys that can be simply customized by the experimenter by including open-ended and closed-ended questions investigating thoughts, current context (activity, persons present and location), appraisals of the current situation and mood. HR and activity data are acquired from a wireless electrocardiogram (Shimmer Research™) equipped with a three-axial accelerometer. The wearable sensor platform includes a board that allows the transduction, amplification and pre-processing of raw sensor signals, and a Bluetooth transmitter to wirelessly send the processed data. The unit is mounted on a soft-textile chest strap designed to seamlessly adapt to the user's body shape, allowing full freedom of movement. Sensed data are transmitted to the mobile phone's Bluetooth receiver and gathered by the PsychLog computing module, which stores and processes the signals for the extraction of relevant features.

Serino and colleagues (Serino et al., 2013) tested the use of PsychLog to investigate the fluctuation of individuals' experience and to detect, on the basis of psychophysiological real-time assessment, stressful events that normally occur during daily activities and situations. Promising results led the authors to consider PsychLog a valid tool to detect and offer real-time and effective interventions.

## POSITIVE TECHNOLOGY INTERVENTIONS FOR STRESS MANAGEMENT

The emerging convergence of technology and health care is offering new methods and tools not only to assess but also to cope with stress. According to Botella and colleagues (Botella et al., 2012), the potentiality of technologies for psychological interventions has been demonstrated in several technological domains, including computer-assisted therapy (e.g., (Carr, Ghosh, & Marks, 1988; Proudfoot et al., 2004), virtual reality applications (e.g., (Glanz, Rizzo, & Graap, 2003; Riva, 2009b), the Internet and its evolution—Web 2.0 (e.g., Andersson, 2009; Gorini, Gaggioli, Vigna, & Riva, 2008) and mobile devices (e.g., Free et al., 2013; Phillips, Felix, Galli, Patel, & Edwards, 2010).

Specifically, there is growing empirical support for the use of these technologies for stress management training (Gorini et al., 2008; Preziosa, Grassi, Gaggioli, & Riva, 2009; Riva, 2009a).

If Positive Psychology identifies three constituents of well-being—namely positive emotions/pleasure, engagement/actualization and meaning/connectedness—positive technologies could be classified according to their effect in promoting these three features (Riva, Banos, et al., 2012):

1. **Hedonic Level:** Technologies used to induce and/or enhance positive and pleasant experiences;
2. **Eudaimonic Level:** Technologies used to support individuals in reaching engaging and self-actualizing experiences;
3. **Social and Interpersonal Level:** Technologies used to support and improve social integration and/or connectedness between individuals and groups.

These levels led to the manipulation of crucial features aimed to help people manage their stress through different positive technologies. Specifically, within this chapter we will focus on the hedonic and eudaimonic experiences supported by technologies in terms of inducing positive affective states and supporting personal growth by teaching strategies to reduce stress and enhance well-being.

## Using Technologies to Foster Positive Emotional States

The first level of Positive Technology concerns how to use technology to foster positive emotional states.

Emotions occur at many levels of user experience, and positive emotions have the potential to trigger an upward spiral of flourishing (Fredrickson & Losada, 2005). According to Fredrickson (Frederickson, 2009), even though a positive emotional state is only momentary, its benefits can last in the form of traits, social bonds and abilities that endure well into the future.

The first step is to clarify the construct we are dealing with because it is essentially diffuse and conceptually difficult to define. Specifically, we want to delineate how we are using the term "emotions" and how we see it relative to related constructs such as mood and affect, according to many theorists and researchers (Batson, Shaw, & Oleson, 1992). Emotions are usually described as intense, short-lived affective states in response to particular stimuli. Moods, by contrast, are more diffuse and longer lasting, and it is often more difficult for an individual to describe the particular cause of his or her mood. The terms "affect" and "affective state" are broader and more inclusive, encompassing emotions, mood and some aspects of motivational processes.

Here we talk about positive emotions with a focus on relaxation as a positive psychological state. To induce positive emotional states in mediated experience, a typical approach is based on the exposure of emotion-eliciting materials, such as pictures, music or films (Codispoti, Bradley, & Lang, 2001; Eich, Ng, Macaulay, Percy, & Grebneva, 2007; Gross & Levenson, 1995; Philippot, 1993). A more recent approach is related to the use of Virtual Reality (VR) in inducing positive affective states. In order to develop virtual environments aimed to help people feel relaxed, one of the first aspects to consider is related to the virtual scenario in which participants can live a positive experience. Typically, virtual environments for stress management depict natural settings.

The theory at the base of the use of natural virtual environments is that restoration from stress and from mental fatigue relates to exposure to nature (Hartig, Evans, Jamner, Davis, & Gärling, 2003). Natural environments protect people against the impact of environmental stressors and offer physiological, emotional and attention restoration. Restorative environments are natural places that allow a shift towards more positively-toned emotional states and positive changes in physiological activity levels, behavior and cognitive functioning (Kaplan, 1995). In particular, immersion in a virtual computer-generated nature setting has been found to be a valid therapeutic aid in the treatment of anxiety disorders, as well as an effective tool in stress management and relaxation (Kahn, Severson, & Ruckert, 2009; Villani, Riva, & Riva, 2007). Plante and colleagues (Plante et al., 2003; Plante, Cage, Clements, & Stover, 2006) reported that individuals who interacted in a mediated environment enriched with a variety of positive visual and auditory stimulation reported greater improvement in self-efficacy and mood. Recently, computer-generated nature of VR has been demonstrated to promote restorative effects (Valtchanov, Barton, & Ellard, 2010).

Riva and Colleagues tested the potentiality of VR in inducing specific emotional responses, including positive moods (Riva et al., 2007). Results suggested the efficacy of VR as an affective medium: the relaxing virtual environments induced relaxation. Within the EMMA Project (Engaging Media for Mental Health Applications), some VR environments (Emotional Parks) were developed to induce positive states (Rosa María Baños et al., 2004; Rosa M Baños et al., 2008; Rosa María Baños et al., 2006). The strategies used to induce positive affective states within the experience in the virtual Emotional Parks combined Velten's self-statement (Velten, 1968), affective images from IAPS (Lang, Bradley, & Cuthbert, 1997) and music. The VR scenario experience was vivid and real and induced a high sense of presence that affected relaxation and the emotional response (Riva et al., 2007).

Villani and colleagues compared the efficacy of structured experiences provided through different technologies (video, audio and VR) for inducing relaxing states (Villani et al., 2007). Results of this experiment showed a significant reduction in anxiety and a significant improvement in positive emotional states, measured through self-report questionnaires and physiological parameters, but there was no difference among the media conditions. However, these results suggested two applied directions: when the goal is to produce a positive experience inducing positive emotions, the context (media form) plays the critical role; when the goal is to use the virtual experience to influence the affect, for example helping participants to cope with a problem, the content (media content) plays the critical role. This means that the virtual scenario and the technological devices can be helpful in affecting short-term psychological states, while the content of the experience plays a critical role in supporting the development of psychological skills useful to cope with real stressful situations. Participants may feel more engaged if they consider the experience to be crucial to their needs and goals (Scherer, 2001), and this is also true for mediated experiences (Villani, Repetto, Cipresso, & Riva, 2012; Villani et al., 2007; Villani & Riva, 2012). Thus, it is important to select people that recognize the importance of the proposed intervention for their well-being.

## Using Technologies to Learn Strategies to Reduce Stress and Enhance Well-Being

As decribed before, the acquisition of specific skills of stress management during the mediated experience can promote a sense of personal self-efficacy and prepare people to cope with real stressful situations. According to Bandura's (Bandura, 1977) theory, once established, self-efficacy tends to generalize to other situations. Indeed, once acquired, these competencies assigned to internal factors become a means to the management of stressful situations, and they can be transferred and applied to other contexts.

According to this view, three approaches aimed to enhance well-being and strengthen specific mental abilities to cope with stress have attracted some interest: relaxation practices, meditation and stress management training.

## Guided Relaxation Practices

The use of positive mediated interactive experiences to help people manage stress represents an innovative perspective. In this view, several studies have been carried out in the last ten years to verify the effectiveness of relaxation protocol supported by new technologies.

In a pilot study, Villani et al. (Villani et al., 2007) found that, after a brief protocol of two sessions where the virtual experience was accompanied by a relaxing narrative, people could learn relaxation strategies. These results led the authors to develop an extended stress management protocol (six sessions) that integrated other strategies. To develop the extended protocol, Villani and Riva (Villani & Riva, 2012) considered stress as having multiple components that typically involve cognitive, experiential, physiological and behavioral response systems that require multiple levels of analysis (Folkman, 2009). In accordance with Murphy (Murphy, 1996), authors combined different strategies used in cognitive-behavioral therapy (CBT) to yield better stress management than single-strategy programs. Specifically, the protocol aimed to increase emotional awareness (Greenberg, 2004), to learn to control emotions and to relax (Borkovec & Costello, 1993), to induce positive emotions (Folkman, 2008; Fredickson, 2001) and to substitute negative emotions through the imagination process (Roemer & Orsillo, 2002). Relaxation practices included in the training were autogenic training (Schultz & Luthe, 1969), Progressive Muscular Relaxation (Jacobson, 1938) and breathing techniques. Authors demonstrated that interactive media could be usefully used to reduce stress.

Recently, Gaggioli and colleagues (Gaggioli et al., 2014) carried out a block randomized controlled trial involving participants recruited from two different worker populations—teachers and nurses—that are recognized as highly exposed to psychological stress. The experimental group received a 5-week treatment course based on the Interreality paradigm that combines experiential virtual scenarios with real-time monitoring and support using advanced technologies (see the last paragraph of the chapter for a deeper description of the Interreality approach). Relaxation was induced through immersion in a natural scenario selected by the subjects where they could move and interact (see Figure 1).

The experience also integrated different pre-recorded audio narratives describing the specific setting and guiding the execution of different progressive muscle relaxation/deep breathing exercises. The con-

*Figure 1. The natural interactive scenario*

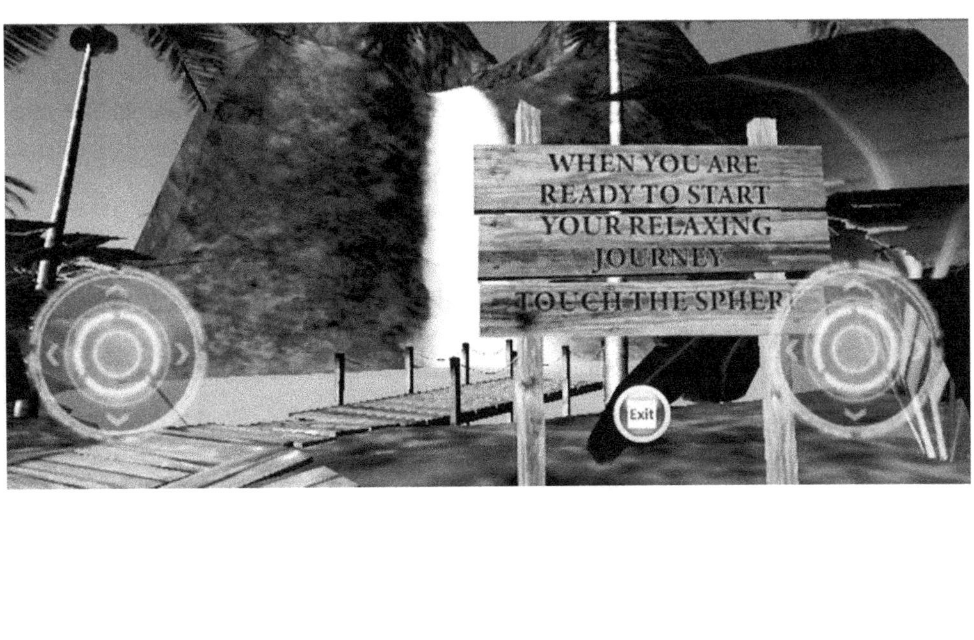
WHEN YOU ARE
READY TO START
YOUR RELAXING
JOURNEY
TOUCH THE SPHER
Exit

trol group received five weeks of traditional stress management training based on cognitive-behavioral therapy (CBT), and the waitlist group was reassessed and compared with the two other groups five weeks after the initial evaluation.

Although both treatments were able to significantly reduce perceived stress better than the waitlist group, only experimental group participants reported a significant reduction in chronic trait anxiety and a significant increase in the emotional support skill. These studies suggest the importance of integrating relaxation practices with other strategies in stress management interventions supported by new technologies.

## Online and Mobile Meditation and Mindfulness

Many people use meditation to treat stress and stress-related conditions and to promote general health (Goyal et al., 2010). Interest in meditation, which comes from Eastern traditions that emphasise lifelong growth, has rapidly grown during the past 30 years in Western. The umbrella of meditation covers various methods whose backgrounds and techniques are quite different. Thus, meditation refers to a family of techniques that have in common a conscious attempt to focus attention in a non-analytical way (Shapiro Jr, 2008).

According to a recent review (Goyal et al., 2014), meditation programs can reduce the negative dimensions of psychological stress more than they can improve the positive dimensions of health and well-being. Uncertainty remains about the role of the specific features of the different meditation techniques in actually influencing psychosocial stress outcomes (Chiesa & Malinowski, 2011; Sedlmeier et al., 2012).

All forms of meditation imply that more time spent meditating will yield larger effects. Thus, long-term trials may be optimal to examine the effect of meditation on many health outcomes.

Among the meditation approaches, mindfulness meditation can be described as a process of present-focused awareness or mindfulness (Bishop et al., 2004; Kabat-Zinn, 1990; Kabat-Zinn, 2003). Several interventions using the Mindfulness-Based Stress Reduction protocol demonstrated good results in reducing levels of stress, anxiety and depression in both clinical and nonclinical populations (Chiesa, Calati, & Serretti, 2011; Eberth & Sedlmeier, 2012; Hofmann, Sawyer, Witt, & Oh, 2010; J. J. Miller, Fletcher, & Kabat-Zinn, 1995; Shapiro, Schwartz, & Bonner, 1998; Shonin, Van Gordon, & Griffiths, 2013).

Despite the efficacy of these programs, the commitment required could cause barriers to its widespread application (Carmody & Baer, 2009). In fact, these programs are time-intensive and require both in- and out-of-session practice; they are also sometimes difficult for people with minimal experience with meditation.

To overcome these limitations, both online interventions and mobile applications offer several advantages, and both can provide helpful mental health resources that may be inaccessible otherwise. The Internet and mobile apps allow providers to deliver interventions, with reduced cost to the health services and to patients, to complete courses in their own comfortable, familiar surroundings (Powell et al., 2013; Zetterqvist, Maanmies, Ström, & Andersson, 2003).

There is growing evidence for online mindfulness courses being as effective as other face-to-face interven- tions (Glück & Maercker, 2011; Krusche, Cyhlarova, King, & Williams, 2012; Morledge et al., 2013). In this view, Krusche and colleagues (Krusche, Cyhlarova, & Williams, 2013) investigated the feasibility and effectiveness of an online mindfulness course for perceived stress, anxiety and depression. The programme consisted of 10 sessions, guided meditation videos and automated emails with elements of Mindfulness-Based Stress Reduction and Mindfulness-Based Cognitive Therapy. Participants could complete the programme at a pace that suited them individually (minimum length of four weeks), and the study evaluated the amount of practice as a mediator of change. Authors found that participants who were more stressed, depressed and anxious at baseline tended to practice less and take more time to complete the course. A longer course time predicted less of a change in stress, anxiety and depression, while more mindfulness practice significantly improved stress, anxiety and depression outcomes when accounting for baseline severity. Results for the effectiveness and feasibility of online mindfulness courses look promising.

Recently, brief mindfulness meditation protocols have also been integrated in self-help interventions supported by new technologies and mobile apps (Ahtinen et al., 2013; Cavanagh et al., 2013; Ly et al., 2014; Warnecke, Quinn, Ogden, Towle, & Nelson, 2011). The efficacy of brief mindfulness meditation protocols have been confirmed for nonclinical populations also at risk for stress-related health problems (Klatt, Buckworth, & Malarkey, 2009; Olivo, Dodson-Lavelle, Wren, Fang, & Oz, 2009).

Although a wide selection of mindfulness-based mobile apps (MBMAs) are available on the market (Plaza, Demarzo, Herrera-Mercadal, & Garcia-Campayo, 2013), the effectiveness of self-help intervention aimed toward helping people practice mindfulness techniques has not been broadly studied yet.

Recently, the effectiveness of a mobile app focused on a specific technique called thought distancing (i.e., a mindfulness technique that requires a person not to react in response to one's own thoughts but to be aware of them and observe them while they go away), which aims to enable decentering, has been tested (Chittaro & Vianello, 2014). Good results have been obtained in terms of achieved mindfulness, perceived level of difficulty and degree of pleasantness.

Carissoli and colleagues (Carissoli, Villani, & Riva, 2015) tested the effectiveness of a brief self-help protocol inspired by mindfulness meditation and delivered through a smartphone app in reducing stress for the nonclinical population. Authors used a controlled pragmatic trial that represents a trial typically designed to test the effectiveness of interventions in real life in order to maximize their applicability and generalizability (Patsopoulos, 2011). Sitting meditation was the focus, consisting of different exercises, such as mindful breathing and thought distancing. Authors found a reduction in hyperactivity and accelerated behaviors, which is consistent with meditation practice as mindfulness is a type of meditative technique that emphasizes an observant and nonreactive stance toward one's thoughts, emotions, and body states. Nevertheless, authors suggested that participants would need more time to become confident with the meditation approach—more time spent meditating could yield larger effects (Goyal et al., 2014).

## Cyber-Stress Inoculation Training

SIT, or stress inoculation training (Donald Meichenbaum, 1977; D. Meichenbaum, 1985), represents a validated short, semistructured and active approach to managing psychological stress (for a review, see Stetz et al., 2007). SIT is a type of training conceived to prepare individuals for stressful events by helping them diminish the potential for a negative cognitive, psychological and behavioral reaction.

SIT is based on the premise that to effectively manage stress, it is crucial to change the way people see the events and how they use their own coping skills. Thus, SIT is generally implemented through gradual and repeated exposure to the elements previously identified as stressors. The clinical rationale behind this approach is to ''inoculate'' the stressor in a person's experience, in combination with the acquisition of effective coping skills, so that people could be prepared when they inevitably encounter similar situations in daily life.

The general objectives of SIT are threefold and related to the three phases of the protocol. First, SIT aims to change the maladaptive stress response of the individual, thanks to the acquisition of active coping strategies. Thus, the first phase, named conceptualization, aims at making individuals aware of the transactional nature of psychological stress (Lazarus & Folkman, 1987) by giving them general information about the main effects and symptoms that could appear in different stressful situations. Second, SIT aims to develop the activity of self-regulation. Thus, the second phase, named skill acquisition and rehearsal, aims at teaching individuals to manage emotions and maladaptive behaviors, as well as learn new active coping skills. Third, SIT aims to explore and modify dysfunctional cognitive appraisal related to stressful events. Thus, the last phase, named application and follow-through, aims at increasing self-efficacy (Bandura, 1998) by helping individuals use the acquired coping skills in real contexts. Typical techniques used in this phase are imaginative rehearsal (in which an individual has to image stressful scenarios and think about coping strategies), behavioral rehearsal (role-playing) and the graded in vivo exposure.

The main objectives and three stages of SIT have been recently implemented in cyber-interventions based on SIT methodology (cyber-SIT), which utilise advanced technologies to create simulations to teach individuals how to effectively cope with psychological stress (Stetz et al., 2007; Wiederhold & Wiederhold, 2006).

In a recent review, Serino and colleagues (Serino et al., 2014) intended to outline the state-of-the-art of cyber-SIT interventions. According to the results of this systematic review, cyber-SIT appears to be a promising clinical approach, and there are interesting researches that effectively combined traditional SIT clinical protocol within advanced technologies. However, at the moment it is an emerging field of research. Thus there are still few studies in the literature meeting the requirement of using cyber-SIT in all its clinical elements and phases. Authors found that two main groups of technologies have been used for delivering cyber-SIT: virtual-interactive environments and mobile technologies. Villani and colleagues tested the effectiveness of a cyber-SIT delivered through mobile phones by comparing it with a control group (neutral video through mobile phones) in a sample of oncology nurses (Villani et al., 2013). Results showed psychological improvement of the experimental group in terms of anxiety state, anxiety trait reduction and coping skills acquisition.

Furthermore, up to now, cyber-SIT interventions have been applied to different contexts, targeting both chronic stress (such as PTSD) and acute stress related to a specific situation (such as stress experienced before an examination). For this reason, Serino and colleagues (Serino et al., 2014) suggested the importance of critically choosing the sampling strategies and defining the inclusion/exclusion criteria according to the specific aim of the protocol.

Practically, how may advanced technologies efficiently support all three phases of SIT? As far as the conceptualization phase, the interactive virtual worlds can use motivation to teach users about the transactional nature of stress, its main causes and effects (Riva, Vigna, et al., 2012). Furthermore, thanks to multimedia presentations where information is enriched and distributed through several channels, new technologies could enhance both the reception of instructional material and also the profound understanding of it (Mayer, 2009).

As far as the skill acquisition and rehearsal phase, advanced technologies can help individuals in acquiring effective coping skills, such as relaxation and meditation strategies. Bandura (Bandura, 2004) suggested that interactive features are the greatest strength of new media. Thus, computer-based feedback can be specified to accommodate the individual's motivations, current self-efficacy levels, unique obstacles and setbacks and progress toward specific goals and positive reinforcements (Bordnick, Traylor, Carter, & Graap, 2011; Fox & Bailenson, 2009).

Finally, as far as the application and follow-through phase, digital environments can be used for patients' exposure to stressful stimuli. Researches demonstrated that the exposure to multimedia/virtual contents has therapeutic benefits for participants (Emmelkamp et al., 2002). Within a cyber-SIT, this could be particularly useful in the last phase by creating controlled, graded and safe simulations of stressful scenarios to allow participants to use the acquired coping skills.

Beyond the exposure, there are currently other techniques used to consolidate the acquired coping skills, such as self-attribution procedures, relapse prevention procedures, helping others with similar problems and booster sessions (Donald Meichenbaum, 1977; Meichenbaum, 1985).

## Frontiers of Biofeedback

Several studies showed interesting results that support the feasibility of detecting affective states through psychophysiological data acquisition and analysis (Giakoumis et al., 2012; Magagnin et al., 2010). Led by Rosalind Picard, a computing group at MIT published several studies that highlighted the use of psychophysiological measures to deduce and classify emotional states while study participants were performing different kinds of PC activities (Mauri et al., 2010; Picard, 2000).

The potential capacity of sensor technologies to augment the mediated experience (through objective, automatic monitoring and feedback) has attracted some interest (Alcañiz, Botella, Banos, Zaragoza, & Guixeres, 2009). Thus, offering individuals the technology with which to monitor certain biological signals, known to be associated with stress, both over time and in real-time biofeedback, might serve to promote engagement with a mediated program for stress management.

Specifically, to detect changes in the physiological and affective states of subjects, researchers highlighted the usefulness of wearable biosensors in mobile platforms, virtual reality environments (Pallavicini, Cipresso, et al., 2013; Raspelli et al., 2012; Villani et al., 2012), or both (Repetto et al., 2013). This can be essential for situations in mobile clinical settings to share that information with the subject and, eventually, interested caregivers, such as professional medical staff, relatives, or even friends (see Figure 2).

An accurate electrocardiogram (ECG) analysis algorithm can be developed to elaborate and process signals generated from the wearable biosensors for effective real-time biofeedback. The QRS complex needs to be detected to generate heart rate and RR intervals. Thus, an accurate QRS detector is important in order to extract reliable HR or RR intervals to make meaningful HRV analysis and a correlation to mental stress. However, an accurate QRS complex detection may be difficult due to the physiological variability of the QRS complex and various types of noise that can be present in the ECG signal. Typical noise artifacts in ECG signals include power line interference, electrode contact noise, motion artifacts, and baseline drift (Friesen et al., 1990). Wearable monitoring systems used for out-of-clinic daily activity tracking utilise motion artifacts the most, where it is important to measure physiological signals accurately anytime and anywhere.

There are numerous detection methods for QRS complexes, including the Pan-Tompkins method (Pan & Tompkins, 1985). Moreover, morphological approaches were developed for baseline correction and noise suppression in clinical ECG signals (Sun, Chan, & Krishnan, 2002).

HRV measures provide a great opportunity to treat stress by using biofeedback based on relevant indexes. In a controlled clinical trial, Gaggioli and colleagues (Gaggioli et al., 2013) specifically tested HRV biofeedback for stress training and found results supporting the idea that it works very well when

*Figure 2. Biofeedback screenshots*

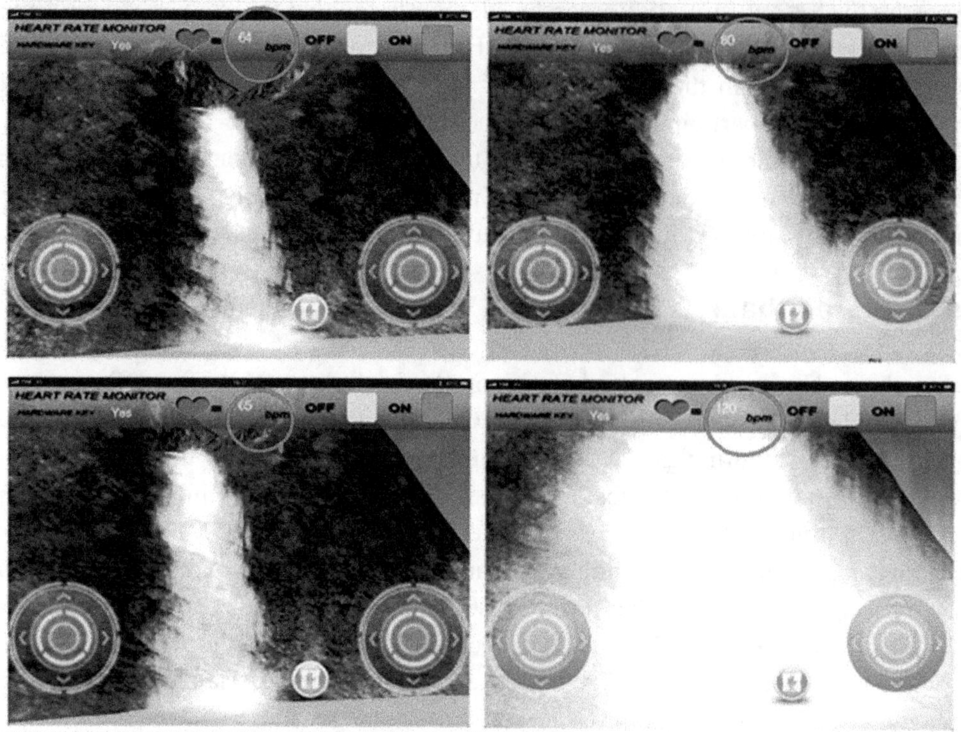


used alongside cognitive behavioral therapy. Furthermore, they found that specific indexes can be used for stressed patients—in particular temporal indexes, such as NN50, RMSSD, and spectral indexes, such as LF/HF (Malik, 1996). The combined use of respiration techniques and biofeedback would help in developing cognitive strategies for cardiorespiratory interventions aimed to reduce stress levels. Moreover, the use of LF/HF index gives patients indirect access to their sympathovagal balance information, which could greatly improve the impact of treatment for high stress levels.

Another interesting challenge that could be further investigated is represented by electroencephalography (EEG), and, in particular, the use of neurofeedback. Asymmetry on frontal brain activation can be measured through Alpha waves from the EEG, which be used as neurofeedback for stress patients (Millings et al., 2015).

## COMBINING ASSESSMENT AND INTERVENTION: THE INTERREALITY APPROACH

Assessment and intervention are inseparable parts of one general process and represent a dynamic spiral across time. To better integrate each other, Riva and colleagues (Pallavicini, Gaggioli, et al., 2013; Riva, 2009a; Silvia Serino et al., 2013) suggested the use of the "Interreality" paradigm (IR), which combines assessment and intervention within a hybrid environment and connects the physical and virtual worlds. The basic idea of IR intervention is to bridge mediated experiences with real experiences. In the IR strategy, behaviour in the physical world influences experiences in the virtual one, and behaviour in the virtual world influences the experience in the real one.

The assessment is conducted continuously in the virtual and real worlds through the tracking of individuals' behavioural and emotional status over time in the context of realistic task challenges. At the same time, the information is constantly used to improve both the appraisal and the coping skills of the patient through a conditioned association between effective performance state and task execution behaviors.

Within a recently funded European project "INTERSTRESS – Interreality in the management and treatment of stress-related disorders," a stress management protocol based on the Interreality paradigm has been proposed. The INTERSTRESS Project is intended to help individuals effectively manage psychological stress through the acquisition of techniques like relaxation and coping strategies within six weeks' treatment supported by advanced pervasive sensors and computing. Specifically, Gaggioli et al. (Andrea Gaggioli et al., 2014) evaluated the efficacy of Interreality for the management and prevention of psychological stress and compared it with a similar non-technological protocol based on the CBT approach. In that case, the main feature of Interreality was a twofold link between the virtual and the real world achieved through experiential virtual scenarios (fully controlled by the therapist and used to learn coping skills and improve self-efficacy) with real-time monitoring and support (identifying critical situations and assessing clinical change) using advanced technologies (virtual worlds, wearable biosensors, and smartphones). Findings provide initial evidence that a technology-enhanced IR protocol provides better outcomes than the traditionally accepted gold standard for psychological stress treatment, CBT, in terms of reduction of chronic trait anxiety and improvement of emotion-related coping skills.

Stressed people can be continuously assessed in the virtual and real worlds by tracking their behavioural and emotional status in the context of challenging tasks (customization of the intervention according to the individual characteristics), and feedback is continuously provided to improve individuals' skills (improvement of self-efficacy).

It is possible to identify two potential clinical advantages of the IR strategy. First, the integrated and quantitative assessment of the user's stress level using biosensors: the level of stress is continuously assessed in the virtual world and in the real world by recording the participant's behavioural and emotional status for the decision support system. Second, the provision of warnings and motivating feedback to improve self-awareness, compliance and long-term outcomes: on the basis of the decision support system, participants constantly receive feedback to improve their appraisal and coping skills in an entertaining and motivating manner both in clinical and mobile settings (Pallavicini, Gaggioli, et al., 2013; Riva, 2009a).

To better understand the potential of the IR approach, it is helpful to take another example—not specifically linked to a clinical scenario—such as the job interview, where individuals can be effectively helped to cope with stress (Villani, Cipresso, & Repetto, 2014). Typically, applicants feel anxious and stressed both because talking to strangers could provoke anxiety and because they could perceive a lack of control of the situation. Mediated interventions based on the different protocols (see previous paragraphs) can give applicants useful information, help them in acquiring effective coping skills, such as relaxation strategies, and let them experience, with controlled, graded and safe simulations, their competence to cope with a job interview. Applicants can do this training anytime and anywhere thanks to mobile technologies. Thanks to psycho-physiological assessment enabled by biosensors, the applicant's emotional states can be monitored during training to tailor the proposed experiences, to provide real time feedback and to administer positive reinforcement of good conduct. Furthermore, this assessment is possible until just a few minutes before undertaking a job interview. If biosensors reveal a high level of anxiety, the system could increase the comfort level by proposing ad hoc relaxation exercises and, by lessening anxiety, the system can support the applicant's performance.

The IR approach constitutes a sound foundation and rationale for future researches in technology-enhanced protocols for psychological stress management.

## FUTURE RESEARCH DIRECTIONS

Despite the opportunities described in the chapter about how integrating technology in positive psychology can help people cope with stress, we have to consider important challenges that need to be dealt with.

First, as described in the chapter, it's easier to focus on the hedonic dimension of the experience by inducing positive emotional states such as relaxation, instead of developing the eudaimonic dimension by improving coping skills and promoting resilience. Nevertheless, as previously shown, if the goal is to promote self-empowerment, the better strategy is to work on both levels.

Second, to our knowledge there are still few studies that tested the effectiveness of experiences supported by technology and compared it with traditional methods. Because many stress management apps, blogs and digital tools are already available in the market, and the popularity of these services is increasing among people, trials showing the effectiveness of these approaches are needed. Pragmatic trials, typically designed to test the effectiveness of interventions in real life in order to maximize their applicability and generalizability (Patsopoulos, 2011), are encouraged.

Third, most apps and tools have been developed thanks to the support of research funding. As a consequence, they are focused on the rationale underlying the proposed content, but too often they don't have adequate usability features. Future researches should test and enhance the user experience of stress management apps and technological tools.

Finally, over the potential opportunities, it will be important to conduct more research on the possible inconvenience of using technology in daily routines so as to preclude constant accessibility and overuse (Thomee, Harenstam, & Hagberg, 2011).

## CONCLUSION

This chapter aimed to describe how positive technologies could be involved in helping people cope with stress.

On the one hand, thanks to the combination of traditional assessment measures of stress and the analysis of physiological correlates of this experience, it is possible to overcome limitations related to self-reported data and move towards self-tracking. Self-tracking is a fast-growing trend in the field of e-health that involves the collection of biological, physical, behavioural or environmental information that can be integrated within a feedback loop of introspection and self-experimentation. The fecund convergence between ICTs and wearable biosensors allows personal health data to be collected, aggregated, visualized, collated into reports and shared (A. Stone, Shiffman, Atienza, & Nebeling, 2007).

On the other hand, the emerging convergence of technology and health care is offering new methods and tools not only to assess but also to cope with stress. In this view, there is growing empirical support for the use of several technologies for stress management protocols.

This chapter focused on the hedonic and eudaimonic experiences supported by technologies in terms of inducing positive affective states and supporting personal growth by teaching strategies to reduce stress and enhance well-being. If natural virtual scenarios and technological devices can be helpful in inducing positive emotions, the content of the experience plays a critical role in changing the affective component and in supporting the development of psychological skills useful to coping with real stressful situations. To reach this goal, three approaches aimed to enhance well-being and strengthen specific mental abilities to cope with stress (such as guided relaxation practices, online and mobile meditation and mindfulness and cyber-stress inoculation training) have been described.

Assessment and intervention are inseparable parts of one general process and represent a dynamic spiral across time. The "Interreality" paradigm (IR) allows the combination of both and a connection between mediated experiences with real experiences.

To conclude, the positive technology approach offers researchers and clinicians new effective opportunities for the assessment and treatment of psychological stress in several contexts.

## AKNOWLEDGMENT

This work was partially supported by the Italian funded project "VRehab. Virtual Reality in the Assessment and TeleRehabilitation of Parkinson's Disease and Post-Stroke Disabilities" - RF-2009-1472190.

## REFERENCES

Ahtinen, A., & Mattila, E., VÃ¤lkkynen, P., Kaipainen, K., Vanhala, T., Ermes, M.,... Lappalainen, R. (2013). Mobile Mental Wellness Training for Stress Management: Feasibility and Design Implications Based on a One-Month Field Study. *Journal of Medical Internet Research, 15*(7). PMID:25100683

Alcañiz, M., Botella, C., Banos, R., Zaragoza, I., & Guixeres, J. (2009). The Intelligent e-Therapy system: A new paradigm for telepsychology and cybertherapy. *British Journal of Guidance & Counselling, 37*(3), 287–296. doi:10.1080/03069880902957015

Andersson, G. (2009). Using the Internet to provide cognitive behaviour therapy. *Behaviour Research and Therapy, 47*(3), 175–180. doi:10.1016/j.brat.2009.01.010 PMID:19230862

Antonovsky, A. (1979). *Health, stress, and coping. New perspective on mental and physical well-being.* San Francisco, CA: Jossey-Bass.

Antonovsky, A. (1987). The salutogenic perspective: Toward a new view of health and illness. *Advances, 4*(1), 47–75.

Antonovsky, A. (1996). The salutogenic model as a theory to guide health promotion. *Health Promotion International, 11*(1), 11–18. doi:10.1093/heapro/11.1.11

Bandura, A. (1977). Self-efficacy: Toward a unifying theory of behavioral change. *Psychological Review, 84*(2), 191–215. doi:10.1037/0033-295X.84.2.191 PMID:847061

Bandura, A. (1998). Health promotion from the perspective of social cognitive theory. *Psychology & Health, 13*(4), 623–649. doi:10.1080/08870449808407422

Bandura, A. (2004). Health promotion by social cognitive means. *Health Education & Behavior, 31*(2), 143–164. doi:10.1177/1090198104263660 PMID:15090118

Baños, R. M., Botella, C., Alcañiz, M., Liaño, V., Guerrero, B., & Rey, B. (2004). Immersion and emotion: Their impact on the sense of presence. *Cyberpsychology & Behavior, 7*(6), 734–741. doi:10.1089/cpb.2004.7.734 PMID:15687809

Baños, R. M., Botella, C., Rubió, I., Quero, S., García-Palacios, A., & Alcañiz, M. (2008). Presence and emotions in virtual environments: The influence of stereoscopy. *Cyberpsychology & Behavior, 11*(1), 1–8. doi:10.1089/cpb.2007.9936 PMID:18275306

Baños, R. M., Liaño, V., Botella, C., Alcañiz, M., Guerrero, B., & Rey, B. (2006). *Changing induced moods via virtual reality Persuasive Technology* (pp. 7–15). Springer.

Batson, C. D., Shaw, L. L., & Oleson, K. C. (1992). Differentiating affect, mood, and emotion: Toward functionally based conceptual distinctions. In M.S. Clark (Eds.), Emotion. Review of personality and social psychology (Vol. 13, pp. 294-326). Thousand Oaks, CA, US: Sage Publications.

Berntson, G. G., & Cacioppo, J. T. (2004). Heart rate variability: Stress and psychiatric conditions. In M. M. A. J. Camm (Ed.), *Dynamic electrocardiography* (pp. 56–63). New York: Futura. doi:10.1002/9780470987483.ch7

Bishop, S. R., Lau, M., Shapiro, S., Carlson, L., Anderson, N. D., Carmody, J., & Velting, D. et al. (2004). Mindfulness: A proposed operational definition. *Clinical Psychology: Science and Practice, 11*(3), 230–241. doi:10.1093/clipsy.bph077

Bordnick, P. S., Traylor, A. C., Carter, B. L., & Graap, K. M. (2011). A feasibility study of virtual reality-based coping skills training for nicotine dependence. *Research on Social Work Practice*, 22(3), 293-300. PMID:25484549

Borkovec, T., & Costello, E. (1993). Efficacy of applied relaxation and cognitive-behavioral therapy in the treatment of generalized anxiety disorder. *Journal of Consulting and Clinical Psychology, 61*(4), 611–619. doi:10.1037/0022-006X.61.4.611 PMID:8370856

Botella, C., Riva, G., Gaggioli, A., Wiederhold, B. K., Alcaniz, M., & Banos, R. M. (2012). The present and future of positive technologies. *Cyberpsychology, Behavior, and Social Networking, 15*(2), 78–84. doi:10.1089/cyber.2011.0140 PMID:22149078

Carissoli, C., Villani, D., & Riva, G. (2015). Does a meditation protocol supported by a mobile application help people reduce stress? Suggestions from a controlled pragmatic trial. *Cyberpsychology, Behavior, and Social Networking, 18*(1), 46–53. doi:10.1089/cyber.2014.0062 PMID:25584730

Carmody, J., & Baer, R. A. (2009). How long does a mindfulness-based stress reduction program need to be? A review of class contact hours and effect sizes for psychological distress. *Journal of Clinical Psychology, 65*(6), 627–638. doi:10.1002/jclp.20555 PMID:19309694

Carr, A., Ghosh, A., & Marks, I. M. (1988). Computer-supervised exposure treatment for phobias. *Canadian Journal of Psychiatry*, *33*(2), 112–117. PMID:3365636

Cavanagh, K., Strauss, C., Cicconi, F., Griffiths, N., Wyper, A., & Jones, F. (2013). A randomised controlled trial of a brief online mindfulness-based intervention. *Behaviour Research and Therapy*, *51*(9), 573–578. doi:10.1016/j.brat.2013.06.003 PMID:23872699

Chiesa, A., Calati, R., & Serretti, A. (2011). Does mindfulness training improve cognitive abilities? A systematic review of neuropsychological findings. *Clinical Psychology Review*, *31*(3), 449–464. doi:10.1016/j.cpr.2010.11.003 PMID:21183265

Chiesa, A., & Malinowski, P. (2011). Mindfulness-based approaches: Are they all the same? *Journal of Clinical Psychology*, *67*(4), 404–424. doi:10.1002/jclp.20776 PMID:21254062

Chittaro, L., & Vianello, A. (2014). Computer-supported mindfulness: Evaluation of a mobile thought distancing application on naive meditators. *International Journal of Human-Computer Studies*, *72*(3), 337–348. doi:10.1016/j.ijhcs.2013.11.001

Cinaz, B., Arnrich, B., La Marca, R., & Tröster, G. (2013). Monitoring of Mental Workload Levels during an Everyday Life Office-Work Scenario. *Personal and Ubiquitous Computing Journal*, *17*(2), 229–239. doi:10.1007/s00779-011-0466-1

Codispoti, M., Bradley, M. M., & Lang, P. J. (2001). Affective reactions to briefly presented pictures. *Psychophysiology*, *38*(3), 474–478. doi:10.1111/1469-8986.3830474 PMID:11352135

Cohen, S. (1986). Contrasting the Hassles Scale and the Perceived Stress Scale: Who's really measuring appraised stress? *The American Psychologist*, *41*(6), 716–718. doi:10.1037/0003-066X.41.6.716

Cohen, S., Janicki-Deverts, D., & Miller, G. E. (2007). Psychological stress and disease. *Journal of the American Medical Association*, *298*(14), 1685–1687. doi:10.1001/jama.298.14.1685 PMID:17925521

Conner, T. S., & Barrett, L. F. (2012). Trends in ambulatory self-report: The role of momentary experience in psychosomatic medicine. *Psychosomatic Medicine*, *74*(4), 327–337. Retrieved from http://www.ncbi.nlm.nih.gov/entrez/query.fcgi?cmd=Retrieve&db=PubMed&dopt=Citation&list_uids=22582330 doi:10.1097/PSY.0b013e3182546f18 PMID:22582330

Csikszentmihalyi, M., & Larson, R. (1987). Validity and reliability of the Experience-Sampling Method. *The Journal of Nervous and Mental Disease*, *175*(9), 526–536. Retrieved from http://www.ncbi.nlm.nih.gov/pubmed/3655778 doi:10.1097/00005053-198709000-00004 PMID:3655778

Davidson, R. J., Jackson, D. C., & Kalin, N. H. (2000). Emotion, plasticity, context, and regulation: Perspectives from affective neuroscience. *Psychological Bulletin*, *126*(6), 890–909. doi:10.1037/0033-2909.126.6.890 PMID:11107881

Di Nuovo, S., Rispoli, L., & Genta, E. (2000). *Misurare lo stress: il test MSP e altri strumenti per una valutazione integrata* (Vol. 19). FrancoAngeli.

Eberth, J., & Sedlmeier, P. (2012). The effects of mindfulness meditation: A meta-analysis. *Mindfulness*, *3*(3), 174–189. doi:10.1007/s12671-012-0101-x

Eich, E., Ng, J. T., Macaulay, D., Percy, A. D., & Grebneva, I. (2007). Combining music with thought to change mood. In J.A. Cohen, & J.J.B. Allen (Eds.), *Handbook of emotion elicitation and assessment* (pp. 124–136). New York: Oxford University Press.

Emmelkamp, P., Krijn, M., Hulsbosch, A., De Vries, S., Schuemie, M., & Van der Mast, C. (2002). Virtual reality treatment versus exposure in vivo: A comparative evaluation in acrophobia. *Behaviour Research and Therapy*, *40*(5), 509–516. doi:10.1016/S0005-7967(01)00023-7 PMID:12038644

Folkman, S. (2008). The case for positive emotions in the stress process. *Anxiety, Stress, and Coping*, *21*(1), 3–14. doi:10.1080/10615800701740457 PMID:18027121

Folkman, S. (2009). Commentary on the special section "theory-based approaches to stress and coping" questions, answers, issues, and next steps in stress and coping research. *European Psychologist*, *14*(1), 72–77. doi:10.1027/1016-9040.14.1.72

Fox, J., & Bailenson, J. N. (2009). Virtual self-modeling: The effects of vicarious reinforcement and identification on exercise behaviors. *Media Psychology*, *12*(1), 1–25. doi:10.1080/15213260802669474

Frederickson, B. (2009). *Positivity: Groundbreaking research reveals how to embrace the hidden strength of positive emotions, overcome negativity, and thrive*. New York: Crown Archetype.

Fredickson, B. (2001). The role of positive emotions in positive psychology. *The American Psychologist*, *56*(3), 218–226. doi:10.1037/0003-066X.56.3.218 PMID:11315248

Fredrickson, B. L., & Losada, M. F. (2005). Positive affect and the complex dynamics of human flourishing. *The American Psychologist*, *60*(7), 678–686. doi:10.1037/0003-066X.60.7.678 PMID:16221001

Free, C., Phillips, G., Felix, L., Galli, L., Patel, V., & Edwards, P. (2010). The effectiveness of M-health technologies for improving health and health services: A systematic review protocol. *BMC Research Notes*, *3*(1), 250. doi:10.1186/1756-0500-3-250 PMID:20925916

Free, C., Phillips, G., Galli, L., Watson, L., Felix, L., Edwards, P., & Haines, A. et al. (2013). The effectiveness of mobile-health technology-based health behaviour change or disease management interventions for health care consumers: A systematic review. *PLoS Medicine*, *10*(1), e1001362. doi:10.1371/journal.pmed.1001362 PMID:23349621

Friesen, G. M., Jannett, T. C., Jadallah, M. A., Yates, S. L., Quint, S. R., & Nagle, H. T. (1990). A comparison of the noise sensitivity of nine QRS detection algorithms. *Biomedical Engineering. IEEE Transactions on*, *37*(1), 85–98.

Gaggioli, A., Pallavicini, F., Morganti, L., Serino, S., Scaratti, C., Briguglio, M., & Bernava, G. et al. (2014). Experiential virtual scenarios with real-time monitoring (interreality) for the management of psychological stress: A block randomized controlled trial. *Journal of Medical Internet Research*, *16*(7), e167. doi:10.2196/jmir.3235 PMID:25004803

Gaggioli, A., Pioggia, G., Tartarisco, G., Baldus, G., Corda, D., Cipresso, P., & Riva, G. (2013). A mobile data collection platform for mental health research. *Personal and Ubiquitous Computing Journal*, *17*(2), 241–251. doi:10.1007/s00779-011-0465-2

Giakoumis, D., Drosou, A., Cipresso, P., Tzovaras, D., Hassapis, G., Gaggioli, A., & Riva, G. (2012). Using activity-related behavioural features towards more effective automatic stress detection. *PLoS ONE*, *7*(9), e43571. doi:10.1371/journal.pone.0043571 PMID:23028461

Glanz, K., Rizzo, A. S., & Graap, K. (2003). Virtual reality for psychotherapy: Current reality and future possibilities. *Psychotherapy (Chicago, Ill.)*, *40*(1-2), 55–67. doi:10.1037/0033-3204.40.1-2.55

Glück, T. M., & Maercker, A. (2011). A randomized controlled pilot study of a brief web-based mindfulness training. *BMC Psychiatry*, *11*(1), 175. doi:10.1186/1471-244X-11-175 PMID:22067058

Gorini, A., Gaggioli, A., Vigna, C., & Riva, G. (2008). A second life for eHealth: Prospects for the use of 3-D virtual worlds in clinical psychology. *Journal of Medical Internet Research*, *10*(3), e21. doi:10.2196/jmir.1029 PMID:18678557

Goyal, M., Haythornthwaite, J., Levine, D., Becker, D., Vaidya, D., Hill-Briggs, F., & Ford, D. (2010). Intensive meditation for refractory pain and symptoms. *Journal of Alternative and Complementary Medicine (New York, N.Y.)*, *16*(6), 627–631. doi:10.1089/acm.2009.0372 PMID:20569029

Goyal, M., Singh, S., Sibinga, E. M., Gould, N. F., Rowland-Seymour, A., Sharma, R., & Shihab, H. M. et al. (2014). Meditation programs for psychological stress and well-being: A systematic review and meta-analysis. *JAMA Internal Medicine*, *174*(3), 357–368. doi:10.1001/jamainternmed.2013.13018 PMID:24395196

Greenberg, L. S. (2004). Emotion–focused therapy. *Clinical Psychology & Psychotherapy*, *11*(1), 3–16. doi:10.1002/cpp.388

Gross, J. J., & Levenson, R. W. (1995). Emotion elicitation using films. *Cognition and Emotion*, *9*(1), 87–108. doi:10.1080/02699939508408966

Hammen, C. (2005). Stress and depression. *Annual Review of Clinical Psychology*, *1*(1), 293–319. doi:10.1146/annurev.clinpsy.1.102803.143938 PMID:17716090

Hartig, T., Evans, G. W., Jamner, L. D., Davis, D. S., & Gärling, T. (2003). Tracking restoration in natural and urban field settings. *Journal of Environmental Psychology*, *23*(2), 109–123. doi:10.1016/S0272-4944(02)00109-3

Hofmann, S. G., Sawyer, A. T., Witt, A. A., & Oh, D. (2010). The effect of mindfulness-based therapy on anxiety and depression: A meta-analytic review. *Journal of Consulting and Clinical Psychology*, *78*(2), 169–183. doi:10.1037/a0018555 PMID:20350028

Hruschka, D. J., Kohrt, B. A., & Worthman, C. M. (2005). Estimating between- and within-individual variation in cortisol levels using multilevel models. *Psychoneuroendocrinology*, *30*(7), 698–714. Retrieved from http://www.ncbi.nlm.nih.gov/entrez/query.fcgi?cmd=Retrieve&db=PubMed&dopt=Citation&list_uids=15854786 doi:10.1016/j.psyneuen.2005.03.002 PMID:15854786

Ice, G. H., Katz-Stein, A., Himes, J., & Kane, R. L. (2004). Diurnal cycles of salivary cortisol in older adults. *Psychoneuroendocrinology, 29*(3), 355-370. doi:S0306453003000349 [pii]

Jackson, J. S., Knight, K. M., & Rafferty, J. A. (2010). Race and unhealthy behaviors: Chronic stress, the HPA axis, and physical and mental health disparities over the life course. *American Journal of Public Health*, *100*(5), 933–939. doi:10.2105/AJPH.2008.143446 PMID:19846689

Jacobs, N., Myin-Germeys, I., Derom, C., Delespaul, P., van Os, J., & Nicolson, N. A. (2007). A momentary assessment study of the relationship between affective and adrenocortical stress responses in daily life. *Biological Psychology*, *74*(1), 60–66. Retrieved from http://www.ncbi.nlm.nih.gov/entrez/query.fcgi?cmd=Retrieve&db=PubMed&dopt=Citation&list_uids=16942831 doi:10.1016/j.biopsycho.2006.07.002 PMID:16942831

Jacobson, E. (1938). Progressive relaxation.

Kabat-Zinn, J. (1990). *Full catastrophe living: Using the wisdom of your body and mind to face stress, pain, and illness*. New York: Delacorte.

Kabat-Zinn, J. (2003). Mindfulness-based interventions in context: Past, present, and future. *Clinical Psychology: Science and Practice*, *10*(2), 144–156. doi:10.1093/clipsy.bpg016

Kahn, P. H. Jr, Severson, R. L., & Ruckert, J. H. (2009). The human relation with nature and technological nature. *Current Directions in Psychological Science*, *18*(1), 37–42. doi:10.1111/j.1467-8721.2009.01602.x

Kahneman, D., Krueger, A. B., Schkade, D. A., Schwarz, N., & Stone, A. A. (2004). A survey method for characterizing daily life experience: the day reconstruction method. *Science, 306*(5702), 1776-1780. doi:306/5702/177610.1126/science.1103572

Kalia, M. (2002). Assessing the economic impact of stress—The modern day hidden epidemic. *Metabolism: Clinical and Experimental*, *51*(6), 49–53. doi:10.1053/meta.2002.33193 PMID:12040542

Kaplan, S. (1995). The restorative benefits of nature: Toward an integrative framework. *Journal of Environmental Psychology*, *15*(3), 169–182. doi:10.1016/0272-4944(95)90001-2

Kiecolt-Glaser, J. K., McGuire, L., Robles, T. F., & Glaser, R. (2002). Psychoneuroimmunology: Psychological influences on immune function and health. *Journal of Consulting and Clinical Psychology*, *70*(3), 537–547. doi:10.1037/0022-006X.70.3.537 PMID:12090368

Kim, D., Seo, Y., Cho, J., & Cho, C. H. (2008). Detection of subjects with higher self-reporting stress scores using heart rate variability patterns during the day. *Paper presented at the Conf Proc IEEE Eng Med Biol Soc*. doi:10.1109/IEMBS.2008.4649244

Kimhy, D., Delespaul, P., Ahn, H., Cai, S., Shikhman, M., Lieberman, J. A.,... Sloan, R. P. (2009). Concurrent measurement of "real-world" stress and arousal in individuals with psychosis: assessing the feasibility and validity of a novel methodology. *Schizophr Bull, 36*(6), 1131-1139. doi:sbp028[pii]10.1093/schbul/sbp028

Kirschbaum, C., & Hellhammer, D. H. (1989). Salivary cortisol in psychobiological research: an overview. *Neuropsychobiology, 22*(3), 150-169. doi:118611[pii]118611

Klatt, M. D., Buckworth, J., & Malarkey, W. B. (2009). Effects of low-dose mindfulness-based stress reduction (MBSR-ld) on working adults. *Health Education & Behavior*, *36*(3), 601–614. doi:10.1177/1090198108317627 PMID:18469160

Krusche, A., Cyhlarova, E., King, S., & Williams, J. M. G. (2012). Mindfulness online: A preliminary evaluation of the feasibility of a web-based mindfulness course and the impact on stress. *BMJ Open*, *2*(3), e000803. doi:10.1136/bmjopen-2011-000803 PMID:22614170

Krusche, A., Cyhlarova, E., & Williams, J. M. G. (2013). Mindfulness online: An evaluation of the feasibility of a web-based mindfulness course for stress, anxiety and depression. *BMJ Open*, *3*(11), e003498. doi:10.1136/bmjopen-2013-003498 PMID:24293203

Lang, P. J., Bradley, M. M., & Cuthbert, B. N. (1997). International affective picture system (IAPS): Technical manual and affective ratings. NIMH Center for the Study of Emotion and Attention, 39-58.

Lazarus, R. S., & Folkman, S. (1987). Transactional theory and research on emotions and coping. *European Journal of Personality*, *1*(3), 141–169. doi:10.1002/per.2410010304

Lemyre, L., & Tessier, R. (1988). Mesure de Stress Psychologique (MSP): Se sentir stressé-e. *Canadian Journal of Behavioural Science/Revue canadienne des sciences du comportement, 20*(3), 302.

Leserman, J., Petitto, J., Gu, H., Gaynes, B., Barroso, J., Golden, R., & Evans, D. et al. (2002). Progression to AIDS, a clinical AIDS condition and mortality: Psychosocial and physiological predictors. *Psychological Medicine*, *32*(06), 1059–1073. doi:10.1017/S0033291702005949 PMID:12214787

Lupien, S. J., McEwen, B. S., Gunnar, M. R., & Heim, C. (2009). Effects of stress throughout the lifespan on the brain, behaviour and cognition. *Nature Reviews. Neuroscience*, *10*(6), 434–445. doi:10.1038/nrn2639 PMID:19401723

Ly, K. H., Truschel, A., Jarl, L., Magnusson, S., Windahl, T., Johansson, R., & Andersson, G. et al. (2014). Behavioural activation versus mindfulness-based guided self-help treatment administered through a smartphone application: A randomised controlled trial. *BMJ Open*, *4*(1), e003440. doi:10.1136/bmjopen-2013-003440 PMID:24413342

Magagnin, V., Mauri, M., Cipresso, P., Mainardi, L., Brown, E. N., Cerutti, S.,... Barbieri, R. (2010). Heart rate variability and respiratory sinus arrhythmia assessment of affective states by bivariate autoregressive spectral analysis. *Paper presented at the Computing in Cardiology.*

Malik, M. (1996). The North American Society of Pacing and Electrophysiology. Heart rate variability: Standards of measurement, physiological interpretation and clinical use. *Circulation*, *93*(5), 1043–1065. doi:10.1161/01.CIR.93.5.1043 PMID:8598068

Mauri, M., Magagnin, V., Cipresso, P., Mainardi, L., Brown, E. N., Cerutti, S.,... Barbieri, R. (2010). Psychophysiological signals associated with affective states. *Paper presented at the 2010 Annual International Conference of the IEEE on Engineering in Medicine and Biology Society (EMBC).* doi:10.1109/IEMBS.2010.5627465

Mayer, R. E. (2009). *Multimedia learning*. Cambridge university press. doi:10.1017/CBO9780511811678

McEwen, B. S. (1998). Stress, adaptation, and disease: Allostasis and allostatic load. *Annals of the New York Academy of Sciences*, *840*(1), 33–44. doi:10.1111/j.1749-6632.1998.tb09546.x PMID:9629234

McEwen, B. S. (2006). Protective and damaging effects of stress mediators: Central role of the brain. *Dialogues in Clinical Neuroscience*, *8*(4), 367. PMID:17290796

McEwen, B. S., & Stellar, E. (1993). Stress and the individual: Mechanisms leading to disease. *Archives of Internal Medicine*, *153*(18), 2093–2101. doi:10.1001/archinte.1993.00410180039004 PMID:8379800

Meichenbaum, D. (1977). Cognitive behaviour modification. *Cognitive Behaviour Therapy*, *6*(4), 185–192.

Meichenbaum, D. (1985). *Stress inoculation training*. New York: Pergamon Press.

Melillo, P., Bracale, M., & Pecchia, L. (2011). Nonlinear Heart Rate Variability features for real-life stress detection. Case study: students under stress due to university examination. *Biomed Eng Online, 10*, 96. doi:1475-925X-10-96 [pii]10.1186/1475-925X-10-96

Miller, G. E., Chen, E., & Zhou, E. S. (2007). If it goes up, must it come down? Chronic stress and the hypothalamic-pituitary-adrenocortical axis in humans. *Psychol Bull, 133*(1), 25-45. doi:2006-23058-00210.1037/0033-2909.133.1.25

Miller, J. J., Fletcher, K., & Kabat-Zinn, J. (1995). Three-year follow-up and clinical implications of a mindfulness meditation-based stress reduction intervention in the treatment of anxiety disorders. *General Hospital Psychiatry*, *17*(3), 192–200. doi:10.1016/0163-8343(95)00025-M PMID:7649463

Millings, A., Morris, J., Rowe, A., Easton, S., Martin, J. K., Majoe, D., & Mohr, C. (2015). *Can the effectiveness of an online stress management program be augmented by wearable sensor technology?* Internet Interventions.

Morey, J. N., Boggero, I. A., Scott, A. B., & Segerstrom, S. C. (2015). Current directions in stress and human immune function. *Current Opinion in Psychology*, *5*, 13–17. doi:10.1016/j.copsyc.2015.03.007 PMID:26086030

Morledge, T. J., Allexandre, D., Fox, E., Fu, A. Z., Higashi, M. K., Kruzikas, D. T., & Reese, P. R. et al. (2013). Feasibility of an online mindfulness program for stress management—a randomized, controlled trial. *Annals of Behavioral Medicine*, *46*(2), 137–148. doi:10.1007/s12160-013-9490-x PMID:23632913

Morris, M. E., Kathawala, Q., Leen, T. K., Gorenstein, E. E., Guilak, F., Labhard, M., & Deleeuw, W. (2010). Mobile therapy: case study evaluations of a cell phone application for emotional self-awareness. *J Med Internet Res, 12*(2), e10. doi:v12i2e1010.2196/jmir.1371

Muaremi, A., Arnrich, B., & Tröster, G. (2013). Towards Measuring Stress with Smartphones and Wearable Devices During Workday and Sleep. *BioNanoScience*, *3*(2), 172–183. doi:10.1007/s12668-013-0089-2 PMID:25530929

Murphy, L. R. (1996). Stress management in work settings: A critical review of the health effects. *American Journal of Health Promotion*, *11*(2), 112–135. doi:10.4278/0890-1171-11.2.112 PMID:10163598

Olivo, E. L., Dodson-Lavelle, B., Wren, A., Fang, Y., & Oz, M. C. (2009). Feasibility and effectiveness of a brief meditation-based stress management intervention for patients diagnosed with or at risk for coronary heart disease: A pilot study. *Psychology Health and Medicine*, *14*(5), 513–523. doi:10.1080/13548500902890087 PMID:19844830

Orsila, R., Virtanen, M., Luukkaala, T., Tarvainen, M., Karjalainen, P., Viik, J., & Nygard, C. H. et al. (2008). Perceived mental stress and reactions in heart rate variability--a pilot study among employees of an electronics company. *International Journal of Occupational Safety and Ergonomics*, *14*(3), 275–283. http://www.ncbi.nlm.nih.gov/entrez/query.fcgi?cmd=Retrieve&db=PubMed&dopt=Citation&list_uids=18954537 doi:10.1080/10803548.2008.11076767 PMID:18954537

Pallavicini, F., Cipresso, P., Raspelli, S., Grassi, A., Serino, S., Vigna, C., & Riva, G. et al. (2013). Is virtual reality always an effective stressors for exposure treatments? Some insights from a controlled trial. *BMC Psychiatry*, *13*(1), 52. doi:10.1186/1471-244X-13-52 PMID:23398927

Pallavicini, F., Gaggioli, A., Raspelli, S., Cipresso, P., Serino, S., Vigna, C., & Riva, G. et al.(2013). Interreality for the management and training of psychological stress: Study protocol for a randomized controlled trial. *Trials*, *14*(1), 191. doi:10.1186/1745-6215-14-191 PMID:23806013

Pan, J., & Tompkins, W. J. (1985). A real-time QRS detection algorithm. *IEEE Transactions on Biomedical Engineering,* 3, 230-236.

Patsopoulos, N. A. (2011). A pragmatic view on pragmatic trials. *Dialogues in Clinical Neuroscience*, *13*(2), 217–224. Retrieved from http://www.ncbi.nlm.nih.gov/pubmed/21842619 PMID:21842619

Philippot, P. (1993). Inducing and assessing differentiated emotion-feeling states in the laboratory. *Cognition and Emotion*, *7*(2), 171–193. doi:10.1080/02699939308409183

Picard, R. W. (2000). *Affective computing*. MIT press.

Plante, T. G., Aldridge, A., Su, D., Bogdan, R., Belo, M., & Kahn, K. (2003). Does Virtual Reality Enhance the Management of Stress When Paired With Exercise? An Exploratory Study. *International Journal of Stress Management*, *10*(3), 203–216. doi:10.1037/1072-5245.10.3.203

Plante, T. G., Cage, C., Clements, S., & Stover, A. (2006). Psychological benefits of exercise paired with virtual reality: Outdoor exercise energizes whereas indoor virtual exercise relaxes. *International Journal of Stress Management*, *13*(1), 108–117. doi:10.1037/1072-5245.13.1.108

Plaza, I., Demarzo, M. M., Herrera-Mercadal, P., & Garcia-Campayo, J. (2013). Mindfulness-based mobile applications: Literature review and analysis of current features. *JMIR Mhealth Uhealth*, *1*(2), e24. doi:10.2196/mhealth.2733 PMID:25099314

Powell, J., Hamborg, T., Stallard, N., Burls, A., McSorley, J., Bennett, K., & Christensen, H. et al. (2013). Effectiveness of a web-based cognitive-behavioral tool to improve mental well-being in the general population: Randomized controlled trial. *Journal of Medical Internet Research*, *15*(1). PMID:23302475

Preziosa, A., Grassi, A., Gaggioli, A., & Riva, G. (2009). Therapeutic applications of the mobile phone. *British Journal of Guidance & Counselling*, *37*(3), 313–325. doi:10.1080/03069880902957031

Proudfoot, J., Ryden, C., Everitt, B., Shapiro, D. A., Goldberg, D., Mann, A., & Gray, J. A. et al. (2004). Clinical efficacy of computerised cognitive–behavioural therapy for anxiety and depression in primary care: Randomised controlled trial. *The British Journal of Psychiatry*, *185*(1), 46–54. doi:10.1192/bjp.185.1.46 PMID:15231555

Raspelli, S., Pallavicini, F., Carelli, L., Morganti, F., Pedroli, E., Cipresso, P., & Silani, V. et al. (2012). Validating the neuro VR-based virtual version of the multiple errands test: Preliminary results. *Presence (Cambridge, Mass.), 21*(1), 31–42. doi:10.1162/PRES_a_00077

Repetto, C., Gaggioli, A., Pallavicini, F., Cipresso, P., Raspelli, S., & Riva, G. (2013). Virtual reality and mobile phones in the treatment of generalized anxiety disorders: A phase-2 clinical trial. *Personal and Ubiquitous Computing*, *17*(2), 253–260. doi:10.1007/s00779-011-0467-0

Riva, G. (2009a). Interreality: A new paradigm for E-health. *Studies in Health Technology and Informatics*, *144*, 3–7. PMID:19592718

Riva, G. (2009b). Virtual reality: An experiential tool for clinical psychology. *British Journal of Guidance & Counselling*, *37*(3), 337–345. doi:10.1080/03069880902957056

Riva, G., Banos, R. M., Botella, C., Wiederhold, B. K., & Gaggioli, A. (2012). Positive technology: Using interactive technologies to promote positive functioning. *Cyberpsychology, Behavior, and Social Networking*, *15*(2), 69–77. doi:10.1089/cyber.2011.0139 PMID:22149077

Riva, G., Mantovani, F., Capideville, C. S., Preziosa, A., Morganti, F., Villani, D., & Alcañiz, M. et al. (2007). Affective interactions using virtual reality: The link between presence and emotions. *Cyberpsychology & Behavior*, *10*(1), 45–56. doi:10.1089/cpb.2006.9993 PMID:17305448

Riva, G., Vigna, C., Grassi, A., Raspelli, S., Cipresso, P., Pallavicini, F.,... Gaggioli, A. (2012). Learning Island: the development of a virtual reality system for the experiential training of stress management. *Paper presented at the MMVR.*

Roemer, L., & Orsillo, S. M. (2002). Expanding our conceptualization of and treatment for generalized anxiety disorder: Integrating mindfulness/acceptance-based approaches with existing cognitive-behavioral models. *Clinical Psychology: Science and Practice*, *9*(1), 54–68. doi:10.1093/clipsy.9.1.54

Rozanski, A., Blumenthal, J. A., & Kaplan, J. (1999). Impact of psychological factors on the pathogenesis of cardiovascular disease and implications for therapy. *Circulation*, *99*(16), 2192–2217. doi:10.1161/01.CIR.99.16.2192 PMID:10217662

Scherer, K. R. (2001). Appraisal considered as a process of multilevel sequential checking. In K.R. Scherer, A. Schorr, & T. Johnstone (Eds.), *Appraisal processes in emotion: Theory, methods, research* (pp. 92-120). Oxford: Oxford University Press.

Schultz, J. H., & Luthe, W. (1969). *Autogenic therapy: Autogenic methods*. New York: Grune & Stratton.

Sedlmeier, P., Eberth, J., Schwarz, M., Zimmermann, D., Haarig, F., Jaeger, S., & Kunze, S. (2012). The psychological effects of meditation: A meta-analysis. *Psychological Bulletin, 138*(6), 1139–1171. doi:10.1037/a0028168 PMID:22582738

Seeman, T. E., Singer, B. H., Rowe, J. W., Horwitz, R. I., & McEwen, B. S. (1997). Price of adaptation—allostatic load and its health consequences: MacArthur studies of successful aging. *Archives of Internal Medicine*, *157*(19), 2259–2268. doi:10.1001/archinte.1997.00440400111013 PMID:9343003

Seligman, M. E., & Csikszentmihalyi, M. (2000). Positive psychology: An introduction. *American Psychological Association, 55*(1), 5-14.

Selye, H. (1956). *The stress of life*. New York, NY, US: McGraw-Hill.

Serino, S., Cipresso, P., Gaggioli, A., & Riva, G. (2013). *The potential of pervasive sensors and computing for positive technology: the interreality paradigm Pervasive and Mobile Sensing and Computing for Healthcare* (pp. 207–232). Springer.

Serino, S., Cipresso, P., Tartarisco, G., Baldus, G., Corda, D., Pioggia, G.,... Riva, G. (2012). An Event-Driven Psychophysiological Assessment for Health Care. *Paper presented at the 2nd International Workshop on Computing Paradigms for Mental Health.*

Serino, S., Cipresso, P., Tartarisco, G., Baldus, G., Corda, D., Pioggia, G., & Riva, G. et al. (2013). Computerized experience-sampling approach for real-time assessment of stress. *EAI Endorsed Transactions, 13*(1-6), e5.

Serino, S., Triberti, S., Villani, D., Cipresso, P., Gaggioli, A., & Riva, G. (2014). Toward a validation of cyber-interventions for stress disorders based on stress inoculation training: A systematic review. *Virtual Reality (Waltham Cross), 18*(1), 73–87. doi:10.1007/s10055-013-0237-6

Shapiro, D. H. Jr. (2008). *Meditation: Self-regulation strategy and altered state of consciousness*. Transaction Publishers.

Shapiro, S. L., Schwartz, G. E., & Bonner, G. (1998). Effects of mindfulness-based stress reduction on medical and premedical students. *Journal of Behavioral Medicine, 21*(6), 581–599. doi:10.1023/A:1018700829825 PMID:9891256

Sheldon, K. M., & King, L. (2001). Why positive psychology is necessary. *The American Psychologist, 56*(3), 216–217. doi:10.1037/0003-066X.56.3.216 PMID:11315247

Shonin, E., Van Gordon, W., & Griffiths, M. D. (2013). Mindfulness-based interventions: Towards mindful clinical integration. *Frontiers in Psychology*, 2013(4). PMID:23616779

Stetz, M. C., Thomas, M. L., Russo, M. B., Stetz, T. A., Wildzunas, R. M., McDonald, J. J., & Romano, J. A. et al. (2007). Stress, mental health, and cognition: A brief review of relationships and countermeasures. *Aviation, Space, and Environmental Medicine*, *78*(Suppl. 1), B252–B260. PMID:17547326

Stone, A., Shiffman, S., Atienza, A., & Nebeling, L. (2007). *The science of real-time data capture: Self-reports in health research.* New York: Oxford University Press.

Stone, A. A., Schwartz, J. E., Schkade, D., Schwarz, N., Krueger, A., & Kahneman, D. (2006). A population approach to the study of emotion: diurnal rhythms of a working day examined with the Day Reconstruction Method. *Emotion, 6*(1), 139-149. doi:2006-04603-013 [pii]10.1037/1528-3542.6.1.139

Strümpfer, D. (1995). The origins of health and strength: From 'salutogenesis' to 'fortigenesis'. *South African Journal of Psychology. Suid-Afrikaanse Tydskrif vir Sielkunde, 25*(2), 81–89. doi:10.1177/008124639502500203

Sun, Y., Chan, K. L., & Krishnan, S. M. (2002). ECG signal conditioning by morphological filtering. *Computers in Biology and Medicine, 32*(6), 465–479. doi:10.1016/S0010-4825(02)00034-3 PMID:12356496

Thayer, J. F., Ahs, F., Fredrikson, M., Sollers, J. J. III, & Wager, T. D. (2012). A meta-analysis of heart rate variability and neuroimaging studies: Implications for heart rate variability as a marker of stress and health. *Neuroscience and Biobehavioral Reviews, 36*(2), 747–756. doi:10.1016/j.neubiorev.2011.11.009 PMID:22178086

Thomee, S., Harenstam, A., & Hagberg, M. (2011). Mobile phone use and stress, sleep disturbances, and symptoms of depression among young adults--a prospective cohort study. *BMC Public Health, 11*(1), 66. doi:10.1186/1471-2458-11-66 PMID:21281471

Valtchanov, D., Barton, K. R., & Ellard, C. (2010). Restorative effects of virtual nature settings. *Cyberpsychology, Behavior, and Social Networking, 13*(5), 503–512. doi:10.1089/cyber.2009.0308 PMID:20950174

Velten, E. Jr. (1968). A laboratory task for induction of mood states. *Behaviour Research and Therapy, 6*(4), 473–482. doi:10.1016/0005-7967(68)90028-4 PMID:5714990

Villani, D., Cipresso, P., & Repetto, C. (2014). Coping with Stress and Anxiety: the Role of Presence in Technology Mediated Environments. In G. Riva, J. A. Waterworth, & D. Murray (Eds.), Interacting with Presence: HCI and the Sense of Presence in Computer-mediated Environments (p. 139). Berlin: De Gruyter Open. Retrieved from www.presence-research. com

Villani, D., Grassi, A., Cognetta, C., Toniolo, D., Cipresso, P., & Riva, G. (2013). Self-help stress management training through mobile phones: An experience with oncology nurses. *Psychological Services, 10*(3), 315–322. doi:10.1037/a0026459 PMID:23937091

Villani, D., Repetto, C., Cipresso, P., & Riva, G. (2012). May I experience more presence in doing the same thing in virtual reality than in reality? An answer from a simulated job interview. *Interacting with Computers, 24*(4), 265–272. doi:10.1016/j.intcom.2012.04.008

Villani, D., Riva, F., & Riva, G. (2007). New technologies for relaxation: The role of presence. *International Journal of Stress Management, 14*(3), 260–274. doi:10.1037/1072-5245.14.3.260

Villani, D., & Riva, G. (2012). Does interactive media enhance the management of stress? Suggestions from a controlled study. *Cyberpsychology, Behavior, and Social Networking, 15*(1), 24–30. doi:10.1089/cyber.2011.0141 PMID:22032797

Warnecke, E., Quinn, S., Ogden, K., Towle, N., & Nelson, M. R. (2011). A randomised controlled trial of the effects of mindfulness practice on medical student stress levels. *Medical Education, 45*(4), 381–388. doi:10.1111/j.1365-2923.2010.03877.x PMID:21401686

Wiederhold, B. K., & Wiederhold, M. D. (2006). From stress inoculation training to posttraumatic stress disorder: developing a continuum of care for the warfighter. *Paper presented at the CyberPsychology & Behavior.*

Zetterqvist, K., Maanmies, J., Ström, L., & Andersson, G. (2003). Randomized controlled trial of internet-based stress management. *Cognitive Behaviour Therapy, 32*(3), 151–160. doi:10.1080/16506070302316 PMID:16291546

## KEY TERMS AND DEFINITIONS

**Biofeedback:** A technique people can use to learn to control their body's functions. With biofeedback, people are connected to electrical sensors that help them receive information (feedback) about their body (bio). In essence, biofeedback helps them focus on making subtle changes in their body; it is often used as a relaxation technique.

**Mindfulness:** A type of meditative technique that emphasizes an observant and nonreactive stance toward one's thoughts, emotions and body states. It involves purposeful attention to daily activities.

**Physiological Signals:** The body generates physiological signals during the functioning of various physiological systems. Hence, physiological signals hold information that can be extracted from these signals to find out the state of the functioning of these physiological systems.

**Relaxation:** Relaxation training can include several strategies that help a person to relax. Relaxation techniques are often employed as one element of a wider stress management program and can decrease muscle tension, lower blood pressure and slow heart and breath rates, among other health benefits.

**Stress Inoculation Training:** Developed by Meichenbaum in the 1960s, SIT is a form of cognitive restructuring. It is a method of changing an individual's thinking patterns about themselves and their lives. It is based on the assumption that people experience stress because they interpret an event or situation in catastrophising ways and their internal dialogue (their thoughts) are negative.

# Chapter 15
# Using the Experience of Evoked Emotion in Virtual Reality to Manage Workplace Stress:
## Affective Control Theory (ACT)

**Jennifer G. Tichon**
*Griffith University, Australia*

**Timothy Mavin**
*Griffith University, Australia*

## ABSTRACT

*This chapter explores how immersion in virtual reality (VR) evokes emotional states similar to those of the real world, and how deliberate immersion in high-stress situations can help teach individuals affective strategies to remain in control of their emotions. Psychological skills training programs teach techniques and strategies to assess, monitor, and adjust thoughts and feelings to cope with stress. VR allows an individual to put these skills to the test through the opportunity to practice coping with their emotional states while immersed in difficult scenarios. Keeping a clear head, ignoring fear when fear isn't useful, learning how to draw on an optimal blend of emotion and reason in times of crisis are all crucial skills for work and life. Affective Control Theory (ACT) proposes that affective strategies that typically strengthen and support performance are skills and that these skills are integral to stress management. Due to its key role in performance, recent research in psychology confirms affect as a crucial variable to consider in interventions in workplace stress.*

## INTRODUCTION

Research identifying the psychological and affective impact of immersion in virtual reality (VR) has enabled a shift from an emphasis on quality of image or graphic perfection to investigations of the emotional experience of the user. As a result, the emotional states that can be evoked in VR are making valuable contributions to stress-management research and training across many domains. In therapeutic settings,

DOI: 10.4018/978-1-4666-9986-1.ch015

VR-based stress-management programs for people with mood disorders such as generalized anxiety disorder typically involve immersion in scenarios that are designed to evoke a positive mood (Dayang, Awang, Suziah, & Halabt, 2011; Riva et al., 2012). Using VR scenarios that induce positive visual and auditory stimulation, the therapist will combine a relaxing narrative with strategies to practice relaxation and cognitive reframing techniques to help the client cope with general stressful situations. Individuals who interact in these environments have reported significantly lowered subjective stress, depression, and anxiety (Shah et al., 2015). In terms of workplace stress, however, stress-invoking experiences are far more content specific than they are for individuals with a mood disorder. VR has been used successfully for many years to prepare personnel to work under high-stress conditions by recreating the emotional experience of coping with worst-case scenarios.

There are clearly many advantages to using VR to teach individuals ways to improve their affective strategies in order to cope with stress in the workplace. For the majority of individuals, physical symptoms of anxiety or stress can result in a range of physical symptoms, such as faster breathing, higher blood pressure, and nausea, which ultimately can interfere with their performance at work. Although the emotions associated with stress are natural—and can at times be motivational and even help people to perform under pressure—they cannot be allowed to manifest to the extent that they interfere with and reduce a person's effectiveness. No matter how difficult or unprecedented the problem, a highly trained professional needs to have the ability to look past emotions and carefully think about the best way to proceed (Lehrer, 2009).

In aviation, pilots have long been taught to practice staying calm (Lehrer, 2009). They are able to do this through the opportunity that VR provides to practice building confidence. Examples of aviation incidents where training in VR environments has come to the fore include United Airlines flight 232, a flight originating from Denver destined for Chicago that suffered a catastrophic center engine failure during flight (the DC-10 aircraft had three engines—two wing-mounted engines and a center engine fixed to the tail). While such a failure would ordinarily be something with which a normal crew would be able to deal, and for which they would have trained, the fact that engine fragments cut essential flight control systems during the disintegration resulted in a high-stress situation. It was only through the actions of the pilots that the aircraft staggered to an emergency landing: "Their actions saved the lives of 185 crew members and passengers" (Salas, Shuffler, & DiazGranados, 2010: 252). More recently, an A320 aircraft departing from New York's LaGuardia Airport decided to ditch in the Hudson River due to bird strikes in both engines. The actions of Captain Sullenberger saved the lives of all those on board. Sullenberger stated after the accident, "It's what we're trained to do" (2010: 250).

Immersion in VR environments that replicate real-world stress has been used for many years to train a range of professionals to control and use their emotions to facilitate their optimal performance. The underlying premise of VR stress training is that a professional's confidence can be strengthened through exposures that provide the opportunity to experience mastery and control under high-stress conditions. However, while reinforcing important professional skills, VR environments also allow trainees to practice something equally important: how to draw on an optimal blend of reason and emotion. Scenarios are designed to allow them to work through fear and successfully translate it into effective performance. They learn how to ignore their fear when fear isn't useful. Indications from VR research are that, through repeated exposure, individuals develop a skill set to control their emotions —best described as affective skills—that they become aware of within themselves and are able to bring to bear to achieve high-demand tasks under stress.

## AFFECTIVE STRATEGIES THAT SUPPORT PERFORMANCE UNDER STRESS

During any difficult task—such as those faced by military personnel in combat situations—controlling emotions and retaining active cognition are not only important, but can be critical to a successful outcome. Clear thinking that supports objective judgment and strong decision making will lead to the optimal outcome for both the overall mission and individual personnel. Clear thinking unclouded by emotions is crucial across all professions and multiple workplaces. The military has therefore long been concerned with identifying strategies that personnel can use to control their affective responses. If they are not controlled, the emotions associated with stress—such as fear, anger and anxiety—can reduce cognition, interfering directly in the prefrontal processes (Russo et al., 2005). Controlling emotion is not something that is easy to predict, as individual differences vary considerably. However, research does suggest that experience plays an important part in emotional control (Tichon, et al., 2014). There has been a considerable amount of research investigating stress in the workplace, with the number of studies increasing over the last 40 years. More specifically, there has been escalating interest in research focusing on *affect* and its impact on performance— both novice and expert (e.g. see Chi, Glaser, & Farr, 1988; Ericsson, Charness, Feltovich, & Hoffman, 2006; Loft et al. 2009). The study into novice versus expert differences has been the focus of attention in both the educational and psychological fields. A key area of concern has been the identification of the methods used to develop expertise to aid in training design. Theoretically, being able identify the fundamental principles, and varying perspectives and mechanisms, of expertise allows for broader theories to be developed, thus allowing for generalizability studies to be conducted in varying professions (Loft, Bolland, Humphreys, & Neal, 2009) such as comparing how an airline captain or surgeon develops expertise.

While studies of expertise that investigate the role of affect have recognized its central role in determining performance outcomes, most work has looked at the *impact* of affect on performance, rather than how affective state and the strategies used to control affective state impact performance. For example, studies have examined the influence on affective states of goal striving during performance (Foo, Uy, & Baron 2009; Koestner, Lekes, Powers, & Chicoine, 2002; Louro, Pieters, & Zeelenberg, 2007). However, this does not answer the questions of how affect impacts an individual's ability to set and achieve goals. Studies have already confirmed that during short-term exercises of approximately two-minutes, an individual's overall performance had a positive correlation with their affective state at the end of the activity (Ballard, 2009). It has been shown in studies underpinned by reinforcement sensitivity theory, that individual performance has the strongest influence on both energetic and tense emotional arousal (Gray, 1990). In control theory, predictions are made of how performance will affect an individual's affective state (see Seo, Barrett, & Bartunek, 2004). When a person experiences an activated affective state—for example, when an airline pilot sees an emergency alert—it is increasingly likely that the individual will increase their effort in order to diagnose and solve a problem.

To summarize these theories, as an individual performs poorly or well, there is a negative or positive correlation respectively—that is, if an individual performs well, there is a corresponding positive experience in affect, such as happiness. Yet, by only focusing on affect as an outcome, theories do not investigate how experts, or more importantly novices (as they are shown to be influenced more), can control their emotions and overall affective state to achieve a stressful task in the workplace setting. For instance, while studying how performance influences affect, Ballard (2009) also investigated how affect shaped goal striving:

*[W]hen an individual is setting a goal, feelings such as alertness or brightness can lead them to engage further and set a more difficult goal. On the other hand, feelings of anxiety or stress can lead them to avoid difficulty by setting a goal that is easier to attain. However, this process changes during goal striving, because once the individual has committed to a goal, the goal becomes more difficult to change. As such when an individual is striving toward their goal, they may respond to feelings of anxiety or stress by increasing their effort in order to regain their progress toward the goal. Ballard (2009: 47)*

Studies consistently show an intricate relationship between the ability to achieve goals and emotional state. As already suggested, and supported by the literature, affect is an outcome of goal performance (e.g. Pekrun, Elliot, & Maier, 2006) and can influence goal pursuit (e.g. Elliot and Thrash, 2002).

Over the years, numerous conceptual and theoretical models have been developed to try to explain the relationship between affect, goal setting and performance (e.g. Linnenbrink & Pintrich, 2002; Pekrun et al., 2006). For instance, one model referred to as a "sequential model" shows how early affective experiences predict goal setting, how goals are able to predetermine individual emotions, and how individual emotions are able to determine achievement (Daniels et al., 2009: 954). For example, constructs such as helplessness or hopefulness that occur early in a task can be related to constructs that occur later in a task, such as anxiety or enjoyment. Furthermore, the model shows how all emotions experienced throughout a task are, to some extent, partially mediated by constructs like expertise, or mastery.

The compensatory control model (Hockey, 1997, 2005) suggests an interreliant relationship between affective and physiological responses, and maintains that these are inherent in the regulatory process. For instance, anxiety can be explained as an output of an individual's action monitor. Here, affect (anxiety) is an outcome of an individual making judgments that goals within a work task are currently not being met. When the model is used to predict performance under high workload or other stressful situations, the model asserts that *positive affect* will decrease under increasing stress. In this model, there is no firm prediction about negative affect under high task demands; however, it suggests that negative emotions are more likely to increase. Thus an individual's adoption of an approach or avoidance orientation may influence the expected affective output of performance goal striving (Fletcher, 2010).

Drawbacks of the models outlined above are that the boundaries imposed by the models themselves are somewhat limiting. They do not entirely explain the totality of possible relationships among affect, goal setting and performance. On the other hand, Affective Control Theory (ACT) may actually provide a new direction.

## AFFECTIVE CONTROL THEORY

ACT theory conceptualizes "affect in mental workload models, models of goal achievement, and goal striving to examining affect in terms of what this variable brings to the relationship between individual appraisal of workload and ultimate achievement of goals" (Tichon, Watson, & Wallis, 2011: 8). Being able to conceptualize affect as a skill, rather than simply as an output construct, may provide a model that not only enables workplaces to predict the affective impact of certain tasks, but also helps them to guide training development for these tasks. Furthermore, being able to measure the affective strategies an individual has developed, both through training and prior experience, will support the prediction of a professional's likelihood of successful performance, helping to identify whether further training is required prior to the task being undertaken. Such measures will assist to reduce stress levels for personnel working under stress (Tichon, Wallis, & Reik, 2010).

Just over 20 years ago, neuroscience convincingly showed interdependence between emotions and activities (Damasio, 1995), demonstrating that emotions are essential for successful performance. Prior to Damasio (1995), it was assumed that performance only required rational thought. In Lazarus's (1966) transactional model of stress, individuals evaluate their own affective resources to cope, along with the actual task itself. Here it could be said that professionals must be able to accurately evaluate emotional resources in addition to the skills required for task completion. So, while the field of psychology continues to investigate affect, limited attention has been paid to affect as a predetermination of performance, how individuals accurately perceive their own affective skills, and how we may go about improving affect as a skill. A model is needed that conceptualizes affect in terms of the degree to which emotion can be used by personnel to ensure a task is successfully completed when working under stress.

In parallel with the development of research on the concept of affect as mainly an output of effort, training via exposure to stress in VR has deliberately been devised to prepare professionals for stressful work situations through focusing on the control and use of emotions. This approach to emotion as an input to effort rather than a final outcome underpins VR training to develop skills in order to effectively control emotions as a way of improving individual work performance. In order for the strengths of affect to provide more applicable training and increase the likelihood of success in working effectively under stress to be best applied in VR, theoretical models must include the role of emotion in preparing for and reacting to work requirements. Training using VR has the aim of strengthening an individual's confidence in their affective skills through providing the opportunity to experience success while working under stress. Yet there seems to be no theoretical modeling to assist in the development of improved training strategies for such approaches.

Some of the approaches proposed by ACT suggest that, in order to strengthen and support performance, affect skills training is integral not only to technical skills, but also to non-technical skills (NTS). For example, in aviation the realization that NTS are fundamental to performance only resulted from investigations into a large number of accidents occurring in the late 1980s and early 1990s. These studies recognized that mere technical proficiency was not a causal factor in many aviation accidents. NTS such as situation awareness (see Endsley, 1988, 1994, 1998), decision-making (Klein 2008), management, teamwork and communication (Flin & Martin, 2001; Flin & Maran, 2004) were fundamental for good team performance. More recently, the separation of technical from non-technical skills has been questioned. Rather than seeing a division, models have been developed that attempt to integrate technical or non-technical skills into relational models rather than reductionist skill sets (Mavin & Dall'Alba, 2010; Mavin & Roth, 2014). If models of performance in aviation are now moving toward the integration of technical and non-technical skills, is it not feasible that affective skills should also be included within such modeling?

The existence of affective skills has long been supported strongly by scientific findings in fields of inquiry such as sports psychology, where "affective intelligence" is the term used to describe the ability to remain emotionally in control during performance. In professional sport, it has been recognized that affective intelligence is not only important, but can be measured as "mental toughness" in athletes. In sport, affective intelligence acknowledges that ideal performance is reliant on an athlete's ability to control emotions, irrespective of obstacles encountered (Connaughton, Wadey, Hanton, & Jones, 2008;

Gucciardi & Gordon, 2009, 2010) and that emotions can deliberately be wielded as a tool to inspire someone to greater performance.

There has been some research demonstrating that an individual's motivation to achieve can only be influenced positively by emotions. Here it is perceived that motivation only occurs under "positive" conditions. Therefore, it is proposed that experiences that are positive facilitate the retrieval of positive self- and task-related information. On the other hand, experiences perceived as "negative" facilitate retrieval of negative self- and task-related information (Daniels et al. 2009; Linnenbrink & Pintrich, 2002). Conversely, unpleasant states have a motivating influence during goal striving, as they lead individuals to mobilize effort (Ballard 2009). Furthermore, individual differences do exist with regard to the evaluation of how negative an experience needs to feel before it will cause a person to lose the motivation to complete their work. The goal of VR stress training for workplaces is to gradually expose individuals to increasing levels of stress until they are able to tolerate significantly higher levels of stress before they quit. The goal of VR exposure to stress is to provide the opportunity, through repetition, for individuals to prove to themselves that they do not need to quit a specific scenario but can continue to work successfully by using their own emotional skills to support their performance.

The ACT ability to conceptualize affect as a skill may play a pivotal role in supporting and improving workplace performance, as it recognizes the role of affect in supporting and strengthening technical skills and NTS. If an individual is unable to control anxiety and fear, this will inevitably degrade their performance, both at the technical and NTS levels. It is proposed that ACT may provide a model that can predict the effect of different affective states and their level of intensity on cognitive processing during the stress of working under high task demands.

The range of impacts that ACT can have in the workplace should not be overlooked. A model that helps to understand the causal relationship between affect, cognition, and performance supports further predictions of the overall emotional readiness of an individual to complete required tasks. If decrements are identified, training in affective skills can be undertaken to closely align their affective strategies to the specific requirements of the task. VR training that enables the replication of the emotional cost of task performance allows the opportunity to more closely align workplace training programs to address the alignment of cognitive and affective reserves with successful performance.

## MEASURING AFFECT

In evaluating the effectiveness of VR training on the development and enhancement of cognitive skills, like situational assessment and decision-making, affective state has become a key area of interest (Tichon, 2010). Yet, as has been the experience in aviation, the assessment of NTS remains challenging. Examples include the difficulty pilots of rank have agreeing on performance assessment measures—an area often referred to as interrater reliability (Mavin, Roth, & Dekker, 2013; Roth & Mavin, 2014), and on how technical and NTS skills should be integrated into training (Mavin, Roth, & Munro, in press). Studies investigating affect/emotion and performance are characterized by one major limitation: the research is currently limited by a need to rely entirely on subjective self-report instruments. Even though technical performance is currently measured using more objective measures, affect and its measurement still rely on combining subjective with objective measures as a way of determining the probable affective states present in what is a very individual experience.

## Subjective Measures

Subjective measures are particularly useful as a means to assess person-environment "fit" based on direct subjective report of stressful experience. However, great caution should be exercised in using subjective self-report measures to assess stress in other domains and purposes. For example, if a researcher is interested in evaluating stress produced by a particular situation, subjective measures may be misleading. An environment perceived as stressful by one individual may not be perceived as stressful to another. (Redden, Sheehy, & Bjorkman, 2004: 554)

Self-reports are generally easier to administer and score than the physiological measures outlined next. They also allow individual assessment, and are relatively inexpensive on a per subject basis.

The Multiple Affect Adjective Checklist (MAACL-R) is a general measure of emotional states that has been used extensively in the investigation of the impact of stress on psychological functioning (Hunsley, 1990) and is currently in use in VR and simulator training evaluations. In studies of acute stress, the Army Research Laboratory (ARL) has found that the Multiple Affect Adjective Checklist–Revised (MACCL–R) reveals temporary stress effects such as anxiety, depression, and hostility. The checklist consists of 132 adjectives that comprise five primary subscales (anxiety, depression, hostility, positive affect, and sensation seeking). The checklist can be completed in approximately five minutes (Redden et al., 2004). The drawback of the scale is that it more easily achieves independence between positive and negative affect rather than between two dimensions of negative affect; however, the items provide a starting point from which to further explore the impact of VR training on individual affective states. Self-report measures can be used in conjunction with one or more of the psycho-physiological measures outlined below.

## Objective Measures

Physiologists demonstrate that high stress levels are accompanied by the symptoms of faster heartbeat, rapid breathing, increased sweating, cool skin, feelings of nausea, tense muscles, and so on (Liao, Zhang, Zhu, Ji, & Gray, 2006). In the past, the military has preferred objective measures for stress. To date, available simple measures have included salivary amylase and salivary cortisol tests. Both are quick, non-intrusive, and inexpensive ways to predict plasma catecholamine levels (e.g. norepinephrine) normally produced under stressful conditions (Chatterton, Vogelsong, Lu, Ellman, & Hudgens, 1996). For instance, the Army Research Laboratory's salivary amylase collection protocol is simple and easy enough to manage in an active field setting (Blewett et al., 1994). Heart rate and blood pressure readings, useful in monitoring stress levels, are again simple to measure using widely available, over-the-counter devices (Redden et al., 2004: 553). As would be expected in battlefield conditions, the military prefers easy to use, light, and non-obtrusive equipment that enables quick measures to be obtained, thus making each of these measures easy to use in a variety of workplaces.

VR provides expanded measurement opportunities. In replicating high-stress work environments and associated work tasks, both safely and realistically, VR also provides the opportunity to use more advanced measures of affective state and levels of intensity. To date, the range of psycho-physiological measures proposed to capture affect include electroencephalography (EEG), cardiac changes (heart rate, blood pressure), ocular events (number and duration of eye blinks), changes in skin response, muscle activity (electromyography, or EMG), and respiration (Redden et al. 2004; Tichon, Wallis, & Reik, 2010). Additionally, an increasing amount of research is investigating behavioral data in the form of facial expressions with or without head movement. These measures may afford increasingly accurate representation of affective state, and therefore are better alternatives to self-report questionnaires, which are subject to bias and require participants to be interrupted during their VR training experience (Reynolds & Picard, 2005; Ahn, Bailenson, Fox, & Jabon, 2009). The application of some of these measures is discussed next.

## Feature Extraction

Feature extraction as an objective measurement tool for recognizing, tracking, and measuring affect and its associated intensity levels has been increasingly investigated as an objective measurement alternative in this field (Bailenson et al., 2008; Liao et al., 2006). It has been determined that observing facial expressions is a significant way to judge a person's affective state (Asthana, Saragih, Wagner, & Goecke, 2009). For instance, raised eyebrows in addition to drawing eyes together and/or stretching lips horizontally to form a rectangular mouth shape can be a sign of fear. Extreme fear can be recognized by raised, tensed upper eyelids that act to widen the eyes (Harrigan & O'Connell, 1996).

Facial recognition uses a bottom-up approach to correlate facial movement with a particular output, such as an emotion or even a behavior. While early research investigated methods for classifying affective states, more recently interest has focused on how affective states may be predicted. For instance, researchers have investigated monitoring affect/emotion as a method of predicting whether a consumer is more or less likely to buy a product and predicting whether a driver will be involved in an accident (Ahn et al., 2009).

Specifically, stress is a variable of interest. Investigations reveal that facial features are highly sensitive to stress, and therefore provide a robust measure of stress (Liao et al., 2006). However, methods that combine facial tracking with other physiological measures concurrently have been proven to be more reliable then single cues alone (Bailenson et al., 2008). Bailenson et al. (2008) developed a model to train coders in assessing and recording changes in facial features. By providing videotapes of subjects' faces, coders were asked to analyze short segments—second by second—to assess sadness or amusement. The results were combined with physiological measurements, including cardiovascular, somatic, and electrodermal responses; all combined to predict emotion. A learning algorithm was then developed to link facial anchor points, as determined by NEVEN vision, which recognizes 53 individual facial features, and physiological responses to the emotional responses rated by the coders. From these data sources, the researchers developed an accurate model of how emotions were expressed in response to the stimuli under study.

Work by El Kaliouby and Robinson (2005) advanced general computational models for facial affect inference, and has been implemented as a real-time system. This approach uses dynamic Bayesian networks that are able to recognize six different classes of complex emotions. Results show that increased reliability occurs where human emotion, measured by facial expression, was analyzed historically over a longer period—although this could be as short as two seconds—rather than attempting to assess affective state during one instant in time. The system was designed to classify emotional states as opposed to emotional intensity. Facial expression recognition is a bottom-up approach in which the correlation between facial movement and the resulting output (an emotion) forms the basis for establishing both a classification and a prediction model (Tichon, Wallis, & Reik, 2010).

In summary, while several studies link feature extraction and emotion, this research has been limited by relying on human subjective coders and the use of passive non-interactive movies to evoke emotion in participants (Bailenson et al., 2008). Immersion in replicated high-stress VR environments provides a far superior research opportunity for progressing investigation into feature extraction and its correlation with affective states.

## Electromyography (EMG)

EMG activity has been reported as a reliable and objective measure of emotion. Yoshie, Kudo and Ohtsuki (2008) investigated the relationship between the negative affect associated with stress and the electromyographic (EMG) activity that occurs during a professional pianist performance. It was shown that agonist as well as antagonist muscle activity increases during performance. This co-contraction of muscles revealed itself as an increase in joint stiffness both during and after performance. The investigation also concluded that the increase in muscle activity also occurred with more force, which often resulted in further observable and recognizable patterns of motor performance (Yoshie et al., 2008).

During a driving task undertaken in a VR scenario, Tichon and colleagues (2011) recorded EMG data at 1000Hz using surface electrodes feeding into a National Instruments analogue recorder controlled by a LabView program running on a central PC (Control PC). Eight synchronous analogue recording channels were available. The muscular contraction associated with anxiety was measured using EMG of the following muscles: jaw clenching (masseter), shoulder tension muscles (upper trapezius), wrist flexing (flexor carpi radialis), calf tension (lateral gastocnemius), and thigh tension (vastus lateralis). Muscle activation patterns of participants revealed an increase in activity associated with anxiety, primarily in the muscles of the leg, with the level of activation increasing by up to 50% above the non-anxious state. Similar patterns were observed through greater amounts of muscle contraction in the jaw, shoulder, and wrist, as well as the thigh and calf muscles, in participants who reported experiencing higher anxiety states during VR immersion.

## Pupilometry

Previous research has identified a number of parameters relating to the eyes and their movement that are influenced by affective state and specifically state anxiety. Blinks, saccades and pupil dilation have all been reported as varying systematically with manipulations to stress or measured anxiety levels. Chapman, Oka, Bradshaw, Jacobson, and Donaldson (1999) conditioned subjects to expect an electrical shock to their fingertip, producing raised levels of anxiety and stress. During periods shortly before a shock, the team recorded increases in the cycling of pupil size (that is, variability in pupil size over time), which they attributed to a rise in anxiety levels. Partla and Surakka (2003) exposed subjects to images designed to produce positive or negative arousal, and reported changes in the maximum, short-term pupil dilatory response, which they termed PSV (pupil size variation). Some tentative links between eye movement and affective state have also been reported for subjects observing static faces portraying a range of emotional expressions. (Susskind et al. 2008). In particular, the authors report increases in peak saccade velocity in response to fearful expressions. Perhaps one of the more widely investigated measures is blink rate. The general consensus is that blinking increases as anxiety levels increase (e.g. Harrigan & O'Connell, 1996); however, the opposite result has also been reported (Liao et al., 2006).

In a study on trainee pilots who were in the early stages of their training, eye movement and pupil size data were recorded using an SR Research EyeLink II head-mounted tracker (Tichon, Mavin, Wallis, Visser, & Riek, 2014). Data collected in real time by the eye-tracker included relative pupil size, eye position, and movement velocity; however, final data also included some derived "events": blinks, fixations, and saccadic movements that were calculated by the eye-tracker host before transferring the results to the final data file. Results of this experimental set-up revealed that fixation duration and saccade rate (total number of saccades during trials in which anxiety was reported) were found to correspond reliably to pilot self-reports of anxiety. Decreases in positive affect also correlated significantly with saccade rate, fixation duration, and mean saccade velocity (average velocity of saccades during trials in which anxiety was reported). Pupil size and saccade amplitude (average amplitude of saccades during trials in which anxiety was reported) did not show a strong comparison with changes in affective state (Tichon, Wallis, & Reik, 2010).

### Electroencephalogram (EEG)

New brain imaging technologies are opening the windows to new ways of looking at affective states (AlZoubi, Calvo, & Stevens, 2009). Some previous studies have used a combination of EEG and other physiological signals, while others have used EEG solely for affect detection. A recent study focusing on the automatic classification techniques that could be used for EEG data showed that accuracies well above the baseline are possible.

## TRAINING AFFECTIVE SKILLS

There are many advantages to being able to train a professional to improve their affective skills in any workplace context. Keeping a clear head when workload or work tasks are causing a significant increase in psychological stress is critical. Many professionals across a multitude of workplaces characterized by high stress, including the military, aviation, police, and accident-response teams face the expectation that they will continue to perform at a high standard. Training higher-order mental abilities for professionals now most often involves VR or computer-driven simulators. The advantage of VR and simulators—both of which have been in widespread use since the early 1980s—is that they allow trainees to practice both worst-case days and individual high-impact scenarios. While reinforcing important technical skills, simulators are also teaching trainees something more important: how to control and use their heightened emotional state to support and enhance both their cognition skills and resultant actions. They learn how to ignore their fear and how to make quick, complicated decisions under the most difficult conditions (Lehrer, 2009). Psychological skills training programs teach techniques and strategies used to assess, monitor, and adjust thoughts and feelings to produce mental states that enhance performance (Vealey, 2007; Gucciardi & Gordon, 2011). Immersion in VR provides the opportunity to put these skills to the test through practicing the completion of tasks while under stress.

In many professions, the most complicated decisions are often required due to unexpected and stressful events; however, no matter how difficult or unprecedented the problem, a highly trained professional has the ability to look past primal emotions and carefully think about how to proceed (Lehrer, 2009). The military reports that the overwhelming majority of combat personnel experience fear before and/or during battle despite training and experience. Often physical symptoms associated with fear—such as nausea and heart palpitations—are reported. Fear is natural, and often important to survival; however, it can't be allowed to manifest to the extent that it interferes with and reduces a professional's effectiveness (Redden et al., 2004). Research indicates that there is in fact a skill set—best described as affective skills—of which professionals are aware within themselves, and that they are able to bring to the fore to achieve high-demand goals. In aviation, pilots have long been taught to practice staying calm (Lehrer, 2009). They are able to do this through the opportunity VR provides to practice building confidence. The pivotal and essential role of affective skills in this workplace is demonstrated in the following quote resulting from an investigation into the decision-making capabilities of flight captains: "I've always believed that flying airplanes is nothing more than an exercise in self-confidence" (Mavin, 2010: 100).

## DISCUSSION

The field of affective computing is still in its infancy. This chapter has introduced a range of physiological measures that, based on prior research, could reasonably be expected to correlate with affective state. Prior literature reveals that there are relatively robust physiological measures that can be monitored during VR training to accurately reflect changes in affective states such as anxiety and stress. By combining standard measures such as blink rate with muscle activation and other eye and head movement data, an objective measure of an individual's affective state while practicing working through high stress in professional contexts is attainable. These combinations of measures can be drawn from commercially available eye-tracking and EMG equipment linked to provide synchronized data acquisition for affect-tracking purposes. The development of an objective measurement tool that formally brings together each of these physiological measures into a real-time affective state-monitoring device would provide an ideal approach to objective measurement of affective skill development for high-stress workplace requirements.

In exploring the relationship between emotion and workplace training in VR, it is apparent that existing theories have limits in terms of explaining the link between affect and performance. The relationship between these two variables does not seem to have been well explained within the context of affectively intense VR or simulator-based training settings. Overwhelmingly, to date, affect has been conceptualized in performance theory as a product of how difficult or dangerous a mission is. Yet training in VR to cope with workplace stress has been targeting the strengthening and control of affective skills to prepare professionals prior to them undertaking difficult high-stress tasks. VR has always been popular in terms of training professionals to "keep a clear head" in times of crisis. The very nature of immersion in VR to prepare personnel makes the case that a professional's affective state is not limited to being a by-product of their work demands. VR has focused on affect because it is acknowledged that intense affect as experienced during stress can negatively impact performance. It can cause overestimation of risks and avoidant choices, and also be a distraction when it provides information or motivation to attend to or act on emotional information at the expense of more important content (Peters, Lipkus, & Diefenbach, 2006). In elite sports, a professional who has developed strategies to control their emotions and to apply them purposefully to achieve optimal performance outcomes is described as being "mentally tough" (Gordon & Gucciardi, 2010; Gucciardi & Gordon, 2009).

A theoretical framework that supports the study of affect and personal strategies to control affect within the context of professional training to prepare for high-stress workplace conditions will assist in the investigation of such questions as: Can a level of "expert affective skill" at which best performance outcomes are achieved on target tasks be ascertained? Can the "expert affective skill" level be used as a benchmark against which a novice's affective performance can be measured to ascertain whether affective levels need to be increased or decreased to support best performance outcomes?

The design of training in VR to support individuals to work through and cope with workplace stress requires a theory that explains the skills and strategies developed as a result of practicing the control and use of emotion. In VR, specific objectives for training are identified, and specialized scripts with events that trigger or evoke specific emotions are developed. The trigger events are designed to elicit a specific affective response from a trainee. The instructor knows, for any given moment in a scenario, what workplace objectives are being trained, what trigger events are about to occur, and what behaviors for managing stress responses are critical to success (Bennett, Schreiber, & Andrews, 2002). Through conceptualizing affect control as an objective measureable professional skill, Affective Control Theory (ACT) fits well within VR training design. It can also be extended to provide a method of representing affective workload at the operational level, and could support the development of a predictive affective workload measure to support workplace operational planning. Predictions of task success can be modeled on the basis of an ability to assess the match between the overall affective requirements of a specific task with the individual affective skill levels of the personnel required to complete it. In practice, this would occur by comparing the individual affective skill level of professionals undertaking the task in a VR environment with predictions made for that same task using a workload prediction model. A number of workload prediction models have been developed, and are in use in assessing VR for workplace stress management training. Predictive workload measures use models that represent workload for the purpose of prediction. These generally analyze a task/workload based on multiple resource theory of human attention, resulting in estimates of the cognitive, psychomotor, affective, and sensory components of workload for each task (Gluck & Gunzelmann, 2013).

The ability to control affect in a manner that uses emotion to improve performance is a trainable skill. Affective skills are integral to success, as affect moderates human performance in ways that are sometimes difficult to predict. The positive or negative effects of a single affective event may depend on operational context, individual perception, or degree. For example, a small amount of fear might encourage a runner to run faster, but a large amount of fear might make them unable to run at all (Redden et al., 2004). The ACT model has significant potential to assist managerial, control, and command personnel to conduct overall workplace planning. For instance, a model of task workload that accounts for affective output (the affective costs of a particular high-stress task) will support the identification of situations in the workplace that will impose high affective task demands on personnel. When an operation has been identified as having high affective demand, the optimal affective level of expertise required of personnel to successfully complete the operation can be estimated. Ultimately, such a theoretical model that facilitates the mapping of affective requirements and cost with task demands could assist in predictions of overall success and in the planning of additional VR training requirements.

In summary, the Affective Skill Theory provides a new approach to comparing an individual's affective skill levels with the requirements of their professional workplace requirements. If the process highlights a mismatch between personnel affective resources and the affective skills or strategies necessary for task success, the framework will in fact pinpoint type and degree of affective training requirements to ensure that a professional's affective skill and workplace responsibilities match.

## FUTURE RESEARCH DIRECTIONS

The recording of objective physiological data during workplace training in VR provides other opportunities for assessing the training impact on affective strategies. VR scene events can be synchronized with emotional responses. Most pupilometry tracking systems will, in addition, also record the scene observed by the participant via a head-mounted camera. With the Eyelink 11, eye-tracking data is rendered onto the camera's video stream as a small fixation cross, and this video is automatically synchronized with the eye-movement data. This allows offline matching of salient visual events (e.g. obstacle appears, target acquired) with the physiological data (Tichon et al., 2014). This information is useful to track because people can learn to distinguish between task-relevant information and task-irrelevant information (Sohn, Douglass, Chen, & Anderson, 2000), with participants learning to pay more attention to on-task regions relative to off-task regions. In VR training, it is useful to know what is happening with participants' perceptual processes at points designed to be stressful within the scene, and what the subsequent impact of evoked emotion is. Future research could monitor individual affective state while simultaneously tracking people's perceptual processing to ascertain the impact of stress at different decision points. It could be expected that higher negative affect levels would negatively influence visual processing of cues within VR scenes. For example, when anxious, a person may focus for less time on an important cue they had spent far longer visually processing during an earlier training session. The ability to synthetically evoke intense emotional states during a complex cognitive task allows accurately timed measurement of user responses, and will help to answer such questions as: Is there an optimal degree of affective intensity that supports the successful completion of a task but over which level the emotional intensity starts to degrade skills? Such insights will assist in the development of VR training scenes specifically targeted at the development of affective control strategies and associated evaluation measures.

## CONCLUSION

Individuals respond to high-stress situations by coordinating their affective strategies to respond—for example, anger prepares the body to fight, and fear prepares it for flight (Matsumoto & Wilson, 2008). Additionally, emotions help individuals to identify associations between event-based triggers and behavioral consequences in order to be better equipped in similar situations in the future (Matsumoto & Wilson, 2008). This chapter has proposed a new theory to account for the role of affect in understanding and evaluating performance under stress. Affective Control Theory proposes that affective strategies that typically strengthen and support performance are "affective skills," and that these skills are as integral to performance and stress management as any other workplace skill—technical or cognitive.

Although affect is widely recognized as a determinant of performance, there is no universal agreement on its conceptualization or role in performance. In ACT, affect is conceptualized as a skill that can be trained prior to undertaking workplace responsibilities. As a skill, affect can also be used as a key variable in evaluating professional success based on the ability to assess the match between the affective skills of personnel with their work-role affective requirements. The theory has the potential to be highly valuable in supporting workplace planning and training through identifying situations in the field that will impose high affective task demands on personnel and support assessment of the optimal affective level of expertise required of personnel in order for them to successfully complete their jobs. This model of human performance conceptualizes affect as an integral component of an individual's professional skills base and, in the same way as a cognitive or physical skill, it contributes to whether a task can be completed successfully when an individual is working under high-stress conditions.

All indications are that affective state should be a key variable for investigation in the development and evaluation of interventions using VR for stress management. In those studies that have included this variable, methods of measuring individual affective states in VR have primarily been subjective—for example, self-report questionnaires or the use of "think aloud" techniques. Having faced a similar problem of overuse of subjective methods, human–machine system design and development have made attempts to move from outcome- to process-measurement approaches. This chapter reviewed approaches to understanding, training, and evaluating affective strategies in VR environments.

## ACKNOWLEDGMENT

The Affective Control Theory (ACT) was developed during a research project investigating physiological measurement of discreet emotional states under grant award #FA2386-10-1-4011 awarded by the US Air Force Asian Office of Aerospace Research & Development.

## REFERENCES

Ahn, S. J., Bailenson, J., Fox, J., & Jabon, M. (2009). Using automated facial expression analysis for emotion and behavior prediction. Paper presented at the annual meeting of the NCA 95th Annual Convention. Retrieved from http://vhil.stanford.edu/pubs/2010/ahn-hemm-facial-expression.pdf

AlZoubi, O., Calvo, R. A., & Stevens, R. H. (2009). Classification of EEG for affect recognition: An adaptive approach. *Proceedings of AI 2009, Advances in Artificial Intelligence* (Vol. *5866*, pp. 52–61).

Asthana, A., Saragih, J., Wagner, M., & Goecke, R. (2009). Evaluating AAM fitting methods for facial expression recognition. *Proceedings of the IEEE International Conference on Affective Computing and Intelligent Interaction ACII2009* (pp. 598–605). Amsterdam: IEEE. doi:10.1109/ACII.2009.5349489

Bailenson, J. N., Pontikakis, E. D., Mauss, I. B., Gross, J. J., Jabon, M. E., Hutcherson, C. A. C., & Oliver, J. et al. (2008). Real-time classification of evoked emotions using facial feature tracking and physiological responses. *International Journal of Human-Computer Studies*, *66*(5), 303–317. doi:10.1016/j.ijhcs.2007.10.011

Ballard, T. J. (2009). The role of affect in goal setting and goal striving: A multilevel analysis [Unpublished Honors thesis]. Brisbane: University of Queensland.

Bennett, W. Jr, Schreiber, B. T., & Andrews, D. (2002). Developing competency-based methods for near-real-time air combat problem solving assessment. *Computers in Human Behavior*, *18*(6), 773–782. doi:10.1016/S0747-5632(02)00030-4

Blewett, W. K., Ramos, G. A., Redmond, D. P., Cadarette, B. S., Hugens, G. A., Fatkin, L. T., & McKiernan, K. (1994). *p2NBC2 test: The effects of microclimate cooling on tactical performance* (Technical Report 148). Aberdeen Proving Ground, MD, US Army Chemical and Biological Defense Agency.

Chapman, C., Oka, S., Bradshaw, D. H., Jacobson, R. C., & Donaldson, G. W. (1999). Phasic pupil dilation response to noxious stimulation in normal volunteers: Relationship to brain evoked potentials and pain report. *Psychophysiology*, *36*(1), 44–52. doi:10.1017/S0048577299970373 PMID:10098379

Chatterton, R. T. Jr, Vogelsong, K. M., Lu, Y., Ellman, A. B., & Hudgens, G. A. (1996). Salivary amylase as a measure of endogenous adrenergic activity. *Clinical Psychologist*, *16*, 433–438. PMID:8842578

Chi, M. T. H., Glaser, R., & Farr, M. J. (Eds.). (1988). *The nature of expertise*. Hillsdale, NJ: Lawrence Erlbaum.

Connaughton, D., Wadey, R., Hanton, S., & Jones, G. (2008). The development and maintenance of mental toughness: Perceptions of elite performers. *Journal of Sports Sciences*, *26*(1), 83–95. doi:10.1080/02640410701310958 PMID:17852671

Damasio, A. R. (1995). *L'erreur de Descartes. La raison des émotions* (O. Jacob, Ed.). Paris: Sciences.

Daniels, L. M., Stupnisky, R. H., Pekrun, R., Haynes, T. L., Perry, R. P., & Newall, N. E. (2009). A longitudinal analysis of achievement goals: From affective antecedents to emotional effects and achievement outcomes. *Journal of Educational Psychology*, *101*(4), 948–963. doi:10.1037/a0016096

Dayang, R., Awang, R., Suziah, S., & Halabt, H. (2011). VReST: An image-based virtual reality stress therapy web application. *Information Technology in Medicine and Education*, *2*, 733–737.

El Kaliouby, R., & Robinson, P. (2005). Real-time inference of complex mental states from facial expressions and head gestures. In B. Kisačanin, V. Pavlović, & T. S. Huang (Eds.), *Real-time vision for human–computer interaction* (pp. 181–200). New York: Springer. doi:10.1007/0-387-27890-7_11

Elliot, A. J., & Thrash, T. M. (2002). Approach-avoidance motivation in personality: Approach and avoidance temperaments and goals. *Journal of Personality and Social Psychology*, *82*(5), 804–818. doi:10.1037/0022-3514.82.5.804 PMID:12003479

Endsley, M. R. (1988). Design and evaluation for situation awareness enhancement. *Proceedings of the Human Factors Society 32nd Annual Meeting* (pp. 97–101). Santa Monica, CA: Human Factors Society. (1994). Situational awareness in dynamic human decision making: Measurement. In R. D. Gilson, D. J. Garland & J. M. Koone (Eds.), *Situational awareness in complex systems* (pp. 79–97). Daytona Beach, FL: Embry-Riddle Aeronautical University Press.

Ericsson, K. A., Charness, N., Feltovich, P. J., & Hoffman, R. R. (2006). *The Cambridge handbook of expertise and expert performance*. Cambridge, UK: Cambridge University Press. doi:10.1017/CBO9780511816796

Fletcher, K. (2010). Towards a computational compensatory control model of mental workload [Unpublished manuscript]. University of Queensland, Brisbane.

Flin, R., & Maran, N. (2004). Identifying and training non-technical skills for teams in acute medicine. *Quality & Safety in Health Care*, *13*(1suppl_1), 80–84. doi:10.1136/qshc.2004.009993 PMID:15465960

Flin, R., & Martin, L. (2001). Behavioural markers for crew resource management: A review of current practice. *The International Journal of Aviation Psychology*, *11*(1), 95–118. doi:10.1207/S15327108IJAP1101_6

Foo, M., Uy, M. A., & Baron, R. A. (2009). How do feelings influence effort? An empirical study of entrepreneurs' affect and venture effort. *The Journal of Applied Psychology*, *94*(4), 1086–1094. doi:10.1037/a0015599 PMID:19594247

Gluck, K. A., & Gunzelmann, G. (2013). Computational process modeling and cognitive stressors: Background and prospects for application in cognitive engineering. In J. D. Lee & A. Kirlik (Eds.), *The Oxford handbook of cognitive engineering* (pp. 424–432). New York: Oxford University Press. doi:10.1093/oxfordhb/9780199757183.013.0029

Gray, J. A. (1990). Brain systems that mediate both emotion and cognition. *Cognition & Emotion. Special Issue: Development of Relationships Between Emotions and Cognition*, *4*(3), 269–288.

Gucciardi, D., & Gordon, S. (2009). Development and preliminary validation of the Cricket Mental Toughness Inventory (CMTI). *Journal of Sports Sciences*, *27*(12), 1293–1310.

Harrigan, J. A., & O'Connell, D. M. (1996). How do you look when feeling anxious? Facial displays of anxiety. *Personality and Individual Differences*, *21*(2), 205–212. doi:10.1016/0191-8869(96)00050-5

Hockey, G. R. J. (1997). Compensatory control in the regulation of human performance under stress and high workload: A cognitive-energetical framework. Biological Psychology, 45, 73–93.

Hunsley, J. (1990). The factor structure of the multiple affect adjective check list-revised (MAACL-R): Some statistical considerations. *Journal of Psychopathology and Behavioral Assessment*, *12*(1), 99–101. doi:10.1007/BF00960457

Klein, G. A. (2008). Naturalistic decision making. *Human Factors*, *50*(3), 456–460. doi:10.1518/001872008X288385 PMID:18689053

Koestner, R., Lekes, N., Powers, T. A., & Chicoine, E. (2002). Attaining personal goals: Self-concordance plus implementation intentions equals success. *Journal of Personality and Social Psychology*, *83*(1), 231–244. doi:10.1037/0022-3514.83.1.231 PMID:12088128

Lazarus, R. S. (1966). *Psychological stress and the coping process*. New York: McGraw-Hill.

Lehrer, J. (2009, January 17). "Deliberate calm" guided US airways crew. *The Los Angeles Times*. Retrieved from http://www.latimes.com/la-oe-lehrer17-2009jan17-story.html

Liao, W., Zhang, W., Zhu, Z., Ji, Q., & Gray, W. D. (2006). Toward a decision-theoretic framework for affect recognition and user assistance. *International Journal of Human-Computer Studies*, *64*(9), 847–873. doi:10.1016/j.ijhcs.2006.04.001

Linnenbrink, E. A., & Pintrich, P. R. (2002). Achievement goal theory and affect: A symmetrical bidirectional model. *Educational Psychologist*, *37*(2), 69–78. doi:10.1207/S15326985EP3702_2

Loft, S., Bolland, S., Humphreys, M., & Neal, A. (2009). A theory and model of conflict detection in air traffic control: Incorporating environmental constraints. *Journal of Experimental Psychology. Applied*, *15*(2), 106–124. doi:10.1037/a0016118 PMID:19586250

Louro, M. J., Pieters, R., & Zeelenberg, M. (2007). Dynamics of multiple-goal pursuit. *Journal of Personality and Social Psychology*, *93*(2), 174–193. doi:10.1037/0022-3514.93.2.174 PMID:17645394

Matsumoto, D., & Wilson, J. (2008). Culture, emotion, and motivation. In R. Sorrentino & S. Yamaguchi (Eds.), *Handbook of Motivation and Cognition Across Cultures* (pp. 541–563). New York: Elsevier. doi:10.1016/B978-0-12-373694-9.00023-4

Mavin, T. J. (2010). Assessing pilots' performance for promotion to airline captain [Unpublished Doctor of Education thesis]. University of Queensland, Brisbane.

Mavin, T. J., & Dall'Alba, G. (2010). A model for integrating technical skills and NTS in assessing pilots' performance. *Proceedings of the 9th International Symposium of the Australian Aviation Psychology*, Sydney (pp. 9–12).

Mavin, T. J., & Roth, W. M. (2014). A holistic view of cockpit performance: An analysis of the assessment discourse of flight examiners. *The International Journal of Aviation Psychology*, *24*(3), 210–227. doi:10.1080/10508414.2014.918434

Mavin, T. J., Roth, W. M., & Dekker, S. (2013). Understanding variance in pilot performance ratings: Two studies of flight examiners, captains, and first officers assessing the performance of peers. *Aviation Psychology and Applied Human Factors*, *3*(2), 53–62. doi:10.1027/2192-0923/a000041

Mavin, T. J., Roth, W. M., & Munro, I. (in press). Models for and practice of continuous professional development for airline pilots: What we can learn from one regional airline. In S. Billett, D. Dymock, & S. Choy (Eds.), *Supporting learning across working life: Models, processes and practices*. New York: Springer.

Partla, T., & Surakka, V. (2003). Pupil size variation as an indication of affective processing. *International Journal of Human-Computer Studies*, *59*(1-2), 185–198. doi:10.1016/S1071-5819(03)00017-X

Pekrun, R., Elliot, A. J., & Maier, M. A. (2006). Achievement goals and discrete emotions: A theoretical model and prospective test. *Journal of Educational Psychology*, *98*(3), 583–597. doi:10.1037/0022-0663.98.3.583

Peters, E., Lipkus, I., & Diefenbach, M. A. (2006). The functions of affect in health communications and in the construction of health preferences. *Journal of Communication*, *56*(s1), s140–s150. doi:10.1111/j.1460-2466.2006.00287.x

Redden, E. S., Sheehy, J. B., & Bjorkman, E. A. (2004). The study and measurement of human performance by military service laboratories. *Advances in Human Performance and Cognitive Engineering Research*, *5*, 517–559. doi:10.1016/S1479-3601(04)05011-8

Reynolds, C., & Picard, R. W. (2005, July 22–27). *Evaluation of affective computing systems from a dimensional metaethical position. Paper presented to 1st Augmented Cognition Conference, in conjunction with the 11th International Conference on Human–Computer Interaction*, Las Vegas.

Riva, G., Vigna, C., Grassi, A., Raspelli, S., Cipresso, P., Pallavicini, F., & Gaggioli, A. et al. (2012). Learning island: The development of a virtual reality system for the experiential training of stress management. *Studies in Health Technology and Informatics*, *173*, 369–371. PMID:22357020

Roth, W.-M., & Mavin, T. J. (2014). Peer assessment of aviation performance: Inconsistent for good reasons. *Cognitive Science*. doi:10.1111/cogs.12152 PMID:25052893

Russo, M. B., Stetz, M. C., & Thomas, M. L. (2005). Monitoring and predicting cognitive state and performance via physiological correlates of neuronal signals. *Aviation, Space, and Environmental Medicine*, *76*(7), C59–C63. PMID:16018331

Salas, E., Shuffler, M. L., & DiazGranados, D. (2010). Team dynamics at 35,000 feet. In E. Salas, F. Jentsch, & D. Maurino (Eds.), *Human factors in aviation* (pp. 249–291). New York: Academic Press.

Seo, M., Barrett, L. F., & Bartunek, J. M. (2004). The role of affective experience in work motivation. *Academy of Management Review*, *29*(3), 423–439. PMID:16871321

Shah, L. B., Torres, S., Kannusamy, P., Chng, C. M., He, H. G., & Klainin-Yobas, P. (2015). Efficacy of the virtual reality-based stress management program on stress-related variables in people with mood disorders: The feasibility study. *Archives of Psychiatric Nursing*, *20*(1), 6–13. doi:10.1016/j.apnu.2014.09.003 PMID:25634868

Sohn, M.-H., Douglass, S. A., Chen, M.-C., & Anderson, J. R. (2000). Eye-movements during unit-task execution in a complex problem-solving situation. *Proceedings of the 44th Annual Meeting of the Human Factors and Ergonomics Society* (pp. 378–381). doi:10.1177/154193120004401113

Susskind, J. M., Lee, D. H., Cusi, A., Feiman, R., Grabski, W., & Anderson, A. K. (2008). Expressing fear enhances sensory acquisition. *Nature Neuroscience*, *11*(7), 843–850. doi:10.1038/nn.2138 PMID:18552843

Tichon, J. (2010). (Manuscript submitted for publication). Evaluation of virtual reality training using affect. *International Journal on E-Learning*.

Tichon, J., Wallis, G., & Reik, S. (2010). *Affective Intensity and its Effects*. Brisbane: University of Queensland. doi:10.1037/e531432011-001

Tichon, J., Watson, G., & Wallis, G. (2011). Using feature extraction and electromyography to evaluate affect during simulation. *International Journal of Human Factors Modeling and Simulation*, *2*(1/2), 149–162. doi:10.1504/IJHFMS.2011.041642

Tichon, J. G., Mavin, T., Wallis, G., Visser, T. A., & Riek, S. (2014). Using pupillometry and electromyography to track positive and negative affect during flight simulation. *Aviation Psychology and Applied Human Factors*, *4*(1), 23–32. doi:10.1027/2192-0923/a000052

Vealey, R. S. (2007). Mental skills training in sport. In G. Tenenbaum & R. C. Eklund (Eds.), *Handbook of sport psychology* (pp. 287–309). Hoboken, NJ: Wiley.

Yoshie, M., Kudo, K., & Ohtsuki, T. (2008, September). Effects of psychological stress on state anxiety, electromyographic activity, and arpeggio performance in pianists. *Medical Problems of Performing Artists*, *23*, 120–132.

## KEY TERMS AND DEFINITIONS

**Affect:** A noun used primarily in psychology to describe feelings and emotions.

**Affective Control:** The ability to flexibly adapt one's emotional responses to attain a specific goal.

**Affective Impact:** Experiences and other stimuli can trigger positive or negative emotional responses that impact on cognitive skills and behavior.

**Affective Skills:** The development of skills to directly improve the manner in which emotions and feelings are processed and controlled.

**Affective Strategy:** A strategy intentionally learned to manage and adapt emotions, both negative and positive.

**Evoked Emotion:** Emotions that are drawn out as a result of being immersed in the virtual experience. A virtual experience is often designed to arouse a specific emotion.

**Immersion:** A person's emotional reaction to the virtual world in terms of feeling as if they are actually a part of the virtual world and physically present in that world.

# Compilation of References


Inghilleri, P., Riva, G., & Riva, E. (Eds.). (2015). Enabling Positive Change. Flow and Complexity in Daily Experience. Berlin: De Gruyter Open. Retrieved from http://www.degruyter.com/view/product/449663 doi:10.2478/9783110410242

Riva, G., Davide, F., & IJsselsteijn, W. A. (Eds.). (2003). Being There: Concepts, effects and measurements of user presence in synthetic environments. Amsterdam: Ios Press. Retrieved from http://www.emergingcommunication.com/volume5.html

Riva, G., Waterworth, J. A., & Murray, D. (Eds.). (2014). Interacting with Presence: HCI and the sense of presence in computer-mediated environments. Berlin: De Gruyter Open. Retrieved from http://www.presence-research.com doi:10.2478/9783110409697

*500m people will be using healthcare mobile applications in 2015* . (2015). Research2guidance. Retrieved from http://research2guidance.com/500m-people-will-be-usinghealthcare-mobile-applications-in-2015/

AARP. (2000). *Fixing to stay: A national survey on housing and home modification issue---Executive summary*. Washington, D.C.: American Assocition for Retired Persons.

Aarsland, D., Brønnick, K., & Fladby, T. (2011). Mild cognitive impairment in Parkinson's disease. *Current Neurology and Neuroscience Reports*, *11*(4), 371–378. doi:10.1007/s11910-011-0203-1 PMID:21487730

ADDA. (2013). Anxiety and Depression Association of America. Screening for Depression. Retrieved from http://www.adaa.org/iving-with-anxiety/ask-and-learn/screenings/screening-depression

Adolfsson, A., Linden, K., Sparud-Lundin, C., Larsson, P. G., & Berg, M. (2014). A web-based support for pregnant women and new mothers with type 1 diabetes mellitus in Sweden (MODIAB-Web): Study protocol for a randomized controlled trial. *Trials*, *15*(1), 513. doi:10.1186/1745-6215-15-513 PMID:25543854

Ahern, N. R., Kiehl, E. M., Sole, M. L., & Byers, J. (2006). A review of instruments measuring resilience. *Issues in Comprehensive Pediatric Nursing*, *29*(2), 103–125. doi:10.1080/01460860600677643 PMID:16772239

Ahn, S. J., Bailenson, J., Fox, J., & Jabon, M. (2009). Using automated facial expression analysis for emotion and behavior prediction. Paper presented at the annual meeting of the NCA 95th Annual Convention. Retrieved from http://vhil.stanford.edu/pubs/2010/ahn-hemm-facial-expression.pdf

Ahn, D., Jin, S. A. A., & Ritterfeld, U. (2012). Sad movies don't always make me cry the cognitive and affective processes underpinning enjoyment of tragedy. *Journal of Media Psychology*, *24*(1), 9–18. doi:10.1027/1864-1105/a000058

Ahn, M. (2004). *Older People's Attitudes toward Residential Technology: The Role of Technology in Aging in Place*. Virginia Polytechnic Institute and State University.

Ahsan, A., & Raihan, A. (2013, December). Understanding m-health impact among Aponjon (MAMA Bangladesh) subscribers through a phone survey in Bangladesh.*Proceedings of the Sixth International Conference on Information and Communications Technologies and Development: Notes*(*Vol. 2,* pp. 1-4). ACM.

Ahtinen, A., Mattila, E., Välkkynen, P., Kaipainen, K., Vanhala, T., Ermes, M., & Lappalainen, R. (2013). Mobile mental wellness training for stress management: Feasibility and design implications based on a one-month field study. *JMIR mHealth and uHealth, 1*(2).

Ahtinen, A., & Mattila, E., VÃ¤lkkynen, P., Kaipainen, K., Vanhala, T., Ermes, M., . . . Lappalainen, R. (2013). Mobile Mental Wellness Training for Stress Management: Feasibility and Design Implications Based on a One-Month Field Study. *Journal of Medical Internet Research, 15*(7). PMID:25100683

Akbarzade, M., Rafiee, B., Asadi, N., & Zare, N. (2015). The Effect of Maternal Relaxation Training on Reactivity of Non-Stress Test, Basal Fetal Heart Rate, and Number of Fetal Heart Accelerations: A Randomized Controlled Trial. *International journal of community based nursing and midwifery, 3*(1), 51.

Albert, M. S. (2011). Changes in cognition. *Neurobiology of Aging, 32*, S58–S63. doi:10.1016/j.neurobiolaging.2011.09.010 PMID:22078174

Alcañiz, M., Baños, R., Botella, C., & Rey, B. (2003). The EMMA project: Emotions as a determinant of presence. *Psychology Journal, 1*(2), 141–150.

Alcañiz, M., Botella, C., Banos, R., Zaragoza, I., & Guixeres, J. (2009). The Intelligent e-Therapy system: A new paradigm for telepsychology and cybertherapy. *British Journal of Guidance & Counselling, 37*(3), 287–296. doi:10.1080/03069880902957015

Aldwin, C. (2007). *Stress, coping, and development: An integrative perspective*. NY: The Guilford Press.

Alexiou, A., Schippers, M., & Oshri, I. (2012). Positive Psychology and Digital Games: The Role of Emotions and Psychological Flow in Serious Games Development. Psychology (Savannah, Ga.), 3(12A), 1243–1247.

Allbeck, J., & Badler, N. (2002). Embodied Autonomous Agents. In K. Stanney (Ed.), *Handbook of Virtual Environments* (pp. 313–332). Lawrence Erlbaum Associates.

Allen, V. L., & Greenberger, D. B. (1978). An Aesthetic Theory of Vandalism. *Crime and Delinquency, 24*(3), 309–321. doi:10.1177/001112877802400305

Alm, N., Astell, A., Gowans, G., Dye, R., Ellis, M., Vaughan, P., & Riley, P. (2009). Engaging multimedia leisure for people with dementia. *Gerontechnology (Valkenswaard), 8*(4), 236–246. doi:10.4017/gt.2009.08.04.006.00

AlZoubi, O., Calvo, R. A., & Stevens, R. H. (2009). Classification of EEG for affect recognition: An adaptive approach. *Proceedings of AI 2009, Advances in Artificial Intelligence* (Vol. *5866*, pp. 52–61).

Amirkhan, J., & Auyeung, B. (2007). Coping with stress across the lifespan: Absolute vs. relative changes in strategy. *Journal of Applied Developmental Psychology, 28*(4), 298–317. doi:10.1016/j.appdev.2007.04.002

Ammaniti, M. (1996). *Maternità e gravidanza: studio delle rappresentazioni materne*. Raffaello Cortina.

Anderson, C., & Bushman, B. J. (2001). Effects of violent video games on aggressive behavior, aggressive cognition, aggressive affect, physiological arousal, and prosocial behavior: a meta-analytic review of the scientific literature. *Psychological Science: A Journal of the American Psychological Society*, 12, 353–359. doi:10.1111/1467-9280.00366

Anderson, C. (2004). An update on the effects of playing violent video games. *Journal of Adolescence, 27*(1), 113–122. doi:10.1016/j.adolescence.2003.10.009 PMID:15013264

Anderson, C. A., Berkowitz, L., Donnerstein, E., Huesmann, L. R., Johnson, J. D., Linz, D., & Neil, M. Malamuth, & Wartella, E. (2003). The influence of media violence on youth. *Psychological Science in the Public Interest*, *4*, 81–110. PMID:26151870

Anderson, C. A., & Dill, K. E. (2000). Video games and aggressive thoughts, feelings, and behavior in the laboratory and in life. *Journal of Personality and Social Psychology*, *78*(4), 772–790. doi:10.1037/0022-3514.78.4.772 PMID:10794380

Anderson, C. A., & Ford, C. M. (1986). Affect of the Game Player: Short-Term Effects of Highly and Mildly Aggressive Video Games. *Personality and Social Psychology Bulletin*, *12*(4), 390–402. doi:10.1177/0146167286124002

Andersson, G. (2009). Using the Internet to provide cognitive behaviour therapy. *Behaviour Research and Therapy*, *47*(3), 175–180. doi:10.1016/j.brat.2009.01.010 PMID:19230862

Andreassi, J. L. (2006). *Psychophysiology: Human behavior and physiological response*. Lawrence Erlbaum Assoc Inc.

Andreu-Mateu, S., Botella, C., Quero, S., Guillén, V., & Baños, R. (2012). La utilización de la realidad virtual y estrategias de psicología positiva en el tratamiento de los trastornos adaptativos. *Behavioral Psychology/Psicología Conductual*, *20*(2), 323-348.

Andrews, F. M., & Withey, S. B. (2012). *Social indicators of well-being: Americans' perceptions of life quality*. New York, NY: Springer Science & Business Media.

Andrews, G., Cuijpers, P., Craske, M., McEvoy, P., & Titov, N. (2010). Computer therapy for the anxiety and depressive disorders is effective, acceptable and practical health care: A meta-analysis. *PLoS ONE*, *5*(10), 131–196. doi:10.1371/journal.pone.0013196 PMID:20967242

Anguera, J., Boccanfuso, J., Rintoul, J. L., Al-Hashimi, O., Faraji, F., Janowich, J., & Gazzaley, A. et al. (2013). Video game training enhances cognitive control in older adults. *Nature*, *501*(7465), 97–101. doi:10.1038/nature12486 PMID:24005416

Anolli, L., Mantovani, F., Confalonieri, L., Ascolese, A., & Peveri, L. (2010). Emotions in Serious Games: From Experience to Assessment. *International Journal of Emerging Technologies in Learning*, *5*, 7–16.

Antonovsky, A. (1979). *Health, stress, and coping. New perspective on mental and physical well-being*. San Francisco, CA: Jossey-Bass.

Antonovsky, A. (1987). The salutogenic perspective: Toward a new view of health and illness. *Advances*, *4*(1), 47–75.

Antonovsky, A. (1996). The salutogenic model as a theory to guide health promotion. *Health Promotion International*, *11*(1), 11–18. doi:10.1093/heapro/11.1.11

Anttonen, J., & Surakka, V. (2005). *Emotions and heart rate while sitting on a chair* (pp. 491–499). ACM. doi:10.1145/1054972.1055040

Argenton, L., Triberti, S., Serino, S., Muzio, M., & Riva, G. (2014). Serious games as positive technologies for individual and group flourishing. In A. L. Brooks et al. (Eds.), *Technologies of Inclusive Well-Being* (pp. 221–244). Berlin, Heidelberg: Springer. doi:10.1007/978-3-642-45432-5_11

Armarego, J. (2002). Advanced software design: a case in problem-based learning.*Proceedings 15th Conference on Software Engineering Education and Training (CSEE&T 2002)* (pp. 57–65). doi:10.1109/CSEE.2002.995197

Asthana, A., Saragih, J., Wagner, M., & Goecke, R. (2009). Evaluating AAM fitting methods for facial expression recognition. *Proceedings of the IEEE International Conference on Affective Computing and Intelligent Interaction ACII2009* (pp. 598–605). Amsterdam: IEEE. doi:10.1109/ACII.2009.5349489

Aue, T., Flykt, A., & Scherer, K. R. (2007). First evidence for differential and sequential efferent effects of stimulus relevance and goal conduciveness appraisal. *Biological Psychology*, *74*(3), 347–357. doi:10.1016/j.biopsycho.2006.09.001 PMID:17052833

Aue, T., & Scherer, K. R. (2008). Appraisal-driven somatovisceral response patterning: Effects of intrinsic pleasantness and goal conduciveness. *Biological Psychology*, *79*(2), 158–164. doi:10.1016/j.biopsycho.2008.04.004 PMID:18495321

Austin, M. P., Tully, L., & Parker, G. (2007). Examining the relationship between antenatal anxiety and postnatal depression. *Journal of Affective Disorders*, *101*(1), 169–174. doi:10.1016/j.jad.2006.11.015 PMID:17196663

Baas, M., De Dreu, C. K., & Nijstad, B. A. (2008). A meta-analysis of 25 years of mood-creativity research: Hedonic tone, activation, or regulatory focus? *Psychological Bulletin*, *134*(6), 779–806. doi:10.1037/a0012815 PMID:18954157

Baccus, J. R., Baldwin, M. W., & Packer, D. J. (2004). Increasing implicit self-esteem through classical conditioning. *Psychological Science*, *15*(7), 498–502. doi:10.1111/j.0956-7976.2004.00708.x PMID:15200636

Baghurst, T., & Kelley, B. C. (2013). An Examination of Stress in College Students Over the Course of a Semester.

Bahar-Fuchs, A., Clare, L., & Woods, B. (2013). Cognitive training and cognitive rehabilitation for mild to moderate Alzheimer's disease and vascular dementia. *Cochrane Database of Systematic Reviews*, 6. PMID:23740535

Bailenson, J. N., Pontikakis, E. D., Mauss, I. B., Gross, J. J., Jabon, M. E., Hutcherson, C. A. C., & Oliver, J. et al. (2008). Real-time classification of evoked emotions using facial feature tracking and physiological responses. *International Journal of Human-Computer Studies*, *66*(5), 303–317. doi:10.1016/j.ijhcs.2007.10.011

Baker, A., Navarro, E. O., & Van Der Hoek, A. (2005). An experimental card game for teaching software engineering processes. *Journal of Systems and Software*, *75*(1-2), 3–16. doi:10.1016/j.jss.2004.02.033

Bala, H., & Venkatesh, V. (2013). Changes in employees' job characteristics during an enterprise system implementation: A latent growth modeling perspective. *Management Information Systems Quarterly*, *37*(4), 1113–1140.

Baldaro, B., Tuozzi, G., Codispoti, M., Montebarocci, O., Barbagli, F., Trombini, E., & Rossi, N. (2004). Aggressive and non-violent videogames: Short-term psychological and cardiovascular effects on habitual players. *Stress and Health*, *20*(4), 203–208. doi:10.1002/smi.1015

Ballard, T. J. (2009). The role of affect in goal setting and goal striving: A multilevel analysis [Unpublished Honors thesis]. Brisbane: University of Queensland.

Ballard, M., & Wiest, R. (1996). Mortal Kombat (tm): The Effects of Violent Videogame Play on Males' Hostility and Cardiovascular Responding. *Journal of Applied Social Psychology*, *26*(8), 717–730. doi:10.1111/j.1559-1816.1996.tb02740.x

Ball, G., & Breese, J. (2000). Emotion and personality in a conversational agent. In *Embodied Conversational Characters. (pp.xx)*. Cambridge, MA: MIT Press.

Bandura, A. (1997). Self-Efficacy: The Exercise of Control. New York: Freeman.

Bandura, A. (1977). Self-efficacy: Toward a unifying theory of behavioral change. *Psychological Review*, *84*(2), 191–215. doi:10.1037/0033-295X.84.2.191 PMID:847061

Bandura, A. (1978). Social learning theory of aggression. *Journal of Communication*, *28*(3), 12–29. doi:10.1111/j.1460-2466.1978.tb01621.x PMID:690254

Bandura, A. (1982). Self-efficacy mechanism in human agency. *The American Psychologist*, *37*(2), 122–147. doi:10.1037/0003-066X.37.2.122

Bandura, A. (1998). Health promotion from the perspective of social cognitive theory. *Psychology & Health, 13*(4), 623–649. doi:10.1080/08870449808407422

Bandura, A. (2004). Health promotion by social cognitive means. *Health Education & Behavior, 31*(2), 143–164. doi:10.1177/1090198104263660 PMID:15090118

Bandura, A., Ross, D., & Ross, S. A. (1963). Imitation of film-mediated aggressive models. *Journal of Abnormal and Social Psychology, 66*(1), 3–11. doi:10.1037/h0048687 PMID:13966304

Baños, R. M., Liaño, V., Botella, C., Alcañiz, M., Guerrero, B., & Rey, B. (2006). Changing Induced Moods via Virtual Reality. In W. Ijsselsteijn, Y. de Kort, C. Midden, B. Eggen & E. van dem Hoven (Eds.), Persuasive Technology, LNCS (Vol. 3962, pp. 7-15). Berlin/Heilderberg: Springer-Verlag.

Baños, R. M., Botella, C., Alcañiz, M., Liaño, V., Guerrero, B., & Rey, B. (2004). Immersion and emotion: Their impact on the sense of presence. *Cyberpsychology & Behavior, 7*(6), 734–741. doi:10.1089/cpb.2004.7.734 PMID:15687809

Baños, R. M., Botella, C., Rubió, I., Quero, S., García-Palacios, A., & Alcañiz, M. (2008). Presence and emotions in virtual environments: The influence of stereoscopy. *Cyberpsychology & Behavior, 11*(1), 1–8. doi:10.1089/cpb.2007.9936 PMID:18275306

Baños, R. M., Etchemendy, E., Castilla, D., García-Palacios, A., Quero, S., & Botella, C. (2012). Positive mood induction procedures for virtual environments designed for elderly people. *Interacting with Computers, 24*(3), 131–138. doi:10.1016/j.intcom.2012.04.002

Baños, R. M., Liaño, V., Botella, C., Alcañiz, M., Guerrero, B., & Rey, B. (2006). *Changing induced moods via virtual reality Persuasive Technology* (pp. 7–15). Springer.

Baños, R., Etchemendy, E., Farfallini, L., García-Palacios, A., Quero, S., & Botella, C. (2014). EARTH of Well-Being system: A pilot study of an Information and Communication Technology-based positive psychology intervention. *The Journal of Positive Psychology, 6*(9), 482–488. doi:10.1080/17439760.2014.927906

Barak, A., & Grohol, J. M. (2011). Current and future trends in internet-supported mental health interventions. *Journal of Technology in Human Services, 29*(3), 155–196. doi:10.1080/15228835.2011.616939

Baranowski, T., Buday, R., Thompson, D. I., & Baranowski, J. (2008). Playing for Real: Video Games and Stories for Health-Related Behavior Change. American Journal of Preventive Medicine, 34(1), 74–82.

Baranowski, T., Lieberman, D., Buday, R., Peng, W., Zimmerli, L., Wiederhold, B., & Kato, P. M. (2013). Videogame Mechanics in Games for Health. Games for Health Journal, 2(4), 194–204. doi:10.1089/g4h.2013.0617 PubMed doi:10.1089/g4h.2013.0617 PMID:26192223

Baranowski, T., Buday, R., Thompson, D., & Baranowski, J. (2008). Playing for real: Video games and stories for health-related behavior change. *American Journal of Preventive Medicine, 34*(1), 74–82. doi:10.1016/j.amepre.2007.09.027 PMID:18083454

Baranowski, T., Buday, R., Thompson, D., Lyons, E. J., Lu, A. S., & Baranowski, J. (2013). Developing games for health behavior change: Getting started. *GAMES FOR HEALTH: Research, Development, and Clinical Applications, 2*(4), 183–190. doi:10.1089/g4h.2013.0048 PMID:24443708

Barclay, L., Everitt, L., Rogan, F., Schmied, V., & Wyllie, A. (1997). Becoming a mother—an analysis of women's experience of early motherhood. *Journal of Advanced Nursing, 25*(4), 719–728. doi:10.1046/j.1365-2648.1997.t01-1-1997025719.x PMID:9104667

Barello, S., & Graffigna, G. (2015). Engaging patients to recover life projectuality: An Italian cross-disease framework. *Quality of Life Research: An International Journal of Quality of Life Aspects of Treatment, Care and Rehabilitation, 24*(5), 1087–1096. doi:10.1007/s11136-014-0846-x PMID:25373927

Barello, S., & Graffigna, G. (2015). Patient engagement in healthcare: Pathways for effective medical decision-making. *Neuropsychogical Trends, 17*, 53–65. doi:10.7358/neur-2015-017-bare

Barello, S., Graffigna, G., & Vegni, E. (2012). Patient engagement as an emerging challenge for healthcare services: Mapping the literature. *Nursing Research and Practice, 2012*, 905-934. doi:10.1155/2012/905934 PMID:23213497

Barello, S., Graffigna, G., Vegni, E., Savarese, M., Lombardi, F., & Bosio, A. C. (2015). 'Engage me in taking care of my heart': A grounded theory study on patient–cardiologist relationship in the hospital management of heart failure. *BMJ Open, 5*(3), e005582. doi:10.1136/bmjopen-2014-005582 PMID:25776041

Barki, H., & Hartwick, J. (1989). Rethinking the concept of user involvement. *Management Information Systems Quarterly, 13*(1), 53–63. doi:10.2307/248700

Barnes, D. E., Yaffe, K., Belfor, N., Jagust, W. J., DeCarli, C., Reed, B. R., & Kramer, J. H. (2009). Computer-based cognitive training for mild cognitive impairment: Results from a pilot randomized, controlled trial. *Alzheimer Disease and Associated Disorders, 23*(3), 205–210. doi:10.1097/WAD.0b013e31819c6137 PMID:19812460

Bartholomew, M. K., Schoppe-Sullivan, S. J., Glassman, M., Kamp Dush, C. M., & Sullivan, J. M. (2012). New parents' Facebook use at the transition to parenthood. *Family Relations, 61*(3), 455–469. doi:10.1111/j.1741-3729.2012.00708.x PMID:23671354

Bartle, R. (2003). *Designing Virtual Worlds*. New Riders Games.

Barton, M., Symborski, C., Quinn, M. M., Morewedge, C. K., Kassam, K. S., & Korris, J. H. (2015, May). The use of theory in designing a serious game for the reduction of cognitive biases. *Proceedings of the 2015 DiGRA International Conference DiGRA '15*, Digital Games Research Association.

Bartsch, A., Vorderer, P., Mangold, R., & Viehoff, R. (2008). Appraisal of Emotions in Media Use: Toward a Process Model of Meta-Emotion and Emotion Regulation. *Media Psychology, 11*(1), 7–27. doi:10.1080/15213260701813447

Bastani, F., Hidarnia, A., Kazemnejad, A., Vafaei, M., & Kashanian, M. (2005). A randomized controlled trial of the effects of applied relaxation training on reducing anxiety and perceived stress in pregnant women. *Journal of Midwifery & Women's Health, 50*(4), e36–e40. doi:10.1016/j.jmwh.2004.11.008 PMID:15973255

Bastani, F., Hidarnia, A., Montgomery, K. S., Aguilar-Vafaei, M. E., & Kazemnejad, A. (2006). Does relaxation education in anxious primigravid Iranian women influence adverse pregnancy outcomes?: A randomized controlled trial. *The Journal of Perinatal & Neonatal Nursing, 20*(2), 138–146. doi:10.1097/00005237-200604000-00007 PMID:16714913

Bastin, C., & Salmon, E. (2014). Early neuropsychological detection of Alzheimer's disease. *European Journal of Clinical Nutrition, 68*(11), 1192–1199. doi:10.1038/ejcn.2014.176 PMID:25182019

Bateman, C. (2014). Empirical game aesthetics. In M. C. Angelides & H. Agius (Eds.), *Handbook of computer game studies* (pp. 411–442). Hoboken, NJ: John Wiley & Sons.

Bateman, C. M. (2007). *Game writing: narrative skills for video games*. Hingham, MA: Charles River Media.

Batson, C. D., Shaw, L. L., & Oleson, K. C. (1992). Differentiating affect, mood, and emotion: Toward functionally based conceptual distinctions. In M.S. Clark (Eds.), Emotion. Review of personality and social psychology (Vol. 13, pp. 294-326). Thousand Oaks, CA, US: Sage Publications.

Baumgartner, T., Valko, L., Esslen, M., et al. (2006). Neural correlate of spatial presence in an arousing and noninteractive virtual reality: an EEG and psychophysiology study. *Cyberpsychology & behavior*, *9*, 30–45.

Baytak, A., Land, S. M. & Smith, B. K. (2011). Children as educational computer game designers: An exploratory study. *Turkish Online Journal of Educational Technology, 10*(4), 84–92.

Beddoe, A. E., & Lee, K. A. (2008). Mind-Body Interventions during Pregnancy. *Journal of Obstetric, Gynecologic, and Neonatal Nursing*, *37*(2), 165–175. doi:10.1111/j.1552-6909.2008.00218.x PMID:18336440

Beebe, K. R., Lee, K. A., Carrieri-Kohlman, V., & Humphreys, J. (2007). The Effects of Childbirth Self-Efficacy and Anxiety during Pregnancy on Prehospitalization Labor. *Journal of Obstetric, Gynecologic, and Neonatal Nursing*, *36*(5), 410–418. doi:10.1111/j.1552-6909.2007.00170.x PMID:17880311

Begy, J., & Consalvo, M. (2011). Achievements, Motivations and Rewards in Faunasphere. Game Studies, 11(1). Retrieved from http://gamestudies.org/1101/articles/begy_consalvo

Belleville, S. (2008). Cognitive training for persons with mild cognitive impairment. *International Psychogeriatrics*, *20*(01), 57–66. doi:10.1017/S104161020700631X PMID:17958927

Belleville, S., Gilbert, B., Fontaine, F., Gagnon, L., Ménard, É., & Gauthier, S. (2006). Improvement of episodic memory in persons with mild cognitive impairment and healthy older adults: Evidence from a cognitive intervention program. *Dementia and Geriatric Cognitive Disorders*, *22*(5-6), 486–499. doi:10.1159/000096316 PMID:17050952

Bellotti, F., Kapralos, B., Lee, K., Moreno-Ger, P., & Berta, R. (2013). Assessment in and of Serious Games: An Overview. *Advances in Human-Computer Interaction*, *4*, 1–11.

Bennett, W. Jr, Schreiber, B. T., & Andrews, D. (2002). Developing competency-based methods for near-real-time air combat problem solving assessment. *Computers in Human Behavior*, *18*(6), 773–782. doi:10.1016/S0747-5632(02)00030-4

Bergeron, B. (2006). *Developing serious games*. Hingham, MA: Charles River Media.

Berntson, G. G., & Cacioppo, J. T. (2004). Heart rate variability: Stress and psychiatric conditions. In M. M. A. J. Camm (Ed.), *Dynamic electrocardiography* (pp. 56–63). New York: Futura. doi:10.1002/9780470987483.ch7

Bersak, D., McDarby, G., Augenblick, N., McDarby, P., McDonnell, D., McDonald, B., & Karkun, R. (2001). Intelligent biofeedback using an immersive competitive environment.*Proceedings of Designing Ubiquitous Computing Games Workshop at UbiComp*.

Bert, F., Gualano, M. R., Brusaferro, S., De Vito, E., de Waure, C., La Torre, G., ... & Carubia, L. (2013). Pregnancy e-health: a multicenter Italian cross-sectional study on Internet use and decision-making among pregnant women. *Journal of epidemiology and community health*, jech-2013.

Bier, N., Grenier, S., Brodeur, C., Gauthier, S., Gilbert, B., Hudon, C., & Belleville, S. et al. (2015). Measuring the impact of cognitive and psychosocial interventions in persons with mild cognitive impairment with a randomized single-blind controlled trial: Rationale and design of the MEMO+ study. *International Psychogeriatrics*, *27*(3), 511–525. doi:10.1017/S1041610214001902 PMID:25268968

Billings, A. G., & Moos, R. H. (1981). The role of coping responses and social resources in attenuating the stress of life events. *Journal of Behavioral Medicine*, *4*(2), 139–157. doi:10.1007/BF00844267 PMID:7321033

Biocca, F., Harms, C., & Burgoon, J. K. (2003). Toward a more robust theory and measure of social presence: Review and suggested criteria. *Presence (Cambridge, Mass.)*, *12*(5), 456–480.

Bishop, S. R., Lau, M., Shapiro, S., Carlson, L., Anderson, N. D., Carmody, J., & Velting, D. et al. (2004). Mindfulness: A proposed operational definition. *Clinical Psychology: Science and Practice*, *11*(3), 230–241. doi:10.1093/clipsy.bph077

Blewett, W. K., Ramos, G. A., Redmond, D. P., Cadarette, B. S., Hugens, G. A., Fatkin, L. T., & McKiernan, K. (1994). *p2NBC2 test: The effects of microclimate cooling on tactical performance* (Technical Report 148). Aberdeen Proving Ground, MD, US Army Chemical and Biological Defense Agency.

Blumberg, F. C., Rosenthal, S. F., & Randall, J. D. (2008). Impasse-driven learning in the context of video games. *Computers in Human Behavior*, *24*(4), 1530–1541. doi:10.1016/j.chb.2007.05.010

Bødker, S. (1996). Applying activity theory to video analysis: how to make sense of video data in human-computer interaction. In B. Nardi (Ed.), *Context and consciousness. Activity theory and human computer interaction* (pp. 147–174). Cambridge, USA: Mit Press.

Bogost, I. (2007). *Persuasive games: The expressive power of videogames*. Cambridge, MA: MIT Press.

Bohil, C. J., Alicea, B., & Biocca, F. A. (2011). Virtual reality in neuroscience research and therapy. *Nature Reviews. Neuroscience*, *12*(12), 752–762. PMID:22048061

Bolier, L., Haverman, M., Kramer, J., Westerhof, G. J., Riper, H., Walburg, J. A., & Bohlmeijer, E. et al. (2013). An Internet-based intervention to promote mental fitness for mildly depressed adults: Randomized controlled trial. *Journal of Medical Internet Research*, *15*(9), e200. doi:10.2196/jmir.2603 PMID:24041479

Bolier, L., Haverman, M., Westerhof, G. J., Riper, H., Smit, F., & Bohlmeijer, E. (2013). Positive psychology interventions: A meta-analysis of randomized controlled studies. *BMC Public Health*, *13*(1), 119. doi:10.1186/1471-2458-13-119 PMID:23390882

Bolier, L., Majo, C., Smit, F., Westerhof, G. J., Haverman, M., Walburg, J. A., & Bohlmeijer, E. et al. (2014). Cost-effectiveness of online positive psychology: Randomized controlled trial. *The Journal of Positive Psychology*, *9*(5), 460–471. doi:10.1080/17439760.2014.910829

Bonawitz, E., Shafto, P., Gweon, H., Goodman, N. D., Spelke, E., & Schulz, L. (2011). The double-edged sword of pedagogy: Instruction limits spontaneous exploration and discovery. *Cognition*, *120*(3), 322–330. doi:10.1016/j.cognition.2010.10.001 PMID:21216395

Bordes, A. et al.. (2005). Fast kernel classifiers with online and active learning. *Journal of Machine Learning Research*, *6*, 1579–1619.

Bordnick, P. S., Traylor, A. C., Carter, B. L., & Graap, K. M. (2011). A feasibility study of virtual reality-based coping skills training for nicotine dependence. *Research on Social Work Practice*, 22(3), 293-300. PMID:25484549

Borkovec, T., & Costello, E. (1993). Efficacy of applied relaxation and cognitive-behavioral therapy in the treatment of generalized anxiety disorder. *Journal of Consulting and Clinical Psychology*, *61*(4), 611–619. doi:10.1037/0022-006X.61.4.611 PMID:8370856

Bosio, C. A., & Graffigna, G. (2014). People Health Engagement: Fra mainstream e nuovo paradigma. *Psicologia della Salute*, *11*(3), 5–10. doi:10.3280/PDS2014-003001

Bostan, B., & Öğüt, S. (2009). In pursuit of optimal gaming experience: Challenges and difficulty levels. *Paper presented at the Entertainment=Emotion Conference*, Spain. Retrieved from https://scholar.google.com/citations?view_op=view_citation&hl=en&user=JDYxzV0AAAAJ&citation_for_view=JDYxzV0AAAAJ:W7OEmFMy1HYC

Botella, C., Etchemendy, E., Castilla, D., Baños, R. M., García-Palacios, A., Quero, S., … Lozano, J. A. (2009). An e-health system for the elderly (Butler Project): a pilot study on acceptance and satisfaction. *Cyberpsychology & Behavior: the impact of the Internet, multimedia and virtual reality on behavior and society, 12*(3), 255-262.

Botella, C., Baños, R. M., Etchemendy, E., García-Palacios, A., & Alcañiz, M. (in press). Psychological countermeasures in manned space missions: "EARTH" system for the Mars-500 project. *Computers in Human Behavior.*

Botella, C., Baños, R., Etchemendy, E., Castilla, D., García-Palacios, A., & Alcañiz, M. (2011). An e-health system for promoting wellbeing in elderly: The Butler System. In Å. Smedberg (Ed.), *E-Health Communities and Online Self-Help Groups: Applications and Usage* (pp. 57–71). Hershey, PA, USA: IGI Global. Doi:10.4018/978-1-60960-866-8

Botella, C., Garcia-Palacios, A., Baños, R. M., & Quero, S. (2009). Cybertherapy: Advantages, Limitations, and Ethical Issues. *PsychNology Journal, 7*(1), 77–100.

Botella, C., Mira, A., Garcia-Palacios, A., Quero, A., Navarro, M. V., Riera López del Amo, T., & Baños, R. M. et al. (2012b). Smiling is fun: A coping with stress and emotion regulation program. Annual Review of Cybertherapy and Telemedicine 2012. Advanced Technologies in the Behavioral. *Social Neuroscience*, 2012, 123–128.

Botella, C., Riva, G., Gaggioli, A., Wiederhold, B. K., Alcaniz, M., & Banos, R. M. (2012). The present and future of positive technologies. *Cyberpsychology, Behavior, and Social Networking, 15*(2), 78–84. doi:10.1089/cyber.2011.0140 PMID:22149078

Boulos, M. N. K., & Wheeler, S. (2007). The emerging Web 2.0 social software: An enabling suite of sociable technologies in health and health care education. *Health Information and Libraries Journal, 24*(1), 2–23. doi:10.1111/j.1471-1842.2007.00701.x PMID:17331140

Bowman, S. L. (2010). *The functions of role-playing games. How partecipants create community, solve problems and explore identity*. London, UK: McFarland & Copany Inc.

Boyle, E. A., Connolly, T. M., Hainey, T., & Boyle, J. M. (2012). Engagement in digital entertainment games: A systematic review. *Computers in Human Behavior, 28*(3), 771–780. doi:10.1016/j.chb.2011.11.020

Boyle, E., Connolly, T. M., & Hainey, T. (2011). The role of psychology in understanding the impact of computer games. *Entertainment Computing, 2*(2), 69–74. doi:10.1016/j.entcom.2010.12.002

Boyle, P. A., Buchman, A. S., Wilson, R. S., Leurgans, S. E., & Bennett, D. A. (2010). Physical Frailty Is Associated with Incident Mild Cognitive Impairment in Comm Community-Based Older Persons. *Journal of the American Geriatrics Society, 58*(2), 248–255. doi:10.1111/j.1532-5415.2009.02671.x PMID:20070417

Breitve, M. H., Chwiszczuk, L. J., Hynninen, M. J., Rongve, A., Brønnick, K., Janvin, C., & Aarsland, D. (2014). A systematic review of cognitive decline in dementia with Lewy bodies versus Alzheimer's. *Alzheimer's Research & Therapy, 6*, 53. PMID:25478024

Breslin, S. (2009). The history and theory of sandbox game play. *Gamasutra*. Retrieved from http://www.gamasutra.com/view/feature/4081/the_history_and_theory_of_sandbox_.php

Breslow, L. (1972). A quantitative approach to the World Health Organization definition of health: Physical, mental and social well-being. *International Journal of Epidemiology, 1*(4), 347–355. doi:10.1093/ije/1.4.347 PMID:4669083

Brewin, C. R. (1989). Cognitive Change Processes in Psychotherapy. *Psychological Review, 96*(3), 379–394. doi:10.1037/0033-295X.96.3.379 PMID:2667012

Brey, P. (2008). Virtual Reality and Computer Simulation. In K. Himma & H. Tavani (Ed.), Handbook of Information and Computer Ethics. John Wiley & Sons. doi:10.1002/9780470281819.ch15

Brezinka, V. (2008). Treasure Hunt – a serious game to support psychotherapeutic treatment of children. In S. K. Andersen, M.C.A. Klein, S. Schulz, J. Aarts, & M.C. Mazzoleni (Eds.), eHealth Beyond the Horizon – Get IT There (pp. 71–76). Amsterdam: IOS Press.

Bribing, G. (1959). Some considerations of the psychological process in pregnancy. *The Psychoanalytic Study of the Child*, *14*, 113–119.

Brigliadori, L., & Brigliadori, R. (2011). *Competing in Gliders. Winning with your mind.* Pivetta Partners, Vedano al Lambro.

Brom, C., Buchtová, M., Šisler, V., Děchtěrenko, F., Palme, R., & Glenk, L. M. (2014). Flow, social interaction anxiety and salivary cortisol responses in serious games: A quasi-experimental study. *Computers & Education*, *79*, 69–100. doi:10.1016/j.compedu.2014.07.001

Brooks, A. L., Brahnam, S., & Jain, L. C. (2014). *Technologies of Inclusive Well-Being. Serious Games, Alternative Realities, and Play Therapy*. New York: Springer. doi:10.1007/978-3-642-45432-5

Broughton, M., Carr, O., Taplin, P., Estival, D., Wark, S., & Lambert, D. (2002). *Conversing with Franco, FOCAL's virtual adviser*. Retrieved from http://www.dominique-estival.net/ConversingWithFranco_final.pdf

Brox, E., Fernandez-Luque, L., & Tøllefsen, T. (2011). Healthy Gaming – Video Game Design to promote Health. *Applied Clinical Informatics*, *2*(2), 128–142. doi:10.4338/ACI-2010-10-R-0060 PMID:23616865

Bryant, F. B. (2003). Savoring beliefs inventory (SBI): A scale for measuring beliefs about savouring. *Journal of Mental Health (Abingdon, England)*, *12*(2), 175–196. doi:10.1080/0963823031000103489

Buckley, K. E., & Anderson, C. A. (2006). A theoretical model of the effects and consequences of playing videogames. In P. Vorderer & J. Bryant (Eds.), Playing video games –motives, responses and consequences (pp. 363–378). Mahwah, NJ: LEA.

Buitelaar, J. K., Huizink, A. C., Mulder, E. J., de Medina, P. G. R., & Visser, G. H. (2003). Prenatal stress and cognitive development and temperament in infants. *Neurobiology of Aging*, *24*, S53–S60. doi:10.1016/S0197-4580(03)00050-2 PMID:12829109

Buntin, M. B., Damberg, C., Haviland, A., Kapur, K., Lurie, N., McDevitt, R., & Marquis, M. S. (2006). Consumer-directed health care: Early evidence about effects on cost and quality. *Health Affairs*, *25*(6), 516–530. doi:10.1377/hlthaff.25.w516 PMID:17062591

Burdea, G., Popescu, V., Hentz, V., & Colbert, K. (2000). Virtual reality-based orthopedic telerehabilitation. *IEEE Transactions on* Rehabilitation Engineering, *8*(3), 430–432.

Burk, D. (2005). Electronic Gaming and the Ethics of Information Ownership. *International Review of Information Ethics*, *4*, 39–45.

Burns, B. D., & Vollmeyer, R. (2002). Goal specificity effects on hypothesis testing in problem solving. *Quarterly Journal of Experimental Psychology*, *55A*(1), 241–261. doi:10.1080/02724980143000262 PMID:11873850

Burns, J. M., Davenport, T. A., Durkin, L. A., Luscombe, G. M., & Hickie, I. B. (2010). The internet as a setting for mental health service utilisation by young people. *The Medical Journal of Australia*, *192*(11), S22–S26. PMID:20528703

Burton, N. W., Pakenham, K. I., & Brown, W. J. (2009). Evaluating the effectiveness of psychosocial resilience training for heart health, and the added value of promoting physical activity: A cluster randomized trial of the READY program. *BMC Public Health*, *9*(1), 247–255. doi:10.1186/1471-2458-9-427 PMID:19930615

Buschert, V., Bokde, A. L. W., & Hampel, H. (2010). Cognitive intervention in Alzheimer disease. *Nature Reviews. Nephrology*, *6*(9), 508–517. PMID:20736983

Bushman, B. J. (2002). Does Venting Anger Feed or Extinguish the Flame? Catharsis, Rumination, Distraction, Anger, and Aggressive Responding. *Personality and Social Psychology Bulletin*, *28*(6), 724–731. doi:10.1177/0146167202289002

Cadore, E. L., Rodríguez-Mañas, L., Sinclair, A., & Izquierdo, M. (2013). Effects of different exercise interventions on risk of falls, gait ability, and balance in physically frail older adults: A systematic review. *Rejuvenation Research*, *16*(2), 105–114. doi:10.1089/rej.2012.1397 PMID:23327448

Cairns, P., Cox, A. L., Day, M., Martin, H., & Perryman, T. (2013). Who but not where: The effect of social play on immersion in digital games. *International Journal of Human-Computer Studies*, *71*(11), 1069–1077. doi:10.1016/j.ijhcs.2013.08.015

Calhoun, A. (2010). A sociopathic comedy of errors, player cruelty in open world games and developer savviness. *Gamasutra*. Retrieved from http://www.gamasutra.com.blogs/AndrewCalhoun/20101018/88273/A_Sociopathic_Comedy_of_Errors_Player_Cruelty_in_ Open_World_Games_and_Developer_Savviness

Calvo, R. A., & Peters, D. (2012). Positive computing: Technology for a wiser world. *Interactions (New York, N.Y.)*, *19*(4), 28–31. doi:10.1145/2212877.2212886

Calvo, R. A., & Peters, D. (2014). *Positive Computing: Technology for Wellbeing and Human Potential*. Cambridge, MA: MIT Press.

Calvo, R. A., & Peters, D. (2014). *Positive Computing: Technology for Well-Being and Human Potential*. MIT Press.

Calvo, R., Peters, D., Johnson, D., & Rogers, Y. (2014). Autonomy in Technology Design. In *CHI'14 Extended Abstracts on Human Factors in Computing Systems*. Toronto: ACM. doi:10.1145/2559206.2560468

Campbell, S. B., Morgan-Lopez, A. A., Cox, M. J., & McLoyd, V. C. (2009). A latent class analysis of maternal depressive symptoms over 12 years and offspring adjustment in adolescence. *Journal of Abnormal Psychology*, *118*(3), 479–493. doi:10.1037/a0015923 PMID:19685946

Carbone, S., Rickwood, D., & Tanti, C. (2011, October). Workforce shortages and their impact on Australian youth mental health service reform. *Advances in Mental Health*, *10*(1), 92–97. doi:10.5172/jamh.2011.10.1.92

Carissoli, C., Villani, D., & Riva, G. (2015). Does a meditation protocol supported by a mobile application help people reduce stress? Suggestions from a controlled pragmatic trial. *Cyberpsychology, Behavior, and Social Networking*, *18*(1), 46–53. doi:10.1089/cyber.2014.0062 PMID:25584730

Carmody, J., & Baer, R. A. (2009). How long does a mindfulness-based stress reduction program need to be? A review of class contact hours and effect sizes for psychological distress. *Journal of Clinical Psychology*, *65*(6), 627–638. doi:10.1002/jclp.20555 PMID:19309694

Carney, D. R., Cuddy, A. J. C., & Yap, A. J. (2010). Power posing: Brief nonverbal displays affect neuroendocrine levels and risk tolerance. *Psychological Science*, *21*(10), 1363–1368. doi:10.1177/0956797610383437 PMID:20855902

Carr, A., Ghosh, A., & Marks, I. M. (1988). Computer-supervised exposure treatment for phobias. *Canadian Journal of Psychiatry*, *33*(2), 112–117. PMID:3365636

Carson, S. L., & Langer, E. J. (2004). Mindful practice for clinicians and patients. In L. Haas (Ed.), *Handbook of primary care psychology* (pp. 173–186). New York, NY, USA: Oxford University Press.

Carson, S. L., & Langer, E. J. (2006). Mindfulness and self-acceptance. *Journal of Rational-Emotive & Cognitive-Behavior Therapy*, *24*(1), 29–43. doi:10.1007/s10942-006-0022-5

Cassell, J., Bickmore, T., Campbell, L., Chang, K., Vilhjàlmsson, H., & Yan, H. (1999). Embodiment in Conversational Interfaces: Rea. *Proceedings ACM SIGCHI* (pp. 520-527). ACM Press.

Castelnuovo, G., Gaggioli, A., Mantovani, F., & Riva, G. (2003). New and old tools in psychotherapy: The use of technology for the integration of traditional clinical treatments. *Psychotherapy (Chicago, Ill.)*, *40*(1-2), 33–44. doi:10.1037/0033-3204.40.1-2.33

Castelnuovo, G., Lo Priore, C., Liccione, D., & Cioffi, G. (2003). Virtual Reality based tools for the rehabilitation of cognitive and executive functions: The V-STORE. *PsychNology Journal*, *1*(3), 311–326. Retrieved from http://www.psychnology.org/pnj311(313)_castelnuovo_lopriore_liccione_cioffi_abstract.htm

Castiello, U., Lusher, D., Mari, M., Edwards, M. G., & Humphreys, G. W. (2002). Observing a human or a robotic hand grasping an object: Differential motor priming effects. In W. Prinz & B. Hommel (Eds.), *Attention and performance XIX* (pp. 314–334). Cambridge, MA: MIT Press.

Castilla, D., García-Palacios, A., Bretón-López, J., Etchemendy, E., Farfallini, L., & Botella, C. (2011). Process of design and usability evaluation of a technology web and virtual reality system for the elderly: Butler. *International Journal of Human-Computer Studies*, *71*(3), 350–362. doi:10.1016/j.ijhcs.2012.10.017

Cavanagh, K., Strauss, C., Cicconi, F., Griffiths, N., Wyper, A., & Jones, F. (2013). A randomised controlled trial of a brief online mindfulness-based intervention. *Behaviour Research and Therapy*, *51*(9), 573–578. doi:10.1016/j.brat.2013.06.003 PMID:23872699

Centers for Disease Control and Prevention. (2006). *Health, United States, 2006, with chartbook on trends in the health of Americans*. Hyattsville, MD: U.S. Department of Health and Human Services, Centers for Disease Control and Prevention, National Center for Health Statistics.

Chanowitz, B., & Langer, E. J. (1981). Premature cognitive commitment. *Journal of Personality and Social Psychology*, *41*(6), 1051–1063. doi:10.1037/0022-3514.41.6.1051 PMID:6975812

Chantry, J., & Dunford, C. (2010). How do computer assistive technologies enhance participation in childhood occupations for children with multiple and complex disabilities? A review of the current literature. *British Journal of Occupational Therapy*, *73*(8), 351–365. doi:10.4276/030802210X12813483277107

Chapman, C., Oka, S., Bradshaw, D. H., Jacobson, R. C., & Donaldson, G. W. (1999). Phasic pupil dilation response to noxious stimulation in normal volunteers: Relationship to brain evoked potentials and pain report. *Psychophysiology*, *36*(1), 44–52. doi:10.1017/S0048577299970373 PMID:10098379

Chapman, S. B., Aslan, S., Spence, J. S., Hart, J. J., Bartz, E. K., Didehbani, N., & DeFina, L. F. et al. (2015). Neural mechanisms of brain plasticity with complex cognitive training in healthy seniors. *Cerebral Cortex*, *25*(2), 396–405. doi:10.1093/cercor/bht234 PMID:23985135

Charness, N., Best, R., & Souders, D. (2012). Memory function and supportive technology. *Gerontechnology (Valkenswaard)*, *11*(1). doi:10.4017/gt.2012.11.01.006.00 PMID:24379752

Chatterton, R. T. Jr, Vogelsong, K. M., Lu, Y., Ellman, A. B., & Hudgens, G. A. (1996). Salivary amylase as a measure of endogenous adrenergic activity. *Clinical Psychologist*, *16*, 433–438. PMID:8842578

Chiesa, A., Calati, R., & Serretti, A. (2011). Does mindfulness training improve cognitive abilities? A systematic review of neuropsychological findings. *Clinical Psychology Review*, *31*(3), 449–464. doi:10.1016/j.cpr.2010.11.003 PMID:21183265

Chiesa, A., & Malinowski, P. (2011). Mindfulness-based approaches: Are they all the same? *Journal of Clinical Psychology*, *67*(4), 404–424. doi:10.1002/jclp.20776 PMID:21254062

Chi, M. T. H., Glaser, R., & Farr, M. J. (Eds.). (1988). *The nature of expertise*. Hillsdale, NJ: Lawrence Erlbaum.

Chi, M. T. H., Roscoe, R. D., Slotta, J. D., Roy, M., & Chase, C. C. (2011). Misconceived causal explanations for emergent processes. *Cognitive Science*, *36*(1), 1–61. doi:10.1111/j.1551-6709.2011.01207.x PMID:22050726

Chittaro, L., & Vianello, A. (2014). Computer-supported mindfulness: Evaluation of a mobile thought distancing application on naive meditators. *International Journal of Human-Computer Studies*, *72*(3), 337–348. doi:10.1016/j.ijhcs.2013.11.001

Cho, J., Martin, P., & Poon, L. W. (2014). Successful Aging and Subjective Well-Being Among Oldest-Old Adults. *The Gerontologist*, *55*(1), 132–143. doi:10.1093/geront/gnu074 PMID:25112594

Chou, C., & Tsai, M.-J. (2007). Gender differences in Taiwan high school students' computer game playing. *Computers in Human Behavior*, *23*(1), 812–824. doi:10.1016/j.chb.2004.11.011

Christensen, H., Griffiths, K. M., & Farrer, L. (2009). Adherence in internet interventions for anxiety and depression. *Journal of Medical Internet Research*, *11*(2), e13. doi:10.2196/jmir.1194 PMID:19403466

Christensen, H., & Hickie, I. B. (2010). E-mental health: A new era in delivery of mental health services. *The Medical Journal of Australia*, *192*(11), S2. PMID:20528702

Chunchu, K., Mauksch, L., Charles, C., Ross, V., & Pauwels, J. (2012). A patient centered care plan in the EHR: Improving collaboration and engagement. *Families, Systems & Health*, *30*(3), 199–209. doi:10.1037/a0029100 PMID:22866953

Cinaz, B., Arnrich, B., La Marca, R., & Tröster, G. (2013). Monitoring of Mental Workload Levels during an Everyday Life Office-Work Scenario. *Personal and Ubiquitous Computing Journal*, *17*(2), 229–239. doi:10.1007/s00779-011-0466-1

Cipresso, P., Albani, G., Serino, S., Pedroli, E., Pallavicini, F., Mauro, A., & Riva, G. (2014). Virtual multiple errands test (VMET): A virtual reality-based tool to detect early executive functions deficit in Parkinson's disease. *Frontiers in Behavioral Neuroscience*. PMID:25538578

Cipresso, P., Gaggioli, A., Serino, S., Raspelli, S., Vigna, C., & Pallavicini, F. et al.. (2012). Inter-Reality in the Evaluation and Treatment of Psychological Stress Disorders: The INTERSTRESS Project. *Studies in Health Technology and Informatics*, *181*, 8–11. PMID:22954818

Clare, L., Linden, D. E. J., Woods, R. T., Whitaker, R., Evans, S. J., Parkinson, C. H., & Rugg, M. D. et al. (2010). Goal-oriented cognitive rehabilitation for people with early-stage Alzheimer disease: A single-blind randomized controlled trial of clinical efficacy. *The American Journal of Geriatric Psychiatry*, *18*(10), 928–939. doi:10.1097/JGP.0b013e3181d5792a PMID:20808145

Clare, L., & Woods, B. (2003). Cognitive rehabilitation and cognitive training for early-stage Alzheimer's disease and vascular dementia. *Cochrane Database of Systematic Reviews*, (4): CD003260. PMID:14583963

Clark, D., Tanner-Smith, E., & Killingsworth, S. (2014). *Digital games, design and learning: A systematic review and meta-analysis (executive summary)*. Menlo Park, CA: SRI International.

Clarke, G., & Yarborough, B. J. (2013). Evaluating the promise of health IT to enhance/expand the reach of mental health services. *General Hospital Psychiatry*, *35*(4), 339–344. doi:10.1016/j.genhosppsych.2013.03.013 PMID:23701698

Cline, R. J., & Haynes, K. M. (2001). Consumer health information seeking on the Internet: The state of the art. *Health Education Research*, *16*(6), 671–692. doi:10.1093/her/16.6.671 PMID:11780707

Clough, P. (2003). Old and new challenges in automatic plagiarism detection. *National Plagiarism Advisory Service, 2003.* Retrieved from http://ir.shef.ac.uk/cloughie/index.html

Codispoti, M., Bradley, M. M., & Lang, P. J. (2001). Affective reactions to briefly presented pictures. *Psychophysiology, 38*(3), 474–478. doi:10.1111/1469-8986.3830474 PMID:11352135

Cogill, S. R., Caplan, H. L., Alexandra, H., Robson, K. M., & Kumar, R. (1986). Impact of maternal postnatal depression on cognitive development of young children. *BMJ, 292*(6529), 1165–1167. doi:10.1136/bmj.292.6529.1165 PMID:3085767

Cohen, S. (1986). Contrasting the Hassles Scale and the Perceived Stress Scale: Who's really measuring appraised stress? *The American Psychologist, 41*(6), 716–718. doi:10.1037/0003-066X.41.6.716

Cohen, S., Janicki-Deverts, D., & Miller, G. E. (2007). Psychological stress and disease. *Journal of the American Medical Association, 298*(14), 1685–1687. doi:10.1001/jama.298.14.1685 PMID:17925521

Cohen, S., Kamarck, T., & Mermelstein, R. (1983). A global measure of perceived stress. *Journal of Health and Social Behavior, 24*(4), 385–396. doi:10.2307/2136404 PMID:6668417

Coleman, J. S. (1988). Social Capital in the creation of human capital. *American Journal of Sociology, 94*, S95–S120. doi:10.1086/228943

Cole, S., Yoo, D., & Knutson, B. (2012). Interactivity and reward-related neural activation during a serious videogame. *PLoS ONE, 7*(3), e33909. doi:10.1371/journal.pone.0033909 PMID:22442733

Coller, B. D., & Scott, M. J. (2009). Effectiveness of using a video game to teach a course in mechanical engineering. *Computers & Education, 53*(3), 900–912. doi:10.1016/j.compedu.2009.05.012

Collin, P. J., Metcalf, A. T., Stephens-Reicher, J. C., Blanchard, M. E., Herrman, H. E., Rahilly, K., & Burns, J. M. (2011, October). ReachOut.com: The role of an online service for promoting help-seeking in young people. *Advances in Mental Health, 10*(1), 39–51. doi:10.5172/jamh.2011.10.1.39

Collins, N. L., Dunkel-Schetter, C., Lobel, M., & Scrimshaw, S. C. (1993). Social support in pregnancy: Psychosocial correlates of birth outcomes and postpartum depression. *Journal of Personality and Social Psychology, 65*(6), 1243–1258. doi:10.1037/0022-3514.65.6.1243 PMID:8295121

Colwell, J., & Payne, J. (2000). Negative correlates of computer game play in adolescents. *British Journal of Psychology, 91*(3), 295–310. doi:10.1348/000712600161844 PMID:10958576

Compas, B. E., Connor-Smith, J. K., Saltzman, H., Thomsen, A. H., & Wadsworth, M. E. (2001). Coping with stress during childhood and adolescence: Problems, progress, and potential in theory and research. *Psychological Bulletin, 127*(1), 87–127. doi:10.1037/0033-2909.127.1.87 PMID:11271757

Connaughton, D., Wadey, R., Hanton, S., & Jones, G. (2008). The development and maintenance of mental toughness: Perceptions of elite performers. *Journal of Sports Sciences, 26*(1), 83–95. doi:10.1080/02640410701310958 PMID:17852671

Conner, T. S., & Barrett, L. F. (2012). Trends in ambulatory self-report: The role of momentary experience in psychosomatic medicine. *Psychosomatic Medicine, 74*(4), 327–337. Retrieved from http://www.ncbi.nlm.nih.gov/entrez/query.fcgi?cmd=Retrieve&db=PubMed&dopt=Citation&list_uids=22582330 doi:10.1097/PSY.0b013e3182546f18 PMID:22582330

Connolly, T. M., Boyle, E. A., MacArthur, E., Hainey, T., & Boyle, J. M. (2012). A systematic literature review of empirical evidence on computer games and serious games. *Computers & Education, 59*(2), 661–686. doi:10.1016/j.compedu.2012.03.004

Conrad, D., & Kellar-Guenther, Y. (2006). Compassion fatigue, burnout, and compassion satisfaction among Colorado child protection workers. *Child Abuse & Neglect*, *30*(10), 1071–1080. doi:10.1016/j.chiabu.2006.03.009 PMID:17014908

Cook, C., Goodman, N. D., & Schulz, L. E. (2011). Where science starts: Spontaneous experiments in preschoolers' exploratory play. *Cognition*, *120*(3), 341–349. doi:10.1016/j.cognition.2011.03.003 PMID:21561605

Cooper, P. J., Tomlinson, M., Swartz, L., Landman, M., Molteno, C., Stein, A., & Murray, L. et al. (2009). Improving quality of mother-infant relationship and infant attachment in socioeconomically deprived community in South Africa: Randomised controlled trial. *BMJ (Clinical Research Ed.)*, *338*(Apr. 14), b974. doi:10.1136/bmj.b974 PMID:19366752

Cornoni-Huntley, J., Brock, D. B., Ostfeld, A. M., Taylor, J. O., & Wallace, R. B. (1986). *Established populations for epidemiologic studies of the elderly resource data book*. Washington, DC: U.S. Government Printing Office.

Corrigan, S., Zon, G. D. R., Maij, A., McDonald, N., & Mårtensson, L. (2014). An approach to collaborative learning and the serious game development. *Cognition Technology and Work*, *17*(2), 269–278. doi:10.1007/s10111-014-0289-8

Costa, D. D., Rippen, N., Dritsa, M., & Ring, A. (2003). Self-reported leisure-time physical activity during pregnancy and relationship to psychological well-being. *Journal of Psychosomatic Obstetrics and Gynaecology*, *24*(2), 111–119. doi:10.3109/01674820309042808 PMID:12854395

Coughlin, J. F., D'Ambrosio, L. A., Reimer, B., & Pratt, M. R. (2007, August). Older adult perceptions of smart home technologies: implications for research, policy & market innovations in healthcare. *Proceedings of the 29th Annual International Conference of the IEEE on Engineering in Medicine and Biology Society EMBS '07* (pp. 1810-1815). IEEE. doi:10.1109/IEMBS.2007.4352665

Cowley, B., Charles, D., Black, M., & Hickey, R. (2008). Toward an understanding of flow in video games. *Computers in Entertainment*, *6*(2), 1. doi:10.1145/1371216.1371223

Coyle, H., Traynor, V., & Solowij, N. (2014). Computerized and virtual reality cognitive training for individuals at high risk of cognitive decline: Systematic review of the literature. *The American Journal of Geriatric Psychiatry*, *23*(4), 335–359. doi:10.1016/j.jagp.2014.04.009 PMID:24998488

Coyne, J. C., Lazarus, R. S., Kutash, I. L., & Schlesinger, L. B. (1980). *Handbook on stress and anxiety*. San Francisco: Jossey-Bass.

Crockett, L. J., Iturbide, M. I., Stone, R. A. T., McGinley, M., Raffaelli, M., & Carlo, G. (2007). Acculturative stress, social support, and coping: Relations to psychological adjustment. *Cultural Diversity & Ethnic Minority Psychology*, *13*(4), 347–355. doi:10.1037/1099-9809.13.4.347 PMID:17967103

Crowe, M., Andel, R., Pedersen, N. L., Johansson, B., & Gatz, M. (2003). Does Participation in Leisure Activities Lead to Reduced Risk of Alzheimer's Disease? A Prospective Study of Swedish Twins. *The Journals of Gerontology. Series B, Psychological Sciences and Social Sciences*, *58*(5), 249–P255. doi:10.1093/geronb/58.5.P249 PMID:14507930

Csikszentmihalyi, I., & Csikszentmihalyi, M. (1988). Optimal experience: Psychological studies of flow in consciousness. New York, NY: Cambridge University Press. doi:10.1017/CBO9780511621956 doi:10.1017/CBO9780511621956

Csikszentmihalyi, M. (1975). Beyond boredom and anxiety. San Francisco, CA: Jossey-Bass.

Csikszentmihalyi, M. (1975). *Beyond Boredom and Anxiety*. San Francisco: Jossey-Bass.

Csikszentmihalyi, M. (1988). The flow experience and its significance for human psychology. In M. Csikszentmihalyi & I. S. Csikszentmihalyi (Eds.), *Optimal experience: Psychological studies of flow in consciousness*. Cambridge: Cambridge University press. doi:10.1017/CBO9780511621956.002

Csikszentmihalyi, M. (1990). *Flow: The psychology of optimal experience*. New York: HarperCollins.

Csikszentmihalyi, M. (1994). *The evolving self*. New York: Harper Perennial.

Csikszentmihalyi, M. (1997). *Creativity: Flow and the Psychology of Discovery and Invention*. New York: Harper Perennial.

Csikszentmihalyi, M. (2000). Finding Flow. The Psychology of Engagement with Everyday Life. *Journal of Happiness Studies*, *1*(1), 121–123. doi:10.1023/A:1010032312178

Csikszentmihalyi, M. (2002). *Flow: The Classic Work on How to Achieve Happiness*. London: Rider.

Csikszentmihalyi, M., & Larson, R. (1987). Validity and reliability of the Experience-Sampling Method. *The Journal of Nervous and Mental Disease*, *175*(9), 526–536. Retrieved from http://www.ncbi.nlm.nih.gov/pubmed/3655778 doi:10.1097/00005053-198709000-00004 PMID:3655778

Cuijpers, P., Donker, T., van Straten, A., Li, J., & Andersson, G. (2010). Is guided self-help as effective as face-to-face psychotherapy for depression and anxiety disorders? A systematic review and meta-analysis of comparative outcome studies. *Psychological Medicine*, *40*(12), 1943–1957. doi:10.1017/S0033291710000772 PMID:20406528

Cummings, E. M., & Davies, P. T. (1994). Maternal depression and child development. *Journal of Child Psychology and Psychiatry, and Allied Disciplines*, *35*(1), 73–112. doi:10.1111/j.1469-7610.1994.tb01133.x PMID:8163630

Currell, R., Urquhart, C., Wainwright, P., & Lewis, R. (2000). Telemedicine versus face to face patient care: Effects on professional practice and health care outcomes. *Cochrane Database of Systematic Reviews*Cd002098. doi:10.1002/14651858.cd002098 PMID:10796678

Cutrona, C. E. (1984). Social support and stress in the transition to parenthood. *Journal of Abnormal Psychology*, *93*(4), 378–390. doi:10.1037/0021-843X.93.4.378 PMID:6512084

Czaja, S. J., Charness, N., Fisk, A. D., Hertzog, C., Nair, S. N., Rogers, W., & Sharit, J. (2006). Factors predicting the use of technology: Findings from the Center for Research and Education on Aging and Technology Enhancement (CREATE). *Psychology and Aging*, *21*(2), 333–352. doi:10.1037/0882-7974.21.2.333 PMID:16768579

Damasio, A. (1999). *The Feeling of What Happens: Body, Emotion and the Making of Consciousness*. San Diego, CA: Harcourt Brace and Co, Inc.

Damasio, A. R. (1995). *L'erreur de Descartes. La raison des émotions* (O. Jacob, Ed.). Paris: Sciences.

Danaher, B. G., Milgrom, J., Seeley, J. R., Stuart, S., Schembri, C., Tyler, M. S., & Lewinsohn, P. et al. (2013). MomMoodBooster web-based intervention for postpartum depression: Feasibility trial results. *Journal of Medical Internet Research*, *15*(11), e242. doi:10.2196/jmir.2876 PMID:24191345

Dandeneau, S. D., & Baldwin, M. W. (2004). The Inhibition of Socially Rejecting Information Among People with High Versus Low Self-Esteem: The Role of Attentional Bias and the Effects of Bias Reduction Training. *Journal of Social and Clinical Psychology*, *23*(4), 584–603. doi:10.1521/jscp.23.4.584.40306

Daniels, L. M., Stupnisky, R. H., Pekrun, R., Haynes, T. L., Perry, R. P., & Newall, N. E. (2009). A longitudinal analysis of achievement goals: From affective antecedents to emotional effects and achievement outcomes. *Journal of Educational Psychology*, *101*(4), 948–963. doi:10.1037/a0016096

Davenport, T. H. (2013). *Process innovation: reengineering work through information technology*. Harvard Business Press.

David, S., Krantz, B. T., & Kiecolt-Glaser, J. (2014). *How stress affects your health*. American Psychological Association.

Davidson, R. J., Jackson, D. C., & Kalin, N. H. (2000). Emotion, plasticity, context, and regulation: Perspectives from affective neuroscience. *Psychological Bulletin*, *126*(6), 890–909. doi:10.1037/0033-2909.126.6.890 PMID:11107881

Davis, E. P., Glynn, L. M., Schetter, C. D., Hobel, C., Chicz-Demet, A., & Sandman, C. A. (2007). Prenatal exposure to maternal depression and cortisol influences infant temperament. *Journal of the American Academy of Child and Adolescent Psychiatry*, *46*(6), 737–746. doi:10.1097/chi.0b013e318047b775 PMID:17513986

Dayang, R., Awang, R., Suziah, S., & Halabt, H. (2011). VReST: An image-based virtual reality stress therapy web application. *Information Technology in Medicine and Education*, *2*, 733–737.

Dayan, J., Creveuil, C., Herlicoviez, M., Herbel, C., Baranger, E., Savoye, C., & Thouin, A. (2002). Role of anxiety and depression in the onset of spontaneous preterm labor. *American Journal of Epidemiology*, *155*(4), 293–301. doi:10.1093/aje/155.4.293 PMID:11836191

De Grove, F., Van Looy, J., Courtois, C., & De Marez, L. (2010). I play, therefore I learn? Measuring the evolution of perceived learning and game experience in the design flow of a serious game. *Proceedings of meaningful play* (pp. 1–32). East Lansing: Michigan State University.

De Wied, M., Zillman, D., & Ordman, V. (1994). The role of empathic distress in the enjoyment of cinematic tragedy. *Poetics*, *23*(1-2), 91–106. doi:10.1016/0304-422X(94)00010-4

Declercq, E. R., Sakala, C., Corry, M. P., & Applebaum, S. (2007). Listening to Mothers II: Report of the Second National US Survey of Women's Childbearing Experiences: Conducted January–February 2006 for Childbirth Connection by Harris Interactive® in partnership with Lamaze International*. *Journal of Perinatal Education*, *16*(4), 9–14. doi:10.1624/105812407X244769 PMID:18769512

Delgado-Egido, B., & Contreras-Felipe, A. (2009). Desarrollo social y emocional. En B. Delgado Egido (Ed.). (2011). Psicología del desarrollo: desde la infancia a la vejez [Social and emotional development]. (Vol. 2, pp. 35-66). Spain: McGraw-Hill.

Delle Fave, A., Massimini, F., & Bassi, M. (2011). *Psychological selection and optimal experience across cultures: Social empowerment through personal growth* (Vol. 2). Springer. doi:10.1007/978-90-481-9876-4

Dennis, T. A., & O'Toole, L. J. (2014). Mental Health on the Go: Effects of a Gamified Attention-Bias Modification Mobile Application in Trait-Anxious Adults. *Clinical Psychological Science.*

Desai, A. K., Grossberg, G. T., & Chibnall, J. T. (2010). Healthy brain aging: A road map. *Clinics in Geriatric Medicine*, *26*(1), 1–16. doi:10.1016/j.cger.2009.12.002 PMID:20176289

Deterding, S., Dixon, D., Khaled, R., & Nacke, L. (2011). From game design elements to gamefulness: defining gamification.*Proceedings of the 15th International Academic MindTrek Conference: Envisioning Future Media Environments* (pp. 9-15). ACM. doi:10.1145/2181037.2181040

Di Nuovo, S., Rispoli, L., & Genta, E. (2000). *Misurare lo stress: il test MSP e altri strumenti per una valutazione integrata* (Vol. 19). FrancoAngeli.

Diaz-Orueta, U., Alvarado, A., Gutiérrez, D., Climent, G., & Banterla, F. (2012). "Isla Calma", a Novel Virtual Reality Environment for Pain and Anxiety Distraction: Report on Usability, Acceptability, and Subjective Experience. Games for Health Journal, 1(5), 353–361. doi:10.1089/g4h.2012.0037 PubMed doi:10.1089/g4h.2012.0037 PMID:26192002

Diaz-Orueta, U., Banterla, F., & Climent, G. (2014). (in press). Isla Calma: Distracción del miedo al dolor y la ansiedad mediante realidad virtual [Isla Calma: pain and anxiety distraction by means of virtual reality]. Revista de Ansiedad y Estrés, 20(2-3), 127–141.

Diaz-Orueta, U., Facal, D., Nap, H. H., & Ranga, M. M. (2012). What is the key for older people to show interest in playing digital learning games? Initial qualitative findings from the LEAGE project on a multicultural European sample. Games for Health Journal, 1(2), 115–123. doi:10.1089/g4h.2011.0024 PubMed doi:10.1089/g4h.2011.0024 PMID:26193185

Diaz-Orueta, U., Garcia-Lopez, C., Crespo-Eguilaz, N., Sánchez-Carpintero, R., Climent, G., & Narbona, J. (2014). AULA virtual reality test as an attention measure: Convergent validity with Conners' Continuous Performance Test. Child Neuropsychology, 20(3), 328–342. doi:10.1080/09297049.2013.792332 PubMed doi:10.1080/09297049.2013.792332 PMID:23638628

Diaz-Orueta, U., Iriarte, Y., Climent, G., & Banterla, F. (2012). AULA: An ecological virtual reality test with distractors for evaluating attention in children and adolescents. Journal of Virtual Reality, 5(2), 1–20.

Diener, E. (1984). Subjective well-being. *Psychological Bulletin*, *95*(3), 542–575. doi:10.1037/0033-2909.95.3.542 PMID:6399758

Diener, E. (2000). Subjective well-being: The science of happiness and a proposal for a national index. *The American Psychologist*, *55*(1), 34–43. doi:10.1037/0003-066X.55.1.34 PMID:11392863

Diener, E., & Chan, M. Y. (2011). Happy people live longer: Subjective well-being contributes to health and longevity. *Applied Psychology: Health and Well-Being*, *3*(1), 1–43. PMID:26286968

Diener, E., Suh, E. M., Lucas, R. E., & Smith, H. L. (1999). Subjective well-being: Three decades of progress. *Psychological Bulletin*, *125*(2), 276–302. doi:10.1037/0033-2909.125.2.276

Diener, E., Suh, E., & Oishi, S. (1997). Recent findings on subjective well-being. *Indian Journal of Clinical Psychology*, *24*(1), 25–41.

Difede, J., & Hoffman, H. (2002). Virtual reality exposure therapy for World Trade Center Post Traumatic Stress Disorder. Cyberpsychology & Behavior, 5(6), 529–535. doi:10.1089/109493102321018169 PubMed doi:10.1089/109493102321018169 PMID:12556115

Dimaras, H., Kimani, K., Dimba, E. A., Gronsdahl, P., White, A., Chan, H. S., & Gallie, B. L. (2012). Retinoblastoma. *Lancet*, *379*(9824), 1436–1446. doi:10.1016/S0140-6736(11)61137-9 PMID:22414599

DiMarco, C., Covvey, H. D., Bray, P., Cowan, D., DiCiccio, V., Hovy, E., . . . Mulholland, D. (2007). The development of a natural language generation system for personalized e-health information. *Paper presented at the Medinfo 2007: the 12th World Congress on Health (Medical) Informatics; Building Sustainable Health Systems.*

Do Lee, C., Folsom, A. R., & Blair, S. N. (2003). Physical activity and stroke risk a meta-analysis. *Stroke*, *34*(10), 2475–2481. doi:10.1161/01.STR.0000091843.02517.9D PMID:14500932

Doherty, G., Coyle, D., & Sharry, J. (2012, May 5–10). Engagement with online mental health interventions: an exploratory clinical study of a treatment for depression. *Paper presented at theSIGCHI Conference on Human Factors in Computing Systems*, Austin, Texas, USA. doi:10.1145/2207676.2208602

Dover, S. (2012). Study: Number of smartphone users tops 1 billion. *CBSNews.* Retrieved from http://www.cbsnews.com/8301-205_162-57534583/study-numberof-smartphone-users-tops-1-billion

Draganski, B., Gaser, C., Kempermann, G., Kuhn, H. G., Winkler, J., Büchel, C., & May, A. (2006). Temporal and spatial dynamics of brain structure changes during extensive learning. *The Journal of Neuroscience*, *26*(23), 6314–6317. doi:10.1523/JNEUROSCI.4628-05.2006 PMID:16763039

Driskell, J. E., & Johnston, J. H. (1998). Stress exposure training. In J. A. Cannon-Bowers & E. Salas (Eds.), *Making decisions under stress: Implications for individual and team training* (pp. 191–217). Washington, DC: American Psychiatric Association. doi:10.1037/10278-007

Drozd, F., Mork, L., Nielsen, B., Raeder, S., & Bjørkli, C. A. (2014). Better Days – A randomized controlled trial of an internet-based positive psychology intervention. *The Journal of Positive Psychology*, *9*(5), 377–388. doi:10.1080/17439760.2014.910822

Duncan, J. (1986). Disorganziation of behaviour after frontal lobe damage. *Cognitive Neuropsychology*, *3*(2), 271–290. doi:10.1080/02643298608253360

Duncan, J. (1995). Attention, intelligence and the frontal lobes. In M. S. Gazzaniga (Ed.), *The cognitive neurosciences* (pp. 721–733). Cambridge, MA: MIT Press.

Duncan, J., & Owen, A. M. (2000). Common regions of the human frontal lobe recruited by diverse cognitive demands. *Trends in Neurosciences*, *23*(10), 475–483. doi:10.1016/S0166-2236(00)01633-7 PMID:11006464

Duncan, J., Seitz, R. J., Kolodny, J., Bor, D., Herzog, H., Ahmed, A., & Emslie, H. et al. (2000). A neural basis for general intelligence. *Science*, *289*(5478), 457–460. doi:10.1126/science.289.5478.457 PMID:10903207

Duncan, L. G., & Bardacke, N. (2010). Mindfulness-based childbirth and parenting education: Promoting family mindfulness during the perinatal period. *Journal of Child and Family Studies*, *19*(2), 190–202. doi:10.1007/s10826-009-9313-7 PMID:20339571

Dunkel Schetter, C. (2011). Psychological science on pregnancy: Stress processes, biopsychosocial models, and emerging research issues. *Annual Review of Psychology*, *62*(1), 531–558. doi:10.1146/annurev.psych.031809.130727 PMID:21126184

Dunkel-Schetter, C., Sagrestano, L. M., Feldman, P., & Killingsworth, C. (1996). Social support and pregnancy. In Handbook of social support and the family (pp. 375-412). Springer US. doi:10.1007/978-1-4899-1388-3_16

Dunkel-Schetter, C. (1998). Maternal stress and preterm delivery. *Prenatal and Neonatal Medicine*, *3*, 39–42.

Dunn, C., Hanieh, E., Roberts, R., & Powrie, R. (2012). Mindful pregnancy and childbirth: Effects of a mindfulness-based intervention on women's psychological distress and well-being in the perinatal period. *Archives of Women's Mental Health*, *15*(2), 139–143. doi:10.1007/s00737-012-0264-4 PMID:22382281

Dunn, E. W., Aknin, L. B., & Norton, M. I. (2008). Spending money on others promotes happiness. *Science*, *319*(5870), 1687–1688. doi:10.1126/science.1150952 PMID:18356530

Dzhafarova, O. A., Donskaya, O. G., & Zubkov, A. A. (2007). Biofeedback computer games. *Biomedical Engineering*, *41*(4), 186–190. doi:10.1007/s10527-007-0040-3

Eberth, J., & Sedlmeier, P. (2012). The effects of mindfulness meditation: A meta-analysis. *Mindfulness*, *3*(3), 174–189. doi:10.1007/s12671-012-0101-x

Edelman, C. L., Mandle, C. L., & Kudzma, E. C. (2013). *Health Promotion Throughout the Life Span*. Elsevier Health Sciences.

Edery, D., & Mollick, E. (2009). *Changing the game: how video games are transforming the future of business*. Upper Saddle River, NJ: FT Press.

Eich, E., Ng, J. T., Macaulay, D., Percy, A. D., & Grebneva, I. (2007). Combining music with thought to change mood. In J.A. Cohen, & J.J.B. Allen (Eds.), *Handbook of emotion elicitation and assessment* (pp. 124–136). New York: Oxford University Press.

El Kaliouby, R., & Robinson, P. (2005). Real-time inference of complex mental states from facial expressions and head gestures. In B. Kisačanin, V. Pavlović, & T. S. Huang (Eds.), *Real-time vision for human–computer interaction* (pp. 181–200). New York: Springer. doi:10.1007/0-387-27890-7_11

Elderly self-care based on self-check of health conditions and self-fitness at home. (2015). ELF@Home. Retrieved from http://www.elfathome.eu

Elliot, A. J., & Thrash, T. M. (2002). Approach-avoidance motivation in personality: Approach and avoidance temperaments and goals. *Journal of Personality and Social Psychology*, *82*(5), 804–818. doi:10.1037/0022-3514.82.5.804 PMID:12003479

Ellul, J. (1967). *The technological society*. New York: A.A. Knopf.

Emmelkamp, P., Krijn, M., Hulsbosch, A., De Vries, S., Schuemie, M., & Van der Mast, C. (2002). Virtual reality treatment versus exposure in vivo: A comparative evaluation in acrophobia. *Behaviour Research and Therapy*, *40*(5), 509–516. doi:10.1016/S0005-7967(01)00023-7 PMID:12038644

Emmons, R. A., & McCullough, M. E. (2003). Counting blessings versus burdens: An experimental investigation of gratitude and subjective well-being in daily life. *Journal of Personality and Social Psychology*, *84*(2), 377–389. Retrieved from http://www.ncbi.nlm.nih.gov/pubmed/12585811 doi:10.1037/0022-3514.84.2.377 PMID:12585811

Endsley, M. R. (1988). Design and evaluation for situation awareness enhancement. *Proceedings of the Human Factors Society 32nd Annual Meeting* (pp. 97–101). Santa Monica, CA: Human Factors Society. (1994). Situational awareness in dynamic human decision making: Measurement. In R. D. Gilson, D. J. Garland & J. M. Koone (Eds.), *Situational awareness in complex systems* (pp. 79–97). Daytona Beach, FL: Embry-Riddle Aeronautical University Press.

Epel, E., Daubenmier, J., Moskowitz, J. T., Folkman, S., & Blackburn, E. (2009). Can meditation slow rate of cellular aging? Cognitive stress, mindfulness, and telomeres. *Annals of the New York Academy of Sciences*, *1172*(1), 34–53. doi:10.1111/j.1749-6632.2009.04414.x PMID:19735238

Ericsson, K. A., Charness, N., Feltovich, P. J., & Hoffman, R. R. (2006). *The Cambridge handbook of expertise and expert performance*. Cambridge, UK: Cambridge University Press. doi:10.1017/CBO9780511816796

Ermi, L., & Mäyrä, F. (2005). Fundamental Components of the Gameplay Experience: Analysing Immersion. In S. De Castell & J. Jenson (Eds.), *Worlds in Play. International on Digital Games* (pp. 15–27). New York, NY: Peter Lang Publishing.

Etchemendy, E., Baños, R. M., Botella, C., Castilla, D., Alcañiz, M., Rasal, P., & Farfallini, L. (2011). An e-health platform for the elderly population: The Butler system. *Computers & Education*, *56*(1), 275–279. doi:10.1016/j.compedu.2010.07.022

European Commission. (2009). *2009 Ageing report: economic and budgetary projections for the EU-27 Member States (2008–2060)*. Luxembourg: Office for Official Publications of the European Communities.

Eysenbach, G. (2005). The law of attrition. *Journal of Medical Internet Research*, *7*(1), e11. doi:10.2196/jmir.7.1.e11 PMID:15829473

Eysenbach, G., Powell, J., Englesakis, M., Rizo, C., & Stern, A. (2004). Health related virtual communities and electronic support groups: Systematic review of the effects of online peer to peer interactions. *BMJ (Clinical Research Ed.)*, *328*(7449), 1166. doi:10.1136/bmj.328.7449.1166 PMID:15142921

Fagundo, A.B., Santamaría, J.J., Forcano, K., Giner-Bartolomé, C., Jiménez-Murcia, S., Sánchez, I. et al. (2013). Video game therapy for emotional regulation and impulsivity control in a series of treated cases with bulimia nervosa. European Eating Disorders Review: the journal of the Eating Disorders Association, 21(6), 493-499.

Farfallini, L. (2014). Validación de una Intervención Positiva auto-aplicada orientada al bienestar: EARTH of Wellbeing [Doctoral thesis]. Universitat Jaume I.

Feagin, S. L. (1983). The pleasures of tragedy. *American Philosophical Quarterly*, *20*(1), 95–104.

Feldstein, S., Dohm, F., & Crown, C. L. (2001). Gender and speech rate in the perception of competence and social attractiveness. *The Journal of Social Psychology*, *141*(6), 785–806. doi:10.1080/00224540109600588 PMID:11827225

Fernández-Aranda, F., Jiménez-Murcia, S., Santamaría, J. J., Gunnard, K., Soto, A., Kalapanidas, E., . . . Penelo, E. (2012). Video games as a complementary therapy tool in mental disorders: PlayMancer, a European multicentre study. Journal of Mental Health (Abingdon, England), 21(4), 364–374. doi:10.3109/09638237.2012.664302 PubMed doi:10.3109/09638237.2012.664302 PMID:22548300

Ferri, C. P., Prince, M., Brayne, C., Brodaty, H., Fratiglioni, L., Ganguli, M., & Huang, Y. et al. (2006). Global prevalence of dementia: A Delphi consensus study. *Lancet*, *366*(9503), 2112–2117. doi:10.1016/S0140-6736(05)67889-0 PMID:16360788

Field, T. S., Gilman, B. H., Subramanian, S., Fuller, J. C., Bates, D. W., & Gurwitz, J. H. (2005). The costs associated with adverse drug events among older adults in the ambulatory setting. *Medical Care*, *43*(12), 1171–1176. doi:10.1097/01.mlr.0000185690.10336.70 PMID:16299427

Field, T., Diego, M. A., Hernandez-Reif, M., Schanberg, S., & Kuhn, C. (2004). Massage therapy effects on depressed pregnant women. *Journal of Psychosomatic Obstetrics and Gynaecology*, *25*(2), 115–122. doi:10.1080/01674820412331282231 PMID:15715034

Field, T., Diego, M., & Hernandez-Reif, M. (2006). Prenatal depression effects on the fetus and newborn: A review. *Infant Behavior and Development*, *29*(3), 445–455. doi:10.1016/j.infbeh.2006.03.003 PMID:17138297

Field, T., Hemandez-Reif, M., Hart, S., Theakston, H., Schanberg, S., & Kuhn, C. (1999). Pregnant women benefit from massage therapy. *Journal of Psychosomatic Obstetrics and Gynaecology*, *20*(1), 31–38. doi:10.3109/01674829909075574 PMID:10212885

Field, T., Hernandez-Reif, M., Diego, M., Schanberg, S., & Kuhn, C. (2006). Stability of mood states and biochemistry across pregnancy. *Infant Behavior and Development*, *29*(2), 262–267. doi:10.1016/j.infbeh.2005.12.009 PMID:17138281

Finfgeld-Connett, D. (2014). Use of content analysis to conduct knowledge-building and theory-generating qualitative systematic reviews. *Qualitative Research*, *14*(3), 341–352. doi:10.1177/1468794113481790

Fisher, G., Giaccardi, E., Eden, H., Sugimoto, M., & Ye, Y. (2005). Beyond binary choices: Integrating individual and social creativity. *International Journal of Human-Computer Studies*, *12*, 428–512.

Fiske, S. T., Cuddy, A. J. C., Glick, P., & Xu, J. (2002). A model of (often mixed) stereotype content: Competence and warmth respectively follow from perceived status and competition. *Journal of Personality and Social Psychology*, *82*(6), 878–902. doi:10.1037/0022-3514.82.6.878 PMID:12051578

Fjorback, L. O., Arendt, M., Ørnbøl, E., Fink, P., & Walach, H. (2011). Mindfulness-Based Stress Reduction and Mindfulness-Based Cognitive Therapy–a systematic review of randomized controlled trials. *Acta Psychiatrica Scandinavica*, *124*(2), 102–119. doi:10.1111/j.1600-0447.2011.01704.x PMID:21534932

Fleming, M. J., & Rickwood, D. J. (2001). Effects of violent versus non-violent video games on children's arousal, aggressive mood, and positive mood. *Journal of Applied Social Psychology*, *31*(10), 2047–2071. doi:10.1111/j.1559-1816.2001.tb00163.x

Fletcher, K. (2010). Towards a computational compensatory control model of mental workload [Unpublished manuscript]. University of Queensland, Brisbane.

Flin, R., & Maran, N. (2004). Identifying and training non-technical skills for teams in acute medicine. *Quality & Safety in Health Care*, *13*(1suppl_1), 80–84. doi:10.1136/qshc.2004.009993 PMID:15465960

Flin, R., & Martin, L. (2001). Behavioural markers for crew resource management: A review of current practice. *The International Journal of Aviation Psychology*, *11*(1), 95–118. doi:10.1207/S15327108IJAP1101_6

Flores, F., Graves, M., Hartfield, B., & Winograd, T. (1988). Computer systems and the design of organizational interaction. *ACM Transactions on Information Systems*, *6*(2), 153–172. doi:10.1145/45941.45943

Folkman, S. (2008). The case for positive emotions in the stress process. *Anxiety, Stress, and Coping*, *21*(1), 3–14. doi:10.1080/10615800701740457 PMID:18027121

Folkman, S. (2009). Commentary on the special section "theory-based approaches to stress and coping" questions, answers, issues, and next steps in stress and coping research. *European Psychologist*, *14*(1), 72–77. doi:10.1027/1016-9040.14.1.72

Folstein, M. F., Folstein, S. E., & McHugh, P. R. (1975). "Mini-mental state": A practical method for grading the cognitive state of patients for the clinician. *Journal of Psychiatric Research*, *12*(3), 189–198. doi:10.1016/0022-3956(75)90026-6 PMID:1202204

Foo, M., Uy, M. A., & Baron, R. A. (2009). How do feelings influence effort? An empirical study of entrepreneurs' affect and venture effort. *The Journal of Applied Psychology*, *94*(4), 1086–1094. doi:10.1037/a0015599 PMID:19594247

Ford, M., Wyeth, P., & Johnson, D. (2012, November). Self-determination theory as applied to the design of a software learning system using whole-body controls.*Proceedings of the 24th Australian Computer-Human Interaction Conference* (pp. 146-149). ACM. doi:10.1145/2414536.2414562

Fortin, S., Godbout, L., & Braun, C. M. J. (2003). Cognitive structure of executive deficits in frontally lesioned head trauma patients performing activities of daily living. *Cortex*, *39*(2), 273–291. doi:10.1016/S0010-9452(08)70109-6 PMID:12784889

Fox, J., & Bailenson, J. N. (2009). Virtual self-modeling: The effects of vicarious reinforcement and identification on exercise behaviors. *Media Psychology*, *12*(1), 1–25. doi:10.1080/15213260802669474

Frederickson, B. (2009). *Positivity: Groundbreaking research reveals how to embrace the hidden strength of positive emotions, overcome negativity, and thrive*. New York: Crown Archetype.

Fredrickson, B. L. (2000). Cultivating positive emotions to optimize health and well-being. *Prevention & Treatment*, *3*(1). doi:10.1037/1522-3736.3.1.31a

Fredrickson, B. L. (2001). The role of positive emotions in positive psychology. The broaden-and-build theory of positive emotions. *The American Psychologist*, *56*(3), 218–226. doi:10.1037/0003-066X.56.3.218 PMID:11315248

Fredrickson, B. L. (2004). The broaden-and-build theory of positive emotions. *Philosophical Transactions of the Royal Society of London. Series B, Biological Sciences*, *359*(1449), 1367–1378. doi:10.1098/rstb.2004.1512 PMID:15347528

Fredrickson, B. L., Danner, D., & Snowdon, D. (2003). The Value of Positive Emotions. *American Scientist*, *91*(4), 330–335. doi:10.1511/2003.4.330

Fredrickson, B. L., & Losada, M. F. (2005). Positive affect and the complex dynamics of human flourishing. *The American Psychologist*, *60*(7), 678–686. doi:10.1037/0003-066X.60.7.678 PMID:16221001

Free, C., Phillips, G., Felix, L., Galli, L., Patel, V., & Edwards, P. (2010). The effectiveness of M-health technologies for improving health and health services: A systematic review protocol. *BMC Research Notes*, *3*(1), 250. doi:10.1186/1756-0500-3-250 PMID:20925916

Free, C., Phillips, G., Galli, L., Watson, L., Felix, L., Edwards, P., & Haines, A. et al. (2013). The effectiveness of mobile-health technology-based health behaviour change or disease management interventions for health care consumers: A systematic review. *PLoS Medicine*, *10*(1), e1001362. doi:10.1371/journal.pmed.1001362 PMID:23349621

Freeman, D. (2007). Studying and treating schizophrenia using virtual reality: A new paradigm. Schizophrenia Bulletin, 34(4), 605–610. doi:10.1093/schbul/sbn020 PubMed doi:10.1093/schbul/sbn020 PMID:18375568

Freeman, D. (2004). Creating emotion in games. *Computers in Entertainment*, *2*(3), 15. doi:10.1145/1027154.1027179

Fried, L. P., Tangen, C. M., Walston, J., Newman, A. B., Hirsch, C., Gottdiener, J., & Burke, G. et al. (2001). Frailty in older adults evidence for a phenotype. *The Journals of Gerontology. Series A, Biological Sciences and Medical Sciences*, *56*(3), M146–M157. doi:10.1093/gerona/56.3.M146 PMID:11253156

Fried, L. P., Tangen, C. M., Walston, J., Newman, A. B., Hirsch, C., Gottdiener, J., & McBurnie, M. A. et al. (2001). Frailty in older adults: Evidence for a phenotype. *Journal of Gerontology*, *56A*, M146–M156. PMID:11253156

Friedman, B., Kahn, P. H., Jr., & Borning, A. (2006). Value sensitive design and information systems. In Human-computer interaction in management information systems: Foundations (Vol. 4). ME Sharpe.

Friesen, G. M., Jannett, T. C., Jadallah, M. A., Yates, S. L., Quint, S. R., & Nagle, H. T. (1990). A comparison of the noise sensitivity of nine QRS detection algorithms. *Biomedical Engineering. IEEE Transactions on*, *37*(1), 85–98.

Frijda, N. H. (1993). *Appraisal and beyond: Special issue of Cognition and Emotion*. Hillsdale, NJ: Erlbaum.

Frome, J. (2007). Eight Ways Videogames Generate Emotion. *Paper presented at DIGRA,* Tokyo, Japan (pp. 831–835).

Fulleron, T. (2014). *Game Design Workshop: a Playcentric Approach to Creating Innovative Games*. Taylor & Francis Press.

Gable, S. L., Reis, H. T., Impett, E. A., & Asher, E. R. (2004). What do you do when things go right? The intrapersonal and interpersonal benefits of sharing positive events. *Journal of Personality and Social Psychology*, *87*(2), 228–245. doi:10.1037/0022-3514.87.2.228 PMID:15301629

Gaggioli, A. (2004). Optimal Experience in Ambient Intelligence. In G. Riva, F. Vatalaro, F. Davide, & M. Alcañiz (Eds.), Ambient Intelligence: The evolution of technology, communication and cognition towards the future of human-computer interaction (pp. 35–43). Amsterdam: IOS Press. Retrieved from http://www.emergingcommunication.com/volume6.html

Gaggioli, A., Bassi, M., & Delle Fave, A. (2003). Quality of Experience in Virtual Environments. In G. Riva, W. A. IJsselsteijn, & F. Davide (Eds.), Being There: Concepts, effects and measurement of user presence in synthetic environment (pp. 121–135). Amsterdam: Ios Press. Retrieved from http://www.emergingcommunication.com/volume5.html

Gaggioli, A., Milani, L., Mazzoni, E., & Riva, G. (2011). Networked Flow: A Framework for Understanding the Dynamics of Creative Collaboration in Educational and Training Settings. *The Open Education Journal, 4*(Suppl 2:M2), 107-115.

Gaggioli, A., Mazzoni, E., Milani, L., & Riva, G. (2015). The creative link: Investigating the relationship between social network indices, creative performance and flow in blended teams. *Computers in Human Behavior*, *42*, 157–166. doi:10.1016/j.chb.2013.12.003

Gaggioli, A., Milani, L., Mazzoni, E., & Riva, G. (2013). *Networked Flow: Towards an Understanding of Creative Networks*. Dordrecht: Springer. doi:10.1007/978-94-007-5552-9

Gaggioli, A., Morganti, L., Bonfiglio, S., Scaratti, C., Cipresso, P., Serino, S., & Riva, G. (2014). Intergenerational Group Reminiscence: A Potentially Effective Intervention to Enhance Elderly Psychosocial Wellbeing and to Improve Children's Perception of Aging. *Educational Gerontology*, *40*(7), 486–498. doi:10.1080/03601277.2013.844042

Gaggioli, A., Pallavicini, F., Morganti, L., Serino, S., Scaratti, C., Briguglio, M., & Bernava, G. et al. (2014). Experiential virtual scenarios with real-time monitoring (interreality) for the management of psychological stress: A block randomized controlled trial. *Journal of Medical Internet Research*, *16*(7), e167. doi:10.2196/jmir.3235 PMID:25004803

Gaggioli, A., Pioggia, G., Tartarisco, G., Baldus, G., Corda, D., Cipresso, P., & Riva, G. (2013). A mobile data collection platform for mental health research. *Personal and Ubiquitous Computing Journal*, *17*(2), 241–251. doi:10.1007/s00779-011-0465-2

Gaggioli, A., & Riva, G. (2014). Psychological treatments: Smart tools boost mental-health care. *Nature*, *512*(7512), 28. doi:10.1038/512028b PMID:25100471

Gagné. (2014). *Marylene. The Oxford handbook of work engagement, motivation, and self-determination theory*. Oxford University Press.

Gagné, M. (2003). The role of autonomy support and autonomy orientation in prosocial behavior engagement. *Motivation and Emotion*, *27*(3), 199–223. doi:10.1023/A:1025007614869

Gajadhar, B., de Kort, Y. W., & IJsselsteijn, W. (2008). Shared Fun Is Doubled Fun: Player Enjoyment as a Function of Social Setting. In P. Markopoulos, B. de Ruyter, W. IJsselsteijn, & D. Rowland (Eds.), *Fun and Games SE - 11* (Vol. 5294, pp. 106–117). Berlin, Germany: Springer Berlin Heidelberg. doi:10.1007/978-3-540-88322-7_11

Gallagher, P. S., & Prestwich, S. H. (2013). Can game design be leveraged to enhance cognitive adaptability? Electronic Journal of e-Learning, (Special Edition on Games Based Learning).

Gallagher, R., & Jeannerod, M. (2002). From action to interaction. *Journal of Consciousness Studies*, *9*, 3–26.

Gallese, V., Fadiga, L., Fogassi, L., & Rizzolatti, G. (1996). Action recognition in the premotor cortex. *Brain*, *119*(2), 593–609. doi:10.1093/brain/119.2.593 PMID:8800951

Gamberini, L., Barresi, G., Majer, A., & Scarpetta, F. (2008). A game a day keeps the doctor away: A short review of computer games in mental healthcare. Journal of Cyber Therapy and Rehabilitation, 1(2), 127–145.

Gambetti, R., & Quigley, S. (Eds.). (2012). *Managing Corporate Communication: A Cross-cultural Approach. Palgrave*. Macmillan.

Ganglbauer, E., Schrammel, J., Deutsch, S., & Tscheligi, M. (2009). Applying psychophysiological methods for measuring user experience: possibilities, challenges and feasibility. *Proceedings of theWorkshop on user experience evaluation methods in product development*.

Gao, L. L., Larsson, M., & Luo, S. Y. (2013). Internet use by Chinese women seeking pregnancy-related information. *Midwifery*, *29*(7), 730–735. doi:10.1016/j.midw.2012.07.003 PMID:22958935

García García, J., & Larrión Zugasti, J. L. (2007). *Deterioro cognitivo y fragilidad. In J.M.L. Arrieta, & F.J.G. Garcia (Eds.), El anciano con demencia* (pp. 59–83). Madrid: Sociedad Española de Medicina Geriátrica.

García-Betances, R. I., Arredondo Waldmeyer, M. T., Fico, G., & Cabrera-Umpiérrez, M. F. (2015). A succinct overview of virtual reality technology use in Alzheimer's disease. *Name: Frontiers in Aging Neuroscience*, *7*, 80. PMID:26029101

García-Betances, R. I., Jiménez-Mixco, V., Arredondo, M. T., & Cabrera-Umpiérrez, M. F. (2015). Using Virtual Reality for Cognitive Training of the Elderly. *American Journal of Alzheimer's Disease and Other Dementias*, *30*(1), 49–54. doi:10.1177/1533317514545866 PMID:25107931

Gardner, J. E. (1991). Can the Mario Bros. help? Nintendo games as an adjunct in psychotherapy with children. Psychotherapy (Chicago, Ill.), 28(4), 667–670. doi:10.1037/0033-3204.28.4.667 doi:10.1037/0033-3204.28.4.667

Garris, R., Ahlers, R., & Driskell, J. E. (2002). Games, motivation, and learning: A research and practice model. *Simulation & Gaming*, *33*(4), 441–467. doi:10.1177/1046878102238607

Garside, R. (2013). Systematic review and synthesis of qualitative research. In Ziebland S., Coulter A., Calabrese J.D., & Lokock L. (Ed.), Understanding and using health experiences: Improving Patient Care (104-135). USA: Oxford Scholarship Online. doi:10.1093/acprof:oso/9780199665372.003.0011

Gaver, W., Beaver, J., & Benford, S. (2003). Ambiguity as a resource for design. *Paper presented at CHI - Designing Design,* Fort Lauderdale, USA (pp. 233–240). doi:10.1145/642611.642653

Gedde-Dahl, M., & Fors, E. A. (2012). Impact of self-administered relaxation and guided imagery techniques during final trimester and birth. *Complementary Therapies in Clinical Practice*, *18*(1), 60–65. doi:10.1016/j.ctcp.2011.08.008 PMID:22196576

Gee, J. P. (2005). Good Video Games and Good Learning. *Phi Kappa Phi Forum, 85*, 33–37. doi:10.1177/1555412008317309

Gee, J. P. (2003). *What Video Games Have to Teach Us About Learning and Literacy* (2nd ed.). London, UK: Palgrave Macmillan.

Gentile, D. A., & Anderson, C. A. (2003). Violent video games: The newest media violence hazard. *Media Violence and Children*, 131–152.

Gentile, D. A., Lynch, P. J., Linder, J. R., & Walsh, D. A. (2004). The effects of violent video game habits on adolescent hostility, aggressive behaviors, and school performance. *Journal of Adolescence*, *27*(1), 5–22. doi:10.1016/j.adolescence.2003.10.002 PMID:15013257

Ghani, J. A., & Deshpande, S. P. (1994). Task characteristics and the experience of optimal flow in Human-Computer Interaction. *The Journal of Psychology*, *128*(4), 381–391. doi:10.1080/00223980.1994.9712742

Giakoumis, D., Drosou, A., Cipresso, P., Tzovaras, D., Hassapis, G., Gaggioli, A., & Riva, G. (2012). Using activity-related behavioural features towards more effective automatic stress detection. *PLoS ONE*, *7*(9), e43571. doi:10.1371/journal.pone.0043571 PMID:23028461

Gianakis, M., & Carey, T. A. (2011). An interview study investigating experiences of psychological change without psychotherapy. *Psychology and Psychotherapy: Theory, Research and Practice*, *84*(4), 442–457. doi:10.1111/j.2044-8341.2010.02002.x PMID:22903885

Gibson, K. L., Coulson, H., Miles, R., Kakekakekung, C., Daniels, E., & O'donnell, S. (2011). Conversations on telemental health: Listening to remote and rural First Nations communities. *Rural and Remote Health*, *11*(2), 1656–1674. PMID:21553998

Gilleade, K. M., & Dix, A. (2004). Using frustration in the design of adaptive videogames.*Proceedings of the 2004 ACM SIGCHI International Conference on Advances in Computer Entertainment Technology - ACE '04* (pp. 228–232). doi:10.1145/1067343.1067372

Girard, C., Ecalle, J., & Magnan, A. (2013). Serious games as new educational tools: How effective are they? A meta-analysis of recent studies. *Journal of Computer Assisted Learning*, *29*(3), 207–219. doi:10.1111/j.1365-2729.2012.00489.x

Girone, M., Burdea, G., Bouzit, M., Popescu, V., & Deutsch, J. E. (2000). Orthopedic rehabilitation using the" Rutgers ankle" interface. *Studies in Health Technology and Informatics*, 2000, 89–95. PMID:10977590

Glanz, K., Rizzo, A. S., & Graap, K. (2003). Virtual reality for psychotherapy: Current reality and future possibilities. *Psychotherapy (Chicago, Ill.)*, *40*(1-2), 55–67. doi:10.1037/0033-3204.40.1-2.55

Glaser, B., & Strauss, A. (1967). *Grounded Theory: The Discovery of Grounded Theory*. New York: de Gruyter.

Glean, N. (2005). Growing complex games. *Paper presented at DiGRA conference Changing Views: Words in Play*, Vancouver.

Gluck, K. A., & Gunzelmann, G. (2013). Computational process modeling and cognitive stressors: Background and prospects for application in cognitive engineering. In J. D. Lee & A. Kirlik (Eds.), *The Oxford handbook of cognitive engineering* (pp. 424–432). New York: Oxford University Press. doi:10.1093/oxfordhb/9780199757183.013.0029

Glück, T. M., & Maercker, A. (2011). A randomized controlled pilot study of a brief web-based mindfulness training. *BMC Psychiatry*, *11*(1), 175. doi:10.1186/1471-244X-11-175 PMID:22067058

Goetzel, R. Z., & Ozminkowski, R. J. (2008). The health and cost benefits of work site health-promotion programs. *Annual Review of Public Health*, *29*(1), 303–323. doi:10.1146/annurev.publhealth.29.020907.090930 PMID:18173386

Goh, D. H., Ang, R. P., & Tan, H. C. (2008). Strategies for designing effective psychotherapeutic gaming interventions for children and adolescents. Computers in Human Behavior, 24(5), 2217–2235. doi:10.1016/j.chb.2007.10.007 doi:10.1016/j.chb.2007.10.007

Goodman, C. A., Jimison, H. B., & Pavel, M. (2002). Participatory design for home care technology.*Proceedings of the Second Joint* (Vol. 3, pp. 1873-1874). Houston, USA: IEEE.

Gopnik, A., & Schulz, L. E. (2007). *Causal learning: Psychology, philosophy and computation*. Oxford: Oxford University Press. doi:10.1093/acprof:oso/9780195176803.001.0001

Gopnik, A., & Wellman, H. M. (2012). Reconstructing constructivism: Causal models, Bayesian learning mechanisms, and the theory. *Psychological Bulletin*, *138*(6), 1085–1108. doi:10.1037/a0028044 PMID:22582739

Gorini, A., Capideville, C. S., De Leo, G., Mantovani, F., & Riva, G. (2010). The Role of Immersion and Narrative in Mediated Presence: The Virtual Hospital Experience. *Cyberpsychology, Behavior, and Social Networking*. doi:10.1089/cyber.2010.0100 PMID:20649451

Gorini, A., Gaggioli, A., Vigna, C., & Riva, G. (2008). A second life for eHealth: Prospects for the use of 3-D virtual worlds in clinical psychology. *Journal of Medical Internet Research*, *10*(3), e21. doi:10.2196/jmir.1029 PMID:18678557

Goyal, M., Haythornthwaite, J., Levine, D., Becker, D., Vaidya, D., Hill-Briggs, F., & Ford, D. (2010). Intensive meditation for refractory pain and symptoms. *Journal of Alternative and Complementary Medicine (New York, N.Y.)*, *16*(6), 627–631. doi:10.1089/acm.2009.0372 PMID:20569029

Goyal, M., Singh, S., Sibinga, E. M., Gould, N. F., Rowland-Seymour, A., Sharma, R., & Shihab, H. M. et al. (2014). Meditation programs for psychological stress and well-being: A systematic review and meta-analysis. *JAMA Internal Medicine*, *174*(3), 357–368. doi:10.1001/jamainternmed.2013.13018 PMID:24395196

Gozli, D. G., Bavelier, D., & Pratt, J. (2014). The effect of action video game playing on sensorimotor learning: Evidence from a movement tracking task. *Human Movement Science*, *38C*, 152–162. doi:10.1016/j.humov.2014.09.004 PMID:25318081

Graffigna, G. (2009). *Interpersonal exchanges about HIV-Aids through different media: A cross-cultural comparison.* Saarbrücken: VDM Verlag.

Graffigna, G., Barello, S., Bonanomi, A., & Lozza, E. (2015). Measuring patient engagement: Development and psychometric properties of the Patient Health Engagement (PHE) scale. *Frontiers in Psychology*, March, 6. PMID:25870566

Graffigna, G., Barello, S., Libreri, C., & Bosio, C. A. (2014). How to engage type-2 diabetic patients in their own health management: Implications for clinical practice. *BMC Public Health*, *14*(1), 648. doi:10.1186/1471-2458-14-648 PMID:24966036

Graffigna, G., Barello, S., & Riva, G. (2013a). How to make health information technology effective: The challenge of patient engagement. *Archives of Physical Medicine and Rehabilitation*, *94*(10), 2034–2035. doi:10.1016/j.apmr.2013.04.024 PMID:24075414

Graffigna, G., Barello, S., & Riva, G. (2013c). Technologies for patient engagement. *Health Affairs (Project Hope)*, *32*(6), 1172. doi:10.1377/hlthaff.2013.0279 PMID:23733998

Graffigna, G., Barello, S., Riva, G., & Bosio, A. C. (2014). Patient Engagement: The Key to Redesign the Exchange Between the Demand and Supply for Healthcare in the Era of Active Ageing. *Studies in Health Technology and Informatics*, *203*, 85–95. PMID:26630515

Graffigna, G., Barello, S., & Triberti, S. (2015). *Patient Engagement: A consumer-centered model to innovate healthcare.* Warsaw, Poland: De Gruyter Open. doi:10.1515/9783110452440

Graffigna, G., Barello, S., Triberti, S., Wiederhold, B. K., Bosio, A. C., & Riva, G. (2014). Enabling eHealth as a pathway for patient engagement: A toolkit for medical practice. *Studies in Health Technology and Informatics*, *199*, 13–21. PMID:24875682

Graffigna, G., Barello, S., Wiederhold, B. K., Bosio, A. C., & Riva, G. (2013). Positive technology as a driver for health engagement. *Studies in Health Technology and Informatics*, *191*, 9–17. PMID:23792833

Granic, I., Lobel, A., & Engels, R. C. M. E. (2014). The benefits of playing video games. *The American Psychologist*, *69*(1), 66–78. doi:10.1037/a0034857 PMID:24295515

Grant, K. A., McMahon, C., & Austin, M. P. (2008). Maternal anxiety during the transition to parenthood: A prospective study. *Journal of Affective Disorders*, *108*(1), 101–111. doi:10.1016/j.jad.2007.10.002 PMID:18001841

Grasby, P. M., Koepp, M. J., Gunn, R. N., Lawrence, A. D., Cunningham, V. J., Dagher, A., & Bench, C. J. et al. (1998). Evidence for striatal dopamine release during a video game. *Nature*, *393*(6682), 266–268. doi:10.1038/30498 PMID:9607763

Grassi, A., Gaggioli, A., & Riva, G. (2009). The green valley: The use of mobile narratives for reducing stress in commuters. *Cyberpsychology & Behavior*, *12*(2), 155–161. doi:10.1089/cpb.2008.0156 PMID:19275475

Grassi, A., Gaggioli, A., & Riva, G. (2011). New technologies to manage exam anxiety.[Randomized Controlled Trial]. *Studies in Health Technology and Informatics*, *167*, 57–62. PMID:21685642

Gray, J. A. (1990). Brain systems that mediate both emotion and cognition. *Cognition & Emotion. Special Issue: Development of Relationships Between Emotions and Cognition*, *4*(3), 269–288.

Green Paper on mobile-health (mHealth). (2014, June). Brussels, Belgium.

Greenberg, L. S. (2004). Emotion–focused therapy. *Clinical Psychology & Psychotherapy*, *11*(1), 3–16. doi:10.1002/cpp.388

Green, C. S., Pouget, A., & Bavelier, D. (2010). Improved probabilistic inference as a general learning mechanism with action video games. *Current Biology*, *20*(17), 1573–1579. doi:10.1016/j.cub.2010.07.040 PMID:20833324

Greener, I. (2012). Consumerism in Health Policy: Where Did it comes from and how can it work. In A. Hann (Ed.), *Health Policy and Politics* (pp. 57–81). Aschgate, UK: Ashgate.

Greenwood, P. M. (2007). Functional plasticity in cognitive aging: Review and hypothesis. *Neuropsychology*, *21*(6), 657–673. doi:10.1037/0894-4105.21.6.657 PMID:17983277

Greitemeyer, T., Osswald, S., & Brauer, M. (2010). Playing prosocial video games increases empathy and decreases schadenfreude. *Emotion (Washington, D.C.)*, *10*(6), 796–802. doi:10.1037/a0020194 PMID:21171755

Griffiths, K., Farrer, L., & Christensen, H. (2010). The efficacy of internet interventions for depres- sion and anxiety disorders: A review of randomised controlled trials. *The Medical Journal of Australia*, *192*, S4–S11. PMID:20528707

Grodal, T. (2000). Video games and the pleasures of control. In D. Zillman & P. Vorderer (Eds.), *Media entertainment: The psychology of its appeal* (pp. 197–213). Mahwah, NJ: Lawrence Erlbaum.

Grohol, J. M., Anthony, K., Nagel, D. A. N., & Goss, S. (2010). Using Websites, blogs and wikis in mental health. In *The use of technology in mental health applications ethics and practice* (pp. 68-75).

Gross, J. J., & Levenson, R. W. (1995). Emotion elicitation using films. *Cognition and Emotion*, *9*(1), 87–108. doi:10.1080/02699939508408966

Gucciardi, D., & Gordon, S. (2009). Development and preliminary validation of the Cricket Mental Toughness Inventory (CMTI). *Journal of Sports Sciences*, *27*(12), 1293–1310.

Guilford, J. S. (1976). *The Guilford-Zimmerman Temperament Survey handbook*. San Diego, CA: EdITS.

Gulliksen, J., Göransson, B., Boivie, I., Blomkvist, S., Persson, J., & Cajander, Å. (2003). Key principles for user-centred systems design. *Behaviour & Information Technology*, *22*(6), 397–409. doi:10.1080/01449290310001624329

Gunawardena, C. N. (1995). Social Presence Theory and Implications for Interaction and Collaborative Learning in Computer Conferences. *International Journal of Educational Telecommunications*, *1*(2), 147–166.

Gunter, G. A., Kenny, R. F., & Vick, E. H. (2008). Taking educational games seriously: Using the RETAIN model to design endogenous fantasy into standalone educational games. *Educational Technology Research and Development*, *56*(5-6), 511–537. doi:10.1007/s11423-007-9073-2

Guralnik, J. M., Simonsick, E. M., Ferrucci, L., Glynn, R. J., Berkman, L. F., Blazer, D. G., & Wallace, R. B. et al. (1994). A short physical performance battery assessing lower extremity function: Association with self-reported disability and prediction of mortality and nursing home admission. *Journal of Gerontology*, *49*(2), M85–M94. doi:10.1093/geronj/49.2.M85 PMID:8126356

Haber, D. (2013). *Health promotion and aging: Practical applications for health professionals*. New York, NY: Springer Publishing Company Heesen.

Haga, S. M., Drozd, F., Brendryen, H., & Slinning, K. (2013). Mamma mia: a feasibility study of a Web-based intervention to reduce the risk of postpartum depression and enhance subjective well-being. *JMIR research protocols, 2*(2).

Haidt, J. (2000). The Positive emotion of elevation. *Prevention & Treatment*, *3*(1). doi:10.1037/1522-3736.3.1.33c

Haidt, J. (2003). Elevation and the Positive Psychology of Morality. In C. L. M. Keyes & J. Haidt (Eds.), *Flourishing: Positive psychology and the life well-lived*. Washington, DC, USA: American Psychological Association. doi:10.1037/10594-012

Haight, B. K., & Webster, J. D. (1995). *The art and science of reminiscing: Theory, research method, and applications*. Washington, DC: Taylor & Francis.

Hall, R. H., Wilfred, L. M., Higlers, M. G., Leu, M. C., Walker, C. P., & Hortenstine, J. M. (2004). Virtual terrorist attack on the computer science building: Design and evaluation of a research methodology. *Presence-Connect, 4*(4). Retrieved from http://lite.mst.edu/documents/vr_affect_presence_connect_2004.pdf

Halpern, J., & Arnold, R. M. (2008). Affective forecasting: An unrecognized challenge in making serious health decisions. *Journal of General Internal Medicine*, *23*(10), 1708–1712. doi:10.1007/s11606-008-0719-5 PMID:18665428

Hammen, C. (2005). Stress and depression. *Annual Review of Clinical Psychology*, *1*(1), 293–319. doi:10.1146/annurev.clinpsy.1.102803.143938 PMID:17716090

Hancock, P., Pepe, A., & Murphy, L. (2005). Hedonomics: The power of positive and pleasurable emotions. *Ergonomics in Design*, *13*(1), 8–14. doi:10.1177/106480460501300104

Hanich, J., Wagner, V., Shah, M., Jacobsen, T., & Menninghaus, W. (2014). Why we like to watch sad films. The pleasure of being moved in aesthetic experiences. *Psychology of Aesthetics, Creativity, and the Arts*, *8*(2), 130–143. doi:10.1037/a0035690

Happonen, A. P., Mattila, E., Kinnunen, M. L., Ikonen, V., Myllymäki, T., Kaipainen, K., & Korhonen, I. (2009, April). P4Well concept to empower self-management of psychophysiological wellbeing and load recovery. *Paper presented at the3rd International Conference on Pervasive Computing Technologies for Healthcare*, London, UK. doi:10.4108/ICST.PERVASIVEHEALTH2009.6037

Hardyman, W., Daunt, K. L., & Kitchener, M. (2014). (in press). Value Co-Creation through Patient Engagement in Health Care: A micro-level approach and research agenda. *Public Management Review*.

Harrigan, J. A., & O'Connell, D. M. (1996). How do you look when feeling anxious? Facial displays of anxiety. *Personality and Individual Differences*, *21*(2), 205–212. doi:10.1016/0191-8869(96)00050-5

Harrington, T. L., & Harrington, M. K. (2000). *Gerontechnology: Why and How. Herman Bouma Foundation for Gerontechnology*. The Netherlands: Shaker Publishing B.V.

Hartig, T., Evans, G. W., Jamner, L. D., Davis, D. S., & Gärling, T. (2003). Tracking restoration in natural and urban field settings. *Journal of Environmental Psychology*, *23*(2), 109–123. doi:10.1016/S0272-4944(02)00109-3

Hartmann, T. (2011). Not so moral responses to media entertainment? *Media Psychology*, *23*(1), 24–28. doi:10.1027/1864-1105/a000028

Hartmann, T., Toz, E., & Brandon, M. (2010). Just a Game? Unjustified Virtual Violence Produces Guilt in Empathetic Players. *Media Psychology*, *13*(4), 339–363. doi:10.1080/15213269.2010.524912

Hartmann, T., & Vorderer, P. (2010). It's Okay to Shoot a Character: Moral Disengagement in Violent Video Games. *Journal of Communication*, *60*(1), 94–119. doi:10.1111/j.1460-2466.2009.01459.x

Haug, T., Nordgreen, T., Öst, L. G., & Havik, O. E. (2012). Self-help treatment of anxiety disorders: A meta-analysis and meta-regression of effects and potential moderators. *Clinical Psychology Review*, *32*(5), 425–445. doi:10.1016/j.cpr.2012.04.002 PMID:22681915

Hayes, A. M., Laurenceau, J. P., Feldman, G., Strauss, J. L., & Cardaciotto, L. (2007). Change is not always linear: The study of nonlinear and discontinuous patterns of change in psychotherapy. *Clinical Psychology Review*, *27*(6), 715–723. doi:10.1016/j.cpr.2007.01.008 PMID:17316941

Hearn, L., Miller, M., & Lester, L. (2014). Reaching perinatal women online: The Healthy You, Healthy Baby website and app. *Journal of Obesity*, 2014. PMID:24872891

Heeter, C. (1992). Being There: The subjective experience of presence. *Presence (Cambridge, Mass.), 1*(2), 262–271. doi:10.1162/pres.1992.1.2.262

Heeter, C. (2003). Reflections on real presence by a virtual person. *Presence (Cambridge, Mass.), 12*(4), 335–345. doi:10.1162/105474603322391587

Heidegger, M. (1977). *The Question Concerning Technology and Other Essays*. New York, USA: Garland Pub.

Held, R. M., & Durlach, N. I. (1992). Telepresence. *Presence (Cambridge, Mass.), 1*(1), 109–112. doi:10.1162/pres.1992.1.1.109

Helliwell, J. F., & Putnam, R. D. (2004). The social context of well-being. *Philosophical Transactions of the Royal Society of London. Series B, Biological Sciences, 359*(1449), 1435–1446. doi:10.1098/rstb.2004.1522 PMID:15347534

Hernández-Martínez, C., Val, V. A., Murphy, M., Busquets, P. C., & Sans, J. C. (2011). Relation between positive and negative maternal emotional states and obstetrical outcomes. *Women & Health, 51*(2), 124–135. doi:10.1080/03630242.2010.550991 PMID:21476173

Herrick, D. M. (2005). *Consumer driven health care: the changing role of the patient*. Retrieved from http://www.ncpa.org/pub/st276/

Hertzog, C., Kramer, A. F., Wilson, R. S., & Lindenberger, U. (2008). Enrichment effects on adult cognitive development can the functional capacity of older adults be preserved and enhanced? *Psychological Science in the Public Interest, 9*(1), 1–65. PMID:26162004

Hertzog, C., Kramer, A. F., Wilson, R. S., & Lindenberger, U. (2009).. . *Enrichment Effects on Adult Cognitive Development, 9*(1), 1–65.

Hess, T. M., Auman, C., Colcombe, S. J., & Rahhal, T. (2003). The Impact of Stereotype Threat on Age Differences in Memory Performance. *The Journals of Gerontology. Series B, Psychological Sciences and Social Sciences, 58*(1), 3–P11. doi:10.1093/geronb/58.1.P3 PMID:12496296

Higginson, S., & Mansell, W. (2008). What is the mechanism of psychological change? A qualitative analysis of six individuals who experienced personal change and recovery. *Psychology and Psychotherapy: Theory, Research and Practice, 81*(3), 309–328. doi:10.1348/147608308X320125 PMID:18588749

Higginson, S., Mansell, W., & Wood, A. M. (2011). An integrative mechanistic account of psychological distress, therapeutic change and recovery: The Perceptual Control Theory approach. *Clinical Psychology Review, 31*(2), 249–259. doi:10.1016/j.cpr.2010.01.005 PMID:20171771

Hipwell, A. E., Goossens, F. A., Melhuish, E. C., & Kumar, R. (2000). Severe maternal psychopathology and infant–mother attachment. *Development and Psychopathology, 12*(02), 157–175. doi:10.1017/S0954579400002030 PMID:10847622

Hockey, G. R. J. (1997). Compensatory control in the regulation of human performance under stress and high workload: A cognitive-energetical framework. Biological Psychology, 45, 73–93.

Hofer, M., & Wirth, W. (2012). It's Right to Be Sad. *Journal of Media Psychology: Theories, Methods, and Applications, 24*(2), 43–54. doi:10.1027/1864-1105/a000061

Hoffman, H. G., Doctor, J. N., Patterson, D. R., Carrougher, G. J., & Furness, T. A. III. (2000). Virtual reality as an adjunctive pain control during burn wound care in adolescent patients. *Pain, 85*(1), 305–309. doi:10.1016/S0304-3959(99)00275-4 PMID:10692634

Hoffman, S., & Hatch, M. C. (2000). Depressive symptomatology during pregnancy: Evidence for an association with decreased fetal growth in pregnancies of lower social class women. *Health Psychology*, *19*(6), 535–543. doi:10.1037/0278-6133.19.6.535 PMID:11129356

Hofmann, S. G., Sawyer, A. T., Witt, A. A., & Oh, D. (2010). The effect of mindfulness-based therapy on anxiety and depression: A meta-analytic review. *Journal of Consulting and Clinical Psychology*, *78*(2), 169–183. doi:10.1037/a0018555 PMID:20350028

Holmes, E. A., James, E. L., Coode-Bate, T., & Deeprose, C. (2009). Can Playing the Computer Game ''Tetris'' Reduce the Build-Up of Flashbacks for Trauma? A Proposal from Cognitive Science. PLoS ONE, 4(1), e4153. doi:10.1371/journal.pone.0004153 PubMed doi:10.1371/journal.pone.0004153 PMID:19127289

Hommel, B., Müsseler, J., Aschersleben, G., & Prinz, W. (2001). The Theory of Event Coding (TEC): A framework for perception and action planning. *Behavioral and Brain Sciences*, *24*(5), 849–937. doi:10.1017/S0140525X01000103 PMID:12239891

Honka, A., Kaipainen, K., Hietala, H., & Saranummi, N. (2011). Rethinking Health: ICT-Enabled Services to Empower People to Manage Their Health. IEEE Reviews in Biomedical Engineering, 4, 119–139. doi:10.1109/RBME.2011.2174217 PubMed doi:10.1109/RBME.2011.2174217 PMID:22273795

Hopkins, P. (2005). NT Clinical. *Nursing Times*, *101*(32). PMID:16119584

Horne-Moyer, H. L., Moyer, B. H., Messer, D. C., & Messer, E. S. (2014). The Use of Electronic Games in Therapy: A Review with Clinical Implications. Current Psychiatry Reports, 16(12), 520. doi:10.1007/s11920-014-0520-6 PubMed doi:10.1007/s11920-014-0520-6 PMID:25312026

Horner, V., & Whiten, A. (2005). Causal knowledge and imitation/emulation switching in chimpanzees (Pan troglodytes) and children (Homo sapiens). *Animal Cognition*, *8*(3), 164–181. doi:10.1007/s10071-004-0239-6 PMID:15549502

House, J. S., Landis, K. R., & Umberson, D. (1988). Social relationships and health. *Science*, *241*(4865), 540–545. doi:10.1126/science.3399889 PMID:3399889

Hoyt, T., & Pasupathi, M. (2008). Blogging about trauma: Linguistic measures of apparent recovery. *Relaunching soon*, *4*(2), 56.

Hruschka, D. J., Kohrt, B. A., & Worthman, C. M. (2005). Estimating between- and within-individual variation in cortisol levels using multilevel models. *Psychoneuroendocrinology*, *30*(7), 698–714. Retrieved from http://www.ncbi.nlm.nih.gov/entrez/query.fcgi?cmd=Retrieve&db=PubMed&dopt=Citation&list_uids=15854786 doi:10.1016/j.psyneuen.2005.03.002 PMID:15854786

Hsee, C. K., Hastie, R., & Chen, J. (2008). Hedonomics: Bridging Decision Research With Happiness Research. *Perspectives on Psychological Science*, *3*(3), 224–243. doi:10.1111/j.1745-6924.2008.00076.x PMID:26158937

Hsu, C. Y., Tsai, C. C., & Wang, H. Y. (2012). Facilitating third graders' acquisition of scientific concepts through digital game-based learning: The effects of self-explanation principles. *The Asia-Pacific Education Researcher*, *21*(1), 71–82.

Hu, C., Kung, S., Rummans, T. A., Clark, M. M., & Lapid, M. I. (2015). Reducing caregiver stress with internet-based interventions: A systematic review of open-label and randomized controlled trials. *Journal of the American Medical Informatics Association*, *22*(e1), e194–e209. PMID:25125686

Hudson, J., Day, M. C., & Oliver, E. J. (2015). A 'new life' story or 'delaying the inevitable'? Exploring older people's narratives during exercise uptake. *Psychology of Sport and Exercise*, *16*, 112–120. doi:10.1016/j.psychsport.2014.09.004

Huizinga, J. (1950). *Homo Ludens: A study of the play - element in culture. A study of the element of play in culture.* London, UK: Routledge.

Hu, M., Szewczyk-Królikowski, K., Tomlinson, P., Nithi, K., Rolinski, M., Murray, C., & Ben Shlomo, Y. (2014). Predictors of cognitive impairment in an early stage Parkinson's disease cohort. *Movement Disorders*, *29*(3), 351–359. doi:10.1002/mds.25748 PMID:24395708

Humphreys, A., & Grayson, K. (2008). The Intersecting Roles of Consumer and Producer: A Critical Perspective on Co-production, Co-creation and Prosumption. *Social Compass*, *2*(3), 963–980. doi:10.1111/j.1751-9020.2008.00112.x

Hunsley, J. (1990). The factor structure of the multiple affect adjective check list-revised (MAACL-R): Some statistical considerations. *Journal of Psychopathology and Behavioral Assessment*, *12*(1), 99–101. doi:10.1007/BF00960457

Hussain, M. S., Calvo, R. A., Ellis, L., Li, J., Ospina-Pinillos, L., Davenport, T., & Hickie, I. (2015). NLG-Based Moderator Response Generator to Support Mental Health. *Paper presented at the33rd Annual ACM Conference Extended Abstracts on Human Factors in Computing Systems*. doi:10.1145/2702613.2732758

Huta, V., & Ryan, R. M. (2010). Pursuing Pleasure or Virtue: The Differential and Overlapping Well-Being Benefits of Hedonic and Eudaimonic Motives. *Journal of Happiness Studies*, *11*(6), 735–762. doi:10.1007/s10902-009-9171-4

Ice, G. H., Katz-Stein, A., Himes, J., & Kane, R. L. (2004). Diurnal cycles of salivary cortisol in older adults. *Psychoneuroendocrinology, 29*(3), 355-370. doi:S0306453003000349 [pii]

IDATE. (2010): Serious games. A 10 billion euro market in 2015. Idate News, 518. Montpellier, France.

Ijsselsteijn, W. A., & Riva, G. (2003). being there: the experience of presence in mediated environments. In: G. Riva, F. Davide, & W.A. Ijsselsteijn (Eds.), Being there: concepts, effects and measurements of user presence in synthetic environments (pp. 3–16). Amsterdam: Ios press. Retrieved from www.emergingcommunication.com/volume5.html

Ijsselsteijn, W., & Riva, G. (2003). Being There: The experience of presence in mediated environments. *Being There: Concepts. Effects and Measurement of User Presence in Synthetic Environments*, *10*, 14.

Insel, P. A., Amara, S. G., & Blaschke, T. F. (2015). Introduction to the Theme "Precision Medicine and Prediction in Pharmacology". *Annual Review of Pharmacology and Toxicology*, *55*(1), 11–14. doi:10.1146/annurev-pharmtox-101714-123102 PMID:25562643

Isbister, K. (2011). Emotion and motion: Games as inspiration for shaping the future of interface. *Interaction*, *18*(September–October), 24–27. doi:10.1145/2008176.2008184

Isen, A. M., Daubman, K. A., & Nowicki, G. P. (1987). Positive affect facilitates creative problem-solving. *Journal of Personality and Social Psychology*, *52*(6), 1122–1131. doi:10.1037/0022-3514.52.6.1122 PMID:3598858

Israel, B. A., Farquhar, S. A., Schulz, A. J., James, S. A., & Parker, E. A. (2002). The relationship between social support, stress, and health among women on Detroit's East Side. *Health Education & Behavior*, *29*(3), 342–360. PMID:12038743

Ivarsson, M., Anderson, M., Åkerstedt, T., & Lindblad, F. (2013). The effect of violent and nonviolent video games on heart rate variability, sleep, and emotions in adolescents with different violent gaming habits. *Psychosomatic Medicine*, *75*(4), 390–396. doi:10.1097/PSY.0b013e3182906a4c PMID:23645706

Ivory, J. D., & Kalyanaraman, S. (2007). The effects of technological advancement and violent content in video games on players' feelings of presence, involvement, physiological arousal, and aggression. *Journal of Communication*, *57*(3), 532–555. doi:10.1111/j.1460-2466.2007.00356.x

Jackson, J. S., Knight, K. M., & Rafferty, J. A. (2010). Race and unhealthy behaviors: Chronic stress, the HPA axis, and physical and mental health disparities over the life course. *American Journal of Public Health, 100*(5), 933–939. doi:10.2105/AJPH.2008.143446 PMID:19846689

Jackson, L. A., Witt, E. A., Games, A. I., Fitzgerald, H. E., von Eye, A., & Zhao, Y. (2012). Information technology use and creativity: Findings from the Children and Technology Project. *Computers in Human Behavior*, *28*(2), 370–376. doi:10.1016/j.chb.2011.10.006

Jacobs, N., Myin-Germeys, I., Derom, C., Delespaul, P., van Os, J., & Nicolson, N. A. (2007). A momentary assessment study of the relationship between affective and adrenocortical stress responses in daily life. *Biological Psychology*, *74*(1), 60–66. Retrieved from http://www.ncbi.nlm.nih.gov/entrez/query.fcgi?cmd=Retrieve&db=PubMed&dopt=Citation&list_uids=16942831 doi:10.1016/j.biopsycho.2006.07.002 PMID:16942831

Jacobson, E. (1938). Progressive relaxation.

Jansz, J. (2005). The emotional appeal of violent video games for adolescent males. *Communication Theory*, *15*(3), 219–241. doi:10.1111/j.1468-2885.2005.tb00334.x

Jean, L., Bergeron, M. È., Thivierge, S., & Simard, M. (2010). Cognitive intervention programs for individuals with mild cognitive impairment: Systematic review of the literature. *The American Journal of Geriatric Psychiatry*, *18*(4), 281–296. doi:10.1097/JGP.0b013e3181c37ce9 PMID:20220584

Jennett, C., Cox, A. L., Cairns, P., Dhoparee, S., Epps, A., Tijs, T., & Walton, A. (2008). Measuring and defining the experience of immersion in games. *International Journal of Human-Computer Studies*, *66*(9), 641–661. doi:10.1016/j.ijhcs.2008.04.004

Jennings, K. D., Harmon, R. J., Morgan, G. A., Gaiter, J. L., & Yarrow, L. J. (1979). Exploratory play as an index of mastery motivation: Relationships to persistence, cognitive functioning, and environmental measures. *Developmental Psychology*, *15*(4), 386–394. doi:10.1037/0012-1649.15.4.386

Jihye, H., & Iftekhar, S. N. Comparison on the Use of Smartphone Application between International and Korean Pregnant Women.

Jin, S.-A. A. (2012). "Toward Integrative Models of Flow": Effects of Performance, Skill, Challenge, Playfulness, and Presence on Flow in Video Games. *Journal of Broadcasting & Electronic Media*, *56*(2), 169–186. doi:10.1080/08838151.2012.678516

Johnson, M. K., Hashtroudi, S., & Lindsay, D. S. (1993). Source monitoring. *Psychological Bulletin*, *114*(1), 3–28. doi:10.1037/0033-2909.114.1.3 PMID:8346328

Johnson, S. A. (2014). "Maternal Devices", Social Media and the Self-Management of Pregnancy, Mothering and Child Health. *Societies*, *4*(2), 330–350. doi:10.3390/soc4020330

Jones, C. M., Scholes, L., Johnson, D., Katsikitis, M., & Carras, M. C. (2014). Gaming well: Links between videogames and flourishing mental health. Frontiers in Psychology, 5, 1–8. doi:10.3389/fpsyg.2014.00260 PubMed doi:10.3389/fpsyg.2014.00260 PMID:24744743

Jones, L. (2012). Pain management for women in labour: An overview of systematic reviews. *Journal of Evidence-Based Medicine*, *5*(2), 101–102. PMID:22419342

Jones, M. G. (1998). Creating Electronic Learning Environments : Games, Flow, and the User Interface.*Proceedings of Selected Research and Development Presentations at the National Convention of the Association for Educational Communications and Technology (AECT)* (pp. 205–214).

Joyce, K. M. (2009). Enhancing Social Presence in Online Learning: Mediation Strategies Applied to Social Networking Tools. *Online Journal of Distance Learning Administration, 12*(4). Retrieved from http://www.westga.edu/~distance/ojdla/winter124/joyce124.html

Juan, M. C., Baños, R., Botella, C., Pérez, D., Alcaníiz, M., & Monserrat, C. (2006). An Augmented Reality System for the Treatment of Acrophobia: The Sense of Presence Using Immersive Photography. *Presence (Cambridge, Mass.), 15*(4), 393–402. doi:10.1162/pres.15.4.393

Just, M., & Carpenter, P. (1992). A capacity theory of comprehension: Individual differences in working memory. *Psychological Review, 99*(1), 122–149. doi:10.1037/0033-295X.99.1.122 PMID:1546114

Juul, J. (2005). *Half-real: Video games between real rules and fictional worlds*. Cambridge, MA: MIT Press.

Juul, J. (2009). *A Casual Revolution: Reinventing Video Games and Their Players*. Cambridge: MIT Press.

Juul, J. (2013). *The art of failure. An essay on the pain of playing videogames*. Cambridge: MIT Press.

Kabat-Zinn, J. (1990). *Full catastrophe living: Using the wisdom of your body and mind to face stress, pain, and illness*. New York: Delacorte.

Kabat-Zinn, J. (1994). *Wherever you go, there you are: Mindfulness meditation in everyday life*. New York: Hyperion.

Kabat-Zinn, J. (2003). Mindfulness-based interventions in context: Past, present, and future. *Clinical Psychology: Science and Practice, 10*(2), 144–156. doi:10.1093/clipsy.bpg016

Kaci Fairchild, J., & Scogin, F. R. (2010). Training to Enhance Adult Memory (TEAM): An investigation of the effectiveness of a memory training program with older adults. *Aging & Mental Health, 14*(3), 364–373. doi:10.1080/13607860903311733 PMID:20425656

Kahn, J., Ducharme, P., Rotenberg, A., & Gonzalez-Heydrich, J. (2013). "RAGE-Control": A Game to Build Emotional Strength. Games for Health Journal, 2(1), 53–57. doi:10.1089/g4h.2013.0007 PubMed doi:10.1089/g4h.2013.0007 PMID:26196556

Kahneman, D., Krueger, A. B., Schkade, D. A., Schwarz, N., & Stone, A. A. (2004). A survey method for characterizing daily life experience: the day reconstruction method. *Science, 306*(5702), 1776-1780. doi:306/5702/177610.1126/science.1103572

Kahneman, D. (2002). Maps of Bounded Rationality: A Perspective on Intuitive Judgment and Choice. In T. Frängsmyr (Ed.), *The Nobel Prizes 2002* (pp. 449–489). Stockholm: Nobel Foundation.

Kahneman, D., Diener, E., & Schwarz, N. (1999). *Well-being. The foundations of hedonic psychology*. New York, NY: Russell Sage.

Kahn, P. H. Jr, Severson, R. L., & Ruckert, J. H. (2009). The human relation with nature and technological nature. *Current Directions in Psychological Science, 18*(1), 37–42. doi:10.1111/j.1467-8721.2009.01602.x

Kairy, D., Rushton, P. W., Archambault, P., Pituch, E., Torkia, C., El Fathi, A., & Gourdeau, R. (2014). Exploring powered wheelchair users and their caregivers' perspectives on potential intelligent power wheelchair use: A qualitative study. *International Journal of Environmental Research and Public Health, 11*(2), 2244–2261. doi:10.3390/ijerph110202244 PMID:24566051

Kalia, M. (2002). Assessing the economic impact of stress—The modern day hidden epidemic. *Metabolism: Clinical and Experimental, 51*(6), 49–53. doi:10.1053/meta.2002.33193 PMID:12040542

Kaplan, S. (1995). The restorative benefits of nature: Toward an integrative framework. *Journal of Environmental Psychology, 15*(3), 169–182. doi:10.1016/0272-4944(95)90001-2

Kaptelinin, V., & Nardi, B. (2006). *Acting with Technology: Activity Theory and Interaction Design.* Cambridge, MA: MIT Press.

Karavolos, M. H., Spencer, H., Bulmer, D. M., Thompson, A., Winzer, K., Williams, P., & Khan, C. M. et al. (2008). Adrenaline modulates the global transcriptional profile of Salmonella revealing a role in the antimicrobial peptide. *BMC Genomics, 9*(1), 458. doi:10.1186/1471-2164-9-458 PMID:18837991

Kartiko, I., Kavakli, M., & Cheng, K. (2009, August 11-14). The impacts of animated - virtual actors' visual complexity and simulator sickness in virtual reality applications. In B. Werner (Ed.), *Proceedings of the 2009 6th International Conference Computer Graphics, Imaging and Visualization* (pp. 147-152). IEEE Computer Society. doi:10.1109/CGIV.2009.66

Kavakli, M. (2012, July 17-20). Interacting with virtual humans and detection of facial expressions: What makes an avatar more real than real? Proceedings of the IADIS Conference on Game and Entertainment Technologies GET '12, Lisbon, Portugal (pp.1-8).

Kavakli, M., & Chen, Y. L. (2014, October 12-16). Gender Differences in Gesture-based Interaction. *Proceedings of the Seventh International Conference on Advances in Human-oriented and Personalized Mechanisms, Technologies, and ServicesCENTRIC '14*, Nice, France (pp. 1-7).

Kavakli, M., & Kartiko, I. (2007, May 30 - 31). Avatar Construction for Believable Agents. *Proceedings of the tenth international conference on computer graphics and artificial intelligence 3IA '07*, Athens, GREECE (pp. 1-6).

Kavakli, M., Li, M., & Rudra, T. (2012). Towards the development of a virtual counselor to tackle students' exam stress, Transactions of the SDPS. *Journal of Integrated Design and Process Science, 16*(1), 5–26.

Kaye, L. K., & Bryce, J. (2012). Putting the fun factor into gaming: The influence of social contexts on experiences of playing videogames. *International Journal of Internet Science.*

Kelaiditi, E., Cesari, M., Canevelli, M., Van Kan, G. A., Ousset, P. J., Gillette-Guyonnet, S., & Vellas, B. et al. (2013). Cognitive frailty: Rational and definition from an (IANA/IAGG) international consensus group. *The Journal of Nutrition, Health & Aging, 17*(9), 726–734. doi:10.1007/s12603-013-0367-2 PMID:24154642

Keller, H., Schneider, K., & Henderson, B. B. (Eds.). (1994). *Curiosity and exploration.* Berlin: Springer-Verlag. doi:10.1007/978-3-642-77132-3

Keller, J., & Bless, H. (2008). Flow and regulatory compatibility: An experimental approach to the flow model of intrinsic motivation. *Personality and Social Psychology Bulletin, 34*(2), 196–209. doi:10.1177/0146167207310026 PMID:18212330

Kelly, M. E., Loughrey, D., Lawlor, B. A., Robertson, I. H., Walsh, C., & Brennan, S. (2014). The impact of cognitive training and mental stimulation on cognitive and everyday functioning of healthy older adults: A systematic review and meta-analysis. *Ageing Research Reviews, 15*, 28–43. doi:10.1016/j.arr.2014.02.004 PMID:24607830

Keng, S. L., Smoski, M. J., & Robins, C. J. (2011). Effects of mindfulness on psychological health: A review of empirical studies. *Clinical Psychology Review, 31*(6), 1041–1056. doi:10.1016/j.cpr.2011.04.006 PMID:21802619

Kesaniemi, Y. K., Danforth, E. Jr, Jensen, M. D., Kopelman, P. G., Lefèbvre, P., & Reeder, B. A. (2001). Dose-response issues concerning physical activity and health: An evidence-based symposium. *Medicine and Science in Sports and Exercise, 33*(Suppl. 6), S351. PMID:11427759

Keyes, C. L. M. (1998). Social Well-being. *Social Psychology Quarterly, 61*(2), 121–140. doi:10.2307/2787065

Keyes, C. L. M., & Lopez, S. J. (2002). Toward a science of mental health: positive direction in diagnosis and interventions. In C. R. Snyder & S. J. Lopez (Eds.), *Handbook of Positive Psychology*. New York: Oxford University Press.

Khalil, G. E. (2012). When losing means winning: The impact of conflict in a digital game in young adults' intentions to get protected from cancer. *Games for Health Journal*, *1*(4), 279–286. doi:10.1089/g4h.2012.0017 PMID:26191631

Khanna, M. S., & Kendall, P. C. (2010). Computer-Assisted Cognitive Behavioral Therapy for Child Anxiety: Results of a Randomized Clinical Trial. Journal of Consulting and Clinical Psychology, 78(5), 737–745. doi:10.1037/a0019739 PubMed doi:10.1037/a0019739 PMID:20873909

Kickmeier-Rust, M. D., & Albert, D. (2009). Emergence in digital educational games: A world of incidents in a universe of rules. *Proceedings of the 3rd European Conference on Game Based Learning* (p. 220). Academic Conferences Limited.

Kiecolt-Glaser, J. K., McGuire, L., Robles, T. F., & Glaser, R. (2002). Psychoneuroimmunology: Psychological influences on immune function and health. *Journal of Consulting and Clinical Psychology*, *70*(3), 537–547. doi:10.1037/0022-006X.70.3.537 PMID:12090368

Kiili, K., Lainema, T., de Freitas, S., & Arnab, S. (2014). Flow framework for analyzing the quality of educational games. *Entertainment Computing*, *3*, 14–19.

Kiili, K., Perttula, A., Lindstedt, A., Arnab, S., & Suominen, M. (in press). Flow Experience as a Quality Measure in Evaluating Physically Activating Collaborative Serious Games. *International Journal of Serious Games*.

Kilner, J. M., Paulignan, Y., & Blakemore, S. J. (2003). An interference effect of observed biological movement on action. *Current Biology*, *13*(6), 522–525. doi:10.1016/S0960-9822(03)00165-9 PMID:12646137

Kim, D., Seo, Y., Cho, J., & Cho, C. H. (2008). Detection of subjects with higher self-reporting stress scores using heart rate variability patterns during the day. *Paper presented at theConf Proc IEEE Eng Med Biol Soc.* doi:10.1109/IEMBS.2008.4649244

Kim, B., Park, H., & Baek, Y. (2009). Not just fun, but serious strategies: Using meta-cognitive strategies in game-based learning. *Computers & Education*, *52*(4), 800–810. doi:10.1016/j.compedu.2008.12.004

Kimhy, D., Delespaul, P., Ahn, H., Cai, S., Shikhman, M., Lieberman, J. A., . . . Sloan, R. P. (2009). Concurrent measurement of "real-world" stress and arousal in individuals with psychosis: assessing the feasibility and validity of a novel methodology. *Schizophr Bull, 36*(6), 1131-1139. doi:sbp028[pii]10.1093/schbul/sbp028

King, L. A. (2001). The Health Benefits of Writing about Life Goals. *Personality and Social Psychology Bulletin*, *27*(7), 798–807. doi:10.1177/0146167201277003

Kirschbaum, C., & Hellhammer, D. H. (1989). Salivary cortisol in psychobiological research: an overview. *Neuropsychobiology, 22*(3), 150-169. doi:118611[pii]118611

Kite, M. E., & Johnson, B. T. (1988). Attitudes Toward Older and Younger Adults : A Meta-Analysis. *Psychology and Aging*, *3*(3), 233–244. doi:10.1037/0882-7974.3.3.233 PMID:3268264

Kivikangas, J. M., & Ravaja, N. (2013). Emotional responses to victory and defeat as a function of opponent. *IEEE Transactions on Affective Computing*, *4*(2), 173–182. doi:10.1109/T-AFFC.2013.12

Kizony, R., Korman, M., Sinoff, G., Klinger, E., & Josman, N. (2012, September 10-12). Using a virtual supermarket as a tool for training executive functions in people with mild cognitive impairment. *Paper presented at the9th International Conference on Disability, Virtual Reality and Associated Technologies ICDVRAT*, Laval, France.

Klasen, M., Weber, R., Kircher, T., Mathiak, K., & Mathiak, K. (2012). Neural contributions to flow experience during video game playing. *Social Cognitive and Affective Neuroscience*, *7*(4), 485–495. doi:10.1093/scan/nsr021 PMID:21596764

Klatt, M. D., Buckworth, J., & Malarkey, W. B. (2009). Effects of low-dose mindfulness-based stress reduction (MBSR-ld) on working adults. *Health Education & Behavior*, *36*(3), 601–614. doi:10.1177/1090198108317627 PMID:18469160

Klein, G. A. (2008). Naturalistic decision making. *Human Factors*, *50*(3), 456–460. doi:10.1518/001872008X288385 PMID:18689053

Klimmt, C., Rizzo, A., Vorderer, P., Koch, J., & Fischer, T. (2009). Experimental evidence for suspense as determinant of video game enjoyment. *Cyberpsychology & Behavior*, *12*(1), 29–31. doi:10.1089/cpb.2008.0060 PMID:19025464

Kline, F. M. (1981). Catharsis in Healing, Ritual and Drama. *The Journal of Clinical Psychiatry*. doi:10.2307/2068827

Knox, M., Lentini, J., Cummings, T. S., McGrady, A., Whearty, K., & Sancrant, L. (2011). Game-based biofeedback for paediatric anxiety and depression. Mental Health in Family Medicine, 8, 195–203. PubMed PMID:22942901

Kober, S. E., Wood, G., Hofer, D., Kreuzig, W., Kiefer, M., & Neuper, C. (2013). Virtual reality in neurologic rehabilitation of spatial disorientation. *Journal of Neuroengineering and Rehabilitation*, *10*(1), 17.

Koestner, R., Lekes, N., Powers, T. A., & Chicoine, E. (2002). Attaining personal goals: Self-concordance plus implementation intentions equals success. *Journal of Personality and Social Psychology*, *83*(1), 231–244. doi:10.1037/0022-3514.83.1.231 PMID:12088128

Kohlberg, L. (1971). Moral psychology and the study of tragedy. In S. Weintraub & P. Young (Eds.), *Directions in Literary criticisms*. University Park, USA: Pennsylvania State University Press.

Koropeckyj-Cox, T. (2002). Beyond Parental Status. *Psychological Well-Being in Middle and Old Age*, *64*(November), 957–971.

Koster, R. (2004). *Theory of fun for game design*. Paraglyph Press.

Koster, R. (2005). *A theory of fun for game design*. Scottsdale, AZ: Paraglyph Press.

Kottler, J. A. (2014). *Change: What really leads to lasting personal transformation*. New York, NY: Oxford University Press.

Koven, N. S. (2011). Specificity of meta-emotion effects on moral decision-making. *Emotion (Washington, D.C.)*, *11*(5), 1255–1261. doi:10.1037/a0025616 PMID:21942703

Krasny-Pacini, A., Chevignard, M., & Evans, J. (2013). Goal Management Training for rehabilitation of executive functions: A systematic review of effectiveness in patients with acquired brain injury. *Disability and Rehabilitation*. doi:10.3109/09638288.2013.777807 PMID:23597002

Krebs, J. (2013). Moral dilemmas in serious games. Proceedings of the 2013 International Conference on Advanced ICT (pp. 232-236).

Kreijns, K., Kirschner, P. A., & Jochems, W. (2003). Identifying the pitfalls for social interaction in computer-supported collaborative learning environments: A review of the research. *Computers in Human Behavior*, *19*(3), 335–353. doi:10.1016/S0747-5632(02)00057-2

Kreijns, K., Kirschner, P. A., & Jochems, W. M. G. (2002). The sociability of computer-supported collaborative learning environments. *Journal of Educational Technology & Society*, *5*, 8–22.

Krusche, A., Cyhlarova, E., King, S., & Williams, J. M. G. (2012). Mindfulness online: A preliminary evaluation of the feasibility of a web-based mindfulness course and the impact on stress. *BMJ Open*, *2*(3), e000803. doi:10.1136/bmjopen-2011-000803 PMID:22614170

Krusche, A., Cyhlarova, E., & Williams, J. M. G. (2013). Mindfulness online: An evaluation of the feasibility of a web-based mindfulness course for stress, anxiety and depression. *BMJ Open*, *3*(11), e003498. doi:10.1136/bmjopen-2013-003498 PMID:24293203

Kvedar, J., Coye, M. J., & Everett, W. (2014). Connected health: A review of technologies and strategies to improve patient care with telemedicine and telehealth. *Health Affairs*, *33*(2), 194–199. doi:10.1377/hlthaff.2013.0992 PMID:24493760

Lagan, B. M., Sinclair, M., & George Kernohan, W. (2010). Internet Use in Pregnancy Informs Women's Decision Making: A Web-Based Survey. *Birth (Berkeley, Calif.)*, *37*(2), 106–115. doi:10.1111/j.1523-536X.2010.00390.x PMID:20557533

Lagan, B. M., Sinclair, M., & Kernohan, W. G. (2011). What Is the Impact of the Internet on Decision-Making in Pregnancy? A Global Study. *Birth (Berkeley, Calif.)*, *38*(4), 336–345. doi:10.1111/j.1523-536X.2011.00488.x PMID:22112334

Lagiewka, K. (2012). European innovation partnership on active and healthy ageing: Triggers of setting the headline target of 2 additional healthy life years at birth at EU average by 2020. *Archives of Public Health*, *70*(1), 1–8. doi:10.1186/0778-7367-70-23 PMID:23088612

Lai, C.-H., Peng, C.-W., Chen, Y.-L., Huang, C.-P., Hsiao, Y.-L., & Chen, S.-C. (2013). Effects of interactive video-game based system exercise on the balance of the elderly. *Gait & Posture*, *37*(4), 511–515. doi:10.1016/j.gaitpost.2012.09.003 PMID:23177921

Lampit, A., Hallock, H., & Valenzuela, M. (2014). Computerized Cognitive Training in Cognitively Healthy Older Adults: A Systematic Review and Meta-Analysis. *PLoS Medicine*, *11*(11), e1001756. doi:10.1371/journal.pmed.1001756 PMID:25405755

Lancaster, C. A., Gold, K. J., Flynn, H. A., Yoo, H., Marcus, S. M., & Davis, M. M. (2010). Risk factors for depressive symptoms during pregnancy: A systematic review. *American Journal of Obstetrics and Gynecology*, *202*(1), 5–14. doi:10.1016/j.ajog.2009.09.007 PMID:20096252

Lancia, F. (2012a). *T-LAB 8.0 – User's Manual*. Retrieved from http://www.tlab.it/en/download.php

Lancia, F. (2012b). *T-LAB pathways to thematic analysis*. Retrieved from http://www.tlab.it/en/tpatways.php

Lancia, F. (2004). *Strumenti per l'Analisi di Testi. Introduzione all'Uso di T-LAB* [Tools for Text Analysis. An Introduction to the Use of T-LAB]. Milano, Italy: Angeli.

Landgraf, S., Krebs, M. O., Olié, J. P., Committeri, G., van der Meer, E., Berhtoz, A., & Amado, I. (2010). Real world referencing and schizophrenia: Are we experiencing the same reality? Neuropsychologia, 48(10), 2922–2930. doi:10.1016/j.neuropsychologia.2010.05.034 PubMed doi:10.1016/j.neuropsychologia.2010.05.034 PMID:20540956

Lang, P. J., Bradley, M. M., & Cuthbert, B. N. (1997). International affective picture system (IAPS): Technical manual and affective ratings. NIMH Center for the Study of Emotion and Attention, 39-58.

Langer, E. J. (1989). *Mindfulness*: Addison-Wesley/Addison Wesley Longman.

Langer, E. J. (2000). Mindful learning. *Current Directions in Psychological Science*, *9*(6), 220–223. doi:10.1111/1467-8721.00099

Langer, E. J., & Rodin, J. (1976). Long-term Effects of a Control-relevant Intervention with the Institutionalized Aged. *Journal of Personality and Social Psychology*, *34*(2), 191–198. doi:10.1037/0022-3514.34.2.191 PMID:1011073

Langer, E., & Moldoveanu, M. (2000). The construct of mindfulness. *The Journal of Social Issues*, *56*(1), 1–9. doi:10.1111/0022-4537.00148

Langlois, F., Vu, T. T. M., Kergoat, M. J., Chassé, K., Dupuis, G., & Bherer, L. (2012). The multiple dimensions of frailty: Physical capacity, cognition, and quality of life. *International Psychogeriatrics*, *24*(09), 1429–1436. doi:10.1017/S1041610212000634 PMID:22717010

Lang, P. J., Bradley, M. M., & Cuthbert, B. N. (1995). *International affective picture system (IAPS): Technical manual and affective ratings*. Gainesville: NIMH Center for the Study of Emotion and Attention, University of Florida.

Langston, C. A. (1994). Capitalizing on and coping with daily-life events: Expressive responses to positive events. *Journal of Personality and Social Psychology*, *67*(6), 1112–1125. doi:10.1037/0022-3514.67.6.1112

Larsson, M. (2009). A descriptive study of the use of the Internet by women seeking pregnancy-related information. *Midwifery*, *25*(1), 14–20. doi:10.1016/j.midw.2007.01.010 PMID:17408822

Laver, K., George, S., Thomas, S., Deutsch, J. E., & Crotty, M. (2011). Virtual reality for stroke rehabilitation. *Stroke*, *43*(2), e20–e21. doi:10.1161/STROKEAHA.111.642439

Layous, K., & Lyubomirsky, S. (2012). The how, who, what, when, and why of happiness: Mechanisms underlying the success of positive interventions. In J. Gruber & J. Moscowitz (Eds.), *The light and dark side of positive emotions* (pp. 473–495). New York, NY: Oxford University Press.

Lazarus, R. (1994). *Emotion and adaptation*. New York, USA: Oxford University Press.

Lazarus, R. S. (1966). *Psychological stress and the coping process*. New York: McGraw-Hill.

Lazarus, R. S., & Folkman, S. (1984). *Stress, appraisal, and coping*. New York: Springer.

Lazarus, R. S., & Folkman, S. (1987). Transactional theory and research on emotions and coping. *European Journal of Personality*, *1*(3), 141–169. doi:10.1002/per.2410010304

Lee, R., & Whitley, H. P. (2014). Use of Social Media to Support Patients with Diabetes Mellitus. *The Consultant Pharmacist*, *29*(1), 53–57. doi:10.4140/TCP.n.2014.53 PMID:24413015

Lee, S., & Espelage, D. L.Jun Sung Hong. (2010). An ecological understanding of youth suicide in South Korea. *School Psychology International*, *31*(5), 531–546. doi:10.1177/0143034310382724

Lehrer, J. (2009, January 17). "Deliberate calm" guided US airways crew. *The Los Angeles Times*. Retrieved from http://www.latimes.com/la-oe-lehrer17-2009jan17-story.html

Lehrer, J. (2009.) "Deliberate calm" guided US airways crew. *The Los Angeles Times*. Retrieved from http://www.latimes.com/la-oe-lehrer17-2009jan17-story.html

Leinonen, M., Koivisto, A., Sirkka, A., & Kiili, K. (2012, October). Designing games for well-being; Exergames for elderly people. *Paper presented at the6th European Conference on Games Based Learning*, Cork, Ireland.

Leitenberg, H. (1990). Handbook of Social and Evaluation Anxiety. New York: Springer Science. doi:10.1007/978-1-4899-2504-6 doi:10.1007/978-1-4899-2504-6

Lemyre, L., & Tessier, R. (1988). Mesure de Stress Psychologique (MSP): Se sentir stressé-e. *Canadian Journal of Behavioural Science/Revue canadienne des sciences du comportement, 20*(3), 302.

Leontjev, A. N. (1978). Activity, consciousness, and personality. Englewood, NJ: Prentice-Hall; Retrieved from http://marxists.org/archive/leontev/works/1978/ch3.htm

Leserman, J., Petitto, J., Gu, H., Gaynes, B., Barroso, J., Golden, R., & Evans, D. et al. (2002). Progression to AIDS, a clinical AIDS condition and mortality: Psychosocial and physiological predictors. *Psychological Medicine, 32*(06), 1059–1073. doi:10.1017/S0033291702005949 PMID:12214787

Lessiter, J., Freeman, J., Keogh, E., & Davidoff, J. (2001). A Cross-Media Presence Questionnaire: The ITC-Sense of Presence Inventory. *Presence (Cambridge, Mass.), 10*(3), 282–297. doi:10.1162/105474601300343612

Le, T., Reeder, B., Yoo, D., Aziz, R., Thompson, H. J., & Demiris, G. (2015). An Evaluation of Wellness Assessment Visualizations for Older Adults. *Telemedicine Journal and e-Health, 21*(1), 9–15. doi:10.1089/tmj.2014.0012 PMID:25401414

Levine, B., Robertson, I. H., Clare, L., Carter, G., Hong, J., Wilson, B. A., & Stuss, D. T. et al. (2000). Rehabilitation of executive functioning: An experimental-clinical validation of goal management training. *Journal of the International Neuropsychological Society, 6*(3), 299–312. doi:10.1017/S1355617700633052 PMID:10824502

Levine, B., Schweizer, T. A., O'Connor, C., Turner, G., Gillingham, S., Stuss, D. T., & Robertson, I. H. et al. (2011). Rehabilitation of executive functioning in patients with frontal lobe brain damage with goal management training. *Frontiers in Human Neuroscience, 5.* doi:10.3389/fnhum.2011.00009 PMID:21369362

Levy, B., & Langer, E. (1994). Aging free from negative stereotypes: Successful memory in China and among the American Deaf.

Levy, B. (1996). Improving memory in old age through implicit self-stereotyping. *Journal of Personality and Social Psychology, 71*(6), 1092–1107. doi:10.1037/0022-3514.71.6.1092 PMID:8979380

Li, M., Rudra, T., & Kavakli, M. (2012, April 16-17). E-counsellor - An Avatar for Student Exam Stress Management. *Proceedings of the 3rd International Conference on Information Management and Evaluation ICIME '12,* Atilim University, Ankara, Turkey (pp.185-193).

Liao, W., Zhang, W., Zhu, Z., Ji, Q., & Gray, W. D. (2006). Toward a decision-theoretic framework for affect recognition and user assistance. *International Journal of Human-Computer Studies, 64*(9), 847–873. doi:10.1016/j.ijhcs.2006.04.001

Ligtenberg, A., de Vries, B., Vreenegoor, R., & Bulens, J. (2010). SimLandScape, a sketching tool for collaborative spatial planning. *URBAN DESIGN International.*

Lima-Pereira, P., Bermúdez-Tamayo, C., & Jasienska, G. (2012). Use of the Internet as a source of health information amongst participants of antenatal classes. *Journal of Clinical Nursing, 21*(3-4), 322–330. doi:10.1111/j.1365-2702.2011.03910.x PMID:22093043

Lindgren, K. (2001). Relationships among maternal–fetal attachment, prenatal depression, and health practices in pregnancy. *Research in Nursing & Health, 24*(3), 203–217. doi:10.1002/nur.1023 PMID:11526619

Linnenbrink, E. A., & Pintrich, P. R. (2002). Achievement goal theory and affect: A symmetrical bidirectional model. *Educational Psychologist, 37*(2), 69–78. doi:10.1207/S15326985EP3702_2

Linwall, M., Rennemark, M., Halling, A., Berglund, J., & Hassmén, P. (2006). Depression and exercise in elderly men and women: Findings from the Swedish national study on aging and care. *Journal of Aging and Physical Activity, 15,* 41–55. PMID:17387228

Littlewood, W. (1996). Autonomy: An Anatomy and a Framework. *System, 24*(4), 427–435. doi:10.1016/S0346-251X(96)00039-5

Liu, M., Calvo, R. A., Davenport, T., & Hickie, I. (2013, Nov 26). Moderator Assistant: helping those who help via online mental health support groups. *Paper presented at theJoint Workshop on Smart Health and Social Therapies, OzChi2013,* Adelaide, Australia.

Liu-Ambrose, T., Nagamatsu, L. S., Graf, P., Beattie, B. L., Ashe, M. C., & Handy, T. C. (2010). Resistance training and executive functions: A 12-month randomized controlled trial. *Archives of Internal Medicine*, *170*(2), 170–178. doi:10.1001/archinternmed.2009.494 PMID:20101012

Liu, C. J., & Latham, N. K. (2009). Progressive resistance strength training for improving physical function in older adults. *Cochrane Database of Systematic Reviews*, CD002759. PMID:19588334

Lo Priore, C., Castelnuovo, G., Liccione, D., & Liccione, D. (2003). Experience with V-STORE: Considerations on presence in virtual environments for effective neuropsychological rehabilitation of executive functions. *Cyberpsychology & Behavior*, *6*(3), 281–287. doi:10.1089/109493103322011579 PMID:12855084

Lobel, A., Granic, I., & Engels Rutger, C. M. E. (2014). Stressful Gaming, Interoceptive Awareness, and Emotion Regulation Tendencies: A Novel Approach. *Cyberpsychology, Behavior, and Social Networking*, *17*(4), 222–227. doi:10.1089/cyber.2013.0296

Loeppke, R. R., Schill, A. L., Chosewood, L. C., Grosch, J. W., Allweiss, P., Burton, W. N., & Larson, P. W. et al. (2013). Advancing workplace health protection and promotion for an aging workforce. *Journal of Occupational and Environmental Medicine*, *55*(5), 500–506. doi:10.1097/JOM.0b013e31829613a4 PMID:23657074

Loewenstein, G. (1994). The psychology of curiosity: A review and reinterpretation. *Psychological Bulletin*, *116*(1), 75–98. doi:10.1037/0033-2909.116.1.75

Loft, S., Bolland, S., Humphreys, M., & Neal, A. (2009). A theory and model of conflict detection in air traffic control: Incorporating environmental constraints. *Journal of Experimental Psychology. Applied*, *15*(2), 106–124. doi:10.1037/a0016118 PMID:19586250

Lombard, M., & Ditton, T. (1997). At the heart of it all: The concept of presence. *Journal of Computer-Mediated Communication*, *3*(2). Retrieved from http://onlinelibrary.wiley.com/doi/10.1111/j.1083-6101.1997.tb00072.x/full

Lorentz, P. (2014). Why Failing in Games is a Positive Aspect of Play: A Review of Jesper Juul's The Art of Failure. *Journal of Game Criticism*, *1*(2).

Lorenz, K. (1981). Exploratory behavior or curiosity. In K. Lorenz & R. W. Kickert (Eds.), *The foundations of ethology* (pp. 325–335). New York: Springer-Verlag. doi:10.1007/978-3-7091-3671-3_18

Louro, M. J., Pieters, R., & Zeelenberg, M. (2007). Dynamics of multiple-goal pursuit. *Journal of Personality and Social Psychology*, *93*(2), 174–193. doi:10.1037/0022-3514.93.2.174 PMID:17645394

Løvoll, H. S., & Vittersø, J. (2014). Can Balance be Boring? A Critique of the "Challenges Should Match Skills" Hypotheses in Flow Theory. *Social Indicators Research*, *115*(1), 117–136. doi:10.1007/s11205-012-0211-9

Lowe, N. K. (2002). The nature of labor pain. *American Journal of Obstetrics and Gynecology*, *186*(5), S16–S24. doi:10.1016/S0002-9378(02)70179-8 PMID:12011870

Lu, A. S., Baranowski, T., Thompson, D., & Buday, R. (2012). Story Immersion of Videogames for Youth Health Promotion: A Review of Literature. *Games for Health Journal*, *1*(3), 199–204. doi:10.1089/g4h.2011.0012 PMID:24416639

Lund, S., Nielsen, B. B., Hemed, M., Boas, I. M., Said, A., Said, K., & Rasch, V. (2014). Mobile phones improve antenatal care attendance in Zanzibar: A cluster randomized controlled trial. *BMC Pregnancy and Childbirth*, *14*(1), 29. doi:10.1186/1471-2393-14-29 PMID:24438517

Lupien, S. J., McEwen, B. S., Gunnar, M. R., & Heim, C. (2009). Effects of stress throughout the lifespan on the brain, behaviour and cognition. *Nature Reviews. Neuroscience*, *10*(6), 434–445. doi:10.1038/nrn2639 PMID:19401723

Lupton, D. (1997). Consumerism, reflexivity and the medical encounter. *Social Science & Medicine*, *45*(3), 373–381. doi:10.1016/S0277-9536(96)00353-X PMID:9232732

Luxton, D. D., McCann, R. A., Bush, N. E., Mishkind, M. C., & Reger, G. M. (2011). mHealth for mental health: Integrating smartphone technology in behavioral healthcare. *Professional Psychology, Research and Practice*, *42*(6), 505–512. doi:10.1037/a0024485

Ly, K. H., Trüschel, A., Jarl, L., Magnusson, S., Windahl, T., Johansson, R., & Andersson, G. et al. (2014). Behavioural activation versus mindfulness-based guided self-help treatment administered through a smartphone application: A randomised controlled trial. *BMJ Open*, *4*(1), e003440. doi:10.1136/bmjopen-2013-003440 PMID:24413342

Lyubomirsky, S., Tkach, C., & Sheldon, K. M. (2004). Pursuing sustained happiness through random acts of kindness and counting one's blessings: Tests of two six-week interventions [Unpublished data]. Department of Psychology, University of California, Riverside.

Lyubomirsky, S. (2011). Hedonic adaptation to positive and negative experiences. In S. Folkman (Ed.), *Oxford handbook of stress health and coping* (pp. 200–224). New York, NY: Oxford University Press.

Lyubomirsky, S., Dickerhoof, R., Boehm, J. K., & Sheldon, K. M. (2011). Becoming happier takes both a will and a proper way: An experimental longitudinal intervention to boost well-being. *Emotion (Washington, D.C.)*, *11*(2), 391–402. doi:10.1037/a0022575 PMID:21500907

Lyubomirsky, S., Sheldon, K. M., & Schkade, D. (2005). Pursuing happiness: The architecture of sustainable change. *Review of General Psychology*, *9*(2), 111–131. doi:10.1037/1089-2680.9.2.111

Lyubomirsky, S., Sousa, L., & Dickerhoof, R. (2006). The costs and benefits of writing, talking, and thinking about life's triumphs and defeats. *Journal of Personality and Social Psychology*, *90*(4), 692–708. doi:10.1037/0022-3514.90.4.692 PMID:16649864

Macuco, C. R. M., Batistoni, S. S. T., Lopes, A., Cachioni, M., da Silva Falcão, D. V., Neri, A. L., & Yassuda, M. S. (2012). Mini-Mental State Examination performance in frail, pre-frail, and non-frail community dwelling older adults in Ermelino Matarazzo, São Paulo, Brazil. *International Psychogeriatrics*, *24*(11), 1725–1731. doi:10.1017/S1041610212000907 PMID:22652040

Madeira, F., Arriaga, P., Adrião, J., Lopes, R., & Esteves, F. (2015). Emotional Gaming. In Y. Baek (Ed.), *Psychology of Gaming*. New York, USA: Nova Science Publishers.

Magagnin, V., Mauri, M., Cipresso, P., Mainardi, L., Brown, E. N., Cerutti, S., . . . Barbieri, R. (2010). Heart rate variability and respiratory sinus arrhythmia assessment of affective states by bivariate autoregressive spectral analysis. *Paper presented at the Computing in Cardiology.*

Mahoney, F. I., & Barthel, D. (1965). Functional evaluation: The Barthel Index. *Maryland State Medical Journal*, *14*, 56–61. PMID:14258950

Malbos, E., Rapee, R. M., & Kavakli, M. (2013). A Controlled Study of Agoraphobia and the Independent Effect of Virtual Reality Exposure Therapy. *The Australian and New Zealand Journal of Psychiatry*, *47*(12), 160–168. doi:10.1177/0004867412453626 PMID:22790176

Malik, M. (1996). The North American Society of Pacing and Electrophysiology. Heart rate variability: Standards of measurement, physiological interpretation and clinical use. *Circulation*, *93*(5), 1043–1065. doi:10.1161/01.CIR.93.5.1043 PMID:8598068

Malone, T. W., & Lepper, M. R. (1987). Making learning fun: A taxonomy of intrinsic motivations for Learning. In R. E. Snow & M. J. Farr (Eds.), *Aptitude, learning and instruction: Cognitive and affective process analyses* (pp. 223–253). Hillsdale: Erlbaum.

Mammen, G., & Faulkner, G. (2013). Physical Activity and the Prevention of Depression. *American Journal of Preventive Medicine*, *45*(5), 649–657. doi:10.1016/j.amepre.2013.08.001 PMID:24139780

Mantovani, F., & Castelnuovo, G. (2003). Sense of presence in virtual training: enhancing skills acquisition and transfer of knowledge through learning experience in virtual environments. In G. Riva, F. Davide, & W. A. IJsselsteijn (Eds.), Being There: Concepts, effects and measurement of user presence in synthetic environments (pp. 167–181). Amsterdam: Ios Press.

Manzoni, G. M., Cesa, G. L., Villani, D., Castelnuovo, G., Molinari, E., & Riva, G. (2006). VR-enhanced treatment of anxiety in obese subjects: A follow-up study on trait-anxiety, psychological symptornatology, and generalized self-efficacy. *Cyberpsychology & Behavior*, *9*(6), 699–700.

Manzoni, G. M., Pagnini, F., Gorini, A., Preziosa, A., Castelnuovo, G., Molinari, E., & Riva, G. (2009). Can relaxation training reduce emotional eating in women with obesity? An exploratory study with 3 months of follow-up. *Journal of the American Dietetic Association*, *109*(8), 1427–1432. doi:10.1016/j.jada.2009.05.004 PMID:19631051

Marsh, T. (2003). Staying there: an activity-based approach to narrative design and evaluation as an antidote to virtual corpsing. In G. Riva, F. Davide, & W. A. IJsselsteijn (Eds.), *Being There: Concepts, effects and measurements of user presence in synthetic environments* (pp. 85–96). Amsterdam: IOS Press.

Mathiesen, K. S., Tambs, K., & Dalgard, O. S. (1999). The influence of social class, strain and social support on symptoms of anxiety and depression in mothers of toddlers. *Social Psychiatry and Psychiatric Epidemiology*, *34*(2), 61–72. doi:10.1007/s001270050113 PMID:10189811

Matsumoto, D., & Wilson, J. (2008). Culture, emotion, and motivation. In R. Sorrentino & S. Yamaguchi (Eds.), *Handbook of Motivation and Cognition Across Cultures* (pp. 541–563). New York: Elsevier. doi:10.1016/B978-0-12-373694-9.00023-4

Matthew, A., & Stults-Kolehmainen, R. S. (2013). *The Effects of Stress on Physical Activity and Exercise*. Springer.

Mattila, E., Orsama, A. L., Ahtinen, A., Hopsu, L., Leino, T., & Korhonen, I. (2013). Personal health technologies in employee health promotion: Usage activity, usefulness, and health-related outcomes in a 1-year randomized controlled trial. *Journal of Medical Internet Research*, *1*(2), e16. PMID:25098385

Mauri, M., Magagnin, V., Cipresso, P., Mainardi, L., Brown, E. N., Cerutti, S., . . . Barbieri, R. (2010). Psychophysiological signals associated with affective states. *Paper presented at the 2010 Annual International Conference of the IEEE on Engineering in Medicine and Biology Society (EMBC)*. doi:10.1109/IEMBS.2010.5627465

Mauri, M., Villamira, M., Cipresso, P., Balgera, A., & Riva, G. (2011). Why Is Facebook So Successful? Psychophysiological Measures Describe a Core Flow State While Using Facebook. *Cyberpsychology, Behavior, and Social Networking*, *14*(12), 723–731. doi:10.1089/cyber.2010.0377 PMID:21879884

Mavin, T. J. (2010). Assessing pilots' performance for promotion to airline captain [Unpublished Doctor of Education thesis]. University of Queensland, Brisbane.

Mavin, T. J., & Dall'Alba, G. (2010). A model for integrating technical skills and NTS in assessing pilots' performance. *Proceedings of the 9th International Symposium of the Australian Aviation Psychology*, Sydney (pp. 9–12).

Mavin, T. J., & Roth, W. M. (2014). A holistic view of cockpit performance: An analysis of the assessment discourse of flight examiners. *The International Journal of Aviation Psychology*, *24*(3), 210–227. doi:10.1080/10508414.2014.918434

Mavin, T. J., Roth, W. M., & Dekker, S. (2013). Understanding variance in pilot performance ratings: Two studies of flight examiners, captains, and first officers assessing the performance of peers. *Aviation Psychology and Applied Human Factors*, *3*(2), 53–62. doi:10.1027/2192-0923/a000041

Mavin, T. J., Roth, W. M., & Munro, I. (in press). Models for and practice of continuous professional development for airline pilots: What we can learn from one regional airline. In S. Billett, D. Dymock, & S. Choy (Eds.), *Supporting learning across working life: Models, processes and practices*. New York: Springer.

Mayer, I. S., van Dierendonck, D., van Ruijven, T., & Wenzler, I. (2013, October 23-25). Stealth Assessment of Teams in a Digital Game Environment. *Proceedings of the GALA 2013 Conference,* Paris (pp. 1–13). Springer. doi:10.1007/978-3-319-12157-4_18

Mayer, J. D., & Gaschke, Y. N. (1988). The experience and meta-experience of mood. *Journal of Personality and Social Psychology*, *55*(1), 102–111. doi:10.1037/0022-3514.55.1.102 PMID:3418484

Mayer, R. E. (2009). *Multimedia learning*. Cambridge university press. doi:10.1017/CBO9780511811678

McCallum, S., & Boletsis, C. (2013). Dementia Games: A Literature Review of Dementia-Related Serious Games. Serious Games Development and Applications, LNCS (Vol. 8101, pp. 15–27). doi:10.1007/978-3-642-40790-1_2 doi:10.1007/978-3-642-40790-1_2

McCallum, S. (2012). Gamification and serious games for personalized health. *Studies in Health Technology and Informatics*, *177*, 85–96. PMID:22942036

McClarty, K. L., Orr, A., Frey, P. M., Dolan, R. P., Vassileva, V., & McVay, A. (2012). *A literature review of gaming in education*. Upper Saddle River, NJ: Pearson.

McEwen, B. S. (1998). Stress, adaptation, and disease: Allostasis and allostatic load. *Annals of the New York Academy of Sciences*, *840*(1), 33–44. doi:10.1111/j.1749-6632.1998.tb09546.x PMID:9629234

McEwen, B. S. (2006). Protective and damaging effects of stress mediators: Central role of the brain. *Dialogues in Clinical Neuroscience*, *8*(4), 367. PMID:17290796

McEwen, B. S., & Stellar, E. (1993). Stress and the individual: Mechanisms leading to disease. *Archives of Internal Medicine*, *153*(18), 2093–2101. doi:10.1001/archinte.1993.00410180039004 PMID:8379800

McGee, J. S., van der Zaag, C., Buckwalter, J. G., Thiebaux, M., Van Rooyen, A., Neumann, U., & Rizzo, A. A. et al. (2000). Issues for the assessment of visuospatial skills in older adults using Virtual Environment technology. *Cyberpsychology & Behavior*, *3*(3), 469–482. doi:10.1089/10949310050078931

McGonigal, J. (2010). *Reality is broken*. New York, NY, USA: The Penguin Press.

McGonigal, J. (2011). *Reality Is Broken. Why games make us better and how they can change the world.* New York: The Penguin Press.

McLay, R. N., Graap, K., Spira, J., Perlman, K., Johnston, S., Rothbaum, B. O., . . . Rizzo, A. (2012). Development and Testing of Virtual Reality Exposure Therapy for Post-Traumatic Stress Disorder in Active Duty Service Members Who Served in Iraq and Afghanistan. Military Medicine, 177(6), 635–642. doi:10.7205/MILMED-D-11-00221 PubMed doi:10.7205/MILMED-D-11-00221 PMID:22730837

McLeod, S. A. (2009). Emotion Focused Coping. *Simply Psychology.* Retrieved from www.simplypsychology.org/stress-management.html#em

Mcluhan, M. (1964). The Medium is the Message. *Understanding Media*, *14*, 7–23.

McQuiggan, S. W., Rowe, J. P., Lee, S., & Lester, J. C. (2008). Story-Based Learning: The Impact of Narrative on Learning Experiences and Outcomes. *Intelligent Tutoring System, LNCS* (Vol. *5091*, 530–539). doi:10.1007/978-3-540-69132-7_56

Meevissen, Y. M. C., Peters, M. L., & Alberts, H. J. E. M. (2011). Become more optimistic by imagining a best possible self: Effects of a two week intervention. *Journal of Behavior Therapy and Experimental Psychiatry*, *42*(3), 371–378. doi:10.1016/j.jbtep.2011.02.012 PMID:21450262

Meichenbaum, D. (1977). Cognitive behaviour modification. *Cognitive Behaviour Therapy*, *6*(4), 185–192.

Meichenbaum, D. (1985). *Stress inoculation training*. New York: Pergamon Press.

Melby-Lervåg, M., & Hulme, C. (2012). Is Working Memory Training Effective? A Meta-Analytic Review. *Developmental Psychology*, *49*(2), 270–291. doi:10.1037/a0028228 PMID:22612437

Melillo, P., Bracale, M., & Pecchia, L. (2011). Nonlinear Heart Rate Variability features for real-life stress detection. Case study: students under stress due to university examination. *Biomed Eng Online, 10*, 96. doi:1475-925X-10-96 [pii]10.1186/1475-925X-10-96

Mellou, E. (1994). Play theories: A contemporary review. *Early Child Development and Care*, *102*(1), 91–100. doi:10.1080/0300443941020107

Meltzoff, A. N., & Decety, J. (2003). What imitation tells us about social cognition: A rapprochement between developmental psychology and cognitive neuroscience. *Philosophical Transactions of the Royal Society*, *358*(1431), 491–500. doi:10.1098/rstb.2002.1261 PMID:12689375

Melzer, K., Schutz, Y., Soehnchen, N., Othenin-Girard, V., de Tejada, B. M., Irion, O., & Kayser, B. et al. (2010). Effects of recommended levels of physical activity on pregnancy outcomes. *American Journal of Obstetrics and Gynecology*, *202*(3), 266–e1. doi:10.1016/j.ajog.2009.10.876 PMID:20022583

Menichetti, J., Cipresso, P., Bussolin, D., & Graffigna, G. (2015). Engaging older people in healthy and active lifestyles: A systematic review. *Ageing and Society*, *1*, 1–25. doi:10.1017/S0144686X15000781

Menichetti, J., Libreri, C., Lozza, E., & Graffigna, G. (2014). Giving patients a starring role in their own care: A bibliometric analysis of the on-going literature debate. *Health Expectations*, *4*(11), 1369–7625. PMID:25369557

Mental Health on the go: Reducing anxiety with smartphone app. (2014, March 18). Association for Psychological Science. *ScienceDaily*. Retrieved from www.sciencedaily.com/releases/2014/03/140318111900.htm

Merry, S. N., Stasiak, K., Shepherd, M., Frampton, C., Fleming, T., & Lucassen, M. F. (2012). The effectiveness of SPARX, a computerised self-help intervention for adolescents seeking help for depression: Randomised controlled non-inferiority trial. British Medical Journal, 344(apr18 3), e2598. doi:10.1136/bmj.e2598 PubMed doi:10.1136/bmj.e2598 PMID:22517917

*mHealth App Developer Economics 2014: The State of the Art of mHealth App* . (2014). Research2guidance. Retrieved from http://research2guidance.com/r2g/mHealth-App-Developer-Economics-2014.pdf

mHealth: New Horizons for Health through Mobile Technologies: Based on the Findings of the Second Global Survey on eHealth (Global Observatory for eHealth Series, Volume 3) (2011). World Health Organization.

Michael, D., & Chen, S. (2006). *Serious Games: Games That Educate, Train and Inform*. Boston: Thomson.

Middlebrooks, C. D., McGillivray, S., Murayama, K., & Castel, A. D. (2015). Memory for Allergies and Health Foods: How Younger and Older Adults Strategically Remember Critical Health Information. *The Journals of Gerontology. Series B, Psychological Sciences and Social Sciences*. doi:10.1093/geronb/gbv032 PMID:25975293

Milgram, S. (1963). Behavioral study of obedience. *Psycho J, 67*, 371–378. PMID:14049516

Millennials Continue Urbanization Of America, Leaving Small Towns. (2014). *National Public Radio.* Retrieved from http://www.npr.org/2014/10/21/357723069/millennials-continue-urbanization-of-america-leaving-small-towns

Miller, G. E., Chen, E., & Zhou, E. S. (2007). If it goes up, must it come down? Chronic stress and the hypothalamic-pituitary-adrenocortical axis in humans. *Psychol Bull, 133*(1), 25-45. doi:2006-23058-00210.1037/0033-2909.133.1.25

Miller, A. M., & Iris, M. (2002). Health promotion attitudes and strategies in older adults. *Health Education & Behavior, 29*(2), 249–267. doi:10.1177/1090198102029002009 PMID:11942718

Miller, E. A. (2003). The technical and interpersonal aspects of telemedicine: Effects on doctor–patient communication. *Journal of Telemedicine and Telecare, 9*(1), 1–7. doi:10.1258/135763303321159611 PMID:12641885

Miller, G. (2012). The Smartphone Psychology Manifesto. *Perspectives on Psychological Science, 7*(3), 221–237. doi:10.1177/1745691612441215 PMID:26168460

Miller, J. J., Fletcher, K., & Kabat-Zinn, J. (1995). Three-year follow-up and clinical implications of a mindfulness meditation-based stress reduction intervention in the treatment of anxiety disorders. *General Hospital Psychiatry, 17*(3), 192–200. doi:10.1016/0163-8343(95)00025-M PMID:7649463

Miller, K. J., Adair, B. S., Pearce, A. J., Said, C. M., Ozanne, E., & Morris, M. M. (2014). Effectiveness and feasibility of virtual reality and gaming system use at home by older adults for enabling physical activity to improve health-related domains: A systematic review. *Age and Ageing, 43*(2), 188–195. doi:10.1093/ageing/aft194 PMID:24351549

Miller, V. (2011). Convergence and the Contemporary Media Experience. In D. M. Berry (Ed.), *ED.) Understanding Digital Culture* (pp. 72–94). London, UK: Sage.

Millings, A., Morris, J., Rowe, A., Easton, S., Martin, J. K., Majoe, D., & Mohr, C. (2015). *Can the effectiveness of an online stress management program be augmented by wearable sensor technology?* Internet Interventions.

Milward, P. (2003). The 'grey digital divide': Perception, exclusion, and barriers of access to the Internet for older people. *First Monday, 8*(7). doi:10.5210/fm.v8i7.1066

Mira, A. (2014). Eficacia diferencial de un programa de intervención auto-aplicado a través de Internet para la prevención y el tratamiento de la depresión leve o moderada con apoyo y sin apoyo por parte del terapeuta. [Doctoral thesis]. Universitat Jaume I. Retrieved from http://hdl.handle.net/10803/284396

Mira, A., Botella, C., García-Palacios, A., Bretón-López, J., Moragrega, I., & Riera-López del Amo, A., … Baños, R. M. (2012a). Coping with stress: A program for the prevention of depression. *Proceedings of the 1st Workshop on ICT applied to Mental Health* (pp. 48-52).

Mira, A., Botella, C., García-Palacios, A., Riera, A., Quero, S., Alcañiz, M., & Baños, R. (2012b). An internet-based program to cope with regulating stress and emotion: An example of positive technology. *Cybertherapy & Rehabilitation, 2*(1), 22-23.

Mitchell, A. J., & Shiri-Feshki, M. (2009). Rate of progression of mild cognitive impairment to dementia--meta-analysis of 41 robust inception cohort studies. *Acta Psychiatrica Scandinavica, 119*(4), 252–265. doi:10.1111/j.1600-0447.2008.01326.x PMID:19236314

Mitgutsch, K., & Alvarado, N. (2012, May). Purposeful by design?: a serious game design assessment framework. *Proceedings of the International Conference on the foundations of digital games* (pp. 121-128). doi:10.1145/2282338.2282364

Mitmansgruber, H., Beck, T. N., Höfer, S., & Schüßler, G. (2009). When you don't like what you feel: Experiential avoidance, mindfulness and meta-emotion in emotion regulation. *Personality and Individual Differences*, *46*(4), 448–453. doi:10.1016/j.paid.2008.11.013

Mitra, S., & Dangwal, R. (2010). Limits to self-organising systems of learning—the Kalikuppam experiment. *British Journal of Educational Technology*, *41*(5), 672–688. doi:10.1111/j.1467-8535.2010.01077.x

Mitra, S., & Padman, R. (2012). Exploring social media for health and wellness: A health plan case study. *Journal of Cases on Information Technology*, *14*(2), 42–64. doi:10.4018/jcit.2012040104

Mitzner, T. L., Boron, J. B., Fausset, C. B., Adams, A. E., Czaja, S. J., Dijkstra, K., & Sharit, J. et al. (2010). Older adults talk technology: Technology usage and attitudes. *Computers in Human Behavior*, *26*(6), 1710–1721. doi:10.1016/j.chb.2010.06.020 PMID:20967133

Miyata, K. (2002). Social support for Japanese mothers online and offline. *The internet in everyday life*, 520-548.

Mobile millennials: over 85% of generation Y owns smartphones. (2014). Nielsen. Retrieved from http://www.nielsen.com/us/en/insights/news/2014/mobile-millennials-over-85-percent-of-generation-y-owns-smartphones.html

Mohr, D. C., Burns, M. N., Schueller, S. M., Clarke, G., & Klinkman, M. (2013). Behavioral intervention technologies: Evidence review and recommendations for future research in mental health. *General Hospital Psychiatry*, *35*(4), 332–338. doi:10.1016/j.genhosppsych.2013.03.008 PMID:23664503

Monkong, L., Pongpanich, S., Viwatwongkasem, C., Chantavanich, S., Wongpiromsarn, Y., & Katz, L. S. (2009). The effectiveness of program developed from cognitive experiential self-theory and life skills technique on adolescent coping with stress. *Nepal Medical College Journal*, *11*(4), 225–228. PMID:20635598

Monti, F., Fagandini, P., Agostini, F., Vettori, D., & La Sala, G. B. (2006). *La complessità della nascita: genitorialità e modalità di parto. La Sala GB, Iori V., Monti F., Fagandini P.(a cura di), La "normale" complessità del venire al mondo*. Milano: Guerini Studio.

Mora, F. (2012). The demise of Google Health and the future of personal health records. *International Journal of Healthcare Technology and Management*, *13*(5/6), 363–377. doi:10.1504/IJHTM.2012.052563

Morey, J. N., Boggero, I. A., Scott, A. B., & Segerstrom, S. C. (2015). Current directions in stress and human immune function. *Current Opinion in Psychology*, *5*, 13–17. doi:10.1016/j.copsyc.2015.03.007 PMID:26086030

Morganti, F., & Riva, G. (2004). Ambient Intelligence in Rehabilitation. In G. Riva, F. Davide, F. Vatalaro, & M. Alcañiz (Eds.), *Ambient Intelligence: The evolution of technology, communication and cognition towards the future of the human-computer interaction* (pp. 283–295). Amsterdam: IOS Press.

Morganti, L., Riva, G., Bonfiglio, S., & Gaggioli, A. (2013). Building collective memories on the web: The Nostalgia Bits project. *International Journal of Web Based Communities*, *9*(1), 83–104. doi:10.1504/IJWBC.2013.051373

Morledge, T. J., Allexandre, D., Fox, E., Fu, A. Z., Higashi, M. K., Kruzikas, D. T., & Reese, P. R. et al. (2013). Feasibility of an online mindfulness program for stress management—a randomized, controlled trial. *Annals of Behavioral Medicine*, *46*(2), 137–148. doi:10.1007/s12160-013-9490-x PMID:23632913

Morris, M. E., Kathawala, Q., Leen, T. K., Gorenstein, E. E., Guilak, F., Labhard, M., & Deleeuw, W. (2010). Mobile therapy: case study evaluations of a cell phone application for emotional self-awareness. *J Med Internet Res, 12*(2), e10. doi:v12i2e1010.2196/jmir.1371

Morris, B. J., Corker, S., Zimmerman, C., Gill, D., & Romig, C. (2013). Gaming science: The 'gamification' of scientific thinking. *Frontiers in Psychology*, *4*, 607. doi:10.3389/fpsyg.2013.00607 PMID:24058354

Morris, M. E. (2005). Social networks as health feedback displays. *IEEE Internet Computing*, *9*(5), 29–37. doi:10.1109/MIC.2005.109

Moser, D. K., & Dracup, K. (1995). Psychosocial recovery from a cardiac event : The influence of perceived control. *Heart and Lung: The Journal of Acute and Critical Care*, *24*(4), 273–280. doi:10.1016/S0147-9563(05)80070-6 PMID:7591794

Muaremi, A., Arnrich, B., & Tröster, G. (2013). Towards Measuring Stress with Smartphones and Wearable Devices During Workday and Sleep. *BioNanoScience*, *3*(2), 172–183. doi:10.1007/s12668-013-0089-2 PMID:25530929

Mulsow, M., Caldera, Y. M., Pursley, M., Reifman, A., & Huston, A. C. (2002). Multilevel factors influencing maternal stress during the first three years. *Journal of Marriage and the Family*, *64*(4), 944–956. doi:10.1111/j.1741-3737.2002.00944.x

Murphy, L. R. (1996). Stress management in work settings: A critical review of the health effects. *American Journal of Health Promotion*, *11*(2), 112–135. doi:10.4278/0890-1171-11.2.112 PMID:10163598

Murray, E., Charles, C., & Gafni, A. (2006). Shared decision-making in primary care: Tailoring the model to fit the context of general practice. *Patient Education and Counseling*, *62*(2), 205–211. doi:10.1016/j.pec.2005.07.003 PMID:16139467

Murray, L. (1992). The impact of postnatal depression on infant development. *Journal of Child Psychology and Psychiatry, and Allied Disciplines*, *33*(3), 543–561. doi:10.1111/j.1469-7610.1992.tb00890.x PMID:1577898

Murray, L., Fiori-Cowley, A., Hooper, R., & Cooper, P. (1996). The impact of postnatal depression and associated adversity on early mother-infant interactions and later infant outcome. *Child Development*, *67*(5), 2512–2526. doi:10.2307/1131637 PMID:9022253

Murray, L., Sinclair, D., Cooper, P., Ducournau, P., Turner, P., & Stein, A. (1999). The socioemotional development of 5-year-old children of postnatally depressed mothers. *Journal of Child Psychology and Psychiatry, and Allied Disciplines*, *40*(08), 1259–1271. doi:10.1111/1469-7610.00542 PMID:10604404

Myers, I. B. (1987). *Introduction to Type: A Description of the Theory and Applications of the Myers-Briggs Type Indicator*. Palo Alto: Consulting Psychologists Press.

Mynatt, E. D., & Rogers, W. (2001). Developing technology to support the functional independence of older adults. *Ageing International*, *27*(1), 24–41. doi:10.1007/s12126-001-1014-5

Nacke, L. E., Bateman, C., & Mandryk, R. L. (2011). BrainHex: Preliminary results from a neurobiological gamer typology survey.*Proceedings of the 10th International Conference on Entertainment Computing* (pp. 288–293). Berlin: Springer. doi:10.1007/978-3-642-24500-8_31

Nacke, L., & Lindley, C. (2008). Boredom, Immersion, Flow - A pilot study investigating player experience. *Measurement*, *24*, 1–5.

Nacke, L., & Lindley, C. (2009). Affective ludology, flow, and immersion in a first-person shooter: Measurement of player experience. *The Journal of the Canadian Game Studies Association*, *3*(5), 37–42.

Nakamura, J., & Csikszentmihalyi, M. (2002). The concept of flow. In C. R. Snyder & S. J. Lopez (Eds.), *The handbook of positive psychology*. Oxford: Oxford University Press.

Nap, H. H., & Diaz-Orueta, U. (2014). Rehabilitation Gaming. In J. Bishop (Ed.), Gamification for Human Factors Integration: Social (pp. 122–147). Hershey, PA, USA: Education, and Psychological Issues. doi:10.4018/978-1-4666-5071-8.ch008 doi:10.4018/978-1-4666-5071-8.ch008

Narendran, S., Nagarathna, R., Narendran, V., Gunasheela, S., & Nagendra, H. R. R. (2005). Efficacy of yoga on pregnancy outcome. *Journal of Alternative and Complementary Medicine (New York, N.Y.)*, *11*(2), 237–244. doi:10.1089/acm.2005.11.237 PMID:15865489

Nascimento, B. R., Brant, L. C., Moraes, D. N., & Ribeiro, A. L. (2014). Global health and cardiovascular disease. *Heart (British Cardiac Society)*, *100*(22), 1743–1749. doi:10.1136/heartjnl-2014-306026 PMID:25327515

Nasreen, H. E., Kabir, Z. N., Forsell, Y., & Edhborg, M. (2011). Prevalence and associated factors of depressive and anxiety symptoms during pregnancy: A population based study in rural Bangladesh. *BMC Women's Health*, *11*(1), 22. doi:10.1186/1472-6874-11-22 PMID:21635722

National Survey of Mental Health and Wellbeing Summary of results. (2007). Australian Bureau of Statistics: Australian Bureau of Statistics, Canberra.

Neill, J. T., & Dias, K. L. (2012). Adventure education and resilience: The double-edged sword. *Journal of Adventure Education and Outdoor Learning*, *2*(1), 35–42.

Newman, M. G., Szkodny, L. E., Llera, S. J., & Przeworski, A. (2011). A review of technology-assisted self-help and minimal contact therapies for anxiety and depression: Is human contact necessary for therapeutic efficacy? *Clinical Psychology Review*, *31*(1), 89–103. doi:10.1016/j.cpr.2010.09.008 PMID:21130939

Nickel, C., Lahmann, C., Muehlbacher, M., Pedrosa Gil, F., Kaplan, P., Buschmann, W., & Nickel, M. et al. (2006). Pregnant women with bronchial asthma benefit from progressive muscle relaxation: A randomized, prospective, controlled trial. *Psychotherapy and Psychosomatics*, *75*(4), 237–243. doi:10.1159/000092894 PMID:16785773

Nielsen, J. (1994a, April 24-28). Enhancing the explanatory power of usability heuristics. *Proc. ACM CHI'94 Conf.*, Boston, MA (pp. 152-158).

Norman, D. A. (2004). *Emotional design: Why we love or hate everyday things*. New York: Basic Books.

O'Malley, P. (2010). Resilient subjects: Uncertainty, warfare and liberalism. *Economy and Society*, *39*(4), 488–509. do i:10.1080/03085147.2010.510681

Oakley, A. (1992). Social support in pregnancy: Methodology and findings of a 1-year follow-up study. *Journal of Reproductive and Infant Psychology*, *10*(4), 219–231. doi:10.1080/02646839208403955

Oakley, A., Hickey, D., Rajan, L., & Rigby, A. S. (1996). Social support in pregnancy: Does it have long-term effects? *Journal of Reproductive and Infant Psychology*, *14*(1), 7–22. doi:10.1080/02646839608405855

Oakley, A., Rajan, L., & Grant, A. (1990). Social support and pregnancy outcome. *BJOG: An International Journal of Obstetrics & Gynaecology*, *97*(2), 155–162. doi:10.1111/j.1471-0528.1990.tb01741.x PMID:2317466

O'Connor, T. G., Heron, J., & Glover, V. (2002). Antenatal anxiety predicts child behavioral/emotional problems independently of postnatal depression. *Journal of the American Academy of Child and Adolescent Psychiatry*, *41*(12), 1470–1477. doi:10.1097/00004583-200212000-00019 PMID:12447034

O'Dwyer-O'Brien, A., Coyle, S., Coyle, D., & O' Reilly, G. (2011, July). Gnatenborough's Island: A C-CBT adaption for young people with internalising disorders. Paper presented at the British Association for Behavioural and Cognitive Psychotherapies 39th Annual Conference, UK.

O'Hara, M. W., & Swain, A. M. (1996). Rates and risk of postpartum depression-a meta-analysis. *International Review of Psychiatry (Abingdon, England)*, *8*(1), 37–54. doi:10.3109/09540269609037816

O'Higgins, A., Murphy, O. C., Egan, A., Mullaney, L., Sheehan, S., & Turner, M. J. (2013). The use of digital media by women using the maternity services in a developed country. *Irish Medical Journal*, *107*(10), 313–315. PMID:25556255

Oksanen, K. (2014). Subjective Experience and Sociability in a Collaborative Serious Game. *Simulation & Gaming*, *44*(6), 767–793. doi:10.1177/1046878113513079

Oliver, M. B. (1993). Exploring the Paradox of the Enjoyment of Sad Films. *Communication*, *19*(3), 315–342. doi:10.1111/j.1468-2958.1993.tb00304.x

Oliver, M. B., Bowman, N. D., Woolley, J. K., Rogers, R., Sherrick, B. I., & Chung, M.-Y. (2015). Video games as meaningful entertainment experiences. *Psychology of Popular Media Culture*. Retrieved15May2015. doi:10.1037/ppm0000066

Oliver, M. B., Hartmann, T., & Woolley, J. K. (2012). Elevation in Response to Entertainment Portrayals of Moral Virtue. *Human Communication Research*, *38*(3), 360–378. doi:10.1111/j.1468-2958.2012.01427.x

Olivo, E. L., Dodson-Lavelle, B., Wren, A., Fang, Y., & Oz, M. C. (2009). Feasibility and effectiveness of a brief meditation-based stress management intervention for patients diagnosed with or at risk for coronary heart disease: A pilot study. *Psychology Health and Medicine*, *14*(5), 513–523. doi:10.1080/13548500902890087 PMID:19844830

Optale, G., Capodieci, S., Marin, S., Pastore, M., & Piron, L. (2007). Multimedia memory- training nel declino cognitivo legato all'età, uno studio controllato e in follow-up. *Psicotech*, *2*, 33–45.

Optale, G., Capodieci, S., Pinelli, P., Zara, D., Gamberini, L., & Riva, G. (2001). Music-enhanced immersive virtual reality in the rehabilitation of memory-related cognitive processes and functional abilities: A case report. *Presence (Cambridge, Mass.)*, *10*(4), 450–462. doi:10.1162/1054746011470217

Optale, G., Urgesi, C., Busato, V., Marin, S., Piron, L., Priftis, K., & Bordin, A. et al. (2010). Controlling Memory Impairment in Elderly Adults Using Virtual Reality Memory Training: A Randomized Controlled Pilot Study. *Neurorehabilitation and Neural Repair*, *24*(4), 348–357. doi:10.1177/1545968309353328 PMID:19934445

Orsila, R., Virtanen, M., Luukkaala, T., Tarvainen, M., Karjalainen, P., Viik, J., & Nygard, C. H. et al. (2008). Perceived mental stress and reactions in heart rate variability--a pilot study among employees of an electronics company. *International Journal of Occupational Safety and Ergonomics*, *14*(3), 275–283. http://www.ncbi.nlm.nih.gov/entrez/query.fcgi?cmd=Retrieve&db=PubMed&dopt=Citation&list_uids=18954537 doi:10.1080/10803548.2008.11076767 PMID:18954537

Pacherie, E. (2006). Toward a dynamic theory of intentions. In S. Pockett, W. P. Banks, & S. Gallagher (Eds.), *Does consciousness cause behavior?* (pp. 145–167). Cambridge, MA: MIT Press. doi:10.7551/mitpress/9780262162371.003.0009

Pacherie, E. (2008). The phenomenology of action: A conceptual framework. *Cognition*, *107*(1), 179–217. doi:10.1016/j.cognition.2007.09.003 PMID:17950720

Pacherie, E., & Haggard, P. (2010). What are intentions? In L. Nadel & W. Sinnott-Armstrong (Eds.), *Conscious Will and Responsibility. A tribute to Benjamin Libet* (pp. 70–84). Oxford: Oxford University Press. doi:10.1093/acprof:oso/9780195381641.003.0008

Page, R. C., Martin, J. A., & Loeb, C. F. (2005). The Oral Health Information Suite (OHIS): Its use in the management of periodontal disease. *Journal of Dental Education*, *69*(5), 509–520. PMID:15897333

Pagnini, F., & Phillips, D. (2015). Being mindful about mindfulness. *The Lancet Psychiatry*, *2*(4), 288 - 289. doi:S2215-0366(15)00041-3

Pagnini, F., Di Credico, C., Gatto, R., Fabiani, V., Rossi, G., Lunetta, C., & Amadei, G. et al. (2014). Meditation training for people with amyotrophic lateral sclerosis and their caregivers. *Journal of Alternative and Complementary Medicine (New York, N.Y.)*, *20*(4), 272–275. doi:10.1089/acm.2013.0268 PMID:24328393

Pagnini, F., Phillips, D., Bosma, C., Reece, A., & Langer, E. (2015). Mindfulness, physical impairment and psychological well-being in people with amyotrophic lateral sclerosis. *Psychology & Health*, *30*(5), 503–517. doi:10.1080/08870446.2014.982652 PMID:25361013

Pagnini, F., Phillips, D., & Langer, E. (2014). A mindful approach with end-of-life thoughts. *Frontiers in Psychology*, *5*, 138. doi:10.3389/fpsyg.2014.00138 PMID:24600429

Pallavicini, F., Cipresso, P., Raspelli, S., Grassi, A., Serino, S., Vigna, C., & Riva, G. et al. (2013). Is virtual reality always an effective stressor for exposure treatments? Some insights from a controlled trial. *BMC Psychiatry*, *13*(1), 52. doi:10.1186/1471-244X-13-52 PMID:23398927

Pallavicini, F., Gaggioli, A., Raspelli, S., Cipresso, P., Serino, S., Vigna, C., & Riva, G. et al.(2013). Interreality for the management and training of psychological stress: Study protocol for a randomized controlled trial. *Trials*, *14*(1), 191. doi:10.1186/1745-6215-14-191 PMID:23806013

Pan, J., & Tompkins, W. J. (1985). A real-time QRS detection algorithm. *IEEE Transactions on Biomedical Engineering*, 3, 230-236.

Paras, B. (2005). Game, motivation, and effective learning: An integrated model for educational game design. In *Proceedings of DIGRA 2005 Conference Changing Views – Worlds in Play.*

Parisi, J. M., Stine-Morrow, E. A., Noh, S. R., & Morrow, D. G. (2009). Predispositional engagement, activity engagement, and cognition among older adults. *Neuropsychology, Development, and Cognition. Section B, Aging, Neuropsychology and Cognition*, *16*(4), 485–504. doi:10.1080/13825580902866653 PMID:19468932

Parker, R. M., Dmitrieva, E., Frolov, S., & Gazmararian, J. A. (2012). Text4baby in the United States and Russia: an opportunity for understanding how mHealth affects maternal and child health. *Journal of health communication, 17*(sup1), 30-36.

Parker, S., Jimmieson, N., & Amiot, C. (2009). The Stress buffering effects of control on task satisfaction and perceived goal attainment: An experimental study of the moderating influence of desirability of control. Applied Psychology, 58(4), 622–652. doi:10.1111/j.1464-0597.2008.00367.x doi:10.1111/j.1464-0597.2008.00367.x

Park, H. (2010). The Effect Of Activities In Virtual Worlds As A Communication Environment To Understand Each Other. *Journal of Cyber Therapy and Rehabilitation*, *3*(1), 71–82.

Parks, A. C. (2014). A case for the advancement of the design and study of online positive psychological interventions. *The Journal of Positive Psychology*, *9*(6), 502–508. doi:10.1080/17439760.2014.936969

Parks, A. C., & Biswas-Diener, R. (2013). Positive Interventions: Past, Present, and Future. In T. Kashdan & J. Carriochi (Eds.), *Bridging Acceptance and Commitment Therapy and Positive Psychology: A Practitioners's Guide to a Unifying Framework*. Oakland, CA: New Harbinger.

Parks, A. C., Della Porta, M. D., Pierce, R. S., Zilca, R., & Lyubomirsky, S. (2012). Pursuing happiness in everyday life: The characteristics and behaviors of online happiness seekers. *Emotion (Washington, D.C.)*, *12*(6), 1222–1234. doi:10.1037/a0028587 PMID:22642345

Partla, T., & Surakka, V. (2003). Pupil size variation as an indication of affective processing. *International Journal of Human-Computer Studies*, *59*(1-2), 185–198. doi:10.1016/S1071-5819(03)00017-X

Patsopoulos, N. A. (2011). A pragmatic view on pragmatic trials. *Dialogues in Clinical Neuroscience*, *13*(2), 217–224. Retrieved from http://www.ncbi.nlm.nih.gov/pubmed/21842619 PMID:21842619

Pedroli, E., Cipresso, P., Serino, S., Pallavicini, F., Albani, G., & Riva, G. (2013). Virtual multiple errands test: Reliability, usability and possible applications. *Studies in Health Technology and Informatics, 191*, 38–42. PMID:23792839

Peine, A., Faulkner, A., Jæger, B., & Moors, E. (2014). Science, technology and the "grand challenge" of ageing – Understanding the socio-material constitution of later life. *Technological Forecasting and Social Change, 93*, 1–9. doi:10.1016/j.techfore.2014.11.010

Peine, A., Rollwagen, I., & Neven, L. (2014). The rise of the "innosumer" - Rethinking older technology users. *Technological Forecasting and Social Change, 82*, 199–214. doi:10.1016/j.techfore.2013.06.013

Pekrun, R., Elliot, A. J., & Maier, M. A. (2006). Achievement goals and discrete emotions: A theoretical model and prospective test. *Journal of Educational Psychology, 98*(3), 583–597. doi:10.1037/0022-0663.98.3.583

Pelachaud, C. 2009. Modelling Multimodal Expression of Emotion in a Virtual Agent, *Philosophical Trans. B,* 364, 3539-3548.

Pennebaker, J. W., Francis, M. E., & Booth, R. J. (2001). Linguistic Inquiry and Word Count (LIWC): A computerized text analysis program. Mahwah (NJ), 7.

Perry, R. P., Hladkyj, S., Pekrun, R. H., Clifton, R. A., & Chipperfield, J. G. (2005). Perceived academic control and failure in college students: A three-year study of scholastic attainment. *Research in Higher Education, 46*(5), 535–569. doi:10.1007/s11162-005-3364-4

Peters, D., & Calvo, R. (2014). Compassion vs. empathy: designing for resilience. *interactions, 21*(5), 48-53.

Peters, E., Lipkus, I., & Diefenbach, M. A. (2006). The functions of affect in health communications and in the construction of health preferences. *Journal of Communication, 56*(Suppl. 1), s140–s150. doi:10.1111/j.1460-2466.2006.00287.x

Petersen, R. C. (2004). Mild cognitive impairment as a diagnostic entity. *Journal of Internal Medicine, 256*(3), 183–194. doi:10.1111/j.1365-2796.2004.01388.x PMID:15324362

Petersen, R. C. (2011). Mild cognitive impairment. *The New England Journal of Medicine, 364*(23), 2227–2234. doi:10.1056/NEJMcp0910237 PMID:21651394

Peters, M. L., Meevissen, Y. M. C., & Hanssen, M. M. (2013). Specificity of the Best Possible Self intervention for increasing optimism: Comparison with a gratitude intervention. *Terapia Psicológica, 31*(1), 93–100. doi:10.4067/S0718-48082013000100009

Peterson, C. (2006). *A Primer in Positive Psychology*. New York, NY: Oxford University Press.

Peterson, C., & Park, N. (2009). Classifying and Measuring Strengths of Character. In C. R. Snyder & S. J. Lopez (Eds.), *Handbook of Positive Psychology*. New York, NY: Oxford University Press. doi:10.1093/oxfordhb/9780195187243.013.0004

Peyton, T. (2014, November). Pregnancy Ecologies As Teachable Moments For The Lifecourse: Changing The mHealth Design Paradigm.*Proceedings of the 18th International Conference on Supporting Group Work* (pp. 269-271). ACM. doi:10.1145/2660398.2660438

Peyton, T., Poole, E., Reddy, M., Kraschnewski, J., & Chuang, C. (2014, June). Every pregnancy is different: designing mHealth for the pregnancy ecology.*Proceedings of the 2014 conference on Designing interactive systems* (pp. 577-586). ACM. doi:10.1145/2598510.2598572

Philippot, P. (1993). Inducing and assessing differentiated emotion-feeling states in the laboratory. *Cognition and Emotion, 7*(2), 171–193. doi:10.1080/02699939308409183

Phillips, A., & Pagnini, F. (2014). A mindful approach to chronic illness. In A. Le, C. T. Nguoumen, & E. Langer (Eds.), *The Wiley-Blackwell Handbook of Mindfulness* (pp. 852–863). London: Wiley-Blackwell. doi:10.1002/9781118294895.ch43

Phillips, N. M., Street, M., & Haesler, E. (2014). Measuring patient participation in health care: A comprehensive systematic review protocol. *The JBI Database of Systematic Reviews and Implementation Reports*, *12*(3), 68–88. doi:10.11124/jbisrir-2014-1380

Picard, R. W. (2000). *Affective computing*. MIT press.

Piette, J. D. (2000). Interactive voice response systems in the diagnosis and management of chronic disease. *The American Journal of Managed Care*, *6*(7), 817–827. PMID:11067378

Plante, T. G., Aldridge, A., Su, D., Bogdan, R., Belo, M., & Kahn, K. (2003). Does Virtual Reality Enhance the Management of Stress When Paired With Exercise? An Exploratory Study. *International Journal of Stress Management*, *10*(3), 203–216. doi:10.1037/1072-5245.10.3.203

Plante, T. G., Cage, C., Clements, S., & Stover, A. (2006). Psychological benefits of exercise paired with virtual reality: Outdoor exercise energizes whereas indoor virtual exercise relaxes. *International Journal of Stress Management*, *13*(1), 108–117. doi:10.1037/1072-5245.13.1.108

Plantinga, C. (2009). *Moving viewers: American Film and the Spectator's Experience*. Oakland, USA: University of California Press.

Plaza, I., Demarzo, M. M., Herrera-Mercadal, P., & Garcia-Campayo, J. (2013). Mindfulness-based mobile applications: Literature review and analysis of current features. *JMIR Mhealth Uhealth*, *1*(2), e24. doi:10.2196/mhealth.2733 PMID:25099314

Pluess, M., Wurmser, H., Buske-Kirschbaum, A., Papousek, M., Pirke, K. M., Hellhammer, D., & Bolten, M. (2012). Positive life events predict salivary cortisol in pregnant women. *Psychoneuroendocrinology*, *37*(8), 1336–1340. doi:10.1016/j.psyneuen.2012.01.006 PMID:22309824

Postman, N. (1993). *Technopoly: The Surrender of Culture to Technology*. New York, USA: Vintage.

Powell, J., Hamborg, T., Stallard, N., Burls, A., McSorley, J., Bennett, K., & Christensen, H. et al. (2013). Effectiveness of a web-based cognitive-behavioral tool to improve mental well-being in the general population: Randomized controlled trial. *Journal of Medical Internet Research*, *15*(1). PMID:23302475

Preece, J. (2001). Online communities: Usability, sociabilty, theory and methods. In *Frontiers of human-centered computing, online communities and virtual environments* (pp. 263–277). Springer London. doi:10.1007/978-1-4471-0259-5_18

Prensky, M. (2001). Digital Natives, Digital Immigrants. *On the Horizon*, *9*(5), 1–6. doi:10.1108/10748120110424816

Preschl, B., Maercker, A., Wagner, B., Forstmeier, S., Baños, R. M., Alcañiz, M., & Botella, C. et al. (2012). Life review therapy with computer supplements for depression in the elderly: A randomized controlled trial. *Aging & Mental Health*, *16*(8), 964–974. doi:10.1080/13607863.2012.702726 PMID:22788983

Preziosa, A., Grassi, A., Gaggioli, A., & Riva, G. (2009). Therapeutic applications of the mobile phone. *British Journal of Guidance & Counselling*, *37*(3), 313–325. doi:10.1080/03069880902957031

Prins, P. J., Brink, E. T., Dovis, S., Ponsioen, A., Geurts, H. M., de Vries, M., & van der Oord, S. (2013). "Braingame Brian": Toward an Executive Function Training Program with Game Elements for Children with ADHD and Cognitive Control Problems. Games for Health Journal, 2(1), 44–49. doi:10.1089/g4h.2013.0004 PubMed doi:10.1089/g4h.2013.0004 PMID:26196554

Procci, K., Bowers, C., Wong, C., & Andrews, A. (2013). Minigames for Mental Health: Improving Warfighters' Coping Skills and Awareness of Mental Health Resources. Games for Health Journal, 2(4), 240–246. doi:10.1089/g4h.2013.0014 PubMed doi:10.1089/g4h.2013.0014 PMID:26192227

Prochaska, J. O., & DiClemente, C. C. (1982). Transtheoretical therapy: Toward a more integrative model of change. *Psychotherapy (Chicago, Ill.)*, *19*(3), 212–216.

Prochaska, J. O., & DiClemente, C. C. (1983). Stages and processes of self-change in smoking toward an integrative model of change. *Journal of Consulting and Clinical Psychology*, *5*(3), 390–395. doi:10.1037/0022-006X.51.3.390 PMID:6863699

Prochaska, J. O., DiClemente, C. C., & Norcross, J. C. (1992). In search of how people change. *The American Psychologist*, *47*(9), 1102–1114. doi:10.1037/0003-066X.47.9.1102 PMID:1329589

Proffitt, R., & Lange, B. (2015). Considerations in the efficacy and effectiveness of virtual reality interventions for stroke rehabilitation: Moving the field forward. *Physical Therapy*, *95*(3), 441–448. doi:10.2522/ptj.20130571 PMID:25343960

Proudfoot, J., Ryden, C., Everitt, B., Shapiro, D. A., Goldberg, D., Mann, A., & Gray, J. A. et al. (2004). Clinical efficacy of computerised cognitive–behavioural therapy for anxiety and depression in primary care: Randomised controlled trial. *The British Journal of Psychiatry*, *185*(1), 46–54. doi:10.1192/bjp.185.1.46 PMID:15231555

Przybylski, A. K., Rigby, C. S., & Ryan, R. M. (2010). A motivational model of video game engagement. *Review of General Psychology*, *14*(2), 154–166. doi:10.1037/a0019440

Przybylski, A. K., Ryan, R. M., & Rigby, C. S. (2009). The motivating role of violence in video games. *Personality and Social Psychology Bulletin*, *35*(2), 243–259. doi:10.1177/0146167208327216 PMID:19141627

Przybylski, K., Weinstein, N., Murayama, K., Lynch, M. F., & Ryan, R. M. (2012). The Ideal Self at Play: The Appeal of Video Games That Let You Be All You Can Be. *Psychological Science*, *23*(1), 69–76. doi:10.1177/0956797611418676 PMID:22173739

Psotka, J. (2013). Educational Games and Virtual Reality as Disruptive Technologies. *Journal of Educational Technology & Society*, *16*(2), 69–80.

Quoidbach, J., Berry, E. V., Hansenne, M., & Mikolajczak, M. (2010). Positive emotion regulation and well-being: Comparing the impact of eight savoring and dampening strategies. *Personality and Individual Differences*, *49*(5), 368–373. doi:10.1016/j.paid.2010.03.048

Rahhal, T., Hasher, L., & Colcombe, S. J. (2001). Instructional manipulations and age differences in memory: Now you see them, now you don't. *Psychology and Aging*, *16*(4), 697–706. doi:10.1037/0882-7974.16.4.697 PMID:11766922

Rahmani, E., & Boren, S. A. (2012). Videogames and Health Improvement: A Literature Review of Randomized Controlled Trials. Research, Development, and Clinical Applications, 1(5), 331–341. PubMed PMID:26191999

Ranjbartabar, H., Maddah, A., & Kavakli, M. (2015a, June 28-July 1). eMedicalHelp: A Customized Medical Diagnostic Application: Is a single questionnaire enough to measure stress? *Proceedings of the 2015 IEEE/ACIS 14th International Conference on Computer and Information Science (ICIS)*, Las Vegas, USA. IEEE.

Ranjbartabar, H., Maddah, A., & Kavakli, M. (2015b). An eMental-Health Application and Customised Questionnaires for Stress Measurement. *International Journal of Computer & Information Science*, 16(2), 1-7.

Rantz, M. J., Skubic, M., Miller, S. J., Galambos, C., Alexander, G., Keller, J., & Popescu, M. (2013). Sensor technology to support Aging in Place. *Journal of the American Medical Directors Association*, *14*(6), 386–391. doi:10.1016/j.jamda.2013.02.018 PMID:23562281

Ranzijn, R. (2002). The potential of older adults to enhance community quality of life: Links between positive psychology and productive aging. *Ageing International*, *27*(2), 30–55. doi:10.1007/s12126-002-1001-5

Raspelli, S., Pallavicini, F., Carelli, L., Morganti, F., Pedroli, E., Cipresso, P., & Riva, G. et al. (2012). Validating the Neuro VR-based virtual version of the Multiple Errands Test: Preliminary results. *Presence (Cambridge, Mass.)*, *21*(1), 31–42. doi:10.1162/PRES_a_00077

Raspelli, S., Pallavicini, F., Grassi, A., Cipresso, P., Balgera, A., & Meazzi, D. et al.. (2011). Validation of a narrative as an emotional-induction technique through different non-invasive psychophysiological monitoring devices: Preliminary results. *Journal of Cybertherapy and Rehabiliation*, *4*(2), 261.

Ravaja, N., Saari, T., Laarni, J., Kallinen, K., Salminen, M., Holopainen, J., & Jarvinen, A. (2005). The psychophysiology of video gaming: Phasic emotional responses to game events. Retrieved from http://www.digra.org/wp-content/uploads/digital-library/06278.36196.pdf

Ravaja, N., Turpeinen, M., Saari, T., Puttonen, S., & Keltikangas-Järvinen, L. (2008). The psychophysiology of James Bond: Phasic emotional responses to violent video game events. *Emotion (Washington, D.C.)*, *8*(1), 114–120. doi:10.1037/1528-3542.8.1.114 PMID:18266521

Rebok, G. W., Ball, K., Guey, L. T., Jones, R. N., Kim, H. Y., King, J. W., & Unverzagt, F. W. et al. (2014). Ten-year effects of the advanced cognitive training for independent and vital elderly cognitive training trial on cognition and everyday functioning in older adults. *Journal of the American Geriatrics Society*, *62*(1), 16–24. PMID:24417410

Redden, E. S., Sheehy, J. B., & Bjorkman, E. A. (2004). The study and measurement of human performance by military service laboratories. *Advances in Human Performance and Cognitive Engineering Research*, *5*, 517–559. doi:10.1016/S1479-3601(04)05011-8

Reeves, B., & Read, J. L. (2009). Total engagement: Using games to change the way people work and businesses compete. Boston: Harvard Business School.

Reiter, E. (1999). Natural Language Generation in STOP. Retrieved from http://inf.abdn.ac.uk/research/stop/stop-nlg.htm

Reiter, E., Dale, R., & Feng, Z. (2000). *Building natural language generation systems* (Vol. 33). MIT Press. doi:10.1017/CBO9780511519857

Repetto, C., Gaggioli, A., Pallavicini, F., Cipresso, P., Raspelli, S., & Riva, G. (2013). Virtual reality and mobile phones in the treatment of generalized anxiety disorders: A phase-2 clinical trial. *Personal and Ubiquitous Computing*, *17*(2), 253–260. doi:10.1007/s00779-011-0467-0

Repetto, C., Gorini, A., Vigna, C., Algeri, D., Pallavicini, F., & Riva, G. (2009). The use of biofeedback in clinical virtual reality: The INTREPID project. *Journal of Visualized Experiments*, November, 33. PMID:19915521

Repetto, C., & Riva, G. (2011). From virtual reality to interreality in the treatment of anxiety disorders. *Neuropsychiatry*, *1*(1), 31–43. doi:10.2217/npy.11.5

Resnick, P., & Varian, H. R. (1997). Recommender systems. *Communications of the ACM*, *40*(3), 56–58. doi:10.1145/245108.245121

Reynolds, C., & Picard, R. W. (2005, July 22–27). *Evaluation of affective computing systems from a dimensional metaethical position.Paper presented to 1st Augmented Cognition Conference, in conjunction with the 11th International Conference on Human–Computer Interaction*, Las Vegas.

Rickel, J., Marcella, S., Gratch, J., Hill, R., Traum, D., & Swartout, W. (2002). Toward a new generation of virtual humans for interactive experiences. *IEEE Intelligent Systems*, *17*(4), 32–38. doi:10.1109/MIS.2002.1024750

Rigby, S., & Ryan, R. (2011). *Glued to games: how video games draw us in and hold us spellbound.* New York, USA: ABC-CLIO.

Ritterband, L. M., Gonder-Frederick, L. A., Cox, D. J., Clifton, A. D., West, R. W., & Borowitz, S. M. (2003). Internet interventions: In review, in use, and into the future. *Professional Psychology, Research and Practice, 34*(5), 527–534. doi:10.1037/0735-7028.34.5.527

Riva, G. (2004). The psychology of Ambient Intelligence: Activity, situation and presence. In G. Riva, F. Davide, F. Vatalaro, & M. Alcañiz (Eds.), Ambient Intelligence: The evolution of technology, communication and cognition towards the future of the human-computer interaction (pp. 19–34). Amsterdam: IOS Press. Retrieved from http://www.emergingcommunication.com/volume6.html

Riva, G. (2004). The psychology of ambient intelligence: activity, situation and presence. In G. Riva, F. Davide, F. Vatalaro, & M. Alcañiz (Eds.), *Ambient intelligence: the evolution of technology, communication and cognition towards the future of the human-computer interaction* (pp. 19–34). Amsterdam: Ios Press. Retrieved from www.emergingcommunication.com/volume6.html

Riva, G. (2008). Enacting Interactivity: The Role of Presence. In F. Morganti, A. Carassa, & G. Riva (Eds.), Enacting Intersubjectivity: A cognitive and social perspective on the study of interactions (pp. 97–114). Amsterdam: IOS Press. Retrieved from http://www.emergingcommunication.com/volume10.html

Riva, G., & Gaggioli, A. (2015). Positive Change and Positive Technology. In P. Inghilleri, G.Riva, & R.E. (Eds.), Enabling Positive Change, Flow and Complexity in Daily Experience (pp. 39-49). Warsaw: De Gruyter Open. doi:10.2478/9783110410242.3

Riva, G., & Mantovani, F. (2012a). Being There: Understanding the Feeling of Presence in a Synthetic Environment and its Potential for Clinical Change. In C. Eichenberg (Ed.), Virtual Reality in Psychological, Medical and Pedagogical Applications (pp. 3–34). New York: InTech. Retrieved from http://www.intechopen.com/books/virtual-reality-in-psychological-medical-and-pedagogical-applications/being-there-understanding-the-feeling-of-presence-in-a-synthetic-environment-and-its-potential-for-c doi:10.5772/46411

Riva, G., & Waterworth, J. A. (2003). Presence and the Self: A cognitive neuroscience approach. *Presence-Connect, 3*(1). Retrieved from http://presence.cs.ucl.ac.uk/presenceconnect/articles/Apr2003/jwworthApr72003114532/jwworthApr72003114532.html

Riva, G., Botella, C., Baños, R., Mantovani, F., García-Palacios, A., Quero, S., . . . Gaggioli, A. (2015). Presence-inducing media for mental health applications. In M. Lombard, F. Biocca, J. Freeman, W. Ijsselsteijn, & R. Schaevitz (Eds.), Inmersed in Media: Telepresence Theory, Measurement & Technology (pp. 283–332). New York: Springer. doi:10.1007/978-3-319-10190-3_12 doi:10.1007/978-3-319-10190-3_12

Riva, G., Botella, C., Légeron, P., & Optale, G. (Eds.), (2004). Cybertherapy: Internet and Virtual Reality as Assessment and Rehabilitation Tools for Clinical Psychology and Neuroscience (Vol. 99). Amsterdam: IOS Press.

Riva, G., Vigna, C., Grassi, A., Raspelli, S., Cipresso, P., Pallavicini, F., . . . Gaggioli, A. (2012). Learning Island: the development of a virtual reality system for the experiential training of stress management. *Paper presented at the MMVR.*

Riva, G. (2009a). Interreality: A new paradigm for E-health. *Studies in Health Technology and Informatics, 144*, 3–7. PMID:19592718

Riva, G. (2009a). Is presence a technology issue? Some insights from cognitive sciences. *Virtual Reality (Waltham Cross), 13*(3), 59–69. doi:10.1007/s10055-009-0121-6

Riva, G. (2009c). Presence as Cognitive Process. In D. Benyon, M. Smyth, & I. Helgason (Eds.), *Presence for everyone: A short guide to presence research* (pp. 29–31). Edinburgh, UK: Napier University.

Riva, G. (2009e). Virtual reality: An experiential tool for clinical psychology. *British Journal of Guidance & Counselling, 37*(3), 337–345. doi:10.1080/03069880902957056

Riva, G. (2010). Dall'intenzione, all'azione, all'interazione: il ruolo di "presenza" e "presenza sociale". In F. Morganti, A. Carassa, & G. Riva (Eds.), *Intersoggettività e Interazione: Un dialogo fra scienze cognitive, scienze sociali e neuroscienze* (pp. 136–177). Torino: Bollati Boringhieri.

Riva, G. (2012a). Personal experience in positive psychology may offer a new focus for a growing discipline. *The American Psychologist, 67*(7), 574–575. doi:10.1037/a0029955 PMID:23046310

Riva, G. (2012c). What is Positive Technology and its impact on CyberPsychology. *Studies in Health Technology and Informatics, 181*, 37–41. PMID:22954824

Riva, G., Algeri, D., Pallavicini, F., Repetto, C., Gorini, A., & Gaggioli, A. (2010). The use of advanced technologies in the treatment of psychological stress. *Journal of Cyber Therapy and Rehabilitation, 2*(2), 169–171.

Riva, G., Bacchetta, M., Baruffi, M., Rinaldi, S., & Molinari, E. (1999). Virtual reality based experiential cognitive treatment of anorexia nervosa. *Journal of Behavior Therapy and Experimental Psychiatry, 30*(3), 221–230. doi:10.1016/S0005-7916(99)00018-X PMID:10619546

Riva, G., Banos, R. M., Botella, C., Wiederhold, B. K., & Gaggioli, A. (2012). Positive technology: Using interactive technologies to promote positive functioning. *Cyberpsychology, Behavior, and Social Networking, 15*(2), 69–77. doi:10.1089/cyber.2011.0139 PMID:22149077

Riva, G., Calvo, R. A., & Lisetti, C. (2015). Cyberpsychology Applications of Affective Computing. In R. A. Calvo, S. K. D'Mello, J. Gratch, & A. Kappas (Eds.), *Handbook of Affective Computing*. New York: Oxford University Press.

Riva, G., Castelnuovo, G., & Mantovani, F. (2006). Transformation of flow in rehabilitation: The role of advanced communication technologies. *Behavior Research Methods, 38*(2), 237–244. doi:10.3758/BF03192775 PMID:16956100

Riva, G., & Gaggioli, A. (2009). Rehabilitation as Empowerment: The Role of Advanced Technologies. In A. Gaggioli, E. A. Keshner, P. L. Weiss, & G. Riva (Eds.), *Technologies in Rehabilitation: Empowering Cognitive, Physical, Social and Communicative Skills through Virtual Reality, Robots, Wearable Systems and Brain-Computer Interfaces Advanced* (Vol. 145, pp. 3–22). Amsterdam: IOS Press.

Riva, G., & Gaggioli, A. (2009). Rehabilitation as empowerment: The role of advanced technologies. *Studies in Health Technology and Informatics, 145*, 3–22. PMID:19592783

Riva, G., & Gaggioli, A. (2009). Rehabilitation as Empowerment: The Role of Advanced Technologies. *Studies in Health Technology and Informatics, 145*, 3–22. PMID:19592783

Riva, G., Gaggioli, A., Villani, D., Cipresso, P., Repetto, C., Serino, S., & Graffigna, G. et al. (2014). Positive Technology for Healthy Living and Active Ageing. *Studies in Health Technology and Informatics*, (203): 44–56. PMID:26630511

Riva, G., & Mantovani, F. (2012d). From the body to the tools and back: A general framework for presence in mediated interactions. *Interacting with Computers, 24*(4), 203–210. doi:10.1016/j.intcom.2012.04.007

Riva, G., Mantovani, F., Capideville, C. S., Preziosa, A., Morganti, F., Villani, D., & Alcañiz, M. et al. (2007). Affective interactions using virtual reality: The link between presence and emotions. *Cyberpsychology & Behavior, 10*(1), 45–56. doi:10.1089/cpb.2006.9993 PMID:17305448

Riva, G., Mantovani, F., Capideville, C. S., Preziosa, A., Morganti, F., Villani, D., & Alcaniz, M. et al. (2007). Affective Interactions Using Virtual Reality: The Link between Presence and Emotions. *Cyberpsychology & Behavior*, *10*(1).

Riva, G., Mantovani, F., & Gaggioli, A. (2004). Presence and rehabilitation: Toward second-generation virtual reality applications in neuropsychology. *Journal of Neuroengineering and Rehabilitation*, *1*(1), 9. doi:10.1186/1743-0003-1-9 PMID:15679950

Riva, G., Manzoni, M., Villani, D., Gaggioli, A., & Molinari, E. (2008). Why you really eat? Virtual reality in the treatment of obese emotional eaters. *Studies in Health Technology and Informatics*, *132*, 417–419. PMID:18391333

Riva, G., Marsan, P. A., & Grassi, C. (2014). *Active Ageing and Healthy Living: A Human Centered Approach in Research and Innovation as Source of Quality of Life*. Amsterdam, The Netherlands: IOS Press.

Riva, G., Raspelli, S., Algeri, D., Pallavicini, F., Gorini, A., Wiederhold, B. K., & Gaggioli, A. (2010). Interreality in practice: Bridging virtual and real worlds in the treatment of posttraumatic stress disorders. *Cyberpsychology, Behavior, and Social Networking*, *13*(1), 55–65. doi:10.1089/cyber.2009.0320 PMID:20528294

Riva, G., Vigna, C., Grassi, A., Raspelli, S., Cipresso, P., Pallavicini, F., & Gaggioli, A. et al. (2012). Learning island: The development of a virtual reality system for the experiential training of stress management. *Studies in Health Technology and Informatics*, *173*, 369–371. PMID:22357020

Riva, G., & Waterworth, J. A. (2014). Being present in a virtual world. In M. Grimshaw (Ed.), *The Oxford Handbook of Virtuality* (pp. 205–221). New York: Oxford University Press.

Riva, G., Waterworth, J. A., & Waterworth, E. L. (2004). The Layers of Presence: A bio-cultural approach to understanding presence in natural and mediated environments. *Cyberpsychology & Behavior*, *7*(4), 405–419. doi:10.1089/cpb.2004.7.402 PMID:15331027

Riva, G., Waterworth, J. A., Waterworth, E. L., & Mantovani, F. (2011). From Intention to Action: The role of Presence. *New Ideas in Psychology*, *29*(1), 24–37. doi:10.1016/j.newideapsych.2009.11.002

Rizzo, A., Pair, J., Graap, K., Manson, B., McNerney, P. J., Wiederhold, B., . . .. (2006). A Virtual Reality Exposure Therapy Application for Iraq War Military Personnel with Post Traumatic Stress Disorder: From Training to Toy to Treatment. In M. Roy (Ed.), NATO Advanced Research Workshop on Novel Approaches to the Diagnosis and Treatment of Posttraumatic Stress Disorder (pp. 235-250). Washington DC: IOS Press.

Rizzo, A. S., Schultheis, M. T., & Rothbaum, B. O. (2003). Ethical Issues for the Use of Virtual Reality in the Psychological Sciences. In S. Bush & M. Drexler (Eds.), *Ethical Issues in Clinical Neuropsychology* (pp. 243–280). Lisse, Netherlands: Swets & Zeitlinger Publishers.

Rizzolatti, G., Fadiga, L., Gallese, V., & Fogassi, L. (1996). Premotor cortex and the recognition of motor actions. *Brain Research. Cognitive Brain Research*, *3*(2), 131–141. doi:10.1016/0926-6410(95)00038-0 PMID:8713554

Rizzolatti, G., & Sinigaglia, C. (2006). *So quel che fai. Il cervello che agisce e i neuroni specchio*. Milano: Raffaello Cortina.

Robertson, D. A., Savva, G. M., & Kenny, R. A. (2013). Frailty and cognitive impairment—a review of the evidence and causal mechanisms. *Ageing Research Reviews*, *12*(4), 840–851. doi:10.1016/j.arr.2013.06.004 PMID:23831959

Robertson, I. H. (1996). *Goal management training: A clinical manual*. Cambridge, UK: PsyConsult.

Robinson, J. C. (2005). Managed consumerism in health care. *Health Affairs*, *24*(6), 1478–1489. doi:10.1377/hlthaff.24.6.1478 PMID:16284020

Rodin, J., & Langer, E. J. (1977). Long-term Effects of a Control-relevant Intervention with the Institutionalized Aged. *J. Pers. Soc. Psycho.*, 35(12), 175–179.

Roemer, L., & Orsillo, S. M. (2002). Expanding our conceptualization of and treatment for generalized anxiety disorder: Integrating mindfulness/acceptance-based approaches with existing cognitive-behavioral models. *Clinical Psychology: Science and Practice*, *9*(1), 54–68. doi:10.1093/clipsy.9.1.54

Rogers, E. M. (1983). *Diffusion of Innovations*. New York, NY: Free Press.

Romano, A. M. (2007). A changing landscape: Implications of pregnant women's Internet use for childbirth educators. *Journal of Perinatal Education*, *16*(4), 18–24. doi:10.1624/105812407X244903 PMID:18769519

Roos, A., Faure, S., Lochner, C., Vythilingum, B., & Stein, D. J. (2013). Predictors of distress and anxiety during pregnancy. *The African Journal of Psychiatry*, *16*(2), 118–122. PMID:23595531

Rose, F. D., Brooks, B. M., & Rizzo, A. A. (2005). Virtual reality in brain damage rehabilitation[review]. *Cyberpsychology & Behavior*, *8*(3), 241–262. doi:10.1089/cpb.2005.8.241 PMID:15971974

Rosenblum, L. (2000). Virtual and Augmented Reality 2020. *IEEE Computer Graphics and Applications*, *20*(1), 38–39. doi:10.1109/38.814551

Rosis, F. D., Pelachaud, C., Poggi, I., Carofiglio, V., & Carolis, B. D. (2003). From Greta's mind to her face: Modelling the dynamics of affective states. *Int. Journal of Human-Computer, Studies in Health Technology and Informatics*, *59*(1-2), 81–118.

Ross, S. E., Bradley, N., Heckert, C., & Teresa, M. (1999). Sources of stress among college students.

Rotheram-Borus, M. J., Tomlinson, M., Gwegwe, M., Comulada, W. S., Kaufman, N., & Keim, M. (2012). Diabetes buddies peer support through a mobile phone buddy system. *The Diabetes Educator*, *38*(3), 357–365. doi:10.1177/0145721712444617 PMID:22546740

Rotheram-Borus, M. J., Tomlinson, M., Swendeman, D., Lee, A., & Jones, E. (2012). Standardized functions for smartphone applications: Examples from maternal and child health. *International Journal of Telemedicine and Applications*, *2012*, 21. doi:10.1155/2012/973237 PMID:23304136

Roth, W.-M., & Mavin, T. J. (2014). Peer assessment of aviation performance: Inconsistent for good reasons. *Cognitive Science*. doi:10.1111/cogs.12152 PMID:25052893

Rozanski, A., Blumenthal, J. A., & Kaplan, J. (1999). Impact of psychological factors on the pathogenesis of cardiovascular disease and implications for therapy. *Circulation*, *99*(16), 2192–2217. doi:10.1161/01.CIR.99.16.2192 PMID:10217662

Rubin, K. H. (2001). *The play observation scale (POS)*. Ontario, Canada: University of Waterloo.

Rubin, R. (1984). Maternal Identity and the Maternal Experience. *AJN The American Journal of Nursing*, *84*(12), 1480. doi:10.1097/00000446-198412000-00030

Rudra, T., Kavakli, M., & Tien, D. (2007a, Oct 30–Nov 2). Emotion Detection from Male Speech in Computer Games. *Proceedings of the IEEE TENCON '07*, Taipei International Convention Center, Taiwan (pp. 1-4).

Rudra, T., Kavakli, M., & Tien, D. (2007b, January 15-18). Emotion Detection from Female Speech in Computer Games. *Proceedings of the 4th International Conference on IT and Application ICITA '07*, Harbin, China (pp. 712-716). IEEE.

Rudra, T., Li, M., & Kavakli, M. (2012, January5-7). ESCAP: Towards the Design of an AI Architecture for a Virtual Counselor to Tackle Students' Exam Stress. *Proceedings of theHawaiian International Conference on System Sciences (HICSS)*, Hawaii (pp. 1-10). doi:10.1109/HICSS.2012.249

Ruff, H. A., & Saltarelli, L. M. (1993). Exploratory play with objects: Basic cognitive processes and individual differences. *New Directions for Child and Adolescent Development*, *59*(59), 5–16. doi:10.1002/cd.23219935903 PMID:8483525

Rush, J., Chalmers, I., & Enkin, M. (1991). Care of the new mother and baby. In I. Chalmers, M. Enkin, & M. Kierse (Eds.), *Effective Care in Pregnancy and Childbirth* (Vol. 2, pp. 1333–1346). Oxford: Oxford University Press.

Russell, J. A. (1996). *Agency: Its role in mental development*. Hove: Erlbaum.

Russell, J. A. (2003). Core Affect and the psychological construction of Emotion. *Psychological Review*, *110*(1), 145–172. doi:10.1037/0033-295X.110.1.145 PMID:12529060

Russo, M. B., Stetz, M. C., & Thomas, M. L. (2005). Monitoring and predicting cognitive state and performance via physiological correlates of neuronal signals. *Aviation, Space, and Environmental Medicine*, *76*(7), C59–C63. PMID:16018331

Russoniello, C. V., Fish, M., & O'Brien, K. (2013). The Efficacy of Casual Videogame Play in Reducing Clinical Depression: A Randomized Controlled Study. Games for Health Journal, 2(6), 341–346. doi:10.1089/g4h.2013.0010 PubMed doi:10.1089/g4h.2013.0010 PMID:26197075

Russoniello, C. V., O'brien, K., & Parks, J. M. (2009). EEG, HRV and Psychological Correlates while Playing Bejeweled II: A Randomized Controlled Study. *Annual Review of Cybertherapy and Telemedicine*, *7*(1), 189–192. doi:10.3233/978-1-60750-017-9-189 PMID:19592761

Ryan, E. B., Szechtman, B., & Bodkin, J. (1992). Attitudes toward younger and older adults learning computers. *Journals of Gerontology: Psychological Science*, *47*(2), 96–101. doi:10.1093/geronj/47.2.P96 PMID:1538074

Ryan, R. M., & Deci, E. L. (2000). Self-determination theory and the facilitation of intrinsic motivation, social development and well-being. *The American Psychologist*, *55*(1), 68–78. doi:10.1037/0003-066X.55.1.68 PMID:11392867

Ryan, R. M., & Deci, E. L. (2001). On Happiness and Human Potentials: A Review of Research on Hedonic and Eudaimonic Well-Being. *Annual Review of Psychology*, *52*(1), 141–166. doi:10.1146/annurev.psych.52.1.141 PMID:11148302

Ryan, R. M., Huta, V., & Deci, E. L. (2008). Living well: A self-determination theory perspective on eudaimonia. *Journal of Happiness Studies*, *9*(1), 139–170. doi:10.1007/s10902-006-9023-4

Ryan, R. M., Rigby, C. S., & Przybylski, A. (2006). The motivational pull of video games: A self-determination theory approach. *Motivation and Emotion*, *30*(4), 344–360. doi:10.1007/s11031-006-9051-8

Ryan, R., & Deci, E. (2000). Intrinsic and Extrinsic Motivations: Classic Definitions and New Directions. *Contemporary Educational Psychology*, *25*(1), 54–67. doi:10.1006/ceps.1999.1020 PMID:10620381

Ryff, C. D. (1989). Happiness is everything, or is it? Explorations on the meaning of psychological well-being. *Journal of Personality and Social Psychology*, *57*(6), 1069–1081. doi:10.1037/0022-3514.57.6.1069

Ryff, C. D., & Keyes, C. L. M. (1995). The structure of psychological well-being revisited. *Journal of Personality and Social Psychology*, *69*(4), 719–727. doi:10.1037/0022-3514.69.4.719 PMID:7473027

Ryff, C. D., & Singer, B. (2000). Interpersonal flourishing: A positive health agenda for the new millennium. *Personality and Social Psychology Review*, *4*(1), 30–44. doi:10.1207/S15327957PSPR0401_4

Safran, J. D., & Greenberg, L. S. (1991). *Emotion, psychotherapy, and change*. New York: The Guilford Press.

Salas, E., Shuffler, M. L., & DiazGranados, D. (2010). Team dynamics at 35,000 feet. In E. Salas, F. Jentsch, & D. Maurino (Eds.), *Human factors in aviation* (pp. 249–291). New York: Academic Press.

Salen, K., & Zimmerman, E. (2004). Rules of Play: Game Design Fundamentals. Cambridge: MIT Press.

Salthouse, T. (1996). The processing-speed theory of adult age differences in cognition. *Psychological Review*, *103*(3), 403–428. doi:10.1037/0033-295X.103.3.403 PMID:8759042

Salzer, M. S. (1997). Consumer empowerment in mental health organizations: Concept, benefits, and impediments. *Administration and Policy in Mental Health and Mental Health Services Research*, *24*(5), 425–434. doi:10.1007/BF02042724 PMID:9239946

Sanchez-Vives, M.V., & Slater, M. (2005). From presence to consciousness through virtual reality. nature review neuroscience, 6, 332–339.

Sanders, E. B. (2002). From User-Centered to Participatory Design Approaches. *Design and the social sciences: Making connections*, 1-8.

Santamaría, J. J., Soto, A., Fernández-Aranda, F., Krug, I., Forcano, L., Gunnard, K., . . .. (2011). Serious games as additional psychological support: A review of the literature. Journal of Cyber Therapy and Rehabilitation, 4(4), 469–476.

Santos-Eggimann, B., Cuénoud, P., Spagnoli, J., & Junod, J. (2009). Prevalence of frailty in middle-aged and older community-dwelling Europeans living in 10 countries. *Journal of Gerontology*, *64*, 675–681. PMID:19276189

Santrock, J. (2010). Psicología del desarrollo en la infancia, 7ª Ed [Developmental Psychology in Childhood, 7th Edition –Book In Spanish. Colombia: Mc-Graw Hill Interamericana.

Saposnik, G., & Levin, M. (2011). Virtual reality in stroke rehabilitation a meta-analysis and implications for clinicians. *Stroke*, *42*(5), 1380–1386. doi:10.1161/STROKEAHA.110.605451 PMID:21474804

Sarafino, E. P. (2012). Health Psychology: Biopsychosocial Interactions (7th ed). Asia: Wiley.

Satyapriya, M., Nagendra, H. R., Nagarathna, R., & Padmalatha, V. (2009). Effect of integrated yoga on stress and heart rate variability in pregnant women. *International Journal of Gynaecology and Obstetrics: the Official Organ of the International Federation of Gynaecology and Obstetrics*, *104*(3), 218–222. doi:10.1016/j.ijgo.2008.11.013 PMID:19110245

Sawyer, K. R. (2003). *Group creativity: Music, theatre, collaboration. New York, NY.* New York: Basic Books.

Sawyer, K. R. (2008). *Group genius: The creative power of collaboration.* New York, NY: Oxford University Press.

Schaub, B. G. (1995). Imagery in health care: Connecting with life energy. *Complementary Health Practice Review*, *1*(2), 113–115.

Schell, J. (2008). *The Art of Game Design: A Book of Lenses.* Amsterdam: Elsevier/Morgan Kaufmann.

Scherer, K. R. (2001). Appraisal considered as a process of multilevel sequential checking. In K.R. Scherer, A. Schorr, & T. Johnstone (Eds.), *Appraisal processes in emotion: Theory, methods, research* (pp. 92-120). Oxford: Oxford University Press.

Schneider, E., Lang, A., Shin, M., & Bradley, S. D. (2004). Death with a Story: How Story Impacts Emotional, Motivational, and Physiological Responses to First-Person Shooter Video Games. *Human Communication Research*, *30*(3), 361–375.

Schneider, S. M., & Workman, M. L. (1999). Effects of virtual reality on symptom distress in children receiving chemotherapy. *Cyberpsychology & Behavior*, *2*(2), 125–134. doi:10.1089/cpb.1999.2.125 PMID:19178248

Schneider, W. (2008). The development of metacognitive knowledge in children and adolescents: Major trends and implications for education. *Mind, Brain, and Education*, *2*(3), 114–121. doi:10.1111/j.1751-228X.2008.00041.x

Schramm, H., & Wirth, W. (2010). Exploring the paradox of sad-film enjoyment: The role of multiple appraisals and meta-appraisals. *Poetics*, *38*(3), 319–335. doi:10.1016/j.poetic.2010.03.002

Schueller, S. M. (2010). Preferences for positive psychology exercises. *The Journal of Positive Psychology*, *5*(3), 192–203. doi:10.1080/17439761003790948

Schueller, S. M. (2012). Personality Fit and Positive Interventions: Extraverted and Introverted Individuals Benefit from Different Happiness Increasing Strategies. *Psychology (Savannah, Ga.)*, *3*(12), 1166–1173. doi:10.4236/psych.2012.312A172

Schueller, S. M., & Parks, A. C. (2012). Disseminating self-help: Positive psychology exercises in an online trial. *Journal of Medical Internet Research*, *14*(3), e63. doi:10.2196/jmir.1850 PMID:22732765

Schultheis, M. T., & Rizzo, A. A. (2001). The application of virtual reality technology in rehabilitation. *Rehabilitation Psychology*, *46*(3), 296–311. doi:10.1037/0090-5550.46.3.296

Schultze, U. (2010). Embodiment and presence in virtual worlds: A review. *Journal of Information Technology*, *25*(4), 434–449. doi:10.1057/jit.2010.25

Schultz, J. H., & Luthe, W. (1969). *Autogenic therapy: Autogenic methods*. New York: Grune & Stratton.

Schulz, L. E., Standing, H. R., & Bonawitz, E. B. (2008). Word, thought, and deed: The role of object categories in children's inductive inferences and exploratory play. *Developmental Psychology*, *44*(5), 1266–1276. doi:10.1037/0012-1649.44.5.1266 PMID:18793061

Scozzari, S., & Gamberini, L. (2011). Virtual Reality as a Tool for Cognitive Behavioral Therapy: A Review. In S. Brahnam & L. C. Jain (Eds.), Advanced Computational Intelligence Paradigms in Healthcare 6. Virtual Reality in Psychotherapy, Rehabilitation, and Assessment, SCI (Vol. 337, pp. 63–108). Berlin: Springer-Verlag.

Searle, J. (1983). *Intentionality: An essay in the philosophy of mind*. New York: Cambridge University Press. doi:10.1017/CBO9781139173452

Sedlmeier, P., Eberth, J., Schwarz, M., Zimmermann, D., Haarig, F., Jaeger, S., & Kunze, S. (2012). The psychological effects of meditation: A meta-analysis. *Psychological Bulletin*, *138*(6), 1139–1171. doi:10.1037/a0028168 PMID:22582738

Seeman, T. E., Singer, B. H., Rowe, J. W., Horwitz, R. I., & McEwen, B. S. (1997). Price of adaptation—allostatic load and its health consequences: MacArthur studies of successful aging. *Archives of Internal Medicine*, *157*(19), 2259–2268. doi:10.1001/archinte.1997.00440400111013 PMID:9343003

Seligman, M. E., & Csikszentmihalyi, M. (2000). Positive psychology: An introduction. *American Psychological Association, 55*(1), 5-14.

Seligman, M. E. (2003). Fundamental assumptions. *The Psychologist*, *16*(3), 126.

Seligman, M. E. P. (2002). *Authentic Happiness*. New York, USA: Atria Books.

Seligman, M. E. P. (2002). *Authentic happiness: Using the new positive psychology to realize your potential for lasting fulfillment*. New York Free Press.

Seligman, M. E. P. (2002). *Authentic Happiness: Using the New Positive Psychology to Realize Your Potential for Lasting Fulfillment*. New York, NY: Free Press.

Seligman, M. E. P. (2002). Positive psychology, positive prevention, and positive therapy. In *Handbook of positive psychology* (pp. 3–9). USA: Oxford University Press.

Seligman, M. E. P. (2002). Positive psychology, positive prevention, and positive therapy. In C. R. Snyder & S. J. Lopez (Eds.), *The handbook of positive psychology*. Oxford, United Kingdom: Oxford University Press.

Seligman, M. E. P., & Csikszentmihalyi, M. (2000). *Positive psychology: An introduction* (Vol. 55). American Psychological Association.

Seligman, M. E. P., & Csikszentmihalyi, M. (2000). Positive psychology: An introduction. *The American Psychologist, 55*(1), 5–14. doi:10.1037/0003-066X.55.1.5 PMID:11392865

Seligman, M. E. P., Rashid, T., & Parks, A. C. (2006). Positive psychotherapy. *The American Psychologist, 61*(8), 774–788. doi:10.1037/0003-066X.61.8.774 PMID:17115810

Seligman, M. E. P., Steen, T. A., Park, N., & Peterson, C. (2005). Positive psychology progress: Empirical validation of interventions. *The American Psychologist, 60*(5), 410–421. doi:10.1037/0003-066X.60.5.410 PMID:16045394

Seligman, M. E., & Csikszentmihalyi, M. (2000). Positive psychology: An introduction: Vol. 55. *No. 1* (p. 5). American Psychological Association.

Selye, H. (1956). *The stress of life*. New York, NY, US: McGraw-Hill.

Seo, M., Barrett, L. F., & Bartunek, J. M. (2004). The role of affective experience in work motivation. *Academy of Management Review, 29*(3), 423–439. PMID:16871321

Sergeant, S., & Mongrain, M. (2011). Are positive psychology exercises helpful for people with depressive personality styles? *The Journal of Positive Psychology, 6*(4), 260–272. doi:10.1080/17439760.2011.577089

Serino, S., Cipresso, P., Tartarisco, G., Baldus, G., Corda, D., Pioggia, G., . . . Riva, G. (2012). An Event-Driven Psychophysiological Assessment for Health Care. *Paper presented at the2nd International Workshop on Computing Paradigms for Mental Health.*

Serino, S., Morganti, F., Di Stefano, F., & Riva, G. (2015). Detecting early egocentric and allocentric impairments deficits in Alzheimer's Disease: an experimental study with virtual reality. *Frontiers in Aging Neuroscience*, 7, 88.

Serino, S., Cipresso, P., Gaggioli, A., & Riva, G. (2013). *The potential of pervasive sensors and computing for positive technology: the interreality paradigm Pervasive and Mobile Sensing and Computing for Healthcare* (pp. 207–232). Springer.

Serino, S., Cipresso, P., Gaggioli, A., & Riva, G. (2013). The potential of pervasive sensors and computing for positive technology: the interreality paradigm. In S. Mukhopadhyay & O. Postolache (Eds.), *Pervasive and Mobile Sensing and Computing for Healthcare* (pp. 207–232). New York, USA: Springer.

Serino, S., Cipresso, P., Gaggioli, A., & Riva, G. (2013). The Potential of Pervasive Sensors and Computing for Positive Technology: The Interreality Paradigm. In S. Mukhopadhyay & O. Postolache (Eds.), *Pervasive and Mobile Sensing and Computing for Healthcare. Smart Sensors, Measurement and Instrumentation* (Vol. 2, pp. 207–232). New York, USA: Springer. doi:10.1007/978-3-642-32538-0_10

Serino, S., Cipresso, P., Tartarisco, G., Baldus, G., Corda, D., Pioggia, G., & Riva, G. et al. (2013). Computerized experience-sampling approach for real-time assessment of stress. *EAI Endorsed Transactions, 13*(1-6), e5.

Serino, S., Triberti, S., Villani, D., Cipresso, P., Gaggioli, A., & Riva, G. (2014). Toward a validation of cyber-interventions for stress disorders based on stress inoculation training: A systematic review. *Virtual Reality (Waltham Cross), 18*(1), 73–87. doi:10.1007/s10055-013-0237-6

Serrano, J. P., Latorre, J. M., Gatz, M., & Montanes, J. (2004). Life review therapy using autobiographical retrieval practice for older adults with depressive symptomatology. *Psychology and Aging, 19*(2), 272–277. doi:10.1037/0882-7974.19.2.272 PMID:15222820

Sethi, S., Campbell, A. J., & Ellis, L. A. (2010). The use of computerized self-help packages to treat adolescent depression and anxiety. *Journal of Technology in Human Services*, *28*(3), 144–160. doi:10.1080/15228835.2010.508317

Shafer, R. (2000). *Housing America's Seniors. Executive Summary*. Cambridge, MA: Joint Center for Housing Studies, Harvard University.

Shah, L. B., Torres, S., Kannusamy, P., Chng, C. M., He, H. G., & Klainin-Yobas, P. (2015). Efficacy of the virtual reality-based stress management program on stress-related variables in people with mood disorders: The feasibility study. *Archives of Psychiatric Nursing*, *20*(1), 6–13. doi:10.1016/j.apnu.2014.09.003 PMID:25634868

Shaker, N., Yannakakis, G., & Togelius, J. (2010). Towards Automatic Personalized Content Generation for Platform Games.*Proceedings of AIIDE 2010 - 6th. Digital Entertainment.*

Shallice, T., & Burgess, P. W. (1991). Deficits in strategy application following frontal lobe damage in man. *Brain*, *114*(2), 727–741. doi:10.1093/brain/114.2.727 PMID:2043945

Shandley, K., Austin, D., Klein, B., & Kyrios, M. (2010). An evaluation of "Reach Out Central": An online gaming program for supporting the mental health of young people. *Health Education Research*, *25*(4), 563–574. doi:10.1093/her/cyq002 PMID:20150530

Shandley, K., Klein, B., & Austin, D. (2008). The players' perspective of Reach Out Central: A therapeutic interactive online game. *E-Journal of Applied Psychology*, *4*(2), 51–55. doi:10.7790/ejap.v4i2.132

Shapiro, D. H. Jr. (2008). *Meditation: Self-regulation strategy and altered state of consciousness*. Transaction Publishers.

Shapiro, S. L., Schwartz, G. E., & Bonner, G. (1998). Effects of mindfulness-based stress reduction on medical and premedical students. *Journal of Behavioral Medicine*, *21*(6), 581–599. doi:10.1023/A:1018700829825 PMID:9891256

Sharf, B. F. (1997). Communicating breast cancer on-line: Support and empowerment on the Internet. *Women & Health*, *26*(1), 65–84. doi:10.1300/J013v26n01_05 PMID:9311100

Sharma, V., Bauer, B., Prasad, K., Sood, A., & Schroeder, D. (2012). P02.197 Self help intervention to decrease stress and increase mindfulness: A pilot trial. *BMC Complementary and Alternative Medicine*, *12*(Suppl. 1), 253. doi:10.1186/1472-6882-12-S1-P253 PMID:23237355

Sharry, J., McDermott, M., & Condron, J. (2003). Relax To Win: Treating children with anxiety problems with a bio-feedback video game. Eisteach, 2, 22–26.

Sheldon, K. M., & King, L. (2001). Why positive psychology is necessary. *The American Psychologist*, *56*(3), 216–217. doi:10.1037/0003-066X.56.3.216 PMID:11315247

Sheldon, K. M., & Lyubomirsky, S. (2006). How to increase and sustain positive emotion: The effects of expressing gratitude and visualizing best possible selves. *The Journal of Positive Psychology*, *1*(2), 73–82. doi:10.1080/17439760500510676

Shibli, N., Hasan, I., Shakeel, A., Shakeel, S., Yousaf, S., & Iqbal, M. (2014). Dr. Oz's Anxiety Scale as an Indicator of Test/Examination Anxiety among Male/Female College Students, *Int. Journal of Scientific and Research Publications*, *4*(12).

Shin, M., Heard, R., Suo, C., & Chow, C. M. (2012). Positive Emotions Associated with ''Counter-Strike'' Game Playing. Games for Health Journal, 1(5), 342–347. doi:10.1089/g4h.2012.0010 PubMed doi:10.1089/g4h.2012.0010 PMID:26192000

Shiovitz-Ezra, S., Leitsch, S., Graber, J., & Karraker, A. (2009). Quality of Life and Psychological Health Indicators in the National Social Life, Health, and Aging Project. *The Journals of Gerontology: Series B*, *64*(Suppl. 1), i30–i37. doi:10.1093/geronb/gbn020 PMID:19204071

Shonin, E., Van Gordon, W., & Griffiths, M. D. (2013). Mindfulness-based interventions: Towards mindful clinical integration. *Frontiers in Psychology*, 2013(4). PMID:23616779

Short, J., Williams, E., & Christie, B. (1976). *The social psychology of telecommunications*. London: Wiley.

Sin, N. L., & Lyubomirsky, S. (2009). Enhancing well-being and alleviating depressive symptoms with positive psychology interventions: A practice-friendly meta-analysis. *Journal of Clinical Psychology*, *65*(5), 467–487. doi:10.1002/jclp.20593 PMID:19301241

Slade, T., Johnston, A., Oakley Browne, M. A., Andrews, G., & Whiteford, H. (2009). 2007 National Survey of Mental Health and Wellbeing: Methods and key findings. *Australasian Psychiatry*, *43*(7), 594–605. PMID:19530016

Slager, K., Ligtenberg, A., de Vries, B., & de Waard, R. S. (2007). Simlandscape: Serious Gaming in Participatory Spatial Planning. *Proceedings of the10th AGILE International Conference on Geographic Information Science*.

Slater, M., Antley, A., Davison, A., Swapp, D., Guger, C., Barker, C., & Sanchez-Vives, M. V. et al. (2006). A virtual reprise of the Stanley Milgram obedience experiments. *PLoS ONE*, *1*(1), e39. doi:10.1371/journal.pone.0000039 PMID:17183667

Slater, M., Spanlang, B., Sanchez-Vives, M. V., & Blanke, O. (2010). First person experience of body transfer in virtual reality. *PLoS ONE*, *5*(5), e10564. doi:10.1371/journal.pone.0010564 PMID:20485681

Smedberg, A., & Sandmark, H. S. (2012). Design of a Mobile Phone App Prototype for Reflections on Perceived Stress. *Proceedings of the Fourth International Conference on eHealth, Telemedicine and Social Medicine TELEMED '12*, Valencia, Spain. IARIA.

Smith E.E., & Kosslyn, S.M. (2007). *Cognitive Psychology: Mind and Brain, Chapter11 Motor Cognition and Mental Simulation.* USA: PHI Pearson Higher education.

Smith, A. (2014). *Older Adults and Technology Use*. Retrieved from http://www.pewinternet.org/2014/04/03/older-adults-and-technology-use/

Smith, B. W., Dalen, J., Wiggins, K., Tooley, E., Christopher, P., & Bernard, J. (2008). The brief resilience scale: Assessing the ability to bounce back. *International Journal of Behavioral Medicine*, *15*(3), 194–200. doi:10.1080/10705500802222972 PMID:18696313

Smith, C. A., Levett, K. M., Collins, C. T., & Crowther, C. A. (2011). Relaxation techniques for pain management in labour. *The Cochrane Library*. PMID:22161453

Snyder, C. R. (2010). *Positive psychology: The scientific and practical explorations of human strengths*. Sage Publications.

Sohn, M.-H., Douglass, S. A., Chen, M.-C., & Anderson, J. R. (2000). Eye-movements during unit-task execution in a complex problem-solving situation.*Proceedings of the 44th Annual Meeting of the Human Factors and Ergonomics Society* (pp. 378–381). doi:10.1177/154193120004401113

Spagnolli, A., & Gamberini, L. (2005). A Place for Presence. Understanding the Human Involvement in Mediated Interactive Environments. *PsychNology Journal*, *13*(1), 6–15. Retrieved from http://www.psychnology.org/index.php?page=abstract---volume-13---spagnolli PMID:16190023

Spagnolli, A., Gamberini, L., & Gasparini, D. (2002). Situated Breakdown Analysis for the Evaluation of a Virtual Environment. *PsychNology Journal*, *1*(1), 5–17. PMID:12322671

Spear, H. J., & Kulbok, P. (2001). Autonomy and adolescence: A concept analysis. *Public Health Nursing (Boston, Mass.)*, *21*(2), 144–152. doi:10.1111/j.0737-1209.2004.021208.x PMID:14987214

Sperling, R. A., Aisen, P. S., Beckett, L. A., Bennett, D. A., Craft, S., Fagan, A. M., & Montine, T. J. et al. (2011). Toward defining the preclinical stages of Alzheimer's disease: Recommendations from the National Institute on Aging-Alzheimer's Association workgroups on diagnostic guidelines for Alzheimer's disease. *Alzheimer's & Dementia*, *7*(3), 280–292. doi:10.1016/j.jalz.2011.03.003 PMID:21514248

Sproull, L., & Kiesler, S. (1986). Reducing Social Context Cues: Electronic Mail in Organizational Communication. *Management Science*, *32*(11), 1492–1512. doi:10.1287/mnsc.32.11.1492

Squire, K., Barnett, M., Grant, J. M., & Higginbotham, T. (2004). Electromagnetism supercharged! Learning physics with digital simulation games.*Proceedings of the 6th International Conference on Learning Sciences* (pp. 513–520). Mahwah, NJ: Lawrence Erlbaum.

Stanovich, K. E., & West, R. F. (2000). Individual differences in reasoning: Implications for the rationality debate? *Behavioral and Brain Sciences*, *23*(5), 645–665, discussion 665–726. doi:10.1017/S0140525X00003435 PMID:11301544

Stapleton, A. J. (2004). Serious Games: Serious Opportunities. *Health Care*, *1*, 1–6.

Steiner, I. D. (1972). *Group process and productivity*. New York, NY: Academic Press.

Stephens-Reicher, J., Metcalf, A., Blanchard, M., Mangan, C., & Burns, J. (2011). Reaching the hard-to-reach: How information communication technologies can reach young people at greater risk of mental health difficulties. *Australasian Psychiatry*, *19*(1), S58–S61. doi:10.3109/10398562.2011.583077 PMID:21878021

Stern, D. N., Bruschweiler-Stern, N., & Freeland, A. (1998). *The birth of a mother*. London: Bloomsbury.

Stetz, M. C., Thomas, M. L., Russo, M. B., Stetz, T. A., Wildzunas, R. M., McDonald, J. J., & Romano, J. A. et al. (2007). Stress, mental health, and cognition: A brief review of relationships and countermeasures. *Aviation, Space, and Environmental Medicine*, *78*(Suppl. 1), B252–B260. PMID:17547326

Stewart, B. (2014). *Dynamics vs. mechanics: A pre-analysis of watch dogs*. Retrieved from [REMOVED HYPERLINK FIELD]http://www.gamasutra.com/blogs/BartStewart/20140423/216090/Dynamics_vs_Mechanics_A_PreAnalysis_of_Watch_Dogs.Php

Stice, E., Ragan, J., & Randall, P. (2004). Prospective relations between social support and depression: Differential direction of effects for parent and peer support? *Journal of Abnormal Psychology*, *113*(1), 155–159. doi:10.1037/0021-843X.113.1.155 PMID:14992668

Stiles, W. B., Barkham, M., Mellor-Clark, J., & Connell, J. (2008). Effectiveness of cognitive-behavioural, person-centred, and psychodynamic therapies in UK primary-care routine practice: Replication in a larger sample. *Psychological Medicine*, *38*(5), 677–688. doi:10.1017/S0033291707001511 PMID:17825124

Stiles, W. B., Barkham, M., Twigg, E., Mellor-Clark, J., & Cooper, M. (2006). Effectiveness of cognitive-behavioural, person-centred and psychodynamic therapies as practised in UK National Health Service settings. *Psychological Medicine*, *36*(4), 555–566. doi:10.1017/S0033291706007136 PMID:16476185

Stone, A. A., Schwartz, J. E., Schkade, D., Schwarz, N., Krueger, A., & Kahneman, D. (2006). A population approach to the study of emotion: diurnal rhythms of a working day examined with the Day Reconstruction Method. *Emotion*, *6*(1), 139-149. doi:2006-04603-013 [pii]10.1037/1528-3542.6.1.139

Stone, A., Shiffman, S., Atienza, A., & Nebeling, L. (2007). *The science of real-time data capture: Self-reports in health research*. New York: Oxford University Press.

Strecher, V. (2007). Internet methods for delivering behavioral and health-related interventions (eHealth). *Annual Review of Clinical Psychology*, *3*(1), 53–76. doi:10.1146/annurev.clinpsy.3.022806.091428 PMID:17716048

Street, R. L., Gold, W. R., & Manning, T. R. (2013). *Health promotion and interactive technology: Theoretical applications and future directions*. London, UK: Routledge.

Stress Management Flyer. (2010). University of Melbourne. Retrieved from http://www.services.unimelb.edu.au/asu/download/Study-StressManagement-Flyer.pdf

Stronge, A. J., Rogers, W. A., & Fisk, A. D. (2007). Human factors considerations in implementing telemedicine systems to accommodate older adults. *Journal of Telemedicine and Telecare*, *13*(1), 1–3. doi:10.1258/135763307779701158 PMID:17288650

Strümpfer, D. (1995). The origins of health and strength: From 'salutogenesis' to 'fortigenesis'. *South African Journal of Psychology. Suid-Afrikaanse Tydskrif vir Sielkunde*, *25*(2), 81–89. doi:10.1177/008124639502500203

Subramanian, S., Knaut, L. A., Beaudoin, C., McFadyen, B. J., Feldman, A. G., & Levin, M. F. (2007). Virtual reality environments for post-stroke arm rehabilitation. *Journal of Neuroengineering and Rehabilitation*, *4*(1), 20. doi:10.1186/1743-0003-4-20 PMID:17587441

Sundstrom, P., Stahl, A., & Hook, K. (2005). eMoto-affectively involving both body and mind. Proceedings of CHI 05 extended abstracts. ACM: New York.

Sun, Y., Chan, K. L., & Krishnan, S. M. (2002). ECG signal conditioning by morphological filtering. *Computers in Biology and Medicine*, *32*(6), 465–479. doi:10.1016/S0010-4825(02)00034-3 PMID:12356496

Susi, T., Johanesson, M., & Backlund, P. (2007). *Serious Games - An Overview*. Skövde, Sweden: University of Skövde Press.

Susskind, J. M., Lee, D. H., Cusi, A., Feiman, R., Grabski, W., & Anderson, A. K. (2008). Expressing fear enhances sensory acquisition. *Nature Neuroscience*, *11*(7), 843–850. doi:10.1038/nn.2138 PMID:18552843

Swamynathan, G., Wilson, C., Boe, B., Almeroth, K., & Zhao, B. Y. (2008). Do social networks improve e-commerce?: a study on social marketplaces. *Paper presented at theFirst Workshop on Online Social Networks*, New York, USA. doi:10.1145/1397735.1397737

Sweetser, P. (2008). *Emergence in games*. Boston, MA: Charles River Media.

Sweetser, P., & Wyeth, P. (2005). GameFlow: A Model for Evaluating Player Enjoyment in Games. *Comput. Entertain.*, *3*(3), 1–24. doi:10.1145/1077246.1077253

Sweller, J. (1994). Cognitive load theory, learning difficulty and instructional design. *Learning and Instruction*, *4*(4), 295–312. doi:10.1016/0959-4752(94)90003-5

Swink, S. (2009). *Game feel: A game designer's guide to virtual sensation*. Amsterdam: Morgan Kaufmann/Elsevier.

Szczesna, A., Grudzinski, J., Grudzinski, T., Mikuszewski, R., & Debowski, A. (2011, November 16-18). The Psychology Serious Game Prototype for Preschool Children. Paper presented at the IEEE 1st International Conference on Serious Games and Applications for Health (SeGAH), Braga, Portugal.

Takatalo, J., Nyman, G., & Laaksonen, L. (2008). Components of human experience in virtual environments. *Computers in Human Behavior*, *24*(1), 1–15. doi:10.1016/j.chb.2006.11.003

Tamrat, T., & Kachnowski, S. (2012). Special delivery: An analysis of mHealth in maternal and newborn health programs and their outcomes around the world. *Maternal and Child Health Journal, 16*(5), 1092–1101. doi:10.1007/s10995-011-0836-3 PMID:21688111

Tang, P., & Venables, T. (2000). "Smart" homes and telecare for independent living. *Journal of Telemedicine and Telecare, 6*(1), 8–14. doi:10.1258/1357633001933871 PMID:10824384

Tariman, J. D., Berry, D. L., Cochrane, B., Doorenbos, A., & Schepp, K. (2010). Preferred and actual participation roles during health care decision making in persons with cancer: A systematic review. *Annals of Oncology, 21*(6), 1145–1151. doi:10.1093/annonc/mdp534 PMID:19940010

Taylor, C. B., & Luce, K. H. (2003). Computer-and Internet-based psychotherapy interventions. *Current Directions in Psychological Science, 12*(1), 18–22. doi:10.1111/1467-8721.01214

Taylor, L. M., Maddison, R., Pfaeffli, L. A., Rawstorn, J. C., Gant, N., & Kerse, N. M. (2012). Activity and energy expenditure in older people playing active video games. *Archives of Physical Medicine and Rehabilitation, 93*(12), 2281–2286. doi:10.1016/j.apmr.2012.03.034 PMID:22522217

Teixeira, J., Martin, D., Prendiville, O., & Glover, V. (2005). The effects of acute relaxation on indices of anxiety during pregnancy. *Journal of Psychosomatic Obstetrics and Gynaecology, 26*(4), 271–276. doi:10.1080/01674820500139922 PMID:16457423

Thayer, J. F., Ahs, F., Fredrikson, M., Sollers, J. J. III, & Wager, T. D. (2012). A meta-analysis of heart rate variability and neuroimaging studies: Implications for heart rate variability as a marker of stress and health. *Neuroscience and Biobehavioral Reviews, 36*(2), 747–756. doi:10.1016/j.neubiorev.2011.11.009 PMID:22178086

The World health report: 2001: Mental health: new understanding, new hope. (2001). *World Health Organization.*

Thivierge, S., Jean, L., & Simard, M. (2014). A randomized cross-over controlled study on cognitive rehabilitation of instrumental activities of daily living in Alzheimer disease. *The American Journal of Geriatric Psychiatry, 22*(11), 1188–1199. doi:10.1016/j.jagp.2013.03.008 PMID:23871120

Thomee, S., Harenstam, A., & Hagberg, M. (2011). Mobile phone use and stress, sleep disturbances, and symptoms of depression among young adults--a prospective cohort study. *BMC Public Health, 11*(1), 66. doi:10.1186/1471-2458-11-66 PMID:21281471

Thompson, G. (2007). The meaning of patient involvement and participation in health care consul-tations: A taxonomy. *Social Science & Medicine, 64*(6), 1297–1310. doi:10.1016/j.socscimed.2006.11.002 PMID:17174016

Tichon, J. (2010). (Manuscript submitted for publication). Evaluation of virtual reality training using affect. *International Journal on E-Learning.*

Tichon, J. G., Mavin, T., Wallis, G., Visser, T. A., & Riek, S. (2014). Using pupillometry and electromyography to track positive and negative affect during flight simulation. *Aviation Psychology and Applied Human Factors, 4*(1), 23–32. doi:10.1027/2192-0923/a000052

Tichon, J., & Banks, J. (2006). Virtual reality exposure therapy: 150-degree screen to desktop PC. *Cyberpsychology & Behavior, 9*(4), 480–487. doi:10.1089/cpb.2006.9.480 PMID:16901251

Tichon, J., Hall, R., & Higlers, M. G. (2003). Education and training in virtual environments for disaster management. *Proceedings of the World Conference on Educational Multimedia, Hypermedia & Telecommunications* (pp. 1191–1194). Honolulu.

Tichon, J., & Mavin, T. (in press). Powering up and bouncing back: Videogames teach resilience. *Games for Health Journal.*

Tichon, J., & Wallis, G. (2010). Stress training and simulator complexity: Why sometimes more is less. *Behaviour & Information Technology*, *29*(5), 459–466. doi:10.1080/01449290903420184

Tichon, J., Wallis, G., & Reik, S. (2010). *Affective Intensity and its Effects*. Brisbane: University of Queensland. doi:10.1037/e531432011-001

Tichon, J., Watson, G., & Wallis, G. (2011). Using feature extraction and electromyography to evaluate affect during simulation. *International Journal of Human Factors Modeling and Simulation*, *2*(1/2), 149–162. doi:10.1504/IJHFMS.2011.041642

Tietjen, A. M., & Bradley, C. F. (1985). Social support and maternal psychosocial adjustment during the transition to parenthood. *Revue canadienne des sciences du comportement [Canadian Journal of Behavioural Science]*, *17*(2), 109.

Timmermann, S. (1998). The Role of Information Technology in Older Adult Learning. *New Directions for Adult and Continuing Education*, 1998(77), 61–72.

Toffler, A. (1980). *The Third Wave*. London, UK: Pan Books.

Tornqvist, D. (2014). Exploratory play in simulation sandbox games: A review of what we know about why players act crazy. *International Journal of Game-Based Learning*, *4*(2), 78–95. doi:10.4018/ijgbl.2014040105

Tosa, N., Murakami, K., Kakimoto, M., & Sato, S. (1994). Neuro-Character. *Proceedings of the AAAI '94 Workshop, AI and A-Life and Entertainment.*

Touhey, J. C., & Bandura, A. (1975). Aggression: A Social Learning Analysis. *Contemporary Sociology*, *4*(2), 169. doi:10.2307/2062223

Tragea, C., Chrousos, G. P., Alexopoulos, E. C., & Darviri, C. (2014). A randomized controlled trial of the effects of a stress management programme during pregnancy. *Complementary Therapies in Medicine*, *22*(2), 203–211. doi:10.1016/j.ctim.2014.01.006 PMID:24731890

Triberti, S., & Argenton, L. (2015). Eros, Thanatos e Pixel: lo scandalo nei videogiochi e i suoi effetti psicologici. In L. Papale & F. Alinovi (Eds.), *Virtual Erotico*. Milan, Italy: Unicopli.

Triberti, S., & Liberati, E. G. (2014). Patient Centered Virtual Reality: An Opportunity to Improve the Quality of Patient's Experience. In P. Cipresso & S. Serino (Eds.), *Virtual Reality: Technologies, Medical Applications and Challenges*. New York, USA: Nova Science.

Triberti, S., Repetto, C., & Riva, G. (2014). Psychological factors influencing the effectiveness of virtual reality-based analgesia: A systematic review. *Cyberpsychology, Behavior, and Social Networking*, *17*(6), 335–345. doi:10.1089/cyber.2014.0054 PMID:24892195

Triberti, S., Villani, D., & Riva, G. (2015). Moral positioning in video games and its relation with dispositional traits: The emergence of a social dimension. *Computers in Human Behavior*, *50*, 1–8. doi:10.1016/j.chb.2015.03.069

Tripp, N., Hainey, K., Liu, A., Poulton, A., Peek, M., Kim, J., & Nanan, R. (2014). An emerging model of maternity care: Smartphone, midwife, doctor? *Women and Birth; Journal of the Australian College of Midwives*, *27*(1), 64–67. doi:10.1016/j.wombi.2013.11.001 PMID:24295598

Tronick, E. Z., & Weinberg, K. (1999). *Le madri depresse ei loro bambini: l'insuccesso nella formazione degli stati di coscienza diadici. Murray, L., Cooper, P.(a cura di). Depressione del post-partum e sviluppo del bambino*. Roma: CIC Edizioni Internazionali.

Tu, C.-H., & McIsaac, M. (2002). The Relationship of Social Presence and Interaction in Online Classes. *American Journal of Distance Education*, *16*(3), 131–150. doi:10.1207/S15389286AJDE1603_2

Turk, M., & Robertson, G. (2000). Perceptual user interfaces. *Communications of the ACM*, *43*(3), 33–34. doi:10.1145/330534.330535

Twitchell, J. (1995). *Dreadful Pleasures: An Anatomy of Modern Horror*. Oxford, United Kingdom: Oxford University Press.

U.S. Bureau of the Census. (2010). Retrieved from http://www.census.gov/

Uhlmann, E., & Swanson, J. (2004). Exposure to violent video games increases automatic aggressiveness. *Journal of Adolescence*, *27*(1), 41–52. doi:10.1016/j.adolescence.2003.10.004 PMID:15013259

Ullén, F., de Manzano, Ö., Almeida, R., Magnusson, P. K. E., Pedersen, N. L., Nakamura, J., & Madison, G. et al. (2012). Proneness for psychological flow in everyday life: Associations with personality and intelligence. *Personality and Individual Differences*, *52*(2), 167–172. doi:10.1016/j.paid.2011.10.003

Urech, C., Fink, N. S., Hoesli, I., Wilhelm, F. H., Bitzer, J., & Alder, J. (2010). Effects of relaxation on psychobiological wellbeing during pregnancy: A randomized controlled trial. *Psychoneuroendocrinology*, *35*(9), 1348–1355. doi:10.1016/j.psyneuen.2010.03.008 PMID:20417038

Urizar, G. G. Jr, Milazzo, M., Le, H. N., Delucchi, K., Sotelo, R., & Muñoz, R. F. (2004). Impact of stress reduction instructions on stress and cortisol levels during pregnancy. *Biological Psychology*, *67*(3), 275–282. doi:10.1016/j.biopsycho.2003.11.001 PMID:15294386

Vachiratamporn, V., Legaspi, R., Moriyama, K., Fukui, K., & Numao, M. (2015). An analysis of player affect transitions in survival horror games. *Journal on Multimodal User Interfaces*, *9*(1), 43–54. doi:10.1007/s12193-014-0153-4

Vaez, M., & Laflamme, L. (2008). Experienced stress, psychological symptoms, self-rated health and academic achievement: A longitudinal study of Swedish university students. *Social Behavior and Personality*, *36*(2), 183–196. doi:10.2224/sbp.2008.36.2.183

Valtchanov, D., Barton, K. R., & Ellard, C. (2010). Restorative effects of virtual nature settings. *Cyberpsychology, Behavior, and Social Networking*, *13*(5), 503–512. doi:10.1089/cyber.2009.0308 PMID:20950174

Van Bilsen, H. (2013). *Cognitive behaviour therapy in the real world: Back to basics*. Karnac Books.

Van Den Hoogen, W. M., IJsselsteijn, W. A., & De Kort, Y. A. (2009). Effects of sensory immersion on behavioural indicators of player experience: Movement synchrony and controller pressure. In *Breaking new ground: innovation in games, play, practice and theory.Proceedings of the 2009 Digital Games Research Association Conference* (pp. 1–6). London: Brunel University.

Van Reekum, C. M., Marije, C., Johnstone, T., Banse, R., Etter, A., Wehrle, T., & Scherer, K. R. (2004). Psychophysiological responses to appraisal dimensions in a computer game. *Cognition and Emotion*, *18*(5), 663–688. doi:10.1080/02699930341000167

Van Rooij, A. J., Meerkerk, G.-J., Schoenmakers, T. M., Griffiths, M., & van de Mheen, D. (2010). Video game addiction and social responsibility. *Addiction Research and Theory*, *18*(5), 489–493. doi:10.3109/16066350903168579

Van Rooij, A. J., Schoenmakers, T. M., Vermulst, A. A., Van Den Eijnden, R. J. J. M., & Van De Mheen, D. (2011). Online video game addiction: Identification of addicted adolescent gamers. *Addiction (Abingdon, England)*, *106*(1), 205–212. doi:10.1111/j.1360-0443.2010.03104.x PMID:20840209 van Schijndel, T. J. P., Franse, R. K., & Raijmakers, M. E. J. (2010). The exploratory behavior scale: Assessing young visitors' hands-on behavior in science museums. *Science Education*, *94*(5), 794–809. doi:10.1002/sce.20394

Vancouver, J. B., & Putka, D. J. (2000). Analyzing Goal-Striving Processes and a Test of the Generalizability of Perceptual Control Theory. *Organizational Behavior and Human Decision Processes*, *82*(2), 334–362. doi:10.1006/obhd.2000.2901 PMID:10891301

Vanhala, T., & Surakka, V. (2005). An agent framework for the development of psycho- physiologically interactive systems.*Proceedings of HCI International 2005*, Las Vegas, Nevada, USA.

Vansteenwegen, D. (2011). *Onderzoeksrapport De gelukscoach - een online programma om meer uit je leven te halen en te werken aan geluk (Research report happiness coach)*. Leuven: ISW Limits.

Varges, S., Bieler, H., Stede, M., Faulstich, L. C., Irsig, K., & Atalla, M. (2012, May 23-25). SemScribe: Natural Language Generation for Medical Reports. *Paper presented at theEighth International Conference on Language Resources and Evaluation (LREC)*, Istanbul, Turkey.

Vealey, R. S. (2007). Mental skills training in sport. In G. Tenenbaum & R. C. Eklund (Eds.), *Handbook of sport psychology* (pp. 287–309). Hoboken, NJ: Wiley.

Veenhoven, R. (2008). Sociological theories of subjective well-being. In M. Eid & R. J. Larsen (Eds.), *The science of subjective well-being* (pp. 44–61). New York: Guilford Press.

Velten, E. Jr. (1968). A laboratory task for induction of mood states. *Behaviour Research and Therapy*, *6*(4), 473–482. doi:10.1016/0005-7967(68)90028-4 PMID:5714990

Ventura, M., Shute, V., & Zhao, W. (2013). The relationship between video game use and a performance-based measure of persistence. *Computers & Education*, *60*(1), 52–58. doi:10.1016/j.compedu.2012.07.003

Verghese, J., Levalley, A., Derby, C., Kuslansky, G., Katz, M., Hall, C., … Lipton, R. B. (2006). Leisure activities and the risk of amnestic mild cognitive impairment in the elderly. Neurology, 66(6), 821–827.

Vieten, C., & Astin, J. (2008). Effects of a mindfulness-based intervention during pregnancy on prenatal stress and mood: Results of a pilot study. *Archives of Women's Mental Health*, *11*(1), 67–74. doi:10.1007/s00737-008-0214-3 PMID:18317710

Villani, D., Cipresso, P., & Repetto, C. (2014). Coping with Stress and Anxiety: the Role of Presence in Technology Mediated Environments. In G. Riva, J. A. Waterworth, & D. Murray (Eds.), Interacting with Presence: HCI and the Sense of Presence in Computer-mediated Environments (p. 139). Berlin: De Gruyter Open. Retrieved from www. presence-research. com

Villani, D., Grassi, A., Cognetta, C., Toniolo, D., Cipresso, P., & Riva, G. (2013). Self-help stress management training through mobile phones: An experience with oncology nurses. *Psychological Services*, *10*(3), 315–322. doi:10.1037/a0026459 PMID:23937091

Villani, D., Lucchetta, M., Preziosa, A., & Riva, G. (2006). Narrative versus environment: The role of media content in emotional induction. *Cyberpsychology & Behavior*, *9*(6), 724–725.

Villani, D., Lucchetta, M., Preziosa, A., & Riva, G. (2009). The role of affective media features on the affective response: A virtual reality study. *e-Minds. International Journal of Human-Computer Interaction*, *1*(5), 35–55.

Villani, D., Preziosa, A., Riva, F., & Riva, G. (2006). Presence enhances relaxation: A preliminary controlled study. *Cyberpsychology & Behavior*, *9*(6), 723–724.

Villani, D., Preziosa, A., & Riva, G. (2006). Coping with stress using virtual reality: A new perspective. *Annual Review of Cybertherapy and Telemedicine*, *4*, 25–32.

Villani, D., Repetto, C., Cipresso, P., & Riva, G. (2012). May I experience more presence in doing the same thing in virtual reality than in reality? An answer from a simulated job interview. *Interacting with Computers*, *24*(4), 265–272. doi:10.1016/j.intcom.2012.04.008

Villani, D., Riva, F., & Riva, G. (2007). New technologies for relaxation: The role of presence. *International Journal of Stress Management*, *14*(3), 260–274. doi:10.1037/1072-5245.14.3.260

Villani, D., & Riva, G. (2012). Does interactive media enhance the management of stress? Suggestions from a controlled study. *Cyberpsychology, Behavior, and Social Networking*, *15*(1), 24–30. doi:10.1089/cyber.2011.0141 PMID:22032797

Virtual Doctor can advise on when to go to the ER. (2011). *KCCI*. Retrieved from http://www.kcci.com/Virtual-doctor-can-advise-on-when-to-go-to-ER/3903134

Vittersø, J. (2004). Subjective well-being versus self-actualization: Using the flow-simplex to promote a conceptual clarification of subjective quality of life. *Social Indicators Research*, *65*(3), 299–331. doi:10.1023/B:SOCI.0000003910.26194.ef

Vlasnik, J. J., Aliotta, S. L., & DeLor, B. (2005). Medication adherence: Factors influencing compliance with prescribed medication plans. *The Case Manager*, *16*(2), 47–51. doi:10.1016/j.casemgr.2005.01.009 PMID:15818344

Vliet, H. V., & Andrews, G. (2009). Internet-based course for the management of stress for junior high schools. *The Australian and New Zealand Journal of Psychiatry*, *43*(4), 305–309. doi:10.1080/00048670902721145 PMID:19296285

Voellmin, A., Entringer, S., Moog, N., Wadhwa, P. D., & Buss, C. (2013). Maternal positive affect over the course of pregnancy is associated with the length of gestation and reduced risk of preterm delivery. *Journal of Psychosomatic Research*, *75*(4), 336–340. doi:10.1016/j.jpsychores.2013.06.031 PMID:24119939

Vuoskoski, J. K., & Thompson, W. F. (2012). Who Enjoys Listening to Sad Music and Why? *Music Perception: An Interdisciplinary Journal*, *29*(3), 311–317. doi:10.1525/mp.2012.29.3.311

Wakefield, C. E., Sansom-Daly, U. M., McGill, B. C., McCarthy, M., Girgis, A., Grootenhuis, M., & Cohn, R. J. (2015). Online parent-targeted cognitive-behavioural therapy intervention to improve quality of life in families of young cancer survivors: Study protocol for a randomized controlled trial. *Trials*, *16*(1), 153. doi:10.1186/s13063-015-0681-6 PMID:25872773

Walker, A. (2002). A strategy for active ageing. *International Social Security Review*, *55*(1), 121–139. doi:10.1111/1468-246X.00118

Wang, H.-X., Jin, Y., Hendrie, H. C., Liang, C., Yang, L., Cheng, Y., & Gao, S. et al. (2013). Late life leisure activities and risk of cognitive decline. *The Journals of Gerontology. Series A, Biological Sciences and Medical Sciences*, *68*(2), 205–213. doi:10.1093/gerona/gls153 PMID:22879456

Wang, Z., & Gan, Y. (2010). Coping mediates between social support, neuroticism, and depression after earthquake and examination stress among adolescents. *Anxiety, Stress, and Coping*, 24(3), 343-358. PMID:20865589

Waring, M. E., Simas, T. A. M., Xiao, R. S., Lombardini, L. M., Allison, J. J., Rosal, M. C., & Pagoto, S. L. (2014). Pregnant women's interest in a website or mobile application for healthy gestational weight gain. *Sexual & Reproductive Healthcare*, *5*(4), 182–184. doi:10.1016/j.srhc.2014.05.002 PMID:25433828

Warnecke, E., Quinn, S., Ogden, K., Towle, N., & Nelson, M. R. (2011). A randomised controlled trial of the effects of mindfulness practice on medical student stress levels. *Medical Education*, *45*(4), 381–388. doi:10.1111/j.1365-2923.2010.03877.x PMID:21401686

Washburn, C. A., & Mandrusiak, M. (2010). Campus suicide prevention and intervention: Putting best practice policy into action. *Canadian Journal of Higher Education*, *40*(1), 101–119.

Waterworth, E. L., Waterworth, J. A., Peter, C., & Ballesteros, S. (2012, June 6-8). Seniors in charge of ICT innovation. *Proceedings of the5th Workshop on Affect and Behaviour Related AssistancePETRA 2012*, Crete.

Waterworth, J. A., & Waterworth, E. L. (2014). Altered, expanded and distributed embodiment: the three stages of interactive presence. In G. Riva, J. A. Waterworth, & D. Murray (Eds.), Interacting with Presence: HCI and the sense of presence in computer-mediated environments (pp. 36–50). Berlin: De Gruyter Open. Retrieved from http://www.presence-research.com

Waterworth, E. L., & Waterworth, J. A. (2009). Designing ICT for the over 80s. In *Topo, P. & Östlund, B. (2009), Dementia, Design and Technology: Time to Get Involved.* Amsterdam: IOS Press.

Waterworth, J. A., & Riva, G. (2014). *Feeling Present in the Physical World and in Computer-Mediated Environments.* Basingstoke, UK: Palgrave Macmillan. doi:10.1057/9781137431677

Waterworth, J. A., & Waterworth, E. L. (2012). Presence as a dimension of communication: Context of use and the person *Emerging Communication. Studies in New Technologies and Practices in Communication*, *9*, 80–95.

Waterworth, J. A., Waterworth, E. L., Mantovani, F., & Riva, G. (2010). On Feeling (the) Present: An evolutionary account of the sense of presence in physical and electronically-mediated environments. *Journal of Consciousness Studies*, *17*(1-2), 167–178.

Wattanasoontorn, V., Boada, I., García, R., & Sbert, M. (2013). Serious games for health. *Entertainment Computing*, *4*(4), 231–247. doi:10.1016/j.entcom.2013.09.002

Watterson, J. L., Walsh, J., & Madeka, I. (2015). Using mHealth to Improve Usage of Antenatal Care, Postnatal Care, and Immunization: A Systematic Review of the Literature. *BioMed Research International, 2015.*

Weaver, A. J., & Lewis, N. (2012). Mirrored Morality: An Exploration of Moral Choice in Video Games. *Cyberpsychology, Behavior, and Social Networking*. doi:10.1089/cyber.2012.0235 PMID:23017118

Webb, M., Burns, J., & Collin, P. (2008). Providing online support for young people with mental health difficulties: Challenges and opportunities explored. *Early Intervention in Psychiatry*, *2*(2), 108–113. doi:10.1111/j.1751-7893.2008.00066.x PMID:21352141

Weber, R., Behr, K.-M., Tamborini, R., Ritterfeld, U., & Mathiak, K. (2009). What Do We Really Know About First-Person-Shooter Games? An Event-Related, High-Resolution Content Analysis. *Journal of Computer-Mediated Communication*, *14*(4), 1016–1037. doi:10.1111/j.1083-6101.2009.01479.x

Webster, J. D., & McCall, M. E. (1999). Reminiscence functions across adulthood: A replication and extension. *Journal of Adult Development*, *6*(1), 73–85. doi:10.1023/A:1021628525902

Weinstein, N., Przybylski, A. K., & Ryan, R. M. (2009). Can nature make us more caring? Effects of immersion in nature on intrinsic aspirations and generosity. *Personality and Social Psychology Bulletin*, *35*(10), 1315–1329. doi:10.1177/0146167209341649 PMID:19657048

Wellman, B., & Frank, K. (2001). Network capital in a multilevel world: Getting support from personal communities. *Social capital: Theory and research* (pp. 233-273).

Westerfelhaus, R., & Alan Brookey, R. (2004). At the unlikely confluence of conservative religion and popular culture: Fight club as heteronormative ritual. *Text and Performance Quarterly*, *24*(3-4), 302–326. doi:10.1080/1046293042000312788

White, S. (2013). Meet Ellie, The Virtual Psychologist. *Technology Guide*. Retrieved from http://www.technologyguide.com/news/virtual-psychologist-could-change-the-future-of-mental-health/

WHO. (1948). Preamble to the Constitution of the World Health Organization as adopted by the International Health Conference, New York, 19-22 June, 1946; signed on 22 July 1946 by the representatives of 61 States (*Official Records of the World Health Organization*, no. 2, p. 100) and entered into force on 7 April 1948.

WHO. (2003). *International Classification of Functioning*. Disability and Health.

Wiederhold, B. K., & Wiederhold, M. D. (2003). A New Approach: Using Virtual Reality Psychotherapy in Panic Disorder with Agoraphobia. Psychiatric Times. Retrieved from http://www.psychiatrictimes.com/articles/new-approach-using-virtual-reality-psychotherapy-panic-disorder-agoraphobia

Wiederhold, B. K., & Wiederhold, M. D. (2006). From stress inoculation training to posttraumatic stress disorder: developing a continuum of care for the warfighter. *Paper presented at the CyberPsychology & Behavior*.

Wiederhold, B. K., & Riva, G. (2012). Positive technology supports shift to preventive, integrative health. *Cyberpsychology, Behavior, and Social Networking*, *15*(2), 67–68. doi:10.1089/cyber.2011.1533 PMID:22320253

Wiederhold, B. K., Riva, G., & Graffigna, G. (2013). Ensuring the best care for our increasing aging population: Health engagement and positive technology can help patients achieve a more active role in future healthcare. *Cyberpsychology, Behavior, and Social Networking*, *16*(6), 411–412. doi:10.1089/cyber.2013.1520 PMID:23751102

Wiemer-Hastings, K., Janit, A. S., Wiemer-Hastings, P. M., Cromer, S., & Kinser, J. (2004). Automatic classification of dysfunctional thoughts: A feasibility test. *Behavior Research Methods, Instruments, & Computers*, *36*(2), 203–212. doi:10.3758/BF03195565 PMID:15354685

Wilcox, A. B. (2015). Patient Engagement and Consumerism. In P. R. O. Payne & P. J. Embi (Eds.), *Translational Informatics* (pp. 153–161). London, UK: Springer.

Wilkinson, N., Ang, R. P., & Goh, D. H. (2008). Online video game therapy for mental health concerns: A review. The International Journal of Social Psychiatry, 54(4), 370–382. doi:10.1177/0020764008091659 PubMed doi:10.1177/0020764008091659 PMID:18720897

Williams, C., & Whitfield, G. (2001). Written and computer-based self-help treatments for depression. *British Medical Bulletin*, *57*(1), 133–144. doi:10.1093/bmb/57.1.133 PMID:11719913

Willis, S. L., Tennstedt, S. L., Marsiske, M., Ball, K., Elias, J., Koepke, K. M., & Stoddard, A. M. et al. (2006). Long-term effects of cognitive training on everyday functional outcomes in older adults. *Journal of the American Medical Association*, *296*(23), 2805–2814. doi:10.1001/jama.296.23.2805 PMID:17179457

Wilson, R. S., Bennett, D., Bienias, J. L., Mendes de Leon, C. F., Morris, M. C., & Evans, D. (2003). Cognitive activity and cognitive decline in a biracial community population. *Neurology*, *61*(6), 812–816. doi:10.1212/01.WNL.0000083989.44027.05 PMID:14504326

Wilson, T., & Gilbert, D. (2003). In M. Zanna (Ed.), *Affective forecasting* (pp. 345–411). Advances in experimental social psychologyNew York, NY: Elsevier.

Windle, G., Bennett, K. M., & Noyes, J. (2011). A methodological review of resilience measurement scales. *Health and Quality of Life Outcomes*, *9*(8). Retrieved from http://www.hqlo.com/content/9/1/8 PMID:21294858

Winograd, T., & Flores, F. (1986). *Understanding Computers and Cognition: A New Foundation for Design*. Wilmington, USA: Intellect Books.

Wolfe, B. E. (2002). The Role of Lived Experience in Self- and Relational Observation: A Commentary on Horowitz (2002). *Journal of Psychotherapy Integration*, *12*(2), 147–153. doi:10.1037/1053-0479.12.2.147

Wolinsky, F. D., Vander Weg, M. W., Howren, M. B., Jones, M. P., & Dotson, M. M. (2013). A randomized controlled trial of cognitive training using a visual speed of processing intervention in middle aged and older adults. *PLoS ONE*, *8*(5), e61624. doi:10.1371/journal.pone.0061624 PMID:23650501

Wouters, P., van Nimwegen, C., van Oostendorp, H., & van der Spek, E. D. (2013). A meta-analysis of the cognitive and motivational effects of serious games. *Journal of Educational Psychology*, *105*(2), 249–265. doi:10.1037/a0031311

Wu, Y. C., Xue, Y., & Hu, F. (2014). Embedded Smart Textile Detecting Equipment Base on Flexibility Sensors. *Applied Mechanics and Materials*, *670*, 1218–1221.

Yali, A. M., & Lobel, M. (2002). Stress-resistance resources and coping in pregnancy. *Anxiety, Stress, and Coping*, *15*(3), 289–309. doi:10.1080/1061580021000020743

Yang, S., & Shin, C. S. (2008). Parental attitudes towards education: What matters for children's well-being? *Children and Youth Services Review*, *30*(30), 1328–1335. doi:10.1016/j.childyouth.2008.03.015

Yassuda, M. S., Lopes, A., Cachioni, M., Falcao, D. V. S., Batistoni, S. S. T., Guimaraes, V. V., & Neri, A. L. (2012). Frailty criteria and cognitive performance are related: Data from the FIBRA study in Ermelino Matarazzo, São Paulo, Brazil. *The Journal of Nutrition, Health & Aging*, *16*(1), 55–61. doi:10.1007/s12603-012-0003-6 PMID:22238002

Ybarra, M., & Eaton, W. (2005). Internet-Based Mental Health Interventions. *Mental Health Services Research*, *7*(2), 75–87. doi:10.1007/s11020-005-3779-8 PMID:15974154

Yee, N. (2006). The labor of fun: How video games blur the boundaries of work and play. Games and Culture, 1(1), 68–71. doi:10.1177/1555412005281819 doi:10.1177/1555412005281819

Yee, N. (2006). Motivations for play in online games. *Cyberpsychology & Behavior*, *9*(6), 772–775. doi:10.1089/cpb.2006.9.772 PMID:17201605

Yildirim, S. (2010, June). Serious Game Design for Military Training. Paper presented at the Games Design and Research Conference, Volda University College, Volda, Norway.

Ylvisaker, M., Hanks, R., & Johnson-Greene, D. (2002). Perspectives on rehabilitation of individuals with cognitive impairment after brain injury: Rationale for reconsideration of theoretical paradigms. *The Journal of Head Trauma Rehabilitation*, *17*(3), 191–209. doi:10.1097/00001199-200206000-00002 PMID:12086574

Yoediono, Z., & Snyderman, R. (2008). Proposal for a new health record to support personalized, predictive, preventative and participatory medicine. *Personalized Medicine*, *5*(1), 47–54. doi:10.2217/17410541.5.1.47

Yoo, Y., & Alavi, M. (2001). The Relationship of Social Presence and Interaction in Online Classes. *Management Information Systems Quarterly*, *25*(3), 371–390. doi:10.2307/3250922

Yoshida, A., Hagita, Y., Yamazaki, K., & Yamaguchi, T. (1993). Which do you feel comfortable, interview by a real doctor or by a virtual doctor? A comparative study. *Proceedings of the2nd IEEE International Workshop on Robot and Human Communication* (pp. 370-374)

Yoshie, M., Kudo, K., & Ohtsuki, T. (2008, September). Effects of psychological stress on state anxiety, electromyographic activity, and arpeggio performance in pianists. *Medical Problems of Performing Artists*, *23*, 120–132.

Zahorik, P., & Jenison, R. L. (1998). Presence as being-in-the-world. *Presence (Cambridge, Mass.)*, *7*(1), 78–89. doi:10.1162/105474698565541

Zanbaka, C., Goolkasian, P., & Hodges, L. F. (2006). Can a virtual cat persuade you? The role of gender and realism in speaker persuasiveness. In CHI 2006 proceedings. Montreal Quebec Canada.

Zei Pollerman, B. (2010, March 10-13). Karasek's Demand/Control model, emotions and Health (Poster). *Proceedings of the 68th Annual scientific meeting* (pp. 72).

Zetterqvist, K., Maanmies, J., Ström, L., & Andersson, G. (2003). Randomized controlled trial of internet-based stress management. *Cognitive Behaviour Therapy*, *32*(3), 151–160. doi:10.1080/16506070302316 PMID:16291546

Zillmann, D., Weaver, J. B., Mundorf, N., & Aust, C. F. (1986). Effects of an opposite-gender companion's affect to horror on distress, delight, and attraction. *Journal of Personality and Social Psychology*, *51*(3), 586–594. doi:10.1037/0022-3514.51.3.586

Zyda, M. (2005). From Visual Simulation to Virtual Reality to Games. *Computer*, *38*(9), 25–32. doi:10.1109/MC.2005.297

# About the Contributors

**Daniela Villani**, PhD, is a Researcher in General Psychology at the Faculty of Educational Science, at Università Cattolica del Sacro Cuore in Milan, Italy. She has collaborated as a junior researcher at the ATNP-LAB (I.R.C.C.S. Istituto Auxologico Italiano, Milan, Italy) to the European project ("EMMA" – Engaging Media for Mental Health Applications-IST-2001-39192) aimed to study the emotional impact in virtual environments and she was a three-year scholarship holder for the realization of the Italian project MIUR FIRB "NEUROTIV – Managed Care based on immersive virtual telepresence for the assessment and rehabilitation in neuro psychology and clinical psychology" (RBNE01W8WH) at the same facility. She received some international awards, including the 'Italian E-content Award in the category of E-Health for the product Dream Island (2005) and the "CRC-Clinical CyberPsychology New Investigator Award" for the quality of research methods in "Narrative Versus Environment: The Role of Media Content in Emotional Induction"(2006). Dr. Villani's research has been characterized by a strong interdisciplinary nature, covering the following research topics: 1) the relationships between emotions and new technologies; 2) the use of interactive simulations for the training of psychological skills; 3) the cognitive factors related to the use of mediated technologies in the education/training and clinical domains, with a specific focus on the analysis of the concept of "presence". She is author of contributes at national and international conferences as well as of national and international publications on peer-reviewed journals with impact factor.

**Pietro Cipresso**, Ph.D., is Senior Researcher and Chief Technical Officer at the Applied Technology for Neuro-Psychology Lab - ATN-P Lab, IRCCS Istituto Auxologico Italiano, Milan and Research Fellow in Psychometrics at Università Cattolica del Sacro Cuore, Italy. He graduated at Bocconi University of Milan in economics, major in statistics and operational research, and received his Ph.D. in communication and new technologies, major in psychology, from IULM University of Milan, with a dissertation in computational communication and emotions. Cipresso has been Visiting Research Scholar at Massachusetts Institute of Technology (MIT) and in charge of projects coordination, collaborating in many international and European projects. Pietro Cipresso is author of more than 100 scientific publications and books like "Modeling Emotions at the Edge of Chaos", "Computing Paradigms for Mental Health", "The Psychology of Social Networking" and "Virtual Reality: Technologies, Medical Applications and Challenges", and also editor of the Central European Journal of Medicine (Springer), an Associate Editor in Psychology Open Books program (De Gruyter) and of other international peer-reviewed scientific journals and books. In 2012, Cipresso was awarded with the Canadian Research Chair in Clinical Cyberpsychology New Investigator Award, sponsored by the Université du Québec, Outaouais, Canada, for a presentation of outstanding quality.

**Andrea Gaggioli**, Ph.D. is a Research Professor of General Psychology at the Università Cattolica del Sacro Cuore, Italy; Senior Researcher of the Interactive Communication and Ergonomics of NEw Technologies (ICE-NET) Lab. at the Catholic University of Milan, Italy, and Deputy Head Researcher at the Applied Technology for Neuro-Psychology Laboratory - ATN-P Lab., I.R.C.C.S. Istituto Auxologico Italiano. For over ten years, Gaggioli has investigated the potential role of pervasive technologies in promoting mental and physical wellbeing. His involvement with those research areas has led to the co-authoring of over fifty articles in refereed journals, including these papers published in "Science": (i) Gaggioli A., Riva G., Working the Crowd, Science. 2008 Sep 12;321(5895):1443; (ii) Gorini A, Gaggioli A, Riva G. Virtual Worlds, Real Healing. Science. 2007 Dec 7;318(5856):1549. For his scientific work, Gaggioli has received several international acknowledgements, including the 2005 Annual Prize from the European Academy of Rehabilitation Medicine (http://www.aemr.eu/).

**Giuseppe Riva**, Ph.D., is Director of the Interactive Communication and Ergonomics of NEw Technologies (ICE-NET) Lab. at the Università Cattolica del Sacro Cuore, Italy, and Head Researcher of the the Applied Technology for Neuro-Psychology Laboratory - ATN-P Lab., I.R.C.C.S. Istituto Auxologico Italiano, Verbania Italy. He also is a full professor of General Psychology and Communication Psychology and a member of the steering committee of the Ph.D. programme in Psychology at the Catholic University of Milan, Italy. According to the scientific databases of the ISI Web of Science, PubMed/Medline and PsycInfo, Riva is the scholar who authored the highest number of peer-reviewed scientific publications in the fields of "Virtual Reality" in the world (as of November 2012). He is also 1st in the field of "Interreality" worldwide and within the top 10 in the field of "ambient intelligence" and "telepresence" research. Giuseppe Riva is currently the President of the International Association of CyberPsychology, Training, and Rehabilitation (http://iactor.ning.com/). Riva is also the Scientific Committee Chair of the CyberTherapy and CyberPsychology Conference (http://www.e-therapy.info/), Workshop Organizer at UbiHealth: The International Workshop on Ubiquitous Health and Wellness (http://www.e-therapy.info/) and Organizing Committee Member for the NextMed – Medicine Meets Virtual Reality Conference (http://www.nextmed.com/mmvr_committee.html).

* * *

**Paula Álvarez** is a Nurse of the SGGPA.

**Rosa M. Baños** is a full professor at the University of Valencia, and holds a PhD in Psychology from the University of Valencia since 1987. She is a Psychologist Specialist in Clinical Psychology since 2004. Currently, she is director of "Master in Interdisciplinary Intervention in Eating, Personality and Emotional Disorders" and co-director of Labpsitec research group (Laboratory of Psychology and Technology). She has participated as the principal investigator or collaborator in 60 funded projects (European, national and regional). She has written more than 70 book chapters, 100 publications in impact journals, and participated in 300 international and national congresses. She is part of the editorial board of several scientific journals and external evaluator of numerous scientific publications and organizations. Her research has focused on the field of psychopathology, assessment and treatment of psychological disorders, and the use of Information and Communication Technology (ICT). Her field of research is wide, and she is currently working on the line of Positive Interventions supported by ICT, among others.

**Katherine Berkovitz**, MA, is a Ph.D. student in the Psychology department at Harvard with over 5 years of experience in social-psychological studies of mindfulness in at risk, older populations and in concert with other studies in stress.

**Cristina Botella** is a full professor of Clinical Psychology at Jaume I University (UJI) (Spain). Director of Labpsitec (www.labpsitec.es). Head of one groups CIBER (Centre for Network Biomedical Research) in the area of Biomedicine and Health Sciences. Botella is also director of the Doctorate Programme in Psychology at UJI. She has been principal investigator in more than 40 research projects and published over 150 papers. Her main line of research is in the treatment of psychological disorders, and the use of ICTs (virtual reality, augmented reality the Internet and mobile apps) to promote health and wellbeing. She was president elect of the International Association of CyberPsychology, Training & Rehabilitation in 2009.

**Alba Carrillo-Vega** is a PhD psychology student at the University of Valencia (Spain). She obtained a fellowship from the Government of Spain in 2014 to carry out her thesis on the use of a positive visualization intervention supported by Information and Communication Technologies. She has two master degrees (Advances in Research and Treatments in Psychopathology and Health, and General Health Psychology). She is a member of Labpsitec group (Laboratory of Psychology and Technology), and her main research is focused on the use of Information and Communication Technologies (ICT) applied to psychological interventions, mainly in the field of Positive Psychology.

**Claudia Carissoli** is a PhD student in Education Science at Catholic University of Milan. She graduated in Economics in 1993 and in Psycology in 2013. She is interested in designing and testing Positive Interventions supported by ICT to promote individual resources (managing stress, reducing anxiety, relaxation, positive emotions), such as the mobile app Benessere Mamma, dedicated to Mothers-to-be well-being.

**Juan Luis Carús** has a PhD in Industrial Engineering (2015) from the Spanish University for Distance Education (UNED) and MSc in Telecommunications Engineering (2009) from the University of Oviedo. In 2007, he received the Thesis Award "Telefónica España" for the best record in technical engineering. Since July 2008, he has been a researcher with the R&D&i Area of CTIC – Technology Centre. His interests include ambient intelligence research projects focusing on signal processing, wearable computing and eHealth. He has been also working on projects related with the metal industry focused on signal processing and quality inspection. He has several international publications on the application of techniques of signal processing in different fields.

**Unai Díaz-Orueta**, Ph.D., received his doctorate in psychology from the University of Deusto, Spain in 2006. Since 2000, he has worked as a clinical psychologist in a variety of settings, including the Crownsville Hospital Center, Crownsville, Maryland (EE.UU., 2000-2001), Hospital Psiquiátrico de Bermeo, (Spain, 2001-2002), La Loma Geriatric Residence, Castro-Urdiales (Spain, 2003-2005), and Zutitu Ltd (2005-2006). With a grant from the Oriol-Urquijo University-Foundation, he developed his doctoral dissertation, "Effects of psychological intervention in cognitive decline of residentialized elderly people," published by UMI Dissertation Publishing, Ann Arbor, MI (USA). Additionally, his experience includes teaching courses and workshops in maintenance of cognitive functions, wellbeing, and laugh-therapy for elderly people at IPACE Ltd, Vitoria (Spain, 2007-2008). From 2008-2012, he worked as a research psychologist at Fundación INGEMA, in several projects related to aging and physical disability. Since May 2012, he has been working as a researcher at the R+D+i Department of Nesplora S.L. (Donostia-San Sebastian, Spain), and since May 2014, as a Collaborator Professor for the Neuropsychology and Education Master's Degree of the UNIR -International University of La Rioja (Spain).

**Ernestina Etchemendy** is a member of the research personnel of CIBERobn since 2008. She obtained her PhD on 2011. Her dissertation was focused on the clinical validation of an e-health platform developed for the elderly which was aimed to enhance their quality of life through different positive emotion exercises, sociability, and entertainment, among others. Currently, her main research line is focused on the use of ICTs, well-being and other important factors of psychological protection.

**Sonia García** holds a MSc in Computer Engineering from the Polytechnic School of Engineering of the University of Oviedo (Spain). Since 2007, she has worked in the R&D Department of CTIC Technology Centre. Her research experience includes TV interactive applications, serious games, usability and eHealth, focusing on the prevention of cognitive impairment and active ageing. Several of her works have been published, both at national and European levels.

**José Gutiérrez** is a doctor of Medicine, Geriatrician at Monte Naranco Hospital. He was the past-president of the Asturias Geriatrics Society. Treasurer of the Spanish Geriatric Society.

**Ian Hickie**, AM is a psychiatrist and prominent mental health campaigner. He is a former NHMRC Australia Fellow heading the University of Sydney's Brain and Mind Centre as a Co-Director for Health and Policy, and is one of Australia's first National Mental Health Commissioners. The Commission oversees enhanced accountability for mental health reform in Australia. Professor Hickie is an internationally renowned researcher in clinical psychiatry and a leading voice on mental health issues, with a special interest in youth mental health, and the prevention of and early intervention in emerging mood disorders. He has been instrumental in using clinical, health services and population health data to drive innovations in health services, particularly in primary care. In partnership with Professor Patrick McGorry, he has been at the forefront of developing the youth mental health service headspace: the National Youth Mental Health Foundation. Professor Hickie passionately advocates for enhanced health and social services for those with persistent mental illness and for increased accountability in the delivery of those services. As inaugural CEO of beyondblue: a national depression initiative, he established important depression awareness, prevention and early intervention programs. As Board Member for Research at the Mental Health Council of Australia (2003-2006), he was at the forefront of assessing consumers' and carers' experiences of mental health services. The findings underpinned the COAG agreement of 2006-2011 providing AUD 5.5 billion in additional expenditure for mental health and the introduction of access to psychological services within the Medicare scheme.

**M. Sazzad Hussain**, PhD, is a Research Fellow at CSIRO, Australia. He was a Research Associate at The University of Sydney where this work was carried out. His research interests include e-Health, Human Computer Interaction, Affective Computing, Learning Technologies and systems to support Mental Health. He has a PhD in multimodal Affect and Cognitive Load detection from The University of Sydney and has worked at National ICT Australia (NICTA) as part of his doctoral research. Sazzad was awarded Best Student for his Master of Science degree and had received the prestigious PhD scholarship 'Endeavour Postgraduate Award by Australia Awards'.

**Manolya Kavakli** is an Associate Professor Manolya Kavakli is the Director of the Virtual Reality Lab at the Simulation Hub and is the Director of the Postgraduate Coursework Program for the Department of Computing, Macquarie University, Sydney, Australia. She is an active researcher working on Human Computer Interaction (HCI) with over 150 refereed papers in the last 25 years. She gained her M.Sc. and Ph.D. degrees in 1990 and 1995 from Istanbul Technical University and was awarded a NATO Science Fellowship in 1996 for postdoctoral research. In 1998 she received a Postdoctoral Fellowship from the University of Sydney, Australia. Dr. Kavakli has supervised 7 postdoctoral fellows and 47 postgraduate (11 PhD, 2 MSc, 7 Honours, 18 MIT and 9 French MEng internship) students in HCI. She is the head of the research group VISOR (Virtual and Interactive Simulations of Reality), which was established in 2003. Her group conducted and applied empirical research on human information processing and signal processing. The main application area for the interfaces is to develop training simulations. At present, she has been supervising 6 postgraduate students in this domain. She has been the recipient of 11 awards, including the 3 Best paper awards in the last 3 years. She received more than 30 grants from a number of scientific international organisations including the Australian Research Council, the Scientific and Technical Research Council of Turkey, Turkish Republic State Planning Organization. Her research has been frequently profiled in international media.

**Timothy Mavin** is an associate professor at the Griffith Institute for Educational Research. His interests are in the area of complex skills development, focusing on training and assessment.

**Julia Menichetti**, MS, is trained as a clinical and health psychologist. She received her undergraduate degree in Neuropsychology, and her MS in Clinical Psychology. She is a PhD candidate in the Department of Psychology of Università Cattolica del Sacro Cuore with a funded project entitled: "The potential of technology to actively engage older people in a healthy lifestyle." Julia has conducted qualitative and quantitative research in the area of active and healthy ageing. Her research interests include the development of prevention and intervention strategies for older populations, with a focus on technological solutions.

**David N Milne** is a postdoctoral researcher with the Positive Computing Laboratory at the University of Sydney. His research focuses on text mining and he is currently collaborating with ReachOut.com to improve how young Australians seek help online. Prior to joining the University of Sydney, David worked at CSIRO, where he collaborated with the Black Dog Institute and Amazon AWS to explore how we express our emotions in social media. He has a well-cited research portfolio in Natural Language Processing, and has won international awards for his work in extracting machine-readable knowledge from Wikipedia and applying it to Text Mining and Information Retrieval tasks.

**Kjartan Nordbo** was born in Bergen, Norway, in 1991. He received the B.S. degree in Computer Science from the University of Bergen, in 2014, and a M.Tech. in Information Technology from the University of Sydney in 2015.

**Francesco Pagnini** is Assistant Professor at the Catholic University of Milan and collaborates as post-doctoral fellow with Harvard University. He has completed his Ph.D. in Clinical Psychology from the University of Bergamo. His primary interest is focused on the improvement of psychological well being of people with chronic disease, in particular with interventions that improve mindfulness. He is currently on research about mindfulness both in Milan, in collaboration with Niguarda Ca' Granda Hospital, and Cambridge, MA.

**Elisa Pedroli** holds a B.A. in Psychology from University of Milano Bicocca and a M.A. in Neuropsychology from the University of Roma Sapienza. She is also a last year intern in Neuropsychology advanced school (5 years) at the University of Milano Bicocca. Since 2011, she has been a junior researcher at the Applied Technology for Neuro-Psychology Lab (ATN-P LAB) at the I.R.C.C.S. Istituto Auxologico Italiano, a biomedical research institute located in the Milan area with ten hospitals. Dr. Pedroli's research focuses on neuropsychological aspects of emerging technologies, with particular reference to virtual & augmented reality systems in clinical settings for the assessment and the rehabilitation of neurological patients. She is also interested in developing innovative rehabilitation tools based on the use of virtual & augmented reality.

**Silvia Serino** is a postdoctoral researcher. Her main research focus is on the use of virtual reality to understand how the brain uses egocentric and/or allocentric reference frames to represent the body and peri-personal space. Serino has published more than 20 papers on international scientific journals.

**Jennifer Gay Tichon** is a senior research fellow with the Griffith Institute for Educational Research. Her research interests center on cognitive psychology and virtual environments.

**Dominicus Tornqvist** is a research assistant with the Griffith Institute of Educational Research at Griffith University. His interests are in motivational psychology and mental modelling of emergent game play in software toys.

**Stefano Triberti** is about to obtain his PhD in Psychology at Università Cattolica del Sacro Cuore of Milan, Italy, with a dissertation focusing on the role of intentions in Human-Technology Interaction. Other research interests of him are the use of new technologies to promote well-being (Positive Technologies), eHealth interventions, and the psychological study of video games.

**John Waterworth** is a full Professor of Informatics (since 2001) and a member of the Q-life research group at Umeå University in Sweden. His recent research has focused on actual and potential effects of using ICT on quality of life and health, especially among the elderly. He has a PhD in Experimental Psychology (1984) and is a Chartered Psychologist of the British Psychological Society. With almost 200 publications to his name, he is best known for his work on topics such as information exploration, the experience of presence and creativity in mediated environments.

**Eva Lindh Waterworth** is manager of the Q-Life research group and a full professor of informatics (since 2010) at Umeå University in Sweden. Her own research focuses on the relationship between quality of life and IT, with a particular interest in creating technology that meets the needs of special groups such as the elderly, the young and the physically and mentally disadvantaged. She has a PhD in Informatics (2001), and a first degree in informatics and business administration.

# Index

## P



## R



## S



## T



## U



## V



## W

www.ingramcontent.com/pod-product-compliance
Lightning Source LLC
LaVergne TN
LVHW060355300926
849162LV00006B/1274